THIRD EDITION

Language Development

Foundations, Processes, and Clinical Applications

Edited by

Nina Capone Singleton, PhD, CCC-SLP

Associate Professor
Seton Hall University

Adjunct Associate Professor
Hackensack Meridian School of Medicine
at Seton Hall University
South Orange, New Jersey

Brian B. Shulman, PhD, CCC-SLP,
BCS-CL, ASHA Fellow, FASAHP, FNAP

Dean and Professor
School of Health and Medical Sciences
Seton Hall University

Adjunct Professor of Pediatrics
Hackensack Meridian School of Medicine
at Seton Hall University
South Orange, New Jersey

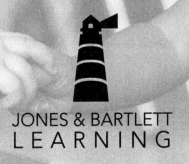

JONES & BARTLETT
LEARNING

World Headquarters
Jones & Bartlett Learning
5 Wall Street
Burlington, MA 01803
978-443-5000
info@jblearning.com
www.jblearning.com

Jones & Bartlett Learning books and products are available through most bookstores and online booksellers. To contact Jones & Bartlett Learning directly, call 800-832-0034, fax 978-443-8000, or visit our website, www.jblearning.com.

Substantial discounts on bulk quantities of Jones & Bartlett Learning publications are available to corporations, professional associations, and other qualified organizations. For details and specific discount information, contact the special sales department at Jones & Bartlett Learning via the above contact information or send an email to specialsales@jblearning.com.

12971-7

Production Credits

VP, Product Management: David D. Cella
Director of Product Management: Matt Kane
Product Manager: Laura Pagluica
Product Assistant: Rebecca Feeney
Production Manager: Carolyn Rogers Pershouse
VMO Manager: Sara Kelly
Vendor Manager: Juna Abrams
Director of Production: Julie Bolduc
Associate Production Editor, Navigate: Rachel DiMaggio
Director of Marketing: Andrea DeFronzo
Marketing Manager: Michael Sullivan
Product Fulfillment Manager: Wendy Kilborn

Composition: codeMantra U.S. LLC
Project Management: codeMantra U.S. LLC
Cover Design: Michael O'Donnell
Text Design: Kristin E. Parker
Director of Rights & Media: Joanna Gallant
Rights & Media Specialist: Thais Miller
Media Development Editor: Troy Liston
Cover Image (Title Page, Chapter Opener):
    © santypan/Shutterstock, Inc.
Printing and Binding: Bang Printing
Cover Printing: Bang Printing

Library of Congress Cataloging-in-Publication Data

Names: Singleton, Nina Capone, editor. | Shulman, Brian B., editor.
Title: Language development: foundations, processes, and clinical applications /
    [edited by] Nina Capone Singleton and Brian B. Shulman.
Other titles: Language development (Shulman)
Description: Third edition. | Burlington, Massachusetts: Jones & Bartlett Learning, [2020] |
    Includes bibliographical references and index.
Identifiers: LCCN 2018016807 | ISBN 9781284129618 (casebound: alk. paper)
Subjects: | MESH: Language Development | Language Development Disorders |
    Speech Disorders | Language | Child
Classification: LCC P118 | NLM WS 105.5.C8 | DDC 401/.93—dc23
LC record available at https://lccn.loc.gov/2018016807

6048

Printed in the United States of America
22 21 20 19 18   10 9 8 7 6 5 4 3 2 1

I dedicate this third edition to my now school-age son, Paul Christopher – a language scientist in the field. Our talks about word meanings, idioms, and his writing journal bring me much joy as he travels through the nuances of higher-level language development.

—Nina Capone Singleton

This book is dedicated to the memory of my father, Millard Shulman, who, along with my mother, Eleanor, taught me to always ask questions and encouraged me to work as hard as I could to achieve the goals I set out for myself.

—Brian B. Shulman

Together, we dedicate this third edition to the next generation of students who will take the knowledge within these pages and apply it to the children whose lives they will influence through evidence-based language assessment and intervention.

Contents

Chapter 13   Multicultural Perspectives: The Road to Cultural Competence................. 255

Luis F. Riquelme and Jason Rosas

Chapter 14   Speech and Language Development of Children Who Were Adopted Internationally 277

Deborah A. Hwa-Froelich

Chapter 15   Children with Language Impairment 293

Liat Seiger-Gardner

Chapter 16   **Listening, Language, and Literacy for Children with Auditory Devices: From Hearing Aids to Cochlear Implants. 313**

Patricia Chute and Mary Ellen Nevins

Chapter 17   **Communication Development in Children with Multiple Disabilities: The Role of Augmentative and Alternative Communication. 329**

Andrea Barton-Hulsey, Melissa A. Cheslock, Rose A. Sevcik and Mary Ann Romski

Foreword

As a student of speech-language pathology, I became interested in the subject of language and language acquisition because of the mystery of it all. The power of language intrigued me. Recognizing that language can take you from the here and now and transport you to the past, to the future, and to imaginary places fascinated me. I realized that just by saying a few words like, "I wish," a thought was considered delivered to the universe. I considered it amazing that while an act, or the absence of an act, could break a promise, merely saying two words, "I promise," creates a bond of intention between two people. I marveled at authors of fiction and nonfiction who are masters of figurative language, symbolism, and perspective, and who use language to create and to describe events that upon reading become shared events between the author and the reader. In contrast, I also developed an awareness that there are children for whom language is an inadequate and an elusive tool.

As a young child listening to fairy tales, few words stirred my imagination as much as my mother reading, "Once upon a time, there was...." As a child, I began to love going to plays, just to have words and actions envelop me for a few captivating hours. As a young teenager, I spent hours on the phone talking with my best friend about everything within our universe. It was our conversations that bonded us—talking about our plans for the future and dissecting every detail of the events of joy and disappointment in junior high and senior high.

I lived in a college town with four universities nearby. Often when famous individuals were invited to speak at these universities, my parents took me to hear them so that I would be exposed to scholarly leaders. While I may not have understood all of what was said at these events, I was struck by the occasion, by the fact that these were people with thoughts and words, and that it was important to get "dressed up" to go to auditoriums, churches, or banquet rooms to hear them speak about their experiences and their views.

Later in the mid-1960s, as editor of my high school newspaper, I took my journalistic responsibility quite seriously, conscious that my fellow students and I were creating a manuscript of our words and our thoughts. I wrote editorials to persuade, to pontificate (yes, I may have been a little pompous), and to motivate. As a high school and college student in the 1960s, language was amazing! Phrases such as "The New Frontier," the "War on Poverty," and "We Shall Overcome" were galvanizing. During the era of activism, words, phrases, and language were vehicles of social, political, and economic change. Language is very powerful.

Thus, with my love for language, as a graduate student of speech-language pathology, I became fascinated with studying the processes of language acquisition and language disorders. As children develop, they progress through the stages of language acquisition without formal instruction and without the benefit of systematic explicit tutelage. The outcome of their marvelous developmental journey is the acquisition of a phonological system, extensive semantic and grammatical systems that convey a myriad of thoughts and communicative functions, the ability to comprehend the language of others, and the capacity to perform executive functions. In literate cultures, children also acquire the milestones of literacy acquisition. Children begin with reflexive vocalizations to which their caregivers give meaning and reply as though there was communicative intent on the part of the baby. This social dance, replete with vocalizations and gestures, over the course of months evolves into intentional communication with a phonology, vocabulary, syntax, and pragmatics that correspond to the young one's linguistic community. This occurs around the globe, in all cultures, and across all socioeconomic circumstances. Given that our world is a social, economic, technological, and commercial village, an understanding and respect for all cultures, languages, and peoples is a requisite for all professionals.

Every year, new information, new theories, and new evidence are published about development to explain the complexities that create and facilitate the language acquisition process. Language and communication are the products of a biological, developmental, and environmental synchrony of various systems, which together produce a linguistically capable and literate human being. In its third edition, this text examines these systems, including the role of biology, child development, and the linguistic input that abounds in the child's environment. In addition to responding to the biology and linguistic interplay, intentional well-formed communication develops when there is efficient hearing and appropriate social-emotional development. The authors who have contributed to this text provide the latest research and perspectives on language development among neurotypical children.

Concern for children who reveal difficulty with the language learning process brings many people to the discipline of communication sciences and disorders. An ever-expanding awareness of typical language learning processes is the foundation for assessment and intervention for young children with language learning disabilities. This edition begins and ends with an awareness of our roles with and responsibilities to children who are challenged in learning to communicate—children whose phonology systems, vocabularies, sensory systems, concept development, syntactic systems, and understanding of language need the expertise of communication disorders specialists if they are to improve. This text bridges biological, environmental, technological, and professional venues to advance the development of professionals and children alike.

**Noma Anderson, PhD, CCC-SLP,
ASHA Fellow, ASHA Honors**
Special Advisor to the University of Tennessee System President on Diversity and Inclusion

2007 President, American Speech-Language-Hearing Association

Preface

▶ Introduction

Welcome to the third edition of this text on language development. Speech-language pathologists, classroom teachers, early childhood educators, psychologists, and linguists are just some of the professionals who study and/or work with the children we describe in our book. This third edition is written in collaboration with several experts across a variety of areas of language development.

▶ Organization

The chapters are organized into three sections—Foundations of Language Development, Domains of Language Development, and Applications of Language Development. Chapter 1 defines language and describes a developmental approach to clinical assessment and treatment of language impairment in children. It now has added policy and developmental milestone information that keeps current with the changing landscape of health care and education. The remaining chapters in Section 1 are dedicated to the nature–nurture factors that influence learning language (Chapter 2), the hearing mechanism (Chapter 3), the comprehension of language (Chapter 4), and how gesture sets the stage for language development (Chapter 5). In summary, Section 1 places the child's language and communication development in the context of his/her overall development.

In Section 2, each of the domains of language has a chapter dedicated to its development: social-emotional (pragmatics; Chapter 6), semantics (Chapter 7), morphology and syntax (grammar; Chapter 8), and phonology (Chapter 9). Chapters 10 and 11 present pre-literacy development and school-age language development, respectively. Of particular note is that Chapter 11 has an emphasis on literacy as well. We rounded the text out with Section 3—Applications of Language Development—with chapters that highlight neurological substrates of language. By this point in your study of language you will be able to connect various language behaviors and development to the brain's structures and functions discussed in Chapter 12. The remaining chapters in Section 3 highlight cultural and linguistic diversity, language impairment, children adopted internationally, and children with hearing impairment—these are children with individual differences encountered in language and communication development.

▶ New and Key Features

This new edition has each of the original chapters updated with new research findings, clinical application activities, and other new components. You will also see chapter format changes and three new chapters—Chapter 12: Mapping Language onto the Brain, Chapter 14: Speech and Language Development of Children Who Were Adopted Internationally, and Chapter 16: Listening, Language, and Literacy for Children with Auditory Devices: From Hearing Aids to Cochlear Implants. We have maintained our key feature of the text, the three primary case studies that are introduced in Chapter 1 and threaded throughout the text: a child who is developing typically and two children who vary from typical development. In subsequent chapters, you will discover that these three case studies are explored further from a variety of perspectives. Be on the lookout for additional case studies. This new edition provides clinical application exercises throughout the printed text and video recording presentations of select content throughout the online version of the text. The video recordings are fun and engaging and illustrate concepts such as how conversations between parents and children are a means of explicit word teaching we may not even be aware of. We hope these video vignettes prompt further discussions between instructor and students and among peers of the processes of language learning across development and contexts as we explore them in this exciting new edition. Speaking of new content, this edition also includes:

- Addition of language sample analyses to the semantic and morpho-syntax chapters
- Updated DSM-5 definitions and ASHA and World Health Organization policy information
- Developmental milestones resources

Whatever your reason for learning about language and communication development, our text presents a broader understanding of this complex, developmental phenomenon within a clinical framework. Understanding language development helps us to understand each child as an individual and to elucidate the individual child's needs within communication contexts.

▶ Instructor Resources

The following resources are available for qualified instructors:

- Test bank
- Slides in PowerPoint format
- Discussion questions
- Videos

Please visit go.jblearning.com/languagedevelopment3e for information on how to access these resources.

About the Authors

NINA CAPONE SINGLETON, PhD, CCC-SLP

Nina Capone Singleton is an Associate Professor in the Department of Speech-Language Pathology and an Adjunct Associate Professor in the Hackensack Meridian School of Medicine at Seton Hall University. Dr. Capone Singleton earned a bachelor of arts degree from Boston University (1990); her master's degree (1997) and PhD (2003) were conferred by Northwestern University.

Dr. Capone Singleton has held clinical positions at the Children's Seashore House of the Children's Hospital of Philadelphia (Philadelphia), Children's Memorial Hospital (Chicago), Bright Futures Early Intervention Clinic (Evanston, Illinois), and the Westchester Institute for Human Development (Valhalla, New York). Clinically, Dr. Capone Singleton evaluates and treats children with language and speech delays, as well as dysphagia. She has extensive experience in the area of pediatric dysphagia. She holds a Certificate of Clinical Competence from the American Speech-Language-Hearing Association and maintains her professional licenses.

Dr. Capone Singleton is the director of the Developmental Language and Cognition Lab at Seton Hall University. In her research, she investigates the relationship between semantic learning and word retrieval as well as the relationship between gesture and language development in children with and without language impairments. She has published in the *Journal of Child Language*, the *Journal of Speech, Language, and Hearing Research*, the *American Journal of Speech-Language Pathology, Pediatric Clinics of North America*, and the journal *Language, Speech, and Hearing Services in the Schools*. She currently serves as an associate editor of the *Folia Phoniatrica et Logopaedica*. She has presented at both national and international conferences.

Dr. Capone Singleton teaches several courses that cover the following topics: language development, language disorders, phonological and other speech disorders, early intervention, and pediatric dysphagia. In addition, Dr. Capone Singleton mentors undergraduate, master's, and doctoral-level students.

BRIAN B. SHULMAN, PhD, CCC-SLP, BCS-CL, ASHA Fellow, FASAHP, FNAP

Brian B. Shulman is Dean of the School of Health and Medical Sciences (SHMS) and Adjunct Professor of Pediatrics in the Hackensack Meridian School of Medicine at Seton Hall University. Dr. Shulman received his Doctor of Philosophy and Master of Arts degrees, both in Speech-Language Pathology, from Bowling Green State University (OH). His Bachelor of Arts degree in Speech-Language Pathology is from the State University of New York College at Cortland. Dr. Shulman holds the rank of Professor in the Department of Speech-Language Pathology at Seton Hall University. He is a Board Certified Specialist in Child Language (BCS-CL) as conferred by the American Board of Child Language and Language Disorders (ABCLLD). A Fellow of the American Speech-Language-Hearing Association (ASHA), the Association of Schools of Allied Health Professions (ASAHP), and the National Academies of Practice (NAP), Dr. Shulman has made numerous invited presentations to professional groups at international, national, state, and local levels. Dr. Shulman has served in a number of leadership positions within ASHA including, but not limited to, Chair of ASHA's Board of Division Coordinators (BDC), a member of ASHA's Council for Clinical Specialty Recognition, and co-chair of two annual ASHA Conventions in 2001 and 2005. Dr. Shulman served a 3-year term from 2006–2008 as ASHA's nationally elected Vice President for Speech-Language Pathology Practice. In that role, he identified national issues, monitored the emergence of new areas of practice, addressed concerns of the work setting, and monitored and facilitated ASHA-related activities designed to promote all practice settings. Dr. Shulman served two 3-year terms as the inaugural Dean Commissioner of the Accreditation Review Commission on Education for the Physician Assistant (ARC-PA). The ARC-PA is the accrediting agency that protects the interests of the public and PA profession by defining the standards for PA education and evaluating PA educational programs within the territorial United States to ensure their compliance with those standards. The ARC-PA is an independent accrediting body authorized to accredit qualified PA educational programs leading to the professional credential, Physician Assistant (PA). Dr. Shulman is the recipient of the 2010 Professional Service Award from the New Jersey Speech-Language-Hearing Association (NJSHA) and is a current member of the Executive Board of the *International Association of Logopedics and Phoniatrics (IALP)* and, in January 2017, became the Treasurer of that association. Dr. Shulman served as Editor of *Pediatric Speech and Language: Perspectives on Interprofessional Practice*, an issue of Pediatric Clinics of North America (Elsevier) published in February 2018.

Acknowledgments

We would like to express our sincere appreciation to our contributors (in alphabetical order): Andrea Barton-Hulsey, Melissa Cheslock, Patricia Chute, Lynn Flahive, Sima Gerber, SallyAnn Giess, Ronald Gillam, Sandra Gillam, William O. Haynes, Barbara Hodson, Deborah Hwa-Froelich, Anthony Koutsoftas, Jamie Mecham, Mary Ellen Nevins, Luis Riquelme, Mary Ann Romski, Jason Rosas, Liat Seiger-Gardner, Rose Sevcik, Carol Ukstins, Lorain Szabo Wankoff, Amy Weiss, Deborah Welling, and Carol Westby. These experts share our view of the importance of linking information on language and communication development to the clinical process. The fact that these contributors represent diverse backgrounds, clinical experiences, and theoretical orientations continues to strengthen this text.

We would also like to extend our gratitude to the following reviewers for their insightful and thoughtful feedback:

Iris Johnson Arnold, Tennessee State University
Meher Banajee, Louisiana State University
Thalia Coleman, Appalachian State University
Claire Edwards, University of Montevallo
Amy J. Hadley, Stockton University
Tobias A. Kroll, Texas Tech University
Henriette W. Langdon, San Jose State University
Hindy Lubinsky, Touro College
Joël Magloire, Bronx Community College
Lesley C. Magnus, Minot State University
Nancy Martino, Xavier University of Louisiana
Amanda B. Miller, California State University
Lekeitha R. Morris, Delta State University
Kerri Phillips, Louisiana Tech University
Siva Priya Santhanam, Metropolitan State University of Denver
Jianliang Zhang, North Carolina Central University

We hope you enjoy the journey of discovering language development as much as we have over the course of our clinical and academic careers!

Nina Capone Singleton, PhD, CCC-SLP

Brian B. Shulman, PhD, CCC-SLP, BCS-CL, ASHA Fellow, FASAHP, FNAP

Contributors

Andrea Barton-Hulsey, PhD, CCC-SLP
Speech-Language Pathologist
Georgia State University

Melissa A. Cheslock, MS, CCC-SLP
Clinic Director/Clinical Supervisor
Department of Communication Science and
    Disorders
University of Montevallo

Patricia Chute, EdD
Provost and Vice President for Academic Affairs
Dalton State College

Lynn K. Flahive, MS, CCC-SLP, BCS-CL
Assistant Professor/Clinic Director
Miller Speech and Hearing Clinic
Texas Christian University

Sima Gerber, PhD, CCC-SLP
Professor
Queens College, The City University of New York

SallyAnn Giess, PhD, CCC-SLP
Speech/Language Pathologist/Adjunct Faculty
California State University, Fullerton

Ronald B. Gillam, PhD, CCC-SLP
Professor
Raymond and Eloise Lillywhite Endowed Chair in
    Speech-Language Pathology
Director
Language, Education and Auditory Processing
    (LEAP) Brain Imaging Laboratory
Emma Eccles Jones Early Childhood Education and
    Research Center
Utah State University

Sandra L. Gillam, PhD, CCC-SLP
Professor
Emma Eccles Jones Early Childhood Education and
    Research Center
Utah State University

William O. Haynes, PhD, CCC-SLP
Professor Emeritus
Department of Communication Disorders
Auburn University

Barbara W. Hodson, PhD, CCC-SLP
Professor
Communication Sciences & Disorders
Wichita State University

Deborah A. Hwa-Froelich, PhD, CCC-SLP
Professor
Saint Louis University
St. Louis, MO

Anthony D. Koutsoftas, PhD, CCC-SLP
Associate Professor
Department of Speech-Language Pathology
Seton Hall University

Jamie Mecham, MS, CCC-SLP
Speech-Language Pathologist
Emma Eccles Jones Early Childhood Education and
    Research Center
Utah State University

Mary Ellen Nevins, EdD
Director
Auditory-Based Intervention Program
University of Arkansas at Little Rock

Luis F. Riquelme, PhD, CCC-SLP, BCS-S
Director, Riquelme & Associates
Associate Professor
Clinical Speech-Language Pathology
New York Medical College

Mary Ann Romski, PhD, CCC-SLP
Regents Professor
Department of Communication
Georgia State University

Jason Rosas, MPhil, MS, CCC-SLP, TSSLD
Assistant Clinic Director
Department of Communication Sciences and
    Disorders
Long Island University—Brooklyn Campus

Liat Seiger-Gardner, PhD, CCC-SLP
Associate Professor and Graduate Program
    Director
Department of Speech-Language-Hearing Sciences
Lehman College, The City University of New York

Rose A. Sevcik, PhD
Professor
Department of Psychology
Georgia State University

Carol A. Ukstins, MS, CCC-A, FAAA
Educational Audiologist
The Newark Public Schools

Lorain Szabo Wankoff, PhD, CCC-SLP
Speech-Language Consultant
Private Practice

Amy L. Weiss, PhD, CCC-SLP
Professor
Department of Communicative Disorders
University of Rhode Island

Deborah R. Welling, AuD, CCC-A, FAAA
Assistant Dean for Dual Degree Programs
Associate Professor, Department of
    Speech-Language Pathology
School of Health and Medical Sciences
Seton Hall University

Carol E. Westby, PhD, CCC-SLP
Language/Literacy Consultant
Bilingual Multicultural Services

SECTION I

History and Foundations of Language Development

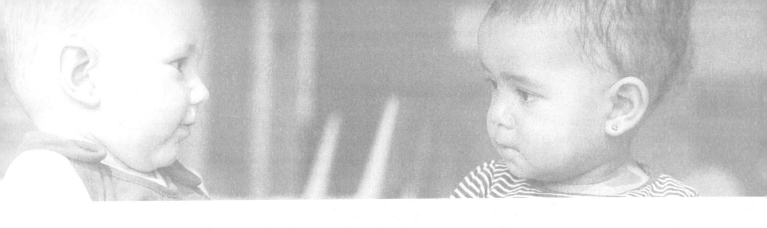

CHAPTER 1

The Development of Language: Definitions, Policy, and Practice

Nina Capone Singleton, PhD, CCC-SLP
Brian B. Shulman, PhD, CCC-SLP, BCS-CL, ASHA Fellow, FASAHP, FNAP

OBJECTIVES

- Define language and its five domains
- Understand the importance of developmental milestones
- Introduce the clinical process of language assessment and intervention
- Introduce agencies that set policy related to language development

KEY TERMS

Assessment
Background history
Evaluation
Formal testing
Functional communication context
Intervention

Language
Milestones
Morphology
Phonology
Pragmatics
Scaffolds

Semantics
Speech-language pathologist
Spontaneous language sampling
Syntax
Treatment
World Health Organization

▶ Introduction

The World Health Organization (WHO) has identified several domains of development that influence early learning and academics. It is likely no surprise to even the beginning student that language development is one of those domains. However, the reader may be interested to know that early language development also plays a role in later "economic participation, social citizenry and health across the lifespan" (p. 15; Irwin, Siddiqi, & Hertzman, 2007). The full list of influential domains on development includes:

- Health
- Physical

- Social/emotional
- Language/cognitive

One strong argument for the early years setting the foundation for lifelong success is *economic efficiency*, and James J. Heckman won a Nobel Prize showing it to be so! For example, Heckman (2008) argued that it was more cost-effective to provide interventions before the age of 5 for disadvantaged children rather than later in childhood. Later interventions included reduced pupil–teacher ratios in school and vocation training. As the result of research like Heckman's, public policy—international, national, state, school district—guides how professionals practice. Professional practice in health care and education can include early screening of the child, referral for evaluation, evaluation, and intervention for the child if needed. **BOXES 1-1** and **1-2** describe agencies at various levels that influence overall child development and, as a by-product (or in some cases, directly), language development.

First, this chapter details the definition of language, each of its domains, its modalities, and the stages of communication that children move through. Second, it reviews the criteria for becoming a speech-language

---

BOX 1-1 Levels of Policy that Influence Professional Practice with Children

WHO International agency http://www.who.int/en/	The WHO directs and coordinates international health within the United Nations. It lists several areas of work, including the promotion of (a) health through the life-course, (b) health systems, and (c) noncommunicable diseases, to name a few.
Center for Disease Control and Prevention (CDC) National agency https://www.cdc.gov/	The U.S. health protection agency, the CDC, is charged with protecting the health, safety, and security of the people in the United States. For example, the CDC provides information regarding diseases and conditions such as autism, birth defects, common cold, flu, and prenatal infections, as well as safety in the home and community (e.g., Sudden Infant Death Syndrome (SIDS)).
American Speech, Language, Hearing Association (ASHA) www.asha.org	ASHA is the professional organization that guides, regulates, and advocates the professions of speech-language pathology and audiology. The national association is responsible for clinical, educational, and research-based policy. For example, it certifies the competencies of clinical practice, accredits graduate programs across the United States, and publishes journals and other publications with cutting-edge research in speech, language, hearing, and swallowing.
State Early Intervention System (EIS) (e.g., in New Jersey, the Department of Health is the lead agency for the NJEIS)	EIS is a state-level system that provides interprofessional assessment and intervention to children between the ages of birth to 3 years of age. **BOX 1-2** elaborates this further.

BOX 1-2 Part C of the Individual with Disabilities Education Act (IDEA, 2004)

All 50 states of the United States, Puerto Rico, and the District of Columbia participate in Child Find and Early Intervention Services. Child Find identifies children from birth to 3 years of age who would benefit from early intervention. Part C of the Individual with Disabilities Education Act (IDEA) recommends these services but they are voluntary at this time, in contrast to the services school systems are required to provide for children from 3 to 21 years of age.

To enroll a child in early intervention, a pediatrician may directly observe or screen a child's need for referral. A parent or legal guardian consents to an evaluation, and the evaluation is completed (1) within a specified period of time and (2) with at least two evaluators who are able to assess five areas of development (motor, cognition, social/emotional, communication, adaptive functioning). If eligible, the family is an integral component of planning and participating in treatment.

pathologist, and third, it delineates the process of evaluating a child and how to proceed if intervention is deemed necessary by the assessment. Finally, three case studies are introduced at the end of this chapter.

▸ What Is Language?

ASHA defines language as a complex and dynamic system of conventional symbols that is used in various modes for thought and communication (ASHA, 1982, p. 1). A variety of symbols express language—for example, the sound symbols heard in speech, the written symbols seen in text, the manual symbols seen in signed languages, and the iconic symbols seen on some augmentative communication devices. Therefore, language is separable from the modality of communication that an individual uses to express himself or herself and to understand others. Everyone in a given community must agree to the same set of symbols for communication to be successful. This need for consistency leads to the "conventional" part of the definition. Language as a dynamic system means that language evolves and changes over time. For example, new vocabulary is added to a language with new technology, as is the case of *email*, *texting*, *blogging*, and *facebooking*. We also now *tweet* and *snapchat* with the advent of new internet platforms.

Domains of Language

Language is a rule-governed behavior, a characteristic that allows it to be generative. Each language has a set of rules. The rules make what is expressed socially appropriate and grammatical within a culture. This set of rules also ensures that communication is successful. For example, in English, subject pronouns are always expressed with the exception of the imperative (e.g., *Call me*). In contrast, in Italian, the subject pronoun can be deleted with multiple verb tenses because case and number are also marked by the verb ending. The idea that language is generative means that there are infinite possibilities in what is said and understood. As a consequence, individuals can express and understand sentences that they have never heard before. They rely on the rule system to generate novel grammatical and socially appropriate sentences in a given language.

Language is described by at least five separable domains: pragmatics, semantics, phonology, morphology, and syntax. These separable domains can be grouped into the form (phonology, morphology, syntax), content (semantics), and use (pragmatics) rules of a language.

The form of the language comes from the sound system (phonology) and the grammar system (morphology and syntax). It is the structural aspect of the language. Phonology is the sound system of the language. It is the smallest unit of language that overlays meaning onto the motor movements of speech. Clinicians use a special notation—the International Phonetic Alphabet (IPA)—to describe the sounds of a language. IPA differs from the orthographic symbols that you are reading now. For example, even though the word *go* consists of two letters and the word *dough* is made up of five letters, each has only two phonemes (i.e., sounds): /g/ and /o/, and /d/ and /o/, respectively. The sound change in /g/ to /d/ from *go* to *dough* is what signals a change in word meaning. However, /g/ and /d/ on their own do not have any meaning.

Go	Dough	Orthography–Word
g–o	d–o–u–g–h	Orthography–Letters
/g/ /o/	/d/ /o/	Phonemes–Sounds

Morphology is the smallest unit of language that expresses meaning. Two types of morphemes are distinguished: bound and free. Bound morphemes must be attached to a root word. Root words are free morphemes because they can stand on their own. Consider three examples: *dogs*, *walks*, and *walked*. Each of these words contains two morphemes. The word *dog/s* contains the free morpheme *dog* and the bound morpheme plural *s*. In this instance, the morpheme plural *s* has the meaning of "more than one." Similarly, the third person singular verb conjugation *s* and the past tense *-ed* in *walk/s* and *walk/ed*, respectively, indicate when an action occurred. The *s* indicates that the action is currently happening and the *-ed* indicates that the action is finished. Even though these morphemes carry meaning, they cannot occur on their own: They are bound to a root word. In contrast, the phoneme /s/ in *soap* expresses no meaning except in how it functions to differentiate the word from other words such as *rope*.

A further distinction made for morphemes is that bound morphemes can be inflectional or derivational. The morphemes just discussed are inflectional morphemes; they indicate the tense of verbs. Tense refers to the timing of an action (present, past, and so on). Derivational morphemes include prefixes (e.g., *re-*, *un-*) and suffixes (e.g., *-ness*, *-ly*). They change the word class of the root morpheme. For example, the morpheme *-ness* changes the word *happy* from an adjective to a noun, *happiness*.

Syntax is the sentence-level structure of language that marks relationships between words and ideas. This domain includes rules for constructing different types of sentences, such as declaratives, interrogatives, negatives, passives, and other complex sentences with conjoined or embedded clauses. See TABLE 1-1 for examples of each sentence type. The structure of phrases falls under the purview of the syntactic domain. Syntactic rules also dictate our choice of words and the order in which those words occur. For example, in English, adjectives are expressed in the noun phrase (e.g., *the friendly dog*), but negation occurs in the verb phrase (e.g., *I am not feeding the friendly dog; I did not feed the dog*). The negative *not* cannot occur in the noun phrase and must be placed between the auxiliary (*am*) and the main verb (*feed*). In English, it is ungrammatical to say *Not, I am feeding the friendly dog*. English also requires a "dummy" *do* verb to be inserted if an auxiliary is not already present. In the second example, *I did not feed the dog*, the affirmative is *I fed the dog*. When this sentence is negated, the *do* verb (*did*) must be used. These sorts of rules fall under the syntactic domain of language. Much of what we understand about the theory and rule system of syntax comes from Noam Chomsky's theory of Universal Grammar (for a review, see Shapiro, 1997).

Semantics is the meaning system of language. It can include the meaning expressed by single vocabulary items (e.g., *dog* = noun, animal, four legs, barks, canine, domesticated) or the proposition expressed by vocabulary items in combination (e.g., *mommy shoe* = the shoe belongs to mommy; *shoe mommy* = a request for the child's shoe). Semantics actually consists of two distinct types of information: lexical and conceptual. Lexical information is the word form that includes the phonological composition of the word, where the word form is referred to as a lexeme. The conceptual information is the meaning associated with the lexeme. For example, the word *dog* comprises three phonemes in sequence /d/, /ɔ/, /g/, which together are expressed as the lexeme /dɔg/. The meaning of dog may include four legs, having a tail, barking, and being a domesticated animal. Children need to develop both lexical and conceptual information of words as well as the link between the two so that they can express and understand language successfully.

Pragmatics refers to how we use the form and content of language. Pragmatic behaviors may include the intention that a spoken utterance or gesture conveys, the way in which we use and understand body language, the social appropriateness of an utterance, and the process of ensuring the appropriate amount of information is provided to a listener. For example, a toddler may point to a cookie and say *gimmie*, or he may say *want cookie*. In both instances, the pragmatic intent of the communication is the same—the child wants the mother to give him the cookie—even though the form of that communication differs. In the first instance, the pointing gesture indicates the object; in the second utterance, the word *cookie* indicates the object. The pragmatic aspect of both utterances is the intention: to request. As another example of pragmatics, rules govern how one varies the language that is used with various listeners. That is, we do not use the same kind of language when speaking to a professor, a supervisor, or a stranger as we do with a parent, a sibling, or a friend. If we were to speak to all of these individuals similarly, one or more could be offended or made to feel uncomfortable.

Another aspect of pragmatics includes how much information is provided to the listener. The information given to a listener has to be sufficient without giving too little or too much information. For example, a speaker cannot use a pronoun (*he*) without having already identified to whom *he* is referring. As another example, speakers must introduce a topic of conversation. If a friend approached you and stated, "*I told the mechanic to rotate my tires,*" you would think this odd. According to pragmatic rules, we generally make

TABLE 1-1 Examples of Sentence Types

Sentence Types	Example
Declarative	My sister walks the dog.
Interrogative	Who is walking the dog?
	What is my sister doing?
Negative	My brother does not walk the dog.
Passive	The dog was fed by my brother.
Conjoined	My brother and sister take turns walking the dog.
	My brother feeds the dog and my sister walks the dog.
Clausal Embedding	My sister walks the dog that lives next door.
	It is our dog that my brother feeds, not our bird.

greetings first and then introduce a topic. Further, we introduce a topic and then expand on details. In fact, we have some explicit language conventions for acknowledging when we violate a rule such as this (e.g., *Oops, I changed lanes*, or *Sidebar*, or *I'm changing topics*). Violations in pragmatics can often be the source of humor between friends. Conversely, it can be problematic when the speaker has no awareness of these rule violations and when they are pervasive in disrupting communication. This problem often arises with children who have overarching language learning delays or disorders specific to the pragmatic domain of language.

Nonverbal behaviors such as eye contact and body gestures also fall under the domain of pragmatics. Nonverbal behaviors communicate information, as the pointing example given earlier illustrates. Consider the message received if a friend says to you, *"It is fine that you forgot to call me."* If the friend says this but also averts her eye gaze and has an angry tone in his/her voice, the nonverbal aspects of this communication let you know the friend is not happy with you. Even though the form of the language expressed understanding, the nonverbal behaviors of eye contact and vocal tone did not. In contrast, if that friend says the same sentence but has a casual tone to his/her voice, then you can assume that no offense occurred. As with the other domains of language, pragmatic rules for nonverbal behavior must be learned, and these rules differ cross-culturally. Thus, it is particularly important for clinicians to fully understand the pragmatic rules (as well as other rule systems) of the language and the culture of their clients.

▶ Receptive Versus Expressive Language

For communication to be successful, language must be produced as well as understood. The ability to understand or comprehend the domains of language is referred to as *receptive language*. The ability to produce or speak (sign, write, and so on) language is referred to as *expressive language*. Following a direction such as "give me your cup" requires the child to understand individual words (*give, cup, me, your*) as well as the relationship between those words. Therefore, knowing the cup for which the child needs to perform the action is dependent on the child understanding the possessive pronoun in combination with the noun. It is the child's cup—not the mother's cup—that needs to be given. If the child throws the cup on the floor instead of handing it over to the mother, they may understand that the *cup* is somehow involved in what was said to them, but they might not understand the

word *give* or the relationship between what they were supposed to do (the action of giving) and the goal of that action (to the mother).

In another example, if you show a child a picture of one shoe and a picture of two shoes and ask them to show you *the shoes* (versus *the shoe*), they should be able to point to the picture of two shoes if they understand the plural *s* morpheme. If the child does not understand the plural morpheme, they will randomly point to either picture.

The child's ability to comprehend a certain level of language often precedes their ability to produce the same language. This phenomenon is observed in both typically developing and language-delayed children. A child may follow a direction correctly but may not produce the same sentence until many months later. Some children with language impairments exhibit more expressive language than an understanding of language; this is not typical of most children's development. It often indicates the child is not truly using language in a meaningful way. Rather, they are expressing in a rote manner the language that they have heard.

▶ Stages of Communication

Three stages of communication have been described: perlocution, illocution, and locution.

The *perlocution stage* refers to the unintentional stage of communication. During this stage, the infant produces behaviors such as burping or vocalizations that have no intended message. This stage typically occurs before approximately 8–10 months of age, although children who demonstrate delays in development may remain in this stage longer. These vegetative or unintentional behaviors are often responded to by adults as if they were intentional communicative acts. The infant may burp and the mother responds, *"Oh, you're full!"*, or the infant may vocalize a sustained /a/ and the father responds, *"Oh, you have something to say?"* These adult responses help the child learn the language and gain a sense of what intentional communication gets them—namely attention and the meeting of needs. It establishes turn-taking interactions, which are also a vehicle for caregivers to provide the child with models of language.

At approximately 10 months of age, the typically developing infant begins to use gestures and nonlinguistic vocalizations (e.g., jargoning) intentionally to communicate. For example, the child may request a cup by pointing to it. This intentional communication without the use of words is referred to as the *illocution stage* of communication.

Soon after, at approximately 12 months of age, the infant produces their first word and enters the *locution stage* of communication. This phase is characterized by intentional communication expressed with words. It is characterized by linguistic (and metalinguistic) communication skills.

Some behaviors first observed during the perlocution and illocution phases of communication are referred to as prelinguistic skills. They are included under the domain of pragmatics and include gestures, eye contact, joint attention, and turn-taking behaviors. The prelinguistic skills of eye contact, joint attention, and taking turns during an interaction are the building blocks of successful communication and language learning. If a child is not looking at you, attending to the activity, and able to take turns, they will miss your language models and will not imitate what you have said or done. Imitation is another skill the infant needs to have in order to learn language. Some children who demonstrate delays in language learning do not engage in these prelinguistic behaviors. If this is the case, these behaviors are appropriate goals of intervention.

The locution phase of communication development can be divided into two types of skills: linguistic and metalinguistic. The term *linguistic* (or language) has already been defined. Language develops throughout one's lifespan. The development of some domains is largely completed by 8 years of age (e.g., phonology), whereas other domains (e.g., semantics) continue to develop throughout adulthood.

The term *metalinguistic* refers to the child's ability to think and talk about language. This skill is necessary if one is to understand the language used in humor, riddles, and metaphors, for example. Higher-level language such as this is often part of academic instruction, social communication, and the culture at large (e.g., advertising). Other examples of metalinguistic skill include a child's ability to identify the first or last sound in a word, express a rhyming word, explain why a joke is funny, and define a word. These tasks require the child to consciously analyze and manipulate language. Proficient reading and writing skills are also considered metalinguistic skills.

▶ Developmental Milestones

Although children have their own temperaments, development is predictable in many ways. In the previous section, the reader reviewed the stages children pass through in communication. Milestones are more behaviors that mark a specific change in development. They emerge in a predictable sequence and

are mastered within a timeline that is consistent for most children. For example, most children speak their first word around their first birthday, combine words around their second birthday, and soon thereafter acquire grammatical endings (e.g., present progressive verb form; *-ing* in *eating*). While on average children speak their first word at 12 months, clinicians should consider a range of 10–14 months for achieving this feat to be typical.

There is also a predictable relationship between developmental areas. Developmental skills fall under broad areas such as motor development (gross motor, fine motor) and cognitive development (play, gesture, memory, attention). Observation in one skill area builds the clinician's expectation about the level of development in other skill areas. For example, some gesture milestones predict the next language milestones. For example, the pointing gesture precedes the child's first words. There are also motor, play, and language skills that develop in parallel. For instance, children walk and say their first word around the same time. When the child is combining words (e.g., *mommy eat*), he or she is also likely to be combining play schemes (e.g., put doll to sleep and pat doll in sequence).

The Center for Disease Control and Prevention (CDC) provides the public with the Milestones in Action website as part of their campaign to *Learn the Signs* and *Act Early*. The Milestones in Action website contains video samples of select milestones across developmental domains from 2 months to 5 years of age (https://www.cdc.gov/ncbddd/actearly/milestones/milestones-in-action.html). In addition, AHSA provides developmental milestones information as part of its campaign to *Identify the Signs* (https://identifythesigns.org/).

A third source of public milestones information is *The First Words Project* (firstwordsproject.com) through Florida State University. The Project offers several 16 by 16™ series Lookbooks. One domain of development that is central to language development is gesture. Before a child participates in the act of communicating with words, he or she is setting the stage by communicating with gestures. Most importantly, gesture and language develop in predictable ways so that if a child has difficulty using language, the clinician still has the child's gestures to interpret. What the child knows is reflected in gestures. Oftentimes, gesture reflects the child's mental representations before speech. The First Words Project offers the 16 Gestures by 16 Months Lookbook. This Lookbook provides caregivers the types of gestures that children use and the timeline of gesture emergence. In essence, children should be developing around one or two gestures each month from 8 months onward.

Knowledge of the milestones that children pass through provides a set of expectations for the caregiver and pediatrician about what children will be doing as they age. The clinician uses these milestones to evaluate the child's performance and functioning and compare it with that of same-age peers. Knowledge of developmental milestones can then guide the clinician in how best to educate parents and make referrals to other professionals.

Comparing the child's current level of functioning and participation in activities with what is expected for his or her age or cognitive level can also help the clinician in determining whether intervention is warranted. If intervention is appropriate, the first step toward intervention is to determine the appropriate goals for the client. Goals are the behaviors or skills that the clinician facilitates the child in learning. Appropriate goals are (1) the milestones that the child should progress to next developmentally and (2) the component skills needed to achieve a more complex milestone. For example, following directions requires the child to attend to the speaker, understand the vocabulary used in the direction, and decode the grammar. When the clinician is well grounded in the normal progression of development, they can determine the appropriate treatment goals, appropriate activity level to target the goals, and the types of scaffolding to provide the child as part of therapy.

Who Is the Speech-Language Pathologist?

Speech-language pathologists are professionals who are trained in the assessment and treatment of disorders in the areas of speech (articulation, voice, and fluency), language, cognition, and eating/swallowing. Speech encompasses the respiratory, laryngeal, velopharyngeal, and oral-motor movements that express language. Speech-language pathologists are also actively involved in elective services, such as training non-native speakers of English to reduce their primary language accent or facilitating gender-preferred speech-language patterns for transgender individuals.

Speech-language pathologists are typically licensed by their state and certified by ASHA, which is the national organization that regulates the professional practice of speech-language pathologists and audiologists. Speech-language pathologists and audiologists are required to earn a graduate degree in speech-language pathology or audiology, respectively; complete a 9-month supervised clinical fellowship after their graduate degree; and pass a national examination (the Praxis examination).

Referral to a Speech-Language Pathologist

Referral to a speech-language pathologist can occur when a parent, teacher, or pediatrician is concerned that a child is delayed in meeting speech, language, or feeding milestones. The number of additional professionals involved in that child's care will depend on what overall difficulties the child is having. ASHA and the WHO have adopted an interprofessional collaborative practice (IPP) framework in multiple settings, including health care and education. BOX 1-3 describes the framework for IPP.

A common context of referral to a speech-language pathologist is during the toddler's visit to his pediatrician. The toddler may be slow to acquire many new words around his or her second birthday. For example, children will typically begin learning words at a rapid rate and combine words into short utterances between 18 and 24 months of age. However, for select children who are developing typically but not meeting

---

BOX 1-3 Interprofessional Education and Interprofessional Collaborative Practice (IPE/IPP)

We focus this text on the beginning journey of the language scientist and/or clinician. This is often the speech-language pathologist. However, ASHA has set this as one of its key objectives in its strategic Pathway to Excellence:

advance interprofessional education and interprofessional collaborative practice
(IPE/IPP) by 2025 (2015; http://www.asha.org/uploadedFiles/ASHA-Strategic-Pathway-to-Excellence.pdf).

ASHA adopts the WHO definition of IPE/IPP as two or more professions effectively collaborating to improve healthcare and educational outcomes. Collaborating professions are learning *about*, *from*, and *with* each other. IPE/IPP promotes a diversity of perspectives. It should bring together a broad range of qualified researchers, clinicians, and/or instructors to meet the needs of consumers, whether they are graduate students of the university studying to be a professional, or the patients they will be serving in the healthcare or educational system.

these vocabulary milestones, parents may notice that their child is not yet saying much or expressing phrases such as *mommy go* or *give me that*. It is at this time that parents will consult with their child's pediatrician. The child may then be referred to an audiologist to rule out a hearing loss and to a speech-language pathologist to evaluate language development. This is not the only context of referral to an audiologist and speech-language pathologist, however. Children may not face difficulty in learning or using language until they enter first grade. Other children may have identifiable developmental disorders or predisposing risk factors in infancy that warrant referral to a speech-language pathologist valid (e.g., autism, Down syndrome, premature birth). Whatever the circumstance, the speech-language pathologist has a broad base of training to address the varied needs of children, including:

- Advocacy
- Prevention
- Screening
- Evaluation
- Intervention
- Consultation

ASHA adopts the WHO model of health and disability—referred to as the International Classification of Functioning—when evaluating and treating children with language delays and disorders. **BOX 1-4** describes the International Classification of Functioning set forth by the WHO.

Initial Contact with a Concerned Caregiver

When the speech-language pathologist first speaks with a concerned caregiver, he or she asks some general questions regarding the child's development to determine whether an evaluation is appropriate. This information includes the parent's main concern, the child's primary medical and developmental diagnoses, and an acquisition timeline of some early developmental milestones. For example, a speech-language pathologist may ask a parent the following questions:

- What concerns you about your child's communication?
- Does the child have any known medical or developmental conditions?
- Has your child's hearing been tested?
- When did your child say their first word?

Organizing an Assessment Protocol for Evaluation of the Child

After it is determined that a language evaluation is appropriate, the speech-language pathologist organizes an assessment protocol. The reader should note that the terms *assessment* and *evaluation* can have slightly different meanings depending on the clinical context in which they are used. However, for the purpose of this chapter, the terms are used interchangeably. Language assessment includes understanding a child's history of development relative to normal developmental milestones as well as the child's functional communication (e.g., conversation) and performance on formal tests. A thorough evaluation of the child can determine whether a delay or disorder exists, and whether the delay/disorder is specific to language or involves multiple areas of development (e.g., cognition, motor skills). The clinician can also hypothesize

---

BOX 1-4 WHO: The International Classification of Functioning, Disability, and Health

The WHO provides the framework to view health and disability. The *International Classification of Functioning, Disability, and Health* (WHO, 2001) defines health and disability by three components: (a) body structures and functions; (b) activities and participation; and (c) contextual factors. Body structures and functions include anatomy, physiology, and mental functions related to communication (e.g., attention, language). Activities and participation include capacity for language under ideal circumstances such as testing in a quiet room and language performance in everyday environments like social contexts, academic environments, and places of vocation. Contextual factors include those of a personal nature—age, gender, education—as well as environmental factors related to physical environment, access to technology, and the attitudes of those with whom the child will come into contact. Contextual factors can create barriers or help facilitate language learning and use.

An evaluation will identify strengths and weaknesses in each of these components. For example, an evaluation should assess the demands of language activities and the child's ability to perform language activities for social, academic, and vocational success. The goal of the intervention will be to facilitate and optimize each of the aforementioned components. In addition, other areas associated with the same underlying skills shared by oral language are examined. These skills include play, emergent literacy, and literacy skills. In addition, social interaction skills are examined for children at all age levels. This framework sets the stage for how we proceed with our intervention.

about the child's prognosis in terms of gains to be made with and without intervention (treatment).

An assessment protocol is a plan of procedures to follow during the evaluation. Some goals of a language evaluation are to answer the following questions:

- Does the child demonstrate delays or a disorder in reaching language milestones?
- What are the child's strengths and weaknesses in language relative to other areas of development (e.g., motor, play) across behavioral domains?
- Can a potential etiology or contributing factors of the delay be determined (e.g., contextual)?
- What is the child's prognosis for gains to be made in development with and without intervention?
- Is intervention warranted for the child? Should this child be monitored?
- What are the appropriate goals of intervention?
- Are referrals to other professionals appropriate (e.g., occupational therapy, physical therapy, developmental pediatrician)?

The evaluation protocol includes gathering details about the child's history of development (background history), testing of language skills (formal testing), and analysis of language skills within a functional communication context (spontaneous language sampling). Discourse (conversational, storytelling) contexts are appropriate for spontaneous language sampling depending on the child's age. For children who function cognitively before the age of 5, discourse samples should be elicited within a play-based context. Patel and

Audiologists are specialists in the area of hearing, which is necessary for oral/aural communication to develop. They are responsible for the assessment of hearing. Intervention (treatment) may be necessary to help an individual learn or maintain language skills in the face of hearing loss or deafness; such intervention is referred to as *aural habilitation* or *aural rehabilitation*. Either an audiologist or a speech-language pathologist may provide intervention for individuals with hearing loss.

Other treatments for individuals with hearing loss may include hearing aids, Frequency Modulation (FM) devices, cochlear implants, and/or environmental manipulations. Cochlear implants are a relatively new surgical treatment for profound hearing loss. They allow sound impulses to reach the brain for processing. Cochlear implants consist of a series of electrodes that replace the part of the cochlea that is not functioning. A surgeon implants the device, but the audiologist is responsible for the programming of the implant once it is placed. Aural habilitation is also necessary for individuals who receive a cochlear implant.

Connaghan (2014) also developed a picture description task—Park Play—that was deemed feasible with children as young as 4 years of age. The benefit of Park Play is that it is an engaging task for young children that elicits consonant and vowel phonemes, as well as prosodic aspects of speech (e.g., altered pitch and loudness variations). The Park Play illustration and its Examiner Response Sheet can be found online in the Supplementary Appendices of Patel and Connaghan (2014).

After an evaluation session is completed, the clinician documents everything in a written report (i.e., the child's history, performance on formal tests, and the clinician's analysis). The clinician synthesizes all information to determine a diagnostic and prognostic statement of how the child is expected to progress with and without intervention. Finally, the report contains recommendations on whether intervention is indicated and what the goals of intervention should be. The next section provides details of the evaluation and report.

▶ Background History

The child's background history is an important feature of the evaluation process because certain events and conditions are known to place a child at risk for language delays. Information is collected about several areas of the child's background. These include prenatal events (i.e., during the mother's pregnancy), birth events, medical/health issues, developmental milestones (gross motor, fine motor, language, play, gesture), caretaking and education information (daycare, schooling, home care), previous evaluations and interventions, and the family's history of speech-language delays. **TABLE 1-2** provides some examples of background history information. Having knowledge of the child's background helps the speech-language pathologist make hypotheses about whether the child is at risk of language delay, why a child may be delayed in language development, and what the child's prognosis may be for making gains in development. For example, children who are born prematurely or are exposed to cocaine or alcohol during the mother's pregnancy are known to be at risk of language delays. Delays in meeting language milestones are also characteristic of some genetic disorders (e.g., Down syndrome). It is also important to be aware of background information in planning the evaluation.

When a child is born prematurely, clinicians must correct the child's age for the remaining gestational months. Development from prenatal to postnatal periods is continuous. Therefore, the child's chronological age of 12 months is calculated from birth regardless of length of gestation, but their adjusted or developmental

TABLE 1-2 Examples of Typical and Remarkable Events Reported in the Background History

Background History	Typical Events	Remarkable Events
Prenatal	Child was born at term after 38–40 weeks' gestation, weighing 6 pounds, 3 ounces	Child was born prematurely, prior to 38 weeks' gestation
Birth	Child was born without difficulty	Child incurred loss of oxygen during the birthing process due to breech birth presentation
Medical/Health	Child has had no ear infections	Child has incurred multiple episodes of otitis media (ear infections)
Developmental	Child sat at 6 months and walked and said first words by 12 months	Child walked at 15 months and is not yet saying first words at 18 months
Education	Child has not received special services for development	Child received early intervention services
Family History	No history of speech-language disorders is reported for family members	Members of child's family have been diagnosed with speech or language disorders (e.g., dyslexia)

age (10 months) takes the gestational age at birth into account. A child who is 12 months of age, chronologically, was born 12 months ago. If the child was born 12 months ago, but this date was 2 months premature (i.e., the child was born at 7 months gestation instead of 9 months gestation), then the child's adjusted age (or developmental age) is 10 months. The expectation for this child is that the child should have the skills of a 10-month-old infant, not the skills of a 12-month old. The issue of correcting a child's age is important in determining whether a child is delayed because the child acquires new skills and meets milestones quite rapidly in the first 2 years of life. Remember that the child typically says the first word at 12 months but will probably not have words at 10 months. A chronological 12-month-old who has an adjusted age of 10 months would not be consideraed delayed if they has not yet spoken their first word. It is common clinical practice to stop adjusting a child's age for prematurity after 2 years of age (chronological age).

▶ Spontaneous Language Sampling

Analysis of a spontaneous language sample is critical to assessing the functional use of language skills for communication and the integrated function of all components of speech and language (Duffy, 2005). Functional communication refers to the child's ability to use each language domain to communicate successfully in their everyday experiences. Analysis of the spontaneous language sample is considered a formal analysis because performance can be compared to the normative data of same-age peers.

The clinician can collect a spontaneous language sample by structuring a developmentally appropriate interaction. For younger children, the clinician can have developmentally appropriate toys available on a mat and include a developmentally appropriate storybook with pictures or talk about the Park Play illustration mentioned above. For older children, the clinician can prepare appropriate topics of conversation about academic, social, hobby, vacation, and sports topics. Marilyn Nippold and colleagues (Nippold, 2014) have developed a task that elicits spontaneous language samples known as the FAVORITE GAME OR SPORT protocol (e.g., Heilmann & Malone, 2014). This protocol prompts children to describe their favorite game or their favorite sport in detail so that a child of the same age but from another country would be able to play. The game cannot be a video game. The sample of the child's language is recorded; later, the clinician can transcribe and analyze the child's language from the recording.

Most formal analyses of language require a sample of 100 utterances that are continuous and considered representative of the child's communication. Often, the child's middle 100 utterances of a language sample are analyzed because this section of the sample is thought to be most representative of the child's skills. This part of the sample occurs after the child has gotten comfortable with the new environment but before they feel fatigued. At this point, the child tends to show their best colors. The same sample can be used to analyze each language domain. The student clinician is wise to keep in mind that children with language impairment (i.e., difficulty learning and using language) will be less likely to produce 100 utterances. A small sample size should be considered diagnostic in its own right, but analysis should still be completed with these fewer utterances.

The book *Guide to Analysis of Language Transcripts* (Retherford, 2000) provides a description of several analyses of semantics, morphology, syntax, and pragmatics. In addition, the manual provides normative data to compare the child's data and interpretation of results. Some examples of common spontaneous language analyses used in clinical practice are the *type:-token ratio* (TTR), the *mean length of utterance* (MLU), and the upper bound length or longest utterance. Each of these analyses is described in later chapters of this text. The MLU and upper bound length are syntactic measures of utterance length in morphemes. The NDW is a semantic measure of how many different vocabulary words the child uses. Formal analyses of discourse and narrative samples are also available (e.g., Applebee's System of Scoring Narrative Stages; Applebee, 1978).

▶ Formal Testing

Formal tests have been developed to survey a child's skills in a variety of areas. These tests allow the clinician to calculate a raw score by adding the points for accuracy. When administering a formal test, the clinician determines the level of skills that the child has, known as the *basal* level of performance, and the upper limit of what the child can accomplish, known as the *ceiling* level of performance. This range from basal to ceiling determines the raw score. The raw score, which is the number of correct items on the test, is statistically converted into a normative scoring system. This normative score is already calculated for the clinician in tables provided in the test's manual.

Two examples of normative scoring systems are the *standard score* and the *percentile*. They are categorized as "normative-referenced" tests because a specific child's performance is compared to a sample of children used to provide a summary of typical (or "normal") development.

The standard score has a mean score and a standard deviation from the mean. For most tests, the mean score is 100 and the standard deviation is 15 points. Thus, a score that falls within the range of either 85–100 or 100–115 is considered to be within one standard deviation of the mean a score that falls within the range of either 70–85 or 115–130 is considered to be within two standard deviations of the mean, and so forth. By current clinical standards, a score that falls within the range of 85–115 is considered typically developing performance. Some subtests of a formal test will use a mean of 10 and a standard deviation of 3 (i.e., typical performance range is a standard score in the range of 7–13). The clinical convention currently used to identify children with a language delay is standard scores that fall below one standard deviation of the mean (i.e., a standard score below 85 or below 7 on an individual subtest).

A percentile score is based on 100% of children sampled and is best understood as how a child performs relative to how many children perform above them and how many children perform below them. For example, if a child's raw score places her at the 90th percentile for her age, 10% of the children at the same chronological age performed better and 89% of same-age children performed more poorly. Using percentile scores, children who fall below the 10th percentile are generally identified as having a delay in the area of development being tested. The standard score of 85 and the 10th–15th percentile roughly coincide. Therefore, whether the clinician uses a standard score or a percentile score should not affect the child's classification as exhibiting a delay in language development.

One benefit to using a standard score or a percentile score is that the child's performance can be compared across formal measures of language and cognitive functioning because many formal tests use these types of normative scoring systems. The child's performance can be characterized as within normal limits (low average, average, high average) or outside of normal limits (above average, below average, or delayed). There is a broad range of skill levels that characterize a child who falls within normal limits. For example, approximately 68% of the population of same-age peers falls within one standard deviation of the mean and approximately 95% of the population falls within two standard deviations of the mean.

Formal tests of language can sample a variety of language domains, or they can test a particular language domain or skill in-depth. Formal tests that sample a variety of language domains provide the clinician with a general language score. For example, the *Preschool Language Scale, Fifth Edition*, (PLS-V;

Another type of formal test is the criterion-referenced test. The criterion-referenced test determines how many skills a child has at a certain age level. The skills surveyed are determined by the normal sequence of developmental milestones. When making a decision regarding the type of formal tests to administer and the normative scores to report, the clinician must be familiar with the policy that governs eligibility of services. For example, in the early intervention system, a child's eligibility for speech-language services is determined by individual states. For preschool, primary school, and secondary school settings, individual school districts determine those criteria under IDEA

Zimmerman, Steiner, & Pond, 2011) tests the child's comprehension and production of a variety of language domains. The language domains are reflected in items that are intermixed throughout the test. This is unlike other formal tests that have separable subtests for each language domain. However, there are two separable subtests: Auditory Comprehension and Expressive Communication. The PLS-V is a normative-referenced test administered to children from birth to 7 years, 11 months. All domains of language are sampled on this test. For example, on the Auditory Comprehension subtest, an item at the 24- to 29-month-old age level surveys a child's ability to follow directions with gesture cues. The child is presented with some objects (e.g., book, duck, teddy bear) and is asked: *Get the book and bring it here.* The clinician also holds out his or her hand. There are four potential directions to complete but the child is credited with accuracy if they complete one of the four correctly. By contrast, on the Expressive Communication subtest, an item at the 30- to 35-month-old age level samples the child's expressive word use for a variety of pragmatic functions (e.g., requesting actions, labeling, getting attention). The child is shown a sealed bag with snack or toys.

The *Rossetti Infant-Toddler Language Scale* (RITLS; Rossetti, 2006) is a criterion-referenced test used to survey the development of children from birth to 36 months of age. The RITLS surveys skills across several skill areas, including interaction/attachment skills, pragmatic skills, gesture skills, play skills, receptive language skills, and expressive language skills. Children are scored as having a percentage of skills achieved under each skill area at each age level. For example, if a child demonstrates four of the five possible skills sampled, they are credited with 80% of the skills at that age level.

There are also formal tests that assess a single domain of language. These tests provide the clinician with a richer picture of the skills in a particular domain. For example, the *Peabody Picture Vocabulary Test, Fourth Edition,* (PPVT-IV; Dunn & Dunn, 2007) is a test of receptive vocabulary. The child is presented with a four-picture array and must identify the correct picture when the clinician says a word label. This test assesses the size of the vocabulary that the child comprehends.

The *Expressive Vocabulary Test* (EVT; Williams, 1997) is a test of expressive vocabulary. The child is presented with a series of single pictures and is asked to name each one. This test assesses the size of the vocabulary that the child expresses.

The *Goldman-Fristoe Test of Articulation, Second Edition,* (GFTA-2; Goldman & Fristoe, 2000) is a test of expressive phonology. The child is presented with a series of single pictures and is asked to name each one. These pictures are different from those used in the EVT because the pictures that make up the GFTA are meant to elicit each consonant or vowel sound of English in different word positions (i.e., initial, medial, final). For example, the phoneme /g/ is tested through naming *girl*, *wagon*, and *frog*. Sound production is also tested in consonant clusters and diphthongs. Consonant clusters occur when two consonants are spoken together with no intervening vowel (e.g., /st/ in *stop*), and diphthongs occur when two vowels are spoken together with no intervening vowel (e.g., /aɪ/ in *eye*).

It should be emphasized here that formal tests alone should never form the sole basis for a speech-language pathologist's determination of a child's performance and subsequent intervention. If they must be used to determine a child's eligibility for services, the formal test data generated must be compared to data obtained through other assessment measures including, but not limited to, spontaneous language sampling.

▶ A Developmental Approach to the Clinical Practice of Speech-Language Pathology

Knowledge of developmental milestones is critical to the practice of speech-language pathology. Clinicians survey several areas of development during an evaluation to understand the child's overall development. Understanding the child's language development within the broader context of the child's overall development enables the clinician:

- To make a more reliable diagnosis
- To make hypotheses about why a child may be delayed in language development

- To predict the child's prognosis for making gains
- To plan an appropriate course of intervention

Assessment

In the context of assessment, if the clinician can gain a sense of the child's cognitive and motor development prior to the language assessment, he or she can plan appropriate tests and activities for the evaluation. This usually occurs while speaking with the caregiver during the initial phone contact prior to evaluation. Similarly, if a clinician has a solid footing in developmental milestones, he or she can make informal observations at the start of the evaluation session and alter the protocol if necessary. Careful planning of the language evaluation (as well as the ability to adapt quickly to the unexpected) ensures that the diagnosis, prognosis, and plan for intervention are valid and reliable.

For example, if the clinician knows ahead of time that a 5-year-old client has cognitive functioning at a younger stage in development, he or she knows that some formal tests used with 5-year-olds cannot be administered to this child. Instead, the clinician may choose a formal test that surveys a broader age range. If a 6-year-old child were functioning more in line with a 30-month-old level of cognition, the spontaneous language sample would be elicited using toys that are more appropriate for the 30-month-old. By contrast, it would be inappropriate to elicit a language sample using a story retell context.

The evaluation is not simply a listing of the things that the child cannot accomplish, but it should rather include a profile of the child's strengths and achieved milestones. By including the child's strengths *and* weaknesses, the clinician presents the child in a broader developmental context and capitalizes on what the child can do to facilitate further development. It is also important for parents to be counseled about their child's strengths so that these strengths can be capitalized.

The clinician who is knowledgeable about developmental milestones will be able to determine whether a child demonstrates development that is considered typical for his/her chronological (or adjusted) age, whether the child is delayed in skills, or whether the child demonstrates development that is atypical. Atypical behaviors are not seen as part of the typical course of development. For example, if a 25-month-old child speaks in only a few one-word utterances, this level of achievement is typical of a 12- to 18-month-old child and can be considered delayed expressive language development. However, if this same child is not exhibiting gesture or communicative eye contact, and/or joint attention, or if the child says more than they understand, the clinician may consider this level to be atypical because eye contact and joint attention are present at the earliest stages of infancy. Also, we know that comprehension precedes production of language in typical development.

Trial Treatment

The clinician can set aside time after testing for trial treatment activities. Trial treatment is also referred to as stimulability. During this period, the clinician assesses the child's response to scaffolding of a few behaviors. A scaffold is formally defined as something to raise or support. In clinical practice, a scaffold refers to the support given to a child that facilitates the next skill level. Scaffolds may include a model of a behavior for the child to imitate (e.g., words, phrases, play schemes, gestures) or providing cues (multimodal hints). The clinician might say "Listen" while touching the child's shoulder to gain their attention prior to giving a direction. Any special accommodations that the clinician makes during the evaluation must be included in the evaluation report. Again, because the clinician will only know the child's areas of delay through the evaluation, he or she must be comfortable with developmental milestones so as to know what to target during trial treatment activities. The child's resulting performance is reported in a section of the evaluation report entitled "Trial Treatment."

The scaffolds to which the child responds (e.g., preparatory sets, cues, prompts, models) are considered by the clinician in his or her final analysis of the child's language development. The clinician's knowledge of the child's developmental level and knowledge of typical developmental milestones dovetail as the clinician begins to plan the child's intervention and hypothesize about the child's prognosis for gains to be made with intervention. For example, if the child produces two-word combinations but is not marking early grammatical morphemes, the clinician will model simple sentences with present progressive verbs (e.g., *dancing*) because the grammatical morpheme *-ing* is expected to emerge next in development. If a 30-month-old child does not produce two-word combinations spontaneously but can imitate combinations when the clinician models them, the child may be at the cusp of that level of language development. Such a child would have a better prognosis of making this gain than a child who is not yet pointing or a child who is not yet able to imitate one- or two-word combinations. The latter child would first need to achieve the precursor gesture and imitation milestones.

Knowledge of developmental milestones across skill areas helps the clinician determine whether a delay is specific to one area of development or whether it involves multiple areas of development. After the evaluation is completed, the speech-language pathologist must integrate, analyze, and interpret the child's history and performance on formal testing, spontaneous communication analyses, and trial treatment. Based on the clinician's interpretation, he or she makes a diagnosis, develops a statement regarding the child's prognosis for gains to be made with (or without) intervention, and recommends the appropriate course of action for intervention.

If multiple areas of development are delayed, the clinician can make hypotheses about which types of goals need to be set for intervention, taking into account the fact that skills in some areas of development are precursors to skills in other areas of development. For example, a child who is not yet sitting up, crawling, or standing may have difficulty exploring objects and the environment. These sensory-motor experiences are the building blocks for early semantic learning and set the stage for many parent–child interactions in which language is modeled and practiced.

An informal observation of the child's skills outside of speech and language domains can lead the clinician to make appropriate referrals to other professionals. In addition to language, the clinician may observe other areas of development, including gross and fine motor skills, gesture, play, sensory regulation, and attention during the evaluation. The clinician may not be able to use a published test to formally assess each of these areas. However, the child's mother may report a delayed milestone, or the clinician may observe the child during the evaluation to be falling behind in a motor milestone (e.g., an 8-month-old child who is not yet sitting independently). A referral to a physical therapist for a gross motor evaluation would be appropriate. Appropriate referrals to other professionals can be made for evaluation of motor, medical, or other cognitive/emotional concerns as they arise. These professionals may include a developmental pediatrician, neurologist, psychologist, audiologist, physical therapist, or occupational therapist.

Prognostic statements can be made based on the known relationships that exist between areas of development. For example, a child who demonstrates a delay in just expressive language is thought to have a better prognosis than a child who has a delay in the expressive language, receptive language, gesture, and play domains.

The assessment process not only leads to a diagnosis, prognosis, and recommendation for intervention, but it also allows the clinician to provide parents education regarding the typical course of development and where their child falls within that framework. A clinician who is facile with developmental milestones is better able to counsel parents about their child and the appropriate expectations caregivers should have for the child.

▶ Setting Goals and the Intervention Process

After the evaluation is complete, the clinician writes a summary of his or her findings in an evaluation report. In some cases, the child may simply need to be monitored over time. If intervention is warranted, however, goals to be targeted in intervention are specified. The overarching goal of intervention is to facilitate development to age-expected or cognitively appropriate levels. Goals are the target behaviors the clinician will facilitate in the intervention process. The target behaviors are those behaviors that the child must evolve to next in development and/or the component skills necessary to reach a particular milestone. In our example of the 30-month-old child who is not yet marking morphemes, an appropriate goal for intervention is that the child will begin marking present progressive verbs ending -ing in two-word combinations (e.g., *mommy eating).* The present progressive is one of the first morphemes to emerge in toddlerhood, so this makes it the appropriate target for therapy. A goal such as marking copula *to be* in short sentences would not be appropriate at this time, as copulas are not mastered until later in the preschool years. Another layer in setting goals for intervention is that they should be functional. What does "functional" mean? For goals to be functional, they must target behaviors and/or skills that are observed in everyday activities in which the child engages. Goals should also be measurable so that progress can be documented.

Three types of goals are developed by the clinician: long term, short term, and session objectives.

- Long-term goals relate to the broadest areas of development or the end product of the intervention. For example, a long-term goal might be "The child will demonstrate developmentally appropriate expressive language skills to support functional communication within academic and social contexts." Success in moving toward the long-term goal does not generally include a percentage of accuracy measure, but rather tends to be measured within the functional context of daily living.

- Short-term goals are the smaller steps taken to achieve the long-term goal. They are meant to be accomplished within weeks to months of setting them. For example, a short-term goal may be "The child will produce grammatical morpheme *-ing* in two- to three-word combinations within play-based activity at least 80% of the time." The target behavior in this case is *-ing*. Limiting the linguistic complexity to a phrase of two to three words is another type of scaffolding the clinician must consider.

- Goals set for a particular treatment session are known as session objectives. A session objective is the smallest step taken to achieve the short-term goal (and ultimately the long-term goal). A session objective may be "The child will produce grammatical morpheme *-ing* in two-word combinations when provided an immediate verbal model and tactile cue by the clinician in 80% of trials." Here, we see that a richer scaffolding (a model and a cue) is provided initially because it will provide the child with the best opportunity to elicit and practice the behavior. As the child gains some mastery over producing the behavior, the clinician can reduce the scaffolding, thereby increasing the child's independence in communication. We would expect this level of independence at a short-term goal interval.

Keep in mind that the session objective and the short-term goal are benchmarks that lead to the accomplishment of the long-term goal. The prognosis for gains to be made toward meeting session objectives, short-term goals, and long-term goals is dependent upon several factors, including the severity of the language impairment, any concomitant disorders, and the family's and child's motivation to participate in the intervention.

Once a set of long-term goals, short-term goals, and session objectives has been determined, the child is ready to embark on the intervention process. During this process, the clinician meets with the child for guided learning and practice. Within the therapy sessions, the clinician continues to use his or her knowledge of development to structure the expectations of the child and the therapeutic environment. As with the assessment process, the appropriate choice of toys, activities, and other materials is critical to the child's success in therapy. The clinician must choose materials that are within the child's developmental functioning so as not to overwhelm the child. The focus of the clinician should be to isolate the skill of difficulty as much as possible. If the child is having difficulty producing present progressive verb tense and the *-ing* form of the verb is targeted during an activity, the child should work only toward imitating the verb form. If an activity is too complex, the child will use their learning resources to complete the activity as well as learn the language form. This dual goal may overwhelm the child, such that they may not be successful.

The new clinician should clearly understand the difference between a goal, any therapeutic scaffolding, and the activity used to target the goal in an intervention session. The *goal* is the language behavior or milestone that the clinician targets during the therapy session (e.g., produce present progressive verb tense *-ing*). The *therapeutic scaffolding* includes models, cues, prompts, feedback, preparatory sets of information, structuring of the amount of language that the child must produce, and any environmental modifications. The *activity* is what the child and clinician engage in to practice the target goal behavior (e.g., playing Go Fish, reading a story and retelling it, playing with miniature toy figures or Play-Doh). The activity is neither the goal, nor is it the scaffold. It is common for young clinicians who are just learning to navigate the clinical process to confuse these three concepts.

Scaffolding

Scaffolding can take many different forms. A verbal model is an exact demonstration of what the clinician wants the child to do. For example, if you want the child to produce the possessive *s*, you might take 10 opportunities during a play activity with *Sesame Street* figures to model *Ernie's car Bert's car, Cookie Monster's car*, and so forth. Always give the child plenty of time to process your model and imitate you. Perhaps the child will repeat *Ernie car* without the possessive *s*. In such a case, the child may need an extra scaffold to make the target morpheme more salient. One scaffold could be a tactile cue. With a tactile cue, the clinician might say *Ernie's car* while running his/her finger along the child's hand while producing the possessive *s*. The tactile cue will highlight the important aspect of the language in a second sensory modality, making it more salient for the child.

In the previous example, the clinician provided a model of the possessive *s* within a phrase—not a sentence or in conversation. Controlling the amount of language surrounding the target scaffolds the child because having more language around the target increases the difficulty of perceiving and producing it.

Feedback as a scaffolding tool helps children see, hear, or feel their own behavior as they practice.

Some feedback tools include a mirror, an iPod with a microphone, or a video recorder. Perhaps the clinician audio-records the child's practice. After each trial, the clinician and the child can then listen to the child's responses together, and the child can determine which trials were accurate or in error. This type of activity would be appropriate for an older child.

Understanding developmental milestones will help the clinician decide which types of cues, prompts, and feedback are appropriate for the child. When a goal is first introduced, the clinician's intention is to provide the most scaffolding needed for a child to produce the behavior. Having the correct level of scaffolding ensures the child practices the accurate behavior or skill as often as possible. It is important to remember that the clinician wants the child to have good practice on most, if not all, of the trials administered.

Accuracy may be measured using one of several conventions, including a percentage of trials (i.e., number of accurate productions ÷ total number of trials administered; 7/10 = 70%), or a frequency count within an interval of time (e.g., five times within a 10-minute activity). If the child is not achieving more than 50% accuracy with a goal, the child is practicing the incorrect behavior just as much (or more) than the desired behavior. This 50% accuracy marker relates to chance levels of performance, as determined statistically. When the child is less than 50–65% accurate, the clinician must reassess the scaffolds, their expectations of the child, and the complexity of the activity being used. One option may be for the clinician to increase or change the type of scaffold provided to the child or to train component parts of the goal. Over time, the scaffolds should fade away so that the child becomes independent in their skills.

Another part of the intervention process is parent training and a home program. Education of the child's parents and other caregivers is ongoing and essential for the child to generalize what they are learning in therapy to his/her daily living environments (e.g., home, school, or the playground).

▶ Case Studies

Three case studies are referred to throughout this text to illustrate the discussions of the various topics in language development. Johnathon, Josephine, and Robert are toddlers who were evaluated because their mothers were concerned about their language development. Each evaluation report reviews the child's background history, clinical findings, diagnosis, prognosis, and recommendations.

Although Johnathon's mother expressed concern regarding her son's development, the evaluation found him to demonstrate typical language development. In contrast, Josephine and Robert each show a language delay. Josephine's delay is characterized predominately by a delay in expressive language, whereas Robert's delay is more encompassing, including delays in receptive and expressive language as well as delays in gesture and play domains. Josephine is considered to have a better prognosis for outgrowing her language delay because she has strengths in receptive language, play, and gesture development. Research shows that children with strengths in these areas tend to fare better than children like Robert, who show delays in the expressive and receptive language, gesture, and play domains.

Although both Josephine and Robert demonstrate delayed language development in their evaluations, their prognosis for developing age-appropriate language later in the preschool years differs. Children who demonstrate language delays like those experienced by Robert are more likely to have persistent language delays in the preschool years and beyond. By 4 years of age, children like Robert are more likely to be diagnosed with Language Disorder (previously referred to as specific language impairment).

🔍 CASE STUDY: JOHNATHON (TD)

Sex: Male
Age: 25 months

Significant History

Johnathon is a 25-month-old boy who was referred to this appointment to assess the status of his speech and language development. His mother was concerned that Johnathon was not yet formulating sentences and questioned his vocabulary development. Johnathon's *prenatal/birth* history was unremarkable. He was born at term weighing 8 pounds, 4 ounces. *Medical* history was fairly unremarkable, with the exception of one ear infection at 12 months and occasional colds. *Developmental* milestones were met in a timely manner. For example, he sat without support by 6 months and walked by 12 months. *Speech-language* history was fairly unremarkable, with first words emerging by 12 months. Johnathon was recently combining words. He followed age-appropriate directions, including those without contextual support (e.g., "Bring me your bottle"). Johnathon ate a full-textured diet. He was enrolled in a daycare program three mornings each week. He was described as interactive and enjoyed playing with a variety of toys. Family history was negative for speech-language disorders.

Clinical Procedures

Tests
MacArthur-Bates Communicative Development Inventories (CDIs)
Rossetti Infant-Toddler Language Scale (RITLS)

Other
Play-based interaction
Spontaneous speech-language sample
Oral mechanism exam
Hearing Screening—Passed prior to attending this session today.

Clinical Findings

General Observations
Johnathon was found to be a pleasant and interactive boy. He readily entered the playroom with his mother and separated without difficulty to explore the room. Breaks in attention generally occurred when a task was more difficult for him to complete, such as those considered more appropriate for an older toddler.

Play
Johnathon's play skills were typical of same-age peers. He demonstrated play skills most typical of a 21- to 24-month-old, with skills continuing to emerge at the 24- to 27-month-old levels on the RITLS. Johnathon used most toys appropriately and chose toys selectively. He readily linked functional play schemes around familiar themes (e.g., doll play) and was observed to use objects symbolically (e.g., he put a toy key to his ear to represent a telephone).

Nonverbal Communication
Johnathon demonstrated communicative eye contact, turn-taking ability, and joint attention during the evaluation. Gestural communication was a strength for him. He demonstrated the prelinguistic gesture sequence of showing, giving, and pointing to objects and often combined these with spoken utterances.

Receptive Language
Johnathon responded to environmental sounds and his name. His attention to verbal requests and comments was inconsistent only when commands were considered more advanced for his age. His performance on the RITLS was most typical of a 21- to 24-month-old toddler with a scatter of skills up to 24- to 27-month age levels. He completed single-step commands (familiar and novel) and chose familiar objects from an array of objects. More complex commands (e.g., two requests with one object, two-step related directives) were followed with gesture cues. His mother reported that Johnathon understands new words rapidly.

Expressive Language
Johnathon's performance on the RITLS was most typical of a child 21–24 months of age, with a scatter of skills up to the 24- to 27-month-old age level. For example, Johnathon used new words, combined words, and produced a self-referent. He was just beginning to use many action words and relate personal experiences. Johnathon used language to fulfill a full range of communicative functions. For example, he initiated interactions verbally with adults, responded to adult utterances, and requested assistance from adults in his environment. On the CDI, Johnathon's mother reported him to have 212 words, which placed him at the 30th percentile for his age. His use of early developing morpho-syntax was also considered to be at the 30th percentile for his age (e.g.,-*ing*, plural *s*).

Phonology
Johnathon was at least 60% intelligible to this unfamiliar listener. His intelligible utterances were predominately single words and word combinations. Attempts at longer utterances resulted in reduced articulatory precision. Jargon was heard infrequently. His phonological repertoire included a full repertoire of stop, nasal, and glide sound classes as well as the early-developing fricatives /h/ and /f/. Consonant substitutions were considered developmentally appropriate

(continues)

(e.g., /θ/ for /s/, reduced lingual tension of /r/). Johnathon produced a full repertoire of singleton vowels and occasional diphthongs. His syllable shape repertoire was predominately restricted to open syllables (CV/maɪ/, VCV/odɛ/, CVCV/wowo/). However, final consonants were emerging. The following phonological processes were heard and considered developmentally appropriate: cluster reduction, stopping of later developing fricatives (/s, z, θ, ð/).

Oral-Motor Examination

Structure, function, and sensation of the oral-facial musculature appeared to be sufficient to support speech and language development.

Diagnosis and Prognosis

Johnathon is a pleasant 25-month-old toddler who presents receptive and expressive language skills that are consistent with a child his age. Play, oral-motor, gesture, and attention skills appear to be age-appropriate and sufficient to support continued language development.

Recommendations

Results from this evaluation were discussed with Johnathon's mother today. Speech-language intervention is not warranted at this time. Johnathon's mother was educated and counseled regarding typical cognitive and language development. She was encouraged to return to this clinic for re-evaluation if at any time she was concerned about subsequent stages of Johnathon's language development. She agreed.

🔍 CASE STUDY: JOSEPHINE (LB)

Sex: Female
Age: 22 months

Significant History

Josephine is a 22-month-old girl who was referred to this appointment due to continued concerns about her limited expressive vocabulary. Josephine's *prenatal/birth* histories were unremarkable. She was born at term weighing 7 pounds, 2 ounces. *Medical/health* history was significant for pneumonia at 19 months and two ear infections since that time. She had known allergies to dust and mold. Josephine's *hearing* was recently evaluated and found to be within normal limits. *Developmental* milestones were reached in a timely manner (e.g., sat at 6 months, walked at 11 months).

Josephine's *speech-language* development was remarkable for limited vocalizations during infancy, including some babbling. Her first word was delayed until 15 months, and her mother believed Josephine to have a small vocabulary for her age. Her primary means of communication were gesturing and attempting to produce phoneme sequences that marked two syllables, but these utterances did not approximate known words. Marking two syllables was a recent accomplishment. Her mother stated that Josephine did not readily imitate words and had isolated instances of accurate word production, but the latter behavior was inconsistent. Josephine was beginning to demonstrate frustration with communication breakdown. Her strengths appeared to be in the domains of play and receptive language. Josephine followed two-step directions that required her to leave the immediate context (e.g., "Go to the family room and get your diaper"). She ate a full diet at the time of this evaluation.

Josephine was evaluated for speech and language previously by her state's early intervention program. Results revealed a delay in expressive language. She was subsequently enrolled in language therapy, once weekly for the past 2 months. Josephine was otherwise cared for by her mother in the home. *Family history* was negative for speech-language disorders.

Clinical Procedures

Tests

MacArthur-Bates Communicative Development Inventories (CDIs)
Rossetti Infant-Toddler Language Scale (RITLS)

Other

Play-based interaction
Spontaneous speech-language sample

Oral mechanism exam
Hearing Screening—Passed prior to attending this session today.

Clinical Findings
General Observations
Josephine was a delightful and interactive child who readily transitioned to the playroom without difficulty. She regulated her behavior well and showed age-appropriate attention to all tasks.

Play
Josephine's play development was well within normal limits (WNL) for her age. She demonstrated a scatter of skills up to at least the 27- to 30-month age level. For example, she readily performed many related activities during play, and she selectively chose and used toys appropriately. Josephine engaged in spontaneous doll play (e.g., covered the doll with a blanket; fed it a bottle, a spoon, and miniature food items; hugged it), and she pretended to talk on the phone and write. She demonstrated symbolic play such as blowing on food during pretend cooking activity.

Nonverbal Communication
Josephine demonstrated the prelinguistic skills of communicative eye contact, joint attention, and turn-taking throughout the evaluation. She often used prelinguistic gestures (show, give, point) and iconic gestures (e.g., hand under cheek to indicate sleeping) to communicate and engage the clinician. Her performance on the RITLS was considered well WNL. Pragmatic skills were limited only by her sparse expressive language. However, nonverbal aspects of pragmatic development were WNL.

Receptive Language
Josephine's comprehension of language was well WNL with a scatter of skills up to at least the 24- to 27-month age level. For example, at this age level, Josephine understood the concept of *one* and recognized family member names. At her age level (21–24 months), she chose one object from a group of five, and followed novel and two-step related commands. She understood new words rapidly by her mother's report. She readily responded to her name.

Expressive Language
Compared to her receptive language abilities, Josephine's expressive language was significantly delayed. On the RITLS, she displayed skills most typical of the 9- to 12-month age level. However, Josephine did not readily engage in spoken imitation or consistently use spontaneous vocalization, babble, or jargon, which typically emerges during that stage of development. The use of routine carrier phrases such as "Ready, get set" facilitated her expression (i.e., /go/). She was not yet using adult-like intonation or using words rather than gesture to communicate. Her strengths were that she used early phonemes (/t, d, n/), woke with a communicative call, shook her head "no" (and "yes"), and combined gesture and vocalization to communicate (12- to 15-month age level). By her mother's report on the CDI, Josephine had seven words in her expressive vocabulary, which is most typical of a 12-month-old at the 50th percentile and consistent with her RITLS performance.

Phonology
Josephine's spontaneous vocalizations were limited in number and were less than 50% intelligible. Given her few spontaneous vocalizations, her phonological repertoire was judged to include the consonants /b, d, g, n, m, j, s, tʃ, ʔ/, the vowels /a, ə, i, o, u/, and the diphthongs /au, ai/. Her syllable shape repertoire included C /s/, CV /do/, CVC /nʌm/, CVCV /daga/, CVCVV /dagau/. She occasionally produced brief periods of reduplicated babble (e.g., /nanoməʔou/). In addition, she produced a prolonged /s/ while playing; /h/ was elicited through playful, nonspeech imitation. Meaningful productions of /g/ were fronted (/do/ for /go/).

Oral-Motor Examination
Structure, function, and sensory aspects of the mechanism appeared to be within functional limits (WFL) and sufficient to support speech development. For example, Josephine displayed neutral jaw posture at rest, good lip rounding for /u/ in spontaneous utterances, and tongue tip elevation for the production of alveolar phonemes /d,n/.

Diagnosis and Prognosis
Josephine is a delightful 22-month-old who demonstrates a mild to moderate delay in expressive language and a moderate delay in speech sound development. Her expressive language delay is characterized by limited vocalizations including babbling, jargoning, or word approximations; a small vocabulary; and a delay in combining words. Her speech sound delay is characterized by a phonological and syllable shape repertoire that are smaller than

(continues)

expected, particularly in terms of her vowel repertoire. Other aspects of language and cognition (prelinguistic skills, receptive language, and play) are well within normal limits.

Prognosis is good and affirms that Josephine will outgrow her expressive language delay given her established prelinguistic skills, strong play and receptive language abilities, reliance on gesture to communicate, and ability to imitate gestures.

Recommendations

Continue to enroll Josephine in speech-language therapy through her state's early intervention program. It is recommended that intervention goals target parent education and training of language facilitation techniques (e.g., recasts, expansion, parallel talk). These techniques can be used throughout the day with Josephine during functional activities. Reevaluate Josephine's speech and language skills through this clinic in 12 months to assess her progress toward age-expected milestones.

🔍 CASE STUDY: ROBERT (LT)

Sex: Male
Age: 27 months

Significant History

Robert is a 27-month-old boy who was referred to this appointment to reassess the status of his speech and language development. Robert's *prenatal/birth* history was significant for maternal preeclampsia and cesarean section delivery at 31 weeks gestation. He was admitted to the neonatal intensive care unit for 3 months after birth. *Medical* history was remarkable for heart murmur, VSD (Ventricular Septal Defect—s/p repair), hypothyroidism (Synthroid prescribed), gastroesophageal reflux (Prevacid prescribed), asthma (Pulmicort and Xopanex prescribed), and failure to thrive. History was negative for ear infections but *audiological testing* revealed questionable unilateral hearing loss in the left ear. An audiological reevaluation was planned for within 6 months.

Developmental milestones were delayed for motor, speech-language, and feeding development. For example, walking was delayed until 17 months (adjusted age), and at the time of this evaluation, he was not yet eating a full diet of textured foods. *Speech-language* history was remarkable for a delay in speaking first words (18 months, adjusted age) and he was not yet combining words. He followed simple directions (e.g., "Sit down"), but his mother believed Robert to have limited attention skills for his age.

Robert had a history of *early intervention*. At the time of this evaluation, he had received physical therapy, occupational therapy, and speech-language therapy through an early intervention program. Robert was enrolled in a daycare program 5 days each week. He was described as happy and enjoyed playing with other children. Family history was remarkable for an uncle diagnosed with Language Disorder as a child.

Clinical Procedures
Tests
MacArthur-Bates Communicative Development Inventories (CDIs)
Rossetti Infant-Toddler Language Scale (RITLS)

Other
Play-based interactions
Spontaneous speech-language sample
Oral mechanism exam

Clinical Findings
General Observations
Robert was an interactive and pleasant boy who readily entered the playroom with his mother. Consistent with his mother's report, Robert displayed limited attention skills for his age. He became easily excitable and disorganized in his behavior. His attention and behavior were more typical of a child approximately 12 months of age. For example, he did not remain engaged in a play activity for very long but preferred to wander around the room or hide under the table. Robert was motivated to interact with adults and imitated adult models. These behaviors were strengths for him.

Play

Robert's performance on the RITLS revealed established play skills at the 9- to 12-month age level, with a scatter of emerging play skills up to the 21- to 24-month age level. His play was characterized predominately by banging/shaking objects and relational play (placing objects within each other). Functional use of objects was emerging, but functional play schemes were not part of his established play repertoire. Robert engaged in simple games, and he showed an emerging ability to perform actions with objects (e.g., throw a ball) and imitate adult actions (e.g., put a key in a door). He was not yet pretending with stuffed animals or dolls.

Nonverbal Communication

Relative to Robert's other skills, his prelinguistic communication was a strength for him. His gesture performance was most typical of a 9- to 12-month-old child on the RITLS, with a scatter of skills up to the 21- to 24-month-old level. He consistently demonstrated communicative eye contact, joint attention, and turn-taking behaviors (both verbal and nonverbal), as well as prelinguistic gestures (e.g., showing objects, giving objects, pointing, requesting). He used gestures to satisfy basic needs (e.g., nods head "no," leads caregiver to desired object, indicates diaper is wet).

Receptive Language

On the RITLS, Robert's comprehension skills were most typical of a 9- to 12-month-old child, with a scatter of skills up to the 21- to 24-month age level. For example, he responded to simple commands (e.g., "Give me"), responded to requests to say words, and chose two objects from an array of objects. However, he did not show an interest in pictures, identifying body parts, or following commands that required him to complete two actions with an object. Robert demonstrated inconsistent attention to his name. He was also inconsistent in attending to gesture cues meant to scaffold his comprehension of spoken language.

Robert had difficulty attending to formal tests of receptive vocabulary, so the CDI: Words and Gestures test was used informally to survey his comprehension of vocabulary. His performance on the CDI revealed a receptive vocabulary of at least 194 items across a variety of categories, including clothing, household items, people, and descriptive words. This vocabulary size is considered typical of toddlers 18–24 months of age (normative range = 150–500 words; Miller & Paul, 1995).

Expressive Language

On the RITLS, Robert's expressive language was assessed to be most typical of a 9- to 12-month-old, with a scatter of skills up to the 15- to 18-month age level. His spontaneous vocalizations were predominately characteristic of reduplicated babbling and emerging variegated babbling (e.g., /mamamo/, /miml/). Robert was not yet jargoning consistently or producing words within jargoned utterances. He was not yet combining pointing with words. Robert used fewer than 10 intelligible words during this session, but those expressed were for imitation (e.g., /nε/ for *night-night*) or spontaneous naming (e.g., /o/ for *telephone*). His mother reported an expressive vocabulary of 14 words. His expressive vocabulary included two sound effects/animal sounds (i.e., *baa, uh oh*), two vehicles (*bus, car*), and several toy and routines items (*night-night, hi, bye*). Early developing morphemes (e.g., *-ing*) and early word combinations were not observed or reported (normative age range for emergence = 18–24 months).

A strength for Robert was his motivation to use spoken vocalizations to interact with others for a variety of pragmatic functions, including protest, response, initiation, and labeling. However, he was not yet engaging in adult-like dialogue or taking turns in conversation. He relied on gesture and vocalizations instead of words.

Phonology

Robert was less than 25% intelligible. His sound and syllable shape repertoires were most typical of a child 12–18 months of age. His phonological repertoire included a restricted set of consonants (/m, n, p, b, d, j, l, v, ?/), vowels (/i, ɪ, ε, e, ʌ, U, o, a/), and a diphthong (/au/). The following phonemes were not heard: /t, k, g, f, æ, u, 3, oɪ/. With immediate verbal models, the diphthong /aɪ/ was elicited in *night-night*. Robert's syllable shape repertoire was restricted to simple open syllables such as CV, V, VCV, and CVCV (e.g., /ba/, /o/, /ʌda/, /mimɪ/). He attempted to imitate words heard in conversation today. His attempts were largely accurate for simple syllables, with the exception of slight vowel distortions or diphthong reductions (e.g., /ba/ for *bye*) and final consonant deletions (e.g., /opε/ for *open*). Spontaneous productions of multisyllable words resulted in phonological simplifications (e.g., /o/ for *telephone*).

(continues)

Oral–Motor Examination

Structure, function, and sensory aspects of the mechanism appeared to be largely within functional limits to support continued speech and language development, with the exception of a reduced range of facial-labial movements for rounded phonemes and slightly reduced strength of facial-labial muscles for full and consistent bilabial plosion.

Diagnosis and Prognosis

Robert is a delightful and engaging 27-month-old who demonstrates mild to moderate delays in speech as well as receptive and expressive language development. In addition, other cognitive areas that affect speech and language development were delayed, including play, gesture, and attention skills. His speech, language, gesture, and play development are most typical of a 12-to 15-month-old child, a scatter of emerging abilities up to the 21-month age level. His speech delay is characterized by reduced intelligibility owing to a small phoneme and syllable shape repertoire, and to a lesser extent by some subtle oral-motor weakness. His expressive language delay is characterized by a small expressive vocabulary, no jargon or use of jargon with words, and delay in combining words. His receptive language delay is characterized by inconsistent attention to spoken language, a small vocabulary, and limited comprehension of age-level directions.

Robert is at risk of continued speech and language delays given his delays in comprehension, play, and gesture. Prognosis for gains to be made with speech-language therapy appears to be good because of his established prelinguistic social skills and his motivation to imitate adult models. Ongoing assessment of his attention development, auditory processing skills, and questionable hearing loss will need to be made to determine the etiology of his comprehension performance.

Recommendations

It is recommended that Robert continue to be enrolled in speech-language therapy. A play-based approach to intervention is most appropriate for him. Gesture and multimodal cueing will facilitate imitation (verbal and nonverbal) and development in a variety of skill areas (speech, language, play). Robert's attention, auditory processing skills, and questionable hearing loss should be continually assessed to determine how each contributes to his comprehension performance. Goals of speech-language intervention should include the following:

Long-Term Goal 1: Robert will demonstrate developmentally appropriate attention skills to support continued social-emotional, cognitive, and language development.
- *Short-Term Goal 1:* Increase intervals of sustained attention to objects, activities, and books.

Long-Term Goal 2: Robert will demonstrate developmentally appropriate play skills to support continued social-emotional, cognitive, and language development.
- *Short-Term Goal 1:* Expand Robert's play repertoire to include object exploration, cause-effect toys, and functional play schemes.
- *Short-Term Goal 2:* Expand Robert's play repertoire to include symbolic play schemes and linking of play schemes for pretend play.

Long-Term Goal 3: Robert will demonstrate developmentally appropriate receptive language skills to support functional communication and pre-academic development.
- *Short-Term Goal 1:* Facilitate Robert's ability to direct attention to language spoken to him.
- *Short-Term Goal 2:* Expand Robert's receptive vocabulary of words that are part of his daily routines.
- *Short-Term Goal 3:* Increase comprehension of unfamiliar one-step directions that include identification of objects.

Long-Term Goal 4: Robert will demonstrate developmentally appropriate expressive language skills to support functional communication and pre-academic development.
- *Short-Term Goal 1:* Increase expressive vocabulary for functional communication that includes naming and requesting. Initial vocabulary targets should be organized around themes such as animals, body parts, household items, doll play, and vehicles.
- *Short-Term Goal 2:* Establish use of personal identification by name (*Robert*) and early pronouns (*me, mine*).
- *Short-Term Goal 3:* Establish Robert's ability to combine words that express early semantic relations.
- *Short-Term Goal 4:* Establish Robert's ability to produce early developing morphemes to mark present progressive tense (*-ing*) and spatial relations (*in, on*).

Long-Term Goal 5: Robert will demonstrate developmentally appropriate speech intelligibility to support functional communication and pre-academic development.
- *Short-Term Goal 1:* Expand Robert's phonological repertoire to include velar stop consonants (/k, g/), alveolar stop /t/, and early-developing fricatives (/f, h/).
- *Short-Term Goal 2:* Expand Robert's syllable shape repertoire to include closed syllable shapes (CVC, CVCVC, VC).

When the speech-language pathologist begins intervention, she or he will need to set session objectives. Session objectives will be measurable goals for the day that include the types of scaffolds discussed previously in this chapter. A session objective may be written to say the following:

Robert will indicate his turn by using gesture and/or spoken self-reference during bubble (or other) play for at least four of five opportunities when provided immediate verbal models and hand-over-hand guidance as needed.

As part of LTG 3, receptive language, a session objective in the home could center around routines such as taking laundry from the clothes dryer to the basket.

Robert will turn his focus of attention to his mother when she says his name and provides a tactile cue (as needed) for four of five opportunities before labeling individual items of clothing coming out of the clothes dryer.

The reader should also keep in mind that goals and session objectives vary in how they are written between clinical work settings—outpatient clinic and early intervention and elementary school.

Study Questions

- Define language and its five domains.
- What are the procedures of a language evaluation?
- How do clinicians use their knowledge of developmental milestones in the clinical practice of speech-language pathology?
- Compare and contrast long-term goals, short-term goals, and session objectives.
- What are some scaffolds that a clinician might use in language therapy?

References

American Speech-Language-Hearing Association. (1982). *Language*. Retrieved from http://www.asha.org/policy

Applebee, A. (1978). *The child's concept of a story: Ages 2 to 17*. Chicago, IL: University of Chicago Press.

Dunn, L. M., & Dunn, D. M. (2007). *The Peabody picture vocabulary test* (4th ed.). Bloomington, MN: NCS Pearson.

Goldman, R., & Fristoe, M. (2000). *Goldman-Fristoe test of articulation* (2nd ed.). Circle Pines, MN: American Guidance Services.

Heckman, J. J. (2008). Schools, skills and synapses. *Economic Inquiry, 46*(3), 289–324.

Heilmann, J., & Malone, T. O. (2014). The rules of the game: Properties of a database of expository language samples. *Language, Speech, and Hearing Services in the Schools, 45,* 277–290.

IDEA. (2004). Individuals with Disabilities Education Act of 2004 (IDEA), Pub. L. No. 108–446, 118 Stat. 2647.

Irwin, L. G., Siddiqi, A., & Hertzman, C. (2007). *Early child development: A powerful equalizer*. Final Report for the World Health Organization's Commission on the Social Determinants of Health.

Miller, J. F., & Paul, R. (1995). *The clinical assessment of language comprehension*. Baltimore, MD: Brookes Publishing.

Nippold, M. A. (2014). *Language sampling with adolescents: Implications for interventions* (2nd ed.). San Diego, CA: Plural.

Patel, R., & Connaghan, K. (2014). Park play: A picture description task for assessing childhood motor speech disorders. *International Journal of Speech Language Pathology, 16*(4), 337–347.

Retherford, K. (2000). *Guide to analysis of language transcripts* (3rd ed.). Eau Claire, WI: Thinking Publications.

Rossetti, L. (2006). *The Rossetti Infant-Toddler language scale*. East Moline, IL: LinguiSystems.

Shapiro, L. (1997). Tutorial: An introduction to syntax. *Journal of Speech, Language and Hearing Research, 40*(2), 254–272.

Williams, K. (1997). *Expressive vocabulary test*. Circle Pines, MN: American Guidance Services.

Zimmerman, I. L., Steiner, V. C., & Pond, R. E. (2011). *Preschool language scale* (5th ed.). San Antonio, TX: Pearson.

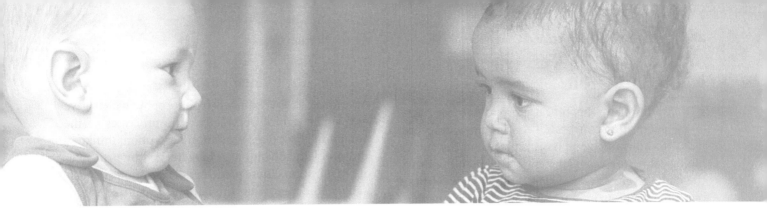

CHAPTER 2

Historical and Contemporary Views of the Nature–Nurture Debate: A Continuum of Perspectives for the Speech-Language Pathologist

Sima Gerber, PhD, CCC-SLP
Lorain Szabo Wankoff, PhD, CCC-SLP

OBJECTIVES

- Explore the continuum of the traditional "nature–nurture" debate as it relates to the acquisition of language
- Understand the historical impact of the nature, nurture, and interactionist perspectives on the field of speech-language pathology
- Describe a contemporary model of language acquisition
- Propose a perspective on using theories of language acquisition to guide the assessment of and intervention for children with language disorders

KEY TERMS

Empiricist theories
Intentionality model
Interactionist perspective

Language acquisition theories
Language assessment
Language intervention

Nature perspective
Nurture perspective
Rationalist theories

▶ Introduction

Traditionally, theoretical approaches to language acquisition constitute a continuum with regard to how much emphasis is placed on the child's biological *nature* versus the environmental input that the child receives (i.e., *nurture*). In contrast to these opposing views, an interactionist approach to language development dovetails the mechanisms internal to the child in concert with the powerful influence of experiential and social factors.

The main objective of this chapter is to review the continuum of nature, nurture, and interactionist perspectives and discuss their impact on the world of speech-language pathology. By tracing the variations of the nativistic, behavioral, and interactionist approaches to the development of language, we can begin to understand how the trends in modern language science have impacted the profession of speech-language pathology over the last 50 or so years. As we consider the status of the nature–nurture debate, the contemporary science of child development expands on this discussion in interesting new ways. In fact, this science suggests that the nature–nurture question, as it relates to child development, is obsolete. As Siegel (1999) suggests, "There is no need to choose between brain or mind, biology or experience, nature or nurture. These divisions are unhelpful and inhibit clear thinking about an important and complex subject: the developing human mind" (p. xii).

▶ Nature, Nurture, and Interactionist Views

Theories of language acquisition are central to the information that speech-language pathologists must learn for several reasons. First, a descriptively adequate theory of language development will provide an outline of what is learned by children when they acquire language. Second, theories of language development that have explanatory adequacy will account for not only the facts of language development, but also the mechanisms of language learning—that is, "how" language is learned (Bohannon & Bonvillian, 2005; Chomsky, 1965).

Different paradigms and their differing perspectives will be described as they relate to two questions:

1. What do children acquire when they acquire language?
2. Which processes account for how children acquire language?

Nature: Rationalist Paradigm

According to the rationalist philosophy, which gave rise to the nature perspective, the processes of the human intellect (e.g., sensation, perception, thinking, and problem-solving) are characterized by principles of organization. These processes of cognition are qualitatively different from the fairly disorganized events that occur in the observable world. The organizing principles and processes that characterize cognition enable humans to make sense of events in the world. From this perspective, speaking and understanding language are considered fundamentally human traits that are biologically determined without direct instruction. In contrast, for example, reading and writing are taught more explicitly (Catts & Kamhi, 2005; Sakai, 2005).

Biological Bases

Although Chomsky was among the first to suggest that humans possess linguistic knowledge at birth, the psychologist Eric Lenneberg (1967) provided much of the groundwork for the view that language is biologically based. He argued that language shows evidence of the following properties:

- *Little variation within the species.* Lenneberg argued that all languages are characterized by a system of phonology, words, and syntax.
- *Specific organic correlates.* Lenneberg argued that like walking but unlike writing, there is a universal timetable for the acquisition of language. He suggested that critical periods exist for second-language learning as well as for rehabilitation after language loss due to injury or insult to brain function.
- *Heredity.* According to Lenneberg, even with environmental deprivation, the capacity for language exists—although it might be manifested in the use of signing, as seen in individuals with hearing impairment.
- *No history within species.* Lenneberg argued that because we have no evidence for a more primitive human language, language must be an inherently human phenomenon.

Recent arguments for the biological basis of language typically refer to data in several related areas. These areas include cerebral asymmetries for the left and right brain dedicated to speech and language processes; critical periods for speech and language development; speech perception processes in infancy; central nervous system development; and genetic evidence from speech and language disorders research

(Sakai, 2005; Werker & Tees, 1984). Furthermore, over the last 30 years, investigators have combined basic research in first-language acquisition with research using brain imaging technology to understand how children become multilingual (Lust, 2007).

Those who argue for the biological basis of language cite data on cerebral asymmetries that are present even at birth in areas of the brain that are critical for language functioning. For example, the Sylvian fissure is longer and the planum temporale is larger on the left side of the brain than on the right side in the majority of fetal and newborn brains. Furthermore, the degree of asymmetry appears to increase as the brain matures, whereas plasticity of the brain decreases over time (Sakai, 2005). Chapter 13 discusses the neurological substrates of language in more detail.

Arguments for the biological basis for speech and language acquisition also find support in research on the growth and development of the central nervous system in the early years of life. These developments include significant increases in brain weight over a relatively short period of time, the formation of myelin sheaths on the axons, and increases in the number of neuronal connectors in the cortex during the first years of life—all of which correlate with advancements in language abilities. Finally, data from genetic studies that show strong patterns of inheritance for family members of children with developmental language disorder (previously called children with specific language impairment, or SLI) also provide support for proponents of a biological basis of language development (Sakai, 2005). Findings from infant speech perception have also lent support for the nature thesis. For example, Eimas, Siqueland, Jusczyk, and Vigorito (1971) demonstrated that the infants modified their suck patterns as they hear changes in speech sound stimuli. Infants as young as 1-month olds perceive the distinctions between /b/ and /p/ in the syllables [ba] and [pa]. The studies that followed this seminal work found that babies make finer phonetic discriminations at 6 months of age than they can at 10 months, when their experience with their own language is more extensive (Trehub, 1976; Werker & Tees, 1984). At 6 months, babies can discriminate between sounds that are not in the native language they have heard, but at 10 months, babies can only discriminate sounds in their own language. In a study by Vouloumanos and Werker (2007), infants also showed a preference for speech over other sound. Infants were presented with isolated syllables of human speech contrasted with nonspeech stimuli that controlled critical spectral and temporal parameters of speech. With similar stimuli, it has previously been demonstrated that infants as young as 2 months of age preferred listening to speech. In the Vouloumanos and Werker (2007) study, newborn babies who were 1–4 days old demonstrated a similar bias for listening to speech versus nonspeech when their contingent sucking responses to speech and nonspeech sounds were compared.

Evidence supporting a critical period for language learning has traditionally come from studies of individuals who have experienced brain injury before puberty rather than after. Rehabilitating the loss of language that occurs prior to puberty has typically been less challenging than when loss occurs after puberty (Sakai, 2005). Similarly, a critical period for learning language is often supported by evidence that second languages are easier to learn before puberty than after. Finally, the unique case of a severely neglected child named Genie illustrated the great difficulties in the acquisition of morphology and syntax when a child is not exposed to language early in life (Curtiss, 1974).

Transformational Generative Grammar—Chomsky

Within the nature perspective, the theory of Noam Chomsky is central. The early versions of Chomsky's Transformational Generative Grammar (1957, 1965) described the innate, generative knowledge that enables the native speaker to produce a potentially infinite number of novel utterances, utterances they have never heard before or spoken, and understand an infinite number of utterances based on knowledge of the rule-system.

According to Chomsky's (1965) early view, the child is born with a language acquisition device (LAD) armed with linguistic universals for the task of language learning. The early and seemingly effortless learning of syntax without explicit parental feedback has been the primary reason for suggesting innate language abilities in children (Chomsky, 1972). The study by Brown and Hanlon in 1970, where parents' overt corrections were in response to semantic errors rather than syntactic ones, has been a frequently cited study to support the notion of innate language abilities (Bohannon & Stanowicz, 1988).

In Chomsky's view, each native speaker-hearer of a language appeared to possess a wealth of knowledge about his or her "grammar." Chomsky termed this knowledge *linguistic competence*. In his account of language acquisition, the LAD was said to enable children to develop a language system fairly rapidly. This language system was sufficiently complex and generative, allowing children to create a potentially infinite number of novel utterances. This capacity was termed *linguistic creativity,* an ability that every native speaker-hearer clearly possessed (Chomsky, 1957, 1965).

Chomsky's description of language acquisition, according to Transformational Generative Grammar, suggested that the child's innate LAD armed with language universal rules could explain not only the rapidity and uniformity of the language acquisition process, but also the complexity of the language knowledge that is acquired (Chomsky, 1982, 1988). Early formulations argued that children were endowed with formal and substantive linguistic universals, such as the three components of the grammar (e.g., syntax, semantics, and phonology) and categories or units of language (e.g., parts of speech or phonological features; McNeil, 1970). Later accounts described the innate capacities as inherent biases or constraints that empowered children to treat linguistic input in particular ways (Wexler, 1999). For example, children learning English might be listening for word order—Subject–Verb–Object, to signal grammatical relations—whereas children learning Hungarian might be listening for noun inflections for that information (Berko-Gleason, 2005; Slobin, 1979).

In response to the early Chomskian accounts of language knowledge, researchers in the early 1960s studied the emerging grammar of the young child while focusing on syntactic rules. In the late 1960s and early 1970s, however, Semantic Generativists focused on the role of semantics in language and language learning (Fillmore, 1968). Developmental psycholinguistic research then shifted from an interest in syntax to an interest in the semantic knowledge that supports the development of syntax. Young children's knowledge of underlying semantic relations (e.g., agent, action, and object) was viewed as the impetus for their developing grammar because semantic relations typically occurred in predictable positions in sentences. For example, in the frequently used declarative sentence type, the agent occupies the initial position and is typically the grammatical subject of the sentence (Schlesinger, 1977).

With the advent of the work of developmental psycholinguists such as Lois Bloom (1970), semantics or the content of child language was considered key to determining the child's grammar. The importance of nonlinguistic context in interpreting the meaning of the child's language was emphasized. Further, the acquisition of semantic categories such as spatial terms, dimensional terms, and semantic features was investigated in an effort to understand the unfolding of the child's semantic knowledge (Clark, 1973).

A revised theory of language by Chomsky, called Government Binding Theory, was formulated in its most comprehensive form in 1982. This account of language described idiosyncratic parameters of particular languages as well as universal principles across different languages. The idiosyncratic patterns of particular languages were captured in the "parameters," which were set differently for different languages with input from the language. For example, the fact that a particular language differs in the direction in which it embeds its clauses to form complex sentences (right or left branching) is captured in the parameter setting of the particular language (Leonard & Loeb, 1988).

According to Transformational Generative Grammar and Principles and Parameters accounts of language acquisition, the child operated as a minilinguist. That is, the child utilized not only the universal features that languages have in common, but would ultimately establish the parameters that make the particular language unique. As the child accrued more and more examples of their own language, they could generate hypotheses about how language works, and these hypotheses would eventually be either confirmed or disconfirmed. Ultimately, the child was said to intuit a finite set of generative rules—that is, rules with the capacity to generate and understand a potentially infinite number of novel utterances.

Cognitive scientists in the 1980s expanded and debated Chomsky's notion of a language faculty by invoking the notion of language as a modular skill or "modularity." Fodor (1983) argued that the human language fits the definition of a module, a specialized encapsulated mental organ that has evolved to handle specific information. Fodor's description of a language module includes at least three claims: (1) language is innate; (2) the function of language is localized in the brain, and (3) language is domain-specific (Bates, 1994). Evidence for modularity was drawn from a number of other sources, including the grammatical profile of children with developmental language disorder (van der Lely, 1997). Children with developmental language disorder are impaired in the domain of language but with the exclusion of impairments in other areas of cognitive, sensory, and motor functioning. This notion has been debated by others, including Elizabeth Bates (1994), who argues that "well-defined regions of the brain may become specialized for a particular function as a result of experience" (p. 138). Although there may be a strong innate predisposition for a domain-specific function, this function may be distributed across various regions of the brain, as in naming ability. Finally, Bates (1994) argues that some systems or functions may be innate and highly localized but not domain-specific as in various attentional systems.

A Contemporary View

In more recent incarnations of the "nature" paradigm, the specialized language faculty triggers the development of linguistic knowledge that uses at least four different mechanisms for conveying semantic relations: hierarchical structure, linear order, agreement, and case (Pinker & Jackendoff, 2005). According to Pinker and Jackendoff (2005), the four mechanisms are sometimes used redundantly. Pinker (2006) addresses the question, "What are the innate mechanisms necessary for language learning to take place?" Certain cognitive accomplishments, such as the representational function (i.e., the ability to represent objects or ideas mentally), are known prerequisites for language to unfold. Furthermore, metacognitive control or executive functioning that serves to monitor the incoming stimuli, the motor output, and the learning that takes place must be accounted for as well. Finally, individuals must operate with an unfolding theory of mind, the ability to attribute mental states such as beliefs, intents, desires, knowledge, pretend to oneself and others, and to understand that others have beliefs, desires, and intentions that are different from one's own (Premack & Woodruff, 1978) as the "language instinct" or the language faculty does its work.

Despite the impact of nature arguments of language acquisition, the limitations of this view are worth noting. For example, contrary to earlier findings, recent evidence suggests that caretakers *do* respond to the language errors of youngsters, including the syntactic ones (Saxton, Galloway, & Backley, 1999). Furthermore, the assumption that language acquisition is essentially completed by 4 or 5 years of age has not been supported, nor has the critical period been clearly identified (Hulit & Howard, 2002). Finally, the notion that language is acquired through a species-specific LAD is controversial, as research into animal communication raises the question of whether language is fully unique to humans (Pinker, 1984).

Implications from a Nature Perspective: Understanding, Assessing, and Treating Children with Language Disorders

From the nature perspective, the assumptions about children who fail to develop language typically include the possibility that the child is experiencing deficits in the innate mechanisms that they bring to the task of learning language and constructing grammar. In fact, these possibilities are often considered most relevant to the discussion of children who are referred to as having a developmental language disorder.

The evidence for a genetic view of SLI has been supported by studies that have found increased rates of speech, language, and reading problems within some families. In fact, the identification of a particular gene, the FOXP2, in one family (KE) with many members who experience speech and language disorders (Vargha-Khadem et al., 1998) was groundbreaking for the genetic line of research with this population.

A subgroup of children with developmental language disorder is often characterized by their difficulties in the acquisition and processing of syntax and grammatical morphology in addition to delays in the acquisition of vocabulary, especially verbs (Seiger-Gardner, 2010). These children seem endowed with many of the developmental capacities that are necessary for learning language, yet they fall behind their typically developing peers in the acquisition of a linguistic system, in particular, the acquisition of the morphosyntactic rules of grammar. In fact, children with SLI often have less well-developed morphosyntactic systems than younger children with comparable mean length of utterance (MLUs), and these differences persist over time. Of interest here are the various explanations for the grammatical limitations that these children experience. For example, the extended optional infinitive account (Rice, Wexler, & Cleave, 1995) suggests that the omission of finiteness markers, such as past *-ed* and third person *-s*, persists for a longer time in children with SLI than in typically developing children. In the computational grammatical complexity view proposed by van der Lely (1998), children with SLI have difficulty with the linguistic representations or computations that are the foundational for structurally complex forms in syntax, morphology, and/or phonology.

In terms of assessment and intervention with children who exhibit language impairments, the nature of hypotheses led the way for many of the hallmarks of the clinical work of a speech-language pathologist. The use of samples of spontaneous language as the data from which to determine children's linguistic knowledge was an example of the methodology learned from linguistic inquiry. For example, assessing children's language to describe their knowledge of the rules of grammar, particularly in terms of morphology and syntax, was clearly an outgrowth of the work of the linguists and psycholinguists of the time. Determining children's mean length of utterance and measuring their linguistic progress relative to this parameter (rather than relative to their chronological age) revolutionized our thinking about the stages and expectations of language acquisition. These assessment goals and procedures brought our clinical evaluations into a new era and have had a lasting impact on our evaluation protocols.

Because of the impact of the nature perspective, language intervention began to focus on determining what children needed to learn about the rules of their language given their stage of language acquisition. The following goals of language therapy were prioritized:

- Addressing syntax
- Expanding the child's length of utterance
- Producing various sentence types
- Developing the use of Brown's (1973) 14 grammatical morphemes

In reference to strategies of language intervention, the notion of enhancing the processing of the informative elements in the linguistic signal can also be traced to our interpretations of the work of the nature perspective. For example, to increase the salience of the linguistic input, a clinician might use prosodic and syntactic bootstrapping techniques. *Bootstrapping* is a term that refers to the child's ability to use the information s/he has to learn new information. Prosodic bootstrapping refers to the placement of target elements at the end of the utterance for greater salience (e.g., a response such as *Yes, she is* might be used to emphasize the copula form). Syntactic bootstrapping refers to the child's use of grammar to learn new language forms. For example, teaching a particular verb form in several linguistic contexts heightens the child's awareness of varied syntactic uses of the form (e.g., *She is pushing me; Who pushed her?; Don't push*) (Nelson, 1998).

Despite the undeniable impact of linguistic theory on the field of speech-language pathology, a clear limitation that followed us into the present is this theory's more narrow focus on the language form. Given that many children who experience difficulties in learning language are challenged in areas such as the development of the precursors to language (e.g., prelinguistic skills such as using gestures), cognitive development (e.g., object permanence), and social–affective development (e.g., eye contact and joint attention with a communication partner), interventions must often override attention to the structure of the language. Nonetheless, by embracing the thinking of linguists, the work of speech-language pathologists moved into the realm of linguistic science.

Nurture: Behaviorist Paradigm

Based on the evidence gathered so far, the nature argument alone is not sufficient to explain the child's accomplishment in developing language. Rather, the relative importance of an innate language faculty versus environmental influence continues to be viewed as controversial.

Historically, the impetus for the nurture argument in learning and language was the "blank slate" philosophy of John Locke (1960/1690). This empiricist approach eventually gave rise to behaviorism in psychology. According to this perspective, explanations of behavior rely only on observable phenomena; in the most radical version of this position, no inferences regarding internal, unobservable events are made. Researchers and theoreticians who focused on the impact of the environment targeted primarily observable and measurable events to explain development.

Classical Conditioning

Classical conditioning was associated with the 20th-century Russian physiologist Pavlov (1902). In his most famous experiment, a dog was given food along with the ringing of a bell. After repeated pairings of the two, the dogs would salivate upon hearing the bell even before the meat powder was introduced. Through classical conditioning, an association (a conditioned response) was formed between the bell and salivation; this association had not previously existed. While the meat powder was termed the "unconditioned stimulus," the bell became the "conditioned stimulus." Salivation was the "unconditioned response" to the meat powder and the "conditioned response" to the bell. The phenomenon of stimulus generalization was observed as well. That is, although the conditioned response would fade or become extinguished with time, before its extinction, some salivation could be elicited by similar bells (Cairns & Cairns, 1975; Pavlov, 1902). Pavlov's classical conditioning paradigm introduced the world of psychology to the concepts of stimulus, response, paired association, and stimulus generalization, all of which are typically integrated into clinical practice with the paradigm of operant conditioning.

Operant Conditioning

The paradigm of operant conditioning, including the notion of verbal operants such as "tacts" (naming behaviors) and "mands" (commands), was developed by Skinner (1957). Proponents of this nurture view argued that although environmental stimuli were not always identifiable, the frequency of certain behaviors or antecedent behaviors could be increased if positive reinforcers (or consequences) were contingent upon the targets.

The principles of operant conditioning were derived from and based on observations made and data collected in animal laboratories. For example, if a rat in a cage received reinforcement with pellets of food for its bar pressing (i.e., bar pressing that was initially accidental), the frequency of its bar pressing was found to increase. Also, the type of response could be shaped through a schedule of reinforcement of successive approximations to the target stimulus.

In these views, explanations for the acquisition of speech and language relied heavily on the role of imitation as well as paired associations between unconditioned stimuli (e.g., food or a bottle) and unconditioned responses (e.g., physiological vocalizations). Invoking principles of classical conditioning, phonological productions or vocalizations would be conditioned responses to the caretaker's vocalizations (i.e., conditioned stimuli) that had been paired with the unconditioned stimuli (e.g., food or bottle).

With the law of effect, the notion that the intensity and frequency of a response will increase with reinforcement, a principle of operant conditioning was utilized to explain the acquisition of the production of words. Language acquisition was viewed as the result of gradual or systematic reinforcement of desirable or target behaviors. Thus, initially, gross approximations of the target (e.g., any vocalization at all) would be reinforced. According to this view, parents would teach children language through both imitation training of words and phrases as well as the shaping of phrases and sentences through successive approximations of adult-like speech.

From the perspective of conditioning, the sentence was described as a chain of associated events. Each word would serve as the response to the preceding word and the stimulus to the following word. According to the argument, grammatical categories and various sentence types could be learned through contextual generalization. In this explanation, children would generalize grammatical categories based on the word position (Braine, 1966).

As with the nature theories, nurture explanations had some limitations. Although selective reinforcement and paired associations could account for certain aspects of sound and word learning, relying solely on principles of behaviorism to explain the acquisition of language knowledge proved inadequate. Stimulus-response explanations could not begin to describe or explain the development of the complex system of language knowledge that the young child acquires in such a short amount of time. Behaviorists were challenged to account for unobservable meaning knowledge, utterance novelty and complexity, and the rapidity with which language was typically acquired. Critics also argued that more typically, parents would give children feedback about their inaccuracies in meaning rather than about their inaccuracies in syntax.

Implications from a Nurture Perspective: Understanding, Assessing, and Treating Children with Language Disorders

Given the constructs of the nurture theories, these concepts ultimately added little to our understanding of the underlying origins of language disorders in children. Nevertheless, the impact of the behavioral paradigm on assessment and intervention has been pervasive in our field.

In reference to assessment protocols, emphasis on the observation of behavior, data-driven descriptions, quantification, and measurement began to define speech-language pathologists' evaluation of language. The use of standardized, formal tests for identifying deficits in all areas of language became, and has continued to be, the anchor of speech and language evaluations. In addition, principles from this approach have been used in Individuals with Disabilities Education Act (IDEA) legislation and its amendments. For example, legal documents such as the individualized education plan and individual family service plan must be generated for children with special needs, including those with language disorders, to assure that these children receive the assessments and services to which they are entitled. These documents identify goals, which are written in terms of observable behaviors, specify mandates for treatment, indicate performance criteria for achieving goals, and clarify the context in which the target behavior is to be elicited. The primary concern is to quantify behavioral change so as to document the treatment efficacy of the intervention used. In this sense, the construct of assessment expanded to include not only the initial evaluation of the child, but also periodic, data-driven reevaluations to determine the extent of the child's progress and learning relative to previously established goals.

Turning to intervention, the use of behavioral programs such as applied behavioral analysis and variations of this methodology was and is reflected in a great deal of the work done within the speech-language pathology field. Early on, language training programs were developed under the aegis of the stimulus-response psychology model (Gray & Ryan, 1973). More than 40 years of research generated from this perspective has documented treatment efficacy in the work done with children with communication and language impairments. The following advances can be attributed to the interest in behavior analysis:

- The identification of antecedent and consequent events in language intervention
- Specification of desired responses
- Determination of effective reinforcers

- Implementation of schedules of reinforcement
- Use of strategies such as imitation, shaping, successive approximations, prompting, modeling, and generalization
- Use of structured adult-directed contexts of learning
- Reliance on preset curricula

Applied behavior analysis (ABA) introduced by Lovaas (1977) was an outgrowth of the operant conditioning paradigm and has continued to be a popular approach to enhancing language development, particularly for children on the autism spectrum. In ABA, an individualized treatment program is developed for each child. Based on the child's strengths and weaknesses, a curriculum focusing on skills such as matching, imitation, play, and receptive and expressive language is developed. Variations of Lovaas' ABA method include the Natural Language Paradigm, Pivotal Response Treatment (Koegel & Koegel, 2006), and the Verbal Behavior Approach (Sundberg, 2008)

Criticisms of behavioral approaches have often centered on the child's difficulty with generalization: that is, using his newly learned behaviors in the contexts of his daily life (e.g., using the utterance *more cookies* to request cookies during snack time at home in addition to during snack time at school, where the utterance was taught.) Milieu or incidental teaching was designed to address this issue by using naturally occurring learning contexts and child-initiated topics in an attempt to enhance generalization (Warren & Kaiser, 1986).

As Nelson (1998) suggests, the irony of using behavioral approaches for language intervention was that "language seems to be too complex a system for some children to master on their own, but breaking it down into manageable pieces does not make it simpler so much as different" (p. 61). Nonetheless, the use of structured approaches to language intervention has held tremendous appeal for speech-language pathologists and policy-makers who are attracted to the science underlying evidence-based practice—that is, treatment approaches that have been supported by well-designed research studies. The significant incongruity between the foundational principles of the nature arguments (role of the child's inborn capacities) and the nurture arguments (role of the child's environment) has presented a dilemma for clinicians who are looking at theoretical paradigms to govern their work. This need for rapprochement of conflicting ideologies has been, and continues to be, a frequently revisited theme in the clinical practice of speech-language pathologists.

Interactionist: Cognitive Interactionist Paradigm

Interactionist models of language development can be discussed relative to two paradigms: cognitive interactionist (Information Processing and Cognitive-Constructivist) and social interactionist (Social-Cognitive, Social-Pragmatic, and Intentionality Model). Within each of these paradigms, various perspectives can be described, all of which presume that the child brings some preexisting information to the task of language learning and that environmental input plays a significant role in language development. The specifics of what the child brings to language learning and how the environment interacts with these innate capacities varies within these views. While they are grouped together as interactionist views in this section, the implications of each perspective for speech-language pathologists are dealt with separately to reflect the unique contribution each has had on the discipline.

Information Processing Models

In a historical description of information processing approaches to language, Klein and Moses (1999) note that in the late 19th century and early 20th century, Broca and Gall were among the first researchers to try to locate language functions in the brain. The connection between brain function and language was studied in victims of brain injury due to stroke, in patients with traumatic war-related injuries, and, ultimately, in children with language disorders and learning disabilities. Descriptions of brain function and modes of language processing as well as perceptual–motor aspects of childhood language disorders were described by Cruickshank (1967) and Johnson and Mykelbust (1967).

An information processing model of language was eventually developed by Osgood (1963). Osgood's model identified the modalities that were said to underlie language functioning, namely visual and auditory memory, auditory discrimination, visual association, visual reception, and auditory closure. Traditional information processing accounts of language development described language processing as a series of steps that were said to occur consecutively or serially, which included attention, sensation, speech perception, lexical search, syntactic processing, and memory storage (Cairns & Cairns, 1975).

More recent information processing accounts of language, which are sometimes referred to as "connectionist," describe parallel processing rather than serial processing of language. According to this view, networks of processors are connected and several operations or decisions may occur simultaneously (Bohannon & Bonvillian, 2005). These multilayered networks of connections function to interpret linguistic input from the exemplars provided to them. The statistical properties of syntactic forms determine their rate of acquisition and cues that consistently signal particular meanings should be acquired first.

Research reported by Bates and MacWhinney (1987) and MacWhinney (1987) has offered support for this view by using data from the acquisition of several languages, including French, English, Italian, Turkish, and Hungarian. For example, Turkish children, whose language has an extremely reliable case-marking system, master case considerably sooner than word order, which has often been considered a universal cue to sentence meaning over other cues (Bohannon & Bonvillian, 2005; Slobin & Bever, 1982).

Critics of the connectionist model include those who question the paradigm on theoretical grounds. While information processing networks might provide neat explanations for describing linguistic rules, they resemble biological systems only superficially (Berko-Gleason, 2005; Fodor & Pylyshyn, 1988; Sampson, 1987). Most importantly, these connectionist accounts omit any mention of social interaction.

Implications from an Information Processing Perspective: Understanding, Assessing, and Treating Children with Language Disorders

The information processing perspective supports the view that the origins of the language-disordered child's difficulties lie in the ability to successfully process the information necessary for learning a language. For example, the child's problems processing auditory signals contribute to their delays in comprehending and/or producing language. This perspective resonates in contemporary arguments that claim that deficits in processing and executive functioning underlie language-learning disabilities. In terms of language assessment, the models described earlier served as the impetus for the development of many tests that continue to be used widely by speech-language pathologists. For example, the Illinois Test of Psycholinguistic Abilities (ITPA) developed by Osgood (1963) reflected the notion of different levels of language functioning (e.g., receptive, expressive, and associative) and different modalities of language (e.g., verbal, auditory, and visual). The idea of discrete components of processing that can be isolated, tested, and ultimately remediated is a familiar construct in

contemporary practice. Use of formal language testing continues to be the accepted protocol for securing speech and language services for children suspected of having language-learning difficulties. The proliferation of speech and language testing materials in the last 40 years speaks to this practice. In fact, the ITPA-3 (Hammill, Mather, & Roberts, 2001), a revision of the earlier test, reflects the continuing interest in this approach to language assessment. In reference to treatment, many speech-language pathologists support the use of intervention programs that are based on processing mechanisms as the underpinnings for language learning. The following advances in the treatment of children with language challenges can be attributed to this view:

- Auditory integration programs
- Processing programs such as *Fast ForWord*
- Programs designed to facilitate the child's development of executive functions such as organization, memory, and retrieval

Information processing models have clearly had far-reaching effects on the field of communication disorders. Our clinical wisdom tells us that this is a productive approach to take with some children who have language-learning difficulties. However, the idea that this perspective describes the challenges faced by *all* children with language disorders and, therefore, represents the approach to be taken with *all* children would be criticized from within the clinical world of speech-language pathology as well as from more contemporary research findings about the relationship between processing and language acquisition (Gillam et al., 2008).

Cognitive-Constructivist Models

Jean Piaget, a Swiss biologist who referred to himself as a genetic epistemologist, became fascinated with the acquisition of knowledge and the "activity" of the body and mind that lead to intellectual growth (Flavell, 1963). His keen observations of children as they engaged in exploration, play, and problem-solving provided the data for his model of functional invariants:

- *Schemas,* or mental structures, correspond to consistencies in the infant's or child's behaviors or actions (e.g., the child who frequently mouths and sucks objects after grasping them is said to be using his or her "sucking" schema).
- *Assimilation* occurs when a child applies a mental schema to an event; it embodies play, exploration, and learning about the environment. The young child will apply his or her sucking schema

to the features inherent in the various objects that are grasped and will repeat the behavior over and over for the sake of play.

- *Accommodation* occurs as a result of the child's new experience with an object, event, or person, and embodies the child's ability to incorporate the new information, resulting in changes in the child's mental schemas. Each time the child applies his or her sucking schema to a different object, the sucking behavior will be slightly modified to incorporate features of the object.
- *Adaptation* consists of assimilation and accommodation (i.e., the mechanisms for the acquisition of knowledge), as described previously (Piaget, 1952).

From a Piagetian perspective, learning is accomplished throughout the lifespan by active participation of infants, children, and adults. For example, children pursue their goals and interests while their mental schemas are adapted to new experiences. Children were said to direct their own learning as they encountered new experiences and challenges during their ongoing interactions in the world (Flavell, 1963).

Piaget (1952) noted that there were qualitative differences in how children would respond to external events over time. These qualitative differences were captured in his account of developmental stages from birth until formal, scientific operational thought, the cornerstone of scientific inquiry.

From a traditional Piagetian view, a direct relationship exists between cognitive achievements and later linguistic attainments. More specifically, Piagetian theory predicts that cognitive prerequisites for early word learning, in the sensorimotor period (i.e., the first 2 years of life) include concepts of object permanence, intentionality, causality, deferred imitation, and symbolic play (Piaget, 1955). These cognitive milestones are necessary for language to develop. For example, without object permanence, the child cannot use a word for an object not in sight. Similarly, without the ability to represent one object for another (e.g., to pretend to drink from a block), the child cannot use the language symbol—a word—to refer to an object.

Implications from a Cognitive-Constructivist Perspective: Understanding, Assessing, and Treating Children with Language Disorders

Given the relationship between language and other cognitive skills presented by Piaget (1955), the notion that children with language disorders might

be exhibiting language delays because of their cognitive deficits was a direct outgrowth of interest in the cognitive-constructivist views. The nature of language disorders was reconsidered from this perspective with an eye toward identifying the cognitive prerequisites to language, from birth through early childhood, as the potential source of the disruption in language learning. In addition, the fact that language was just one of a number of representational behaviors (i.e., the ability to use a word or an object to stand for or represent something else) paved the way for considering language impairments as a reflection of a symbolic disorder rather than a language disorder alone. In fact, this period marked the beginning of a new line of inquiry relative to the cognitive abilities of children with developmental language disorder. The possibility that these children might have unrecognized cognitive deficits led to a reconsideration of what was meant by "normal" cognition and to a new arena for studying the relationship between aspects of cognition and linguistic development (Johnston, 1994).

This view of the cognitive underpinnings to language found a place in the assessment protocols used by speech-language pathologists in a number of ways. First, assessment of the sensorimotor stages of development was now included in language evaluations as clinicians began to assess children's abilities in areas such as:

- *Object permanence*, the ability to understand that an object exists even if it is not present, seen when children search for a hidden object
- *Means-end behavior*, the ability to execute a series of steps to reach a goal, such as pulling a string on a toy to retrieve it
- *Causality*, the ability to understand the connection between a cause and an effect, such as hitting the mobile to start the music

Second, children's play itself was seen as a rich source of information about their ideas and schemas as well as their overall cognitive achievements. The use of developmental paradigms to systematically assess stages of play became a central component of language evaluations and is considered by many to be the heart of the assessment process (Westby, 1980, 2000). The interest in children's symbolic capacity, rather than language alone, moved the assessment process beyond rules of language to the potential foundations of thinking and, therefore, talking.

Regarding intervention, Piaget's theories and the subsequent applications of these theories to the study of language acquisition had a tremendous impact on both the goals and the contexts of language intervention. The notion that children must acquire a broad foundation of ideas and world knowledge prior to talking gave speech-language pathologists license to facilitate development in areas other than language. The view that children were active learners in their developmental processes led speech-language pathologists to encourage children to interact more freely with toys and objects as they explored the world and learned through this exploration. This led to greater use of child-centered intervention contexts rather than those that were adult-directed.

The following advances were a direct result of the introduction of Piagetian thinking into the treatment of children with language disorders:

- The repertoire of goals typically began to include cognitive behaviors, such as the sensorimotor developments mentioned earlier
- The importance of the developmental stage rather than chronological age
- The emphasis on play as both a goal and a context of therapy

Although the relationship between certain types of cognitive achievements and language developments was delineated, the exact nature of this relationship—including the particular cognitive prerequisites to language—was not necessarily agreed upon. Nonetheless, the idea that cognitive foundations support language acquisition and that the two are integrally related throughout the developmental process shifted and broadened the work (and play) of the speech-language pathologist.

Interactionist: Social Interactionist Paradigm

Social-Cognitive Models

Other developmental interactionists who have influenced the language learning research include Vygotsky (1986) and Bruner (1975, 1977). Vygotsky believed that children's cognitive development resulted from interaction between children's innate skills and their social experiences with peers, adults, and the culture in general. In addition, Vygotsky is well known for his description of the "zone of proximal development"—that is, the area between what a child can accomplish independently and what they can accomplish with another person who has greater knowledge, experience, or skill and who provides some scaffolding. When collaborating on a task, the child and the adult engage in a dialogue that is then stored away by the child for future use as "private speech" (e.g., self-directed talk or when a youngster is "talking to himself"). According

to Vygotsky, when language emerges in the form of private speech, it can be used as a tool to guide and direct problem-solving and other cognitive activities.

Similarly, Bruner's work (1975, 1977) was pioneering relative to social interactionist theories of language acquisition. Bruner (1977) suggested that when caregivers and their infants engage in joint referencing, they share a common focus of interest that ultimately contributes to language acquisition. Three mechanisms (indicating, deictic terms, and naming) serve to establish joint reference between a caregiver and a baby, essentially laying the groundwork to enter the language acquisition process. According to Bruner, the caregiver that uses an "indicator" is using gestural, postural, or vocal means to get the baby's attention. With time, these indicators become more conventional symbols as the caregiver adjusts his or her communication to the level of the child. If the child reaches for an object that the caretaker is holding or if the child looks at the caretaker, the child is likely to receive an enthusiastic response from the adult. When the child begins to use gestures and vocalizations to show, point, or give objects, the caregiver will typically respond verbally, vocally, or gesturally to the child. When using "deictic terms" (e.g., *here, there, this, that, you, me*) with changing referents, caregivers incorporate spatial and contextual cues to assist children in comprehending this terminology. "Naming" occurs when the child can associate a label with a referent, which is accomplished receptively before it is accomplished expressively.

Bruner also discussed the notion of scaffolding as one way in which caregivers facilitate language learning and dialogue. Caregivers are said to adjust the degree of linguistic and nonlinguistic support that they offer to children as they are learning language. For example, as the young child becomes more verbal, the caretaker will typically need to provide less nonverbal cuing during conversation (Bruner, 1975, 1977).

In contemporary social-cognitive research, children are said to possess a unique capacity that enables them to learn language by interpreting the intentions of those who interact with them. Social-cognitive views, such as those advocated by Paul Bloom (2000), suggest that children learning language need at least a primitive theory of mind to enable them to adequately interpret the intentions of others. Children's requisite cognitive abilities allow them to process information, while their preformed concepts for entities in the world serve as the basis for word learning and language development. While helpful adults might accelerate or assist in the process of word learning, as long as children can infer the referential intentions of others, no other social support is necessary. Tomasello,

Carpenter, and Liszkowski (2007) support the view that children's inference of intentionality is critical for word and language learning.

According to Tomasello (2003), pointing gestures are an important part of the system of shared intentionality. Prior to language use, pointing not only establishes joint attention, but it also serves to influence the mental states of others by attempting to influence how another thinks, feels, and acts (Tomasello et al., 2007). In support of this view, Goldin-Meadow (2007) suggests that pointing at 14 months is a better predictor of lexical vocabulary than the speech of the caretaker. Pointing serves the child by not only drawing attention to the self, but also to the objects that they find interesting enough to communicate about. The child's use of pointing or gesture with words also helps them segue into syntax. For example, "children combine pointing gestures with words to express sentence-like meanings ('eat' + point at cookie) months before they can express the same meanings in word + word combination ('eat + cookie')" (Goldin-Meadow, 2007, p. 741). From the perspective discussed here, language use originates from shared attention and the interpretation of intentionality. The basic processes that explain language learning in this view are the understanding of intentions and children's general cognitive abilities, including pattern abstraction and category construction. Owing to their unique social capabilities, human infants learn to interpret the communicative intentions of others, communicate their own intentions, and utilize their cognitive resources to create language knowledge that is both interpersonally driven and intrapersonally developed.

Social-Pragmatic Models

Pragmatics in linguistic theory has traditionally been concerned with the functions of language, speaker-listener roles, conversational discourse, presupposition, and Grices's (1975) conversational maxims. Research in the pragmatics of language originated in the work of Austin (1962) and Searle (1969). In terms of the functions of adult language, linguists identified three types of speech acts:

- *Perlocutions* referred to how listeners interpreted the speaker's speech acts.
- *Illocutions* referred to the intentions of the speaker.
- *Locutions* referred to the meanings expressed in the utterance.

In describing how intentionality develops in young children, Bates, Camaioni, and Volterra (1975) used this paradigm of functional categories. During the perlocutionary stage, which was said to extend from birth to 9 months, the child's actions and behaviors are given a communicative intent by the caretaker. For example, the caretaker might interpret a baby's cooing as a sign of happiness or contentment. The illocutionary stage (8–12 months) marks the period of time when children first produce their truly intentional behaviors, either vocally or gesturally. Gestures such as showing, giving, or pointing, perhaps accompanied with vocalizations, are typically used. During this time, children are said to produce the nonlinguistic precursor to the declarative, referred to as the *protodeclarative* (e.g., gesturing or vocalizing to point out an object or event), as well as the nonlinguistic precursor to the imperative, referred to as the *protoimperative* (e.g., gesturing or vocalizing to request an object or an event). The third stage, referred to as the locutionary stage (12 months of age), is characterized by the use of words produced with gestures to convey specific meanings and intentions.

A pragmatic approach to child language was taken by Halliday (1975), who described the functions of his son Nigel's nonlinguistic communication. These functions included satisfying needs, controlling the behaviors of others, interacting, and expressing emotion and interest. With his first words, Nigel could explore and categorize things in his environment, imagine or pretend, and inform others of his experiences.

John Dore (1974, 1975) identified the primitive speech acts of children at the one-word stage of language (e.g., labeling, answering, requesting an action, requesting an answer, calling, greeting, protesting, repeating/imitating, and practicing) as well as the speech acts of children at multiword stages of language development. Beyond such speech acts, research in the area of pragmatics addressed the child's knowledge of presupposition (Greenfield & Smith, 1976) and understanding of conversational protocol, including topic control and conversational turn-taking (Bloom, Rocissano, & Hood, 1976).

One of the research topics that grew out of social-pragmatic views of language was the nature of the adult input to babies and young children. Since the 1970s, researchers in child language have noted that adults speak differently to very young children than they do to other people. These patterns, which have been referred to as "motherese," are characterized by utterances that are shorter in length, simpler in grammatical complexity, and slower in rate of speech. Also typical of motherese is the use of fewer verbs, fewer tense markers, and vocabulary that is less diverse and more concrete (Phillips, 1973; Snow, 1973, 1978, 1999).

In a similar vein, later studies described child-directed speech (CDS) as contextually redundant and perceptually salient. Because most CDS refers to the here and now, that is, it codes an ongoing action or activity within the child's view, it is contextually redundant (Akhtar, Dunham, & Dunham, 1991; Tomasello, 1988). In terms of perceptual salience, CDS typically has an overall higher fundamental frequency, exaggerated stress, a wider range of intonation, more distinct pausing, and, as noted earlier, an overall slower rate (Lund & Duchan, 1993). Researchers suggest that the vocal and grammatical parameters of the primary linguistic data that are provided by the caretaker make semantic, syntactic, phonological, and pragmatic information more accessible to the young infant, who is innately wired to receive this information. Findings from a number of more recent studies have suggested that infant-directed speech facilitates segmentation of the speech stream, which in turn leads to the discovery of phonemes and words (Kuhl, 2004; Saffran, Senghas, & Trueswell, 2001; Thiessen, Hill, & Saffran, 2005).

Taking this one step further, in recent studies of language input to young children, the role of frequency and distributional regularity of grammatical forms in the adult language has been found to influence the child's knowledge of word order. In experimental work by Matthews, Theakston, and Tomasello (2004), younger children were more likely to adopt the experimenter's atypical word order with novel verbs than with more frequent verbs. In contrast, older children were more likely to generalize their knowledge of standard SVO word order to the less familiar verbs.

Finally, it should be emphasized that although CDS has been found in many different cultures and languages throughout the world (e.g., Chinese, Arabic, Spanish, Marathi, and Comanche), CDS is not used to the same extent in all communities (Golinkoff & Hirsh-Pasek, 2000). For example, in the findings reported by Brice-Heath (1983), child-directed speech was not as prevalent in one of the Carolina Piedmont communities studied.

Implications from a Social-Cognitive and Social-Pragmatic Perspective: Understanding, Assessing, and Treating Children with Language Disorders

Some theories of language acquisition have had a profound impact on the study of specific populations of language-impaired children. For example, social-cognitive and social-pragmatic theories, which clarified the relationship between children's capacity for interaction and their capacity to learn to comprehend and produce language, spoke directly to the profiles of children with autism spectrum disorders (ASD).

Children with autism often face challenges in intentionality, both in their own communication and in

their understanding of others' communication. In fact, the difficulty in reading these children's intentions sets them apart from typically developing children and from other groups of children with language impairments. Based on social-cognitive and social-pragmatic views of language acquisition, speech-language pathologists working with children on the autism spectrum began to broaden their understanding of why these children experienced such severe difficulties in the acquisition and use of language. Further, atypical behaviors, such as echolalia, were reconsidered. Using taxonomies of communicative intentions, the ground-breaking work of Prizant and Duchan (1981), as related to the functions of echolalia and delayed echolalia, opened the door for considering that the "inappropriate" behaviors of children with ASD were, in fact, communicative and intentional, albeit in unconventional ways.

Many taxonomies of pragmatic development that focused on nonlinguistic aspects of communication also contributed to expanding the understanding of the nature of communication impairments in children whose deficits went far beyond their linguistic systems. The emphasis on gesture, facial expression, body language, eye gaze, presupposition, and listener perspective as foundations of communicative competence helped us more accurately describe many children's disruptions in language. These taxonomies were eventually adapted for use in assessment as the functions of language and the forms that were used to express these functions (nonlinguistic and linguistic, conventional and unconventional) were analyzed. Simultaneously, taxonomies of conversational skills that addressed speaker-listener roles, topic control, and topic expansion (Prutting & Kirchner, 1987) were included in the battery of assessment tools as the evaluation of language expanded beyond vocabulary, morphology, syntax, and semantics.

These theories of language also had a dramatic effect on the interventions used in children with language disorders. Intervention programs were developed, such as *It Takes Two to Talk* (Pepper & Weitzman, 2004) and *More than Words* (Sussman, 1999), which emphasized parent training, one of the hallmarks of social-pragmatic models. The following were prioritized as goals as a result of social-cognitive and social-pragmatic theories of language acquisition:

- Prelinguistic and nonlinguistic communication
- Functions of language, conversational skills, adjacency and contingency, discourse genres, communication repair, listener adaptation, and, to some extent, the social-emotional underpinnings of the pragmatics of language
- Language and conversational skills needed for successful peer interactions

Intentionality Model

We end this section on interactionist views of language acquisition with a contemporary model that reflects an integrated perspective on the developmental language process. This model has particular resonance and relevance for understanding, assessing, and treating children with language disorders. Models of this type hold great promise for the discipline of speech-language pathology because they provide the kinds of expansive paradigms that anchor our clinical work in the breadth and depth of typical development.

In 1978, Bloom and Lahey proposed a model of language acquisition that revolutionized the work of speech-language pathologists. This view of language as the integration of form (phonology, morphology, syntax), content (semantics), and use (pragmatics) was subsequently translated into assessment and intervention paradigms (Lahey, 1988). The resulting "map" of language development, which traced the child's expression of ideas from single words to complex sentences, provided speech-language pathologists with developmental information that was at once organic, dynamic, and grounded in what was known about typical development.

More recently, Bloom and Tinker (2001) expanded the original model, embedding the development of form, content, and use into two broader developmental domains, *engagement* and *effort*. These authors suggest that the study of language has often resulted in the isolation of a particular aspect of language in an effort to investigate and study it. They remind us that "we need to consider what it means when we take the units of language out of the very fabric of the child's life in which they are necessarily embedded" (p. 4); "Somehow the child has to be kept in the picture as the major player, as the agent of the practices that contribute to the acquisition process" (p. 5). These concerns resonate with speech-language pathologists, who have the awesome task of isolating units of language so as to increase their saliency during the intervention process and, at the same time, trying to connect this process to "the very fabric of the child's life" (p. 4).

Bloom and Tinker's model suggests that a child's intentionality (i.e., the child's goal-directed action as well as their representations of objects, wishes, feelings, and beliefs), contributes to their development in two ways. First, the child's actions in the world (sensorimotor actions, emotional displays, play, and speech) as well as acts of interpretation and expression of language lead to the development of new representations of the mental contents of her mind. Second, the child's participation in a social world depends on and

is promoted by these acts of expression and interpretation between the child and her caregiver.

The child's agency, what they have in mind or their intentional state, is a central theme in this model. In this formulation, the child perceives, apprehends, and constructs intentional states. As the child expresses these states and interprets others' intentional states from their actions and their words, new intentional states and representations are formed. Intentional states include *psychological attitudes* (e.g., beliefs, desires, feelings) directed toward *propositional content* (e.g., persons, objects, and events in the world). Thus, the intentionality model speaks to the interaction between two domains of development, affect (i.e., feelings and emotions) and cognition, in the young child. The child's expression of their intentions is realized through emotion, play, and speech.

Although the intentionality model might be envisioned as a psychological model, Bloom and Tinker (2001) suggest that it embraces the social and cultural world of the child as well. Their treatment of the social world resides in the child's representations of others in their mind. The interaction of the child with the physical and social world and the effects of these interactions on their development lead us to consider this model an example of the interactionist view of development.

A component of the intentionality model (**FIGURE 2-1**) is *engagement,* which refers to "the child's emotional and social directedness for determining what is relevant for learning and the motivation for learning" (Bloom & Tinker, 2001, p. 14). Here, Bloom and Tinker are referring to the intersubjectivity that develops between the child and the parent, which serves as the foundation for the child's relatedness to other persons throughout life. The relationship between the child and the caregivers, the child's relationships with objects and events, and the relationships in the physical world all contribute to the child's development of engagement.

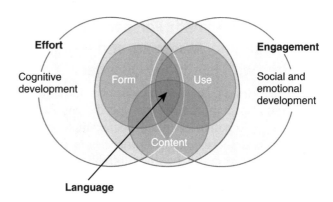

FIGURE 2-1 The intentionality model.

Intentionality Model appearing in Bloom, L., & Tinker, E. (2001). The intentionality model and language acquisition. *Monographs of the Society for Research in Child Development, 66*(4), 267.

The component of *effort* refers to the cognitive processes and the work it takes to acquire language. Early discussions of language acquisition emphasized the ease of learning to talk, as evidenced by the fact that children had accomplished most of this task by 3 years of age. In contrast, Bloom and Tinker (2001) underscore the effort and resources that are required to integrate the various dimensions of expressing (producing) and interpreting (understanding) language. The complexity of these tasks is captured when considering that

> expression, at a minimum, requires the child to construct and hold in mind intentional state representations, retrieve linguistic units and procedures from memory, and articulate words and sentences. For interpretation, at a minimum, the child must connect what is heard to what is already in mind, recall elements from memory that are associated with prior experiences of the words, and form a new intentional state representation.

(Bloom & Tinker, 2001, p. 15)

Effort can also be understood in terms of the complexity of what children are learning simultaneously. For example, children are learning to interpret and express intentions at the same time that they are learning about the world, their emotional lives, and the emotional lives of significant others. In this view, the child's cognitive resources are a real part of the acquisition process and will help us understand what they can and cannot do at different points in time. The implications of this concept for thinking about children with challenges in speech, language, and communication are immediately apparent as we imagine the additional taxing of resources that would result from neurological, psychological, and emotional disruptions.

Implications from the Intentionality Model: Understanding, Assessing, and Treating Children with Language Disorders

By using Bloom and Tinker's (2001) Intentionality Model, disorders of language can be addressed relative to the area or areas of language that are compromised rather than from a categorical or etiological framework. The advantage of using Bloom and Tinker's perspective is that we can begin to view challenges in language from two overarching developmental domains—effort (cognitive development) and engagement (social-emotional development)—in addition to the linguistic domains of form, content, and use. Children with primary problems in effort and those with

primary problems in engagement can be considered relative to these underlying challenges, and the resulting impact of these derailments on the development of form, content, and use can be addressed. In the spirit of Bloom and Lahey (1978) and Lahey (1988), language-disordered children would be classified on the basis of the areas of language and language-related developments that might be considered strengths and challenges rather than using etiological categories such as developmental language disorder, intellectual disability, ASD, and so forth.

For individual assessments of children, Bloom and Tinker's (2001) intentionality model is invaluable. Developmental models of language, which are both broad and integrated, offer speech-language pathologists a rich paradigm from which to assess language in a way that will lead directly to intervention. Using the Intentionality Model, developmental areas such as social, affective, and cognitive domains can be assessed. Assessment based on this thinking leads to more holistic intervention goals and procedures, as the interrelationship between and among the developmental components is recognized and the use of developmental sequences and processes is prioritized (Gerber, 2003). Clearly, for some children, assessments of all the components of the Bloom and Tinker (2001) model will lead to the formulation of intervention priorities in areas such as engagement rather than the more traditional focus on form.

Although Bloom and Tinker's (2001) model does not offer a predetermined set of intervention goals, it anchors the work of speech-language pathologists in a perspective that embraces many of the models of language acquisition that have been discussed in this chapter. The clinician who begins the treatment of any particular child with an integrated understanding of the processes and products of typical language acquisition and then combines this knowledge with an inherent understanding of the interpersonal relationships within which these processes and products unfold will be ready to meet the challenges and joys of facilitating each child's comprehension and production of language. More specifically, intervention goals and strategies that are generated from the Intentionality Model include the following advances:

- Greater attention to the cognitive precursors and co-cursors to language, such as symbolic development
- Focus on the social-emotional precursors and co-cursors to language, such as affective engagement, reciprocity, and joint attention
- Determining goals based on the a model of form, content, and use
- Viewing the parent as the intervention partner

Two Contemporary Models of Child Development

We have considered many theories and models that speak directly to language acquisition and have provided assessment and/or treatment paradigms for children with speech, language, and communication delays. Two additional models of development will be mentioned despite the fact that they have not specifically addressed language development per se. Both provide a view of child development from which all other developments can be considered.

As with the Bloom & Tinker model, emphasis on emotional development, symbolic capacity, the caretaker-child relationship, and developmental process is a hallmark of the Developmental, Individual Differences, Relationship-based approach (DIR) developed by Greenspan, Wieder, and Simons (1998). Although this model of development, assessment, and intervention does not address the acquisition of language, the focus on social-emotional, interpersonal foundations of all development, and the interest in intentionality and communication are consistent with the Bloom and Tinker (2001) model. Unlike the Bloom and Tinker (2001) model, DIR provides a paradigm that integrates developmental threads from many disciplines (mental health, occupational therapy, speech-language therapy, and education) into an assessment and intervention approach that is quite unique. Nine stages of functional emotional development relative to typical development are outlined and used as the basis of understanding where a child is functioning on the emotional-symbolic ladder. This in combination with the interest in the individual processing profile of the child (e.g., sensory and regulatory challenges), embedding the development of speech, language, and communication into the broadest perspective of the child and their family and is completely in sync with contemporary views of child development (Gerber, 2012). Finally, the role of the parent-child dyad as the intervention unit, key in the DIR approach, has now become both a research and clinical model in the treatment of children with ASD.

Many of the broader perspectives that are integral to the DIR model, such as the role of emotional development in the child's life, are considered in the field of interpersonal neurobiology (Siegel, 1999). Although not specifically related to language acquisition, the most contemporary thinking on human development speaks to the interaction between the child's experience with their caregivers and neurological development. As Siegel (2001) has suggested, "the mind develops at the interface between human relationships and the unfolding structure and function of the brain"

(p. 67). In particular, the brain structures that control social and emotional functioning develop during the first years of the child's life as a result, in part, of the child's interpersonal experience.

Relevant to work with children with developmental disabilities is Siegel's point that all adults who play the role of "caregivers" in the child's life can be significant as attachment figures. "Understanding a child's individual needs and style of communicating, taking joy in the child, and being able to soothe the child when he is in distress, are each basic components of the child's relationship with the attachment figure" (p. 78). The following five basic elements speak to how caregivers can foster a secure attachment in the children under their care:

1. Collaboration or contingent communication
2. Reflective dialogues or sharing internal experiences
3. Repair of disrupted communication to reestablish connection
4. Coherent narratives—adults who can integrate their autobiography can provide integrated experiences for their children
5. Emotional communication—interpersonal sharing of positive, joyful experiences

Implications from Contemporary Models of Child Development: Understanding, Assessing, and Treating Children with Language Disorders

The implications of these recent theories and models of child development are yet to be fully realized in understanding children with challenges in language development, assessing them, and treating them. However, there are some trends in these directions. For example, in a recent article related to children with ASD, Singletary (2015) suggests that neurobiological factors interfere with the infant's ability to experience the child-caregiver interactions in the way that typically developing children do. As a result of this disruption, the child is not able to take advantage of "growth-promoting parental input." (p. 81). This in turn results in a kind of social deprivation and isolation, which leads to both psychological and biological stress in the child.

In terms of assessment and intervention, although there are now many programs that prioritize the caregiver-child relationship in the therapeutic context (*More than words*; PACT), speech and language services are still primarily delivered by SLPs, even in contexts where parents are available, as is the case of home-based early intervention. Similarly, the interface

Participants—Small group of students

Ask your professor to provide you with a 20- or 30-minute video of a language intervention session with a young child. After watching this video, discuss which theory or theories of language acquisition you think have motivated the clinician's approach (goals and strategies) and support your answer. If the therapy seems to have several theoretical bases, indicate which aspects of the therapy relate to which theories.

DVD option: Watch the following online materials: https://www.youtube.com/playlist?list= PL25410923E953E679

#6 Visual Reality—Emma's intervention engagement— 2 of 2

Start at 5:35 and go to 13:00.

between emotional development and symbolic development discussed by Greenspan et al. (1998) is not typically represented in the paradigms used for assessment and intervention.

Looking forward, the world of speech, language, and communication disorders in children will hopefully embrace the most recent holistic thinking about child development and, with this step, begin to use this information to provide more integrated intervention services for children and their families.

▸ The Science of Child Development: Broader Perspectives

A contemporary review of the science of language acquisition would not be complete without a discussion of the most recent perspectives on the science of early child development and early intervention. Since 2000, a number of reports have been published that reflect the work of the National Scientific Council on the Developing Child. This interdisciplinary team of scientists and scholars has addressed what the biological and social sciences "do and do not say about early childhood, brain development, and the impact of intervention programs" (National Research Council & Institute of Medicine, 2000, p. 2). The status of the nature–nurture debate comes across loud and clear in the findings and recommendations of this group, as the interactionist view is presented in the most contemporary framework.

The council's analysis of decades of data from a small number of intensive child development programs supports the assumption that it is possible to improve many outcomes for "vulnerable children"; however, it also demonstrates that many programs have not yielded beneficial results. Several of the findings from this analysis of cutting-edge neuroscience, developmental-behavioral research, and program evaluation are particularly relevant to the nature–nurture issue in language acquisition. The review presented in this section puts the topic of language acquisition into a broader scientific context and serves as another source for intervention implications.

> Early experiences determine whether a child's developing brain architecture provides a strong or weak foundation for all future learning, behavior, and health
>
> (National Research Council & Institute of Medicine, 2000, p. 3).

Among the many conclusions that have been drawn from this finding is that a need exists for earlier intervention programs for children at risk. Early intervention has the potential to influence the child's brain circuitry—once again speaking to the interaction between nature and nurture. For speech-language pathologists, this finding supports the benefits provided by early, finely tuned adult input and well-designed interactive experiences and sets the stage for honing the experiences that the young child with language difficulties will receive. For vulnerable children, the plasticity of the brain and the windows of opportunity in early childhood are the keys to ensuring intensity of services and parental participation in the intervention plan.

In fact, the world of communication disorders has a long history of supporting early and intensive intervention for children with developmental delays. Contemporary studies aimed at identifying prelinguistic markers of language and communication disorders speak to the urgency of earlier identification, which will then lead to earlier intervention (Wetherby et al., 2004). Similarly, our growing awareness of the role of the parent-child relationship will, hopefully, result in paradigm shifts relative to determining who the participants are during language intervention sessions (Longtin & Gerber, 2008).

At present, the guiding principles proposed by ASHA speak to what early intervention services should look like for young children with speech, language, and communication disorders. These include services that are:

■ Family-centered and culturally responsive
■ Developmentally supportive and promoting children's participation in their natural environments

- Comprehensive, coordinated, and team-based
- Based on the highest quality internal and external evidence that is available

These principles are based on what is known about early childhood development as well as best practices for intervention. As more early childhood programs embrace these principles, the day-to-day treatment of children with communication disorders will be improved.

> The interactive influences of genes and experience shape the architecture of the child's developing brain
>
> (National Research Council & Institute of Medicine, 2000, p. 8).

In this view, genes dictate when specific brain circuits are formed, whereas experiences shape their formation. Children's inborn drive toward competence and their experience with responsive relationships motivate the developmental process and lead to a healthy brain architecture. Early interactions are key to children's development because they are comprised of mutual and reciprocal exchanges. Therefore, these interactions are key to the construction of intervention goals and strategies. In typical development, a parent or caretaker can provide these opportunities for mutuality and reciprocity to the child, who is an eager and active participant in the process. For children who are developing atypically, the same interactive dance, which may be much harder to choreograph, must nonetheless be prioritized as a step toward shaping the architecture of the child's developing brain.

> Brain architecture and the skills that come with development are built "from the bottom up," with simpler developments serving as the foundations for more advanced ones.
>
> (National Research Council & Institute of Medicine, 2000, p. 8).

Here, the take-home message for speech-language pathologists interested in language acquisition speaks to the importance of a developmental approach when facilitating language learning. It is important to remember that more complex skills build on simpler ones. Although this hierarchy may seem self-evident, the implication of this multilayer structure for professionals developing intervention programs clearly sets the direction of the program content. An extensive and specific understanding of the steps in development within any particular domain (language, affect, cognition) and a commitment to developmentally expanding the child's repertoire of skills with this information in mind is the logical implication of this finding.

> Cognitive, emotional, and social capabilities are inextricably intertwined throughout the life course, and their interactive relationship develops in a continuous process over time
>
> (National Research Council & Institute of Medicine, 2000, p. 10).

This finding presents one of the greatest challenges for professionals working with children who have developmental derailments. The implication here is that to provide the best experiences for promoting development, clinicians must think not only about their particular area of expertise, but also about the relationship and interrelationship of that area with other developmental domains. In fact, the most promising intervention programs are likely to be those that keep the interactive flow between and among developmental threads in view and that plan for each goal with an eye toward the prerequisites and co-requisites of that specific development. Prioritizing a particular area of development, such as language, while honoring the simultaneity and interconnectedness of the child's development in social, affective, cognitive, and regulatory domains, presents an ongoing learning opportunity for clinicians.

▶ How to Use This Information as a Lifelong Student of Language Disorders: A Case Study

In this chapter, we started the discussion with our shared interest in the amazing moment when a child says his first word or, in the case of children with language delays and disorders, the worrisome and unexpected moment when they do not. This can be a defining time in the child's life, and in the life of their parents. A child who begins to talk at 12 months may see in the delighted faces of caretakers that they have accomplished something extraordinary. The parents of this child, in turn, experience the magic of knowing what their baby is thinking and feeling through their use of words.

The scenario is quite different for the child and their family when the first word is not spoken when expected; again, life will change. The child may experience the anxiety or frustration that naturally arises when there is a disconnect between what one knows and what one can express; the child may also sense the caretakers' concern as they wonder what has happened to the precious first words and perhaps begin to question, in worrisome ways, "is my child normal?"

Who are these children who do not speak when we might expect them to? In reality, they represent a continuum, including those children who are initially indistinguishable from their peers, aside from their late start in talking, and who will ultimately move on to typical functioning. The continuum also includes those children who will struggle throughout their lives with developing a linguistic system and with communicating. Distinguishing those children at the extreme ends of the continuum is not difficult; however, our understanding of the developmental components that have been affected in any particular child and the interplay between and among these components can be a challenge to disentangle.

While students of speech-language pathology traditionally begin their study of language development with an exploration of the nature–nurture debate, for many of the children they will work with, there is little debate. Most often, the parents we meet have provided the "good enough" input that we assume is needed to activate language learning and use. Given this fact, we turn to the possibility that this child has come to the world with some disruptions in the biological endowments that lead to talking.

As an example, one of the authors of this chapter saw an 18-month-old child who had many developmental concerns. Timmy was experiencing delays in the following areas:

- Motor development, including difficulty standing, walking, and holding his body upright when sitting
- Emotional development, including a restricted range of affect and few reciprocal interactions
- Language development, including no single words, few sounds, and delayed comprehension
- Social-communication development, including few intentions expressed and minimal responsiveness to others
- Play development, including a limited range of interests in toys and objects

In Timmy's case, the absence of words was merely one of a rather complex composite of developmental derailments. Naturally, the questions Timmy's parents asked were the logical ones: Why wasn't he talking? How could they help him begin to talk? What would Timmy be like when he was 5?

For those of us interested in helping children and parents experience the joys of shared communication, we begin our assessment and subsequently develop an intervention plan by trying to discover what separates the talking child from the nontalking child or, in some cases, the communicating child from the noncommunicating child. As we observe the child's interactions, we typically pose a first set of global diagnostic questions that will help us understand the underpinnings of the child's delay:

- Does the child have the necessary sensory abilities to learn language?
- Does the child have the necessary motor coordination skills needed to produce speech?
- Does the child have the range of ideas and knowledge that serve as the foundations for language?
- Does the child have the social interactive and affective capacities that lead to language?

If the answer to certain questions is "no"—for example, "She doesn't hear well enough to learn language"—we can begin the intervention process by providing the child with what they need (e.g., hearing aids or a cochlear implant) and be confident that this is an appropriate starting point for accelerating the child's process of language learning. When the challenges are more pervasive—for example, limited social-affective capacities—the intervention process becomes less clearly defined. Nonetheless, our starting point for any child is our understanding of their developmental needs and the formulation of an initial program, which will require time and collaboration on the part of the child's educators, therapists, and, to a great extent, her parents.

Although some children we see will have identified biological, neurological, or sensory deficits, Timmy did not. His hearing was within normal limits, his neurological evaluation was unremarkable, and his genetic testing was negative. The possibility that his difficulties had biological underpinnings was inferred from the developmental derailments described previously and the absence of any environmental explanations for his delays.

How can a "student" of speech-language pathology embrace the most current thinking about language development and, at the same time, benefit from the long history of contributions made to our understanding of language acquisition and the influences of these contributions to the field of speech-language pathology? More specifically, how will we determine how to work and play with Timmy and what to encourage as a sound and scientific approach to facilitating his linguistic and communication development?

At this point, we should remind ourselves of the diversity in individual profiles of the children we have seen or will see over our careers. Although the authors of this chapter have seen many children with autism, language impairment, cognitive delays, and language-learning disabilities in their more than

40 years (each!) as speech-language pathologists, they would definitely say they have never seen the same child twice.

This diversity in and of itself gives us a first clue to answering the question "How do I know when to use which theory or model of language?" "It depends" would have to be the honest and informed answer.

Understanding that each child's profile of strengths and challenges is a natural result of their biology and experience and the interplay between the two suggests that the possibilities are endless and relative to the areas of development in which to support, enhance, facilitate, or teach. Perhaps for one child, the inability to learn the linguistic rules of the language will be the roadblock to further language learning; in such a case, understanding and addressing the perceptual, psycholinguistic, and pragmatic aspects of rule-learning will be the charge to their speech-language pathologist. For another child, whose ideas about the world seem to be standing in the way of their development of greater comprehension and production of language, the notions of the child as an active learner of the sensorimotor, symbolic, and ideational underpinnings of language should be reviewed. For a third child, whose social-emotional affective development is derailed, emphasizing caretaker-child interactions, shared attention, reciprocity, and co-construction of meaning would be an excellent starting point.

In the end, what would we advise the new or seasoned speech-language pathologist relative to the question of theories of language acquisition? For sure, each theory has some relevance to the larger puzzle of determining how it is that typically developing children come to comprehend and produce novel utterances with social savvy and an understanding of the interpersonal customs and constraints of their language. Given that reality, plus the fact that no one really knows why a particular child is having difficulty with language and communication, wise speech-language pathologists will keep their eyes and ears open and consider this topic to be a work in progress. Interestingly enough, although speech-language pathologists often think about borrowing from what is known about children who are typically developing, clinical findings about children with challenges in language and the paths to their progress will inform theories and models of language acquisition as well.

For Timmy, considering the range of delays and disruptions that he was experiencing, the speech-language pathologist would do best to encourage his parents to provide support in all aspects of development that relate to language and to find the kind of intervention that speaks to a cohesive, interdisciplinary, broad view of the factors that influence the ability to learn a linguistic system and the pleasures of communication. In fact, this is just what Timmy's parents did. For this child, the result was a very good one: Timmy progressed in his comprehension and production of language, his affective engagement and reciprocity, his social interaction, and his development of ideas. This comprehensive approach fit well with the parents' own philosophy of how to help their son, an aspect of intervention that should not be minimized. Today, Timmy is a 3-year old with lots to say and a growing sense of the joys of interacting. However, should he meet additional challenges along the way, his speech-language pathologist would do well to go back to the theories of language acquisition and look yet again for clues to the nuances and mysteries of development and disorder.

Study Questions

- How does the traditional nature–nurture debate relate to the study of language acquisition?
- Describe how interactionist theories have influenced the field of speech-language pathology
- Describe the components of Bloom and Tinker's (2001) intentionality model.
- Discuss why it is important to use a theoretical model to understand language development in clinical practice.
- With reference to a particular child, describe how this discussion of specific theories would affect your approach to assessment and/or intervention.

References

Akhtar, N., Dunham, F., & Dunham, P. (1991). Directive interactions and early vocabulary development: The role of joint attentional focus. *Journal of Child Language, 18*(1), 41–49.

Austin, J. (1962). *How to do things with words.* London, UK: Oxford University Press.

Bates, E. (1994). Modularity, domain specificity and the development of language. *Discussions in Neuroscience, 10*(1/2), 136–149.

Bates, E., Camaioni, L., & Volterra, V. (1975). The acquisition of performatives prior to speech. *Merrill Palmer Quarterly, 21*(3), 205–216.

Bates, E., & MacWhinney, B. (1987). Competition, variation, and language learning. In B. MacWhinney (Ed.), *Mechanisms of language acquisition* (pp. 157–194). Hillsdale, NJ: Erlbaum.

Berko-Gleason, J. (2005). *The development of language.* Boston, MA: Pearson Education.

Bloom, L. (1970). *Language development: Form and function in emerging grammars.* Cambridge, MA: MIT Press.

Bloom, L., & Lahey, M. (1978). *Language development and language disorders.* New York, NY: John Wiley & Sons.

Bloom, L., Rocissano, L., & Hood, L. (1976). Adult-child discourse: Developmental intervention between information processing and linguistic knowledge. *Cognitive Psychology, 8*, 521–552.

Bloom, L., & Tinker, E. (2001). The intentionality model and language acquisition. *Monographs of the Society for Research in Child Development, 66*(4), 267.

Bloom, P. (2000). *How children learn the meaning of words.* Cambridge, MA: MIT Press.

Bohannon, J. N. III, & Bonvillian, J. D. (2005). Theoretical approaches to language acquisition. In J. Berko Gleason (Ed.), *The development of language* (pp. 230–291). Boston, MA: Pearson Education.

Bohannon, J. N. III, & Stanowicz, L. (1988). The issue of negative evidence: Adult responses to children's language errors. *Developmental Psychology, 24*(5), 684–689.

Braine, M. D. S. (1966). Learning the positions of words relative to a marker element. *Journal of Experimental Psychology, 72*(4), 532–540.

Brice-Heath, S. (1983). *Ways with words.* Cambridge, UK: Cambridge University Press.

Brown, R. (1973). *A first language: The early stages.* Cambridge, MA: Harvard University Press.

Bruner, J. (1975). The ontogenesis of speech acts. *Journal of Child Language, 2*(1), 1–19.

Bruner, J. (1977). Early social interaction and language acquisition. In R. Schaffer (Ed.), *Studies in mother-infant interaction* (pp. 271–289). New York, NY: Academic Press.

Cairns, C., & Cairns, H. (1975). *Psycholinguistics: A cognitive view of language.* New York, NY: Holt, Rinehart & Winston.

Catts, H., & Kamhi, A. (2005). *Language and reading disabilities.* Boston, MA: Pearson Education.

Chomsky, N. (1957). *Syntactic structures.* The Hague, Netherlands: Mouton.

Chomsky, N. (1965). *Aspects of a theory of syntax.* Cambridge, MA: MIT Press.

Chomsky, N. (1972). *Language and mind.* New York, NY: Harcourt Brace Jovanovich.

Chomsky, N. (1972). *Studies on semantics in generative grammar.* The Hague, Netherlands: Mouton.

Chomsky, N. (1982). *Lectures on government and binding.* New York, NY: Foris.

Chomsky, N. (1988). *Language and the problems of knowledge.* Cambridge, MA: MIT Press.

Clark, E. (1973). What's in a word? On the child's acquisition of semantics in his first language. In T. E. Moore (Ed.), *Cognitive development and the acquisition of language* (pp. 65–110). New York, NY: Academic Press.

Cruickshank, W. M. (1967). *The brain-injured child in home, school, and society.* New York, NY: Syracuse University Press.

Curtiss, S. (1974). *Genie: A psycholinguistic study of a modern day "wild" child.* New York, NY: Academic Press.

Dore, J. (1974). A pragmatic description of early language development. *Journal of Psycholinguistic Research, 4*, 343–350.

Dore, J. (1975). Holophrases, speech acts, and language universals. *Journal of Child Language, 2*(1), 21–40.

Eimas, P., Siqueland, E., Jusczyk, P., & Vigorito, J. (1971). Speech perception in infants. *Science, 171*, 303–306.

Fillmore, C. (1968). The case for case. In E. Bach & R. Harmas (Eds.), *Universals in linguistic theory* (pp. 1–90). New York, NY: Holt, Rinehart, & Winston.

Flavell, J. H. (1963). *The developmental psychology of Jean Piaget.* New York, NY: D. Van Nostrand Co.

Fodor, J. (1983). *Modularity of mind.* Cambridge, MA: MIT Press.

Fodor, J., & Pylyshyn, Z. (1988). Connectionism and cognitive architecture: A critical analysis. *Cognition, 28*, 3–71.

Gerber, S. (2003). A developmental perspective on language assessment and intervention for children on the autistic spectrum. *Topics in Language Disorders, 23*(2), 74–95.

Gerber, S. (2012). A contemporary model of assessment and intervention: The integration of developmental language models and the developmental individual difference relationship-based approach. In P. Prelock & R. Mac McCauley (Eds.), *Treatment of autism spectrum disorders: Evidence-based intervention strategies for communication and social interaction.* Baltimore, MD: Brookes Publishing.

Gillam, R. B., Loeb, D. F., Hoffman, L. M., Bohman, T., Champlin, C. A., Thibodeau, L., … Friel-Patti, S. (2008). The efficacy of Fast ForWord language intervention in school-age children with language impairment: A randomized controlled trial. *Journal of Speech, Language, and Hearing Research, 51*, 97–119.

Goldin-Meadow, S. (2007). Pointing sets the stage for learning language—and creating language. *Child Development, 78*(3), 741–745.

Golinkoff, R. M., & Hirsh-Pasek, K. (2000). *How babies talk.* New York, NY: Plume.

Gray, B. B., & Ryan, B. (1973). *A language training program for the non-language child.* Champaign, IL: Research Press.

Greenfield, P., & Smith, J. (1976). *The structure of communication in early language development.* New York, NY: Academic Press.

Greenspan, S., Wieder, S., & Simons, R. (1998). *The child with special needs: Encouraging intellectual and emotional growth.* Reading, MA: Addison Wesley Longman.

Halliday, M. A. K. (1975). *Learning how to mean: Explorations in the development of language.* London, UK: Edward Arnold.

Hammill, D., Mather, N., & Roberts, R. (2001). *Illinois test of psycholinguistic abilities* (3rd ed.). Austin, TX: Pro-Ed.

Hulit, L. M., & Howard, M. R. (2002). *Born to talk* (3rd ed.). Boston, MA: Pearson Education.

Johnson, D. J., & Mykelbust, J. R. (1967). *Learning disabilities: Educational principles and practices.* New York, NY: Grune & Stratton.

Johnston, J. (1994). Cognitive abilities of children with language impairment. In R. Watkins & M. Rice (Eds.), *Specific language impairments in children* (vol. 4, pp. 107–121). Baltimore, MA: Paul H. Brookes.

Klein, H., & Moses, N. (1999). *Intervention planning for children with communication disorders.* Boston, MA: Allyn & Bacon.

Koegel, R., & Koegel, L. (2006). *Pivotal response treatments for autism.* Baltimore, MD: Paul H. Brookes.

Kuhl, P. K. (2004). Early language acquisition: Cracking the speech code. *Neuroscience, 5*(11), 831–843.

Lahey, M. (1988). *Language disorders and language development.* New York, NY: Macmillan.

Lenneberg, E. (1967). *Biological foundations of language.* New York, NY: John Wiley & Sons.

Leonard, L., & Loeb, D. (1988). Government-binding theory and some of its implications: A tutorial. *Journal of Speech and Hearing Research, 31*, 515–524.

Locke, J. (1960/1690). An essay concerning human understanding. In Staff of Columbia College (Ed.), *Introduction to contemporary civilization in the West* (pp. 1010–1069). New York, NY: Columbia University Press.

Longtin, S., & Gerber, S. (2008). Contemporary perspectives on facilitating language acquisition for children on the autistic spectrum: Engaging the parent and the child. *The Journal of Developmental Processes, 3*(1), 38–51.

Lovaas, O. I. (1977). *The autistic child: Language development through behavior modification.* New York, NY: Irvington.

Lund, N. J., & Duchan, J. F. (1993). *Assessing children's language in naturalistic contexts* (3rd ed.). Englewood Cliffs, NJ: Prentice-Hall.

Lust, B. (2007). *Child language: Acquisition and growth.* Cambridge: Cambridge University Press.

MacWhinney, B. (1987). *Mechanisms of language acquisition.* Hillsdale, NJ: Erlbaum.

Matthews, D., Theakston, A., & Tomasello, M. (2004). The role of frequency and distributional regularity in the acquisition of word order. *Proceedings of the 32nd Stanford Child Language Research Forum.*

McNeil, D. (1970). *The acquisition of language: The study of developmental linguistics.* New York, NY: Harper & Row.

National Research Council & Institute of Medicine. (2000). *From neurons to neighborhoods: The science of early childhood development.* Washington, DC: National Academy Press.

Nelson, N. (1998). *Childhood language disorders in context: Infancy through adolescence* (2nd ed.). Boston, MA: Pearson Education.

Osgood, C. (1963). On understanding and creating sentences. *American Psychologist, 18,* 735–751.

Pavlov, I. P. (1902). *The work of the digestive glands.* W. H. Thompson (Trans.). London: Charles Griffin.

Pepper, J., & Weitzman, E. (2004). *It takes two to talk: A practical guide for parents of children with language delays* (3rd ed.). Toronto, ON: The Hanen Center.

Phillips, J. R. (1973). Syntax and vocabulary of mothers' speech to young children: Age and sex comparisons. *Child Development, 44,* 182–185.

Piaget, J. (1952). *Origins of intelligence in children.* New York, NY: International University Press.

Piaget, J. (1955). *The language and thought of the child.* M. Gabain (Trans.). Cleveland, OH: Meridian.

Pinker, S. (1984). *Language, learnability, and language development.* Cambridge, MA: Harvard University Press.

Pinker, S. (2006). The blank slate. *General Psychologist, 41*(1), 1–8.

Pinker, S., & Jackendoff, R. (2005). The faculty of language: What's special about it? *Cognition, 95*(2), 201–236.

Premack, D. G., & Woodruff, G. (1978). Does the chimpanzee have a theory of mind? *Behavioral and Brain Sciences, 1*(4), 515–526.

Prizant, B., & Duchan, J. (1981). The functions of immediate echolalia in autistic children. *Journal of Speech and Hearing Disorders, 46,* 241–250.

Prutting, C., & Kirchner, D. (1987). A clinical appraisal of the pragmatic aspects of language. *Journal of Speech and Hearing Disorders, 52,* 105–119.

Rice, M. L., Wexler, K., & Cleave, P. (1995). Specific language impairment as a period of extended optional infinitive. *Journal of Speech and Hearing Research, 38,* 850–863.

Saffran, J. R., Senghas, A., & Trueswell, J. C. (2001). The acquisition of language by children. *Proceedings of the National Academy of Sciences, 98*(23), 12874–12875.

Sakai, K. L. (2005). Language acquisition and brain development. *Science, 310,* 815–819.

Sampson, G. (1987). Review of *parallel distributed processing: Explorations in the microstructure of cognition, vol. 1:* *Foundations,* by D. Rummelhart, J. McClelland, and PDP Research Group. *Language, 63,* 871–886.

Saxton, M., Galloway, C., & Backley, P. (1999). *Negative evidence and negative feedback: Longer term effects on the grammaticality of child speech.* Paper presented at the VIIIth International Congress for the Study of Child Language, San Sebastian, Spain.

Schlesinger, I. M. (1977). *Production and comprehension of utterances.* Hillsdale, NJ: Lawrence Erlbaum.

Searle, J. R. (1969). *Speech acts.* Cambridge, UK: Cambridge University Press.

Seiger-Gardner, L. (2010). Children with language impairment. In B. Shulman & N. Capone (Eds.), *Language development: Foundations, processes, and clinical applications* (pp. 379–406). Sudbury, MA: Jones & Bartlett Learning.

Siegel, D. (1999). *The developing mind: How relationships and the brain interact to shape who we are.* New York, NY: Guilford Press.

Siegel, D. (2001). Toward an interpersonal neurobiology of the developing mind: Attachment relationships, "mindsight," and neural integration. *Infant Mental Health Journal, 22,* 67–94.

Singletary, W. (2015). An integrative model of autism spectrum disorder: ASD as a neurobiological disorder of experienced environmental deprivation, early life stress and allostatic overload. *Neuropsychoanalysis, 17*(2), 81–119.

Skinner, B. F. (1957). *Verbal behavior.* Upper Saddle River, NJ: Prentice Hall.

Slobin, D. (1979). *Psycholinguistics* (2nd ed.). Glenview, IL: Scott Foresman.

Slobin, D., & Bever, T. (1982). Children use canonical sentence schemas: A crosslinguistic study of word order and infections. *Cognition, 12*(3), 229–265.

Snow, C. (1973). Mother's speech to children learning language. *Child Development, 43,* 549–565.

Snow, C. (1978). The conversational context of language acquisition. In R. Campbell & P. Smith (Eds.), *Recent advances in the psychology of language* (vol. 4a, pp. 253–269). New York, NY: Plenum Press.

Snow, C. (1999). Social perspectives on the emergence of language. In B. MacWhinney (Ed.), *The emergence of language* (pp. 257–276). Mahwah, NJ: Erlbaum.

Sundberg, M. L. (2008). *Verbal behavior milestones assessment and placement program: The VB-MAPP.* Concord, CA: AVB Press.

Sussman, F. (1999). *More than words: Helping parents promote communication and social skills in children with autism spectrum disorders.* Toronto, ON: The Hanen Center.

Thiessen, E. D., Hill, E. A., & Saffran, J. R. (2005). Infant-directed speech facilitates word segmentation. *Infancy, 7*(1), 53–71.

Tomasello, M. (1988). The role of joint attentional processes in early language development. *Language Sciences, 10,* 69–88.

Tomasello, M. (2003). *Constructing a language: A usage-based theory of language acquisition.* Cambridge, MA: Harvard University Press.

Tomasello, M., Carpenter, M., & Liszkowski, U. (2007). A new look at infant pointing. *Child Development, 78*(3), 705–722.

Trehub, S. (1976). The discrimination of foreign speech contrasts by infants and children. *Child Development, 47,* 466–472.

van der Lely, H. K. (1998). SLI in children: Movement, economy, and deficits in the computational-syntactic system. *Language Acquisition, 7*(2–4), 161.

van der Lely, H. K. (1997). Modularity and Innateness: Insight from a grammatical-specific language impairment. In A. Sorace, C. Heycock, & R. Shillcock (Eds.), *Proceedings of the Conference on Language Acquisition.* Edinburgh, Scotland: University of Edinburgh Press.

Vargha-Khadem, F., Watkins, K. E., Price, C. J., Ashburner, J., Alcock, K. J., Connelly, A., ... Passingham, R. E. (1998). Neural basis of an inherited speech and language disorder. *Proceedings of the National Academy of Sciences, USA, 95*(21), 12695–12700.

Vouloumanos, A., & Werker, J. F. (2007). Listening to language at birth: Evidence for a bias for speech in neonates. *Developmental Sciences, 10*(2), 159–171.

Vygotsky, L. S. (1986). *Thought and language.* A. Kozulin (Trans.). Cambridge, MA: MIT Press.

Warren, S. F., & Kaiser, A. P. (1986). Incidental language teaching: A critical review. *Journal of Speech and Hearing Disorders, 51*(4), 291–299.

Werker, J. F., & Tees, R. C. (1984). Cross-language speech perception: Evidence for perceptual reorganization during the first year of life. *Infant Behavior and Development, 7,* 49–64.

Westby, C. (1980). Assessment of cognitive and language abilities through play. *Language, Speech and Hearing Services in the Schools, 11*(3), 154–168.

Westby, C. (2000). A scale for assessing development of children's play. In K. Gitlin-Weiner, A. Sandgun, & C. Schaefer (Eds.), *Play diagnosis and assessment* (pp. 15–27). New York, NY: John Wiley & Sons.

Wetherby, A., Woods, J., Allen, L., Cleary, J., Dickenson, H., & Lord, C. (2004). Early indicators of autism spectrum disorders in the second year of life. *Journal of Autism and Developmental Disorders, 34*(5), 473–493.

Wexler, K. (1999). Maturation and growth of grammar. In W. Ritchie & T. Bhatia (Eds.), *Handbook of child language acquisition* (pp. 55–110). New York, NY: Academic Press.

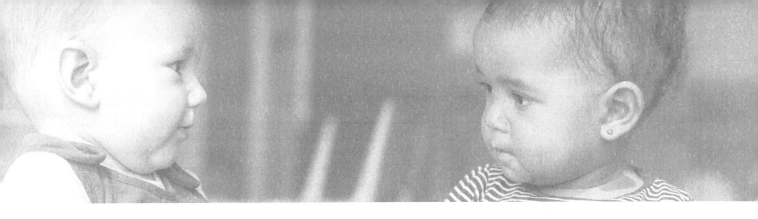

CHAPTER 3

The Hearing Mechanism and Auditory Development

Deborah R. Welling, AuD, CCC-A, FAAA
Carol A. Ukstins, MS, CCC-A, FAAA

OBJECTIVES

- Describe the structure and understand the functional differences between the conductive and sensorineural mechanisms of the ear
- Outline the process of normal auditory development
- Compare and contrast the levels of listening skills, hierarchy
- Identify and describe the different characteristics of the various types of hearing loss
- Understand the basic components of 21st-century listening technology
- Understand the connection between auditory input and communication output

KEY TERMS

Asymmetrical
Auditory attention
Auditory closure
Auditory memory
Cochlea
Cochlear implant
Comprehension level
Conductive hearing loss
Conductive mechanism
Detection level
Discrimination level
Eustachian tube

Feedback
Frequency
Hearing aid
High-frequency sensorineural
   hearing loss
Identification level
Impedance mismatch
Localization
Middle ear transformer function
Mixed hearing loss
Organ of Corti
Ossicular chain

Otitis media
Resonance properties
Resonant frequencies
Reverberation
Sensorineural hearing loss
Sensorineural mechanism
Sound encoding
Traveling wave
Tympanic membrane
Unilateral hearing loss

▶ Introduction

Normal hearing development is perhaps the most important factor in the development of normal speech and language skills. Unfortunately, hearing loss can occur as the result of prenatal factors and be present from the time of birth. Hearing loss can also occur at some later point due to a nearly endless list of events causing hearing to be either temporarily or permanently impaired, thereby impeding the process of normal speech-language development. To make matters more complicated, hearing loss is not an "all or nothing" affair. Rather, hearing ability can range from completely normal to profoundly deaf and anywhere in between.

▶ Anatomy and Physiology of the Peripheral Auditory System

In order to understand how we hear, we must first understand the structure and function of the ear itself. Made up of three parts, the outer ear, the middle ear, and the inner ear (refer to Figure 3-4), our ears are a finely tuned mechanism that processes the acoustic signal. The descriptions of the conductive (outer and middle ear) and sensorineural (inner ear) mechanisms that follow are meant as an introductory look at the basic structures of the peripheral auditory system and how it works. The primary purpose of providing this information is to assist the reader in obtaining a fundamental understanding of the anatomy and physiology of the ear and lay a foundation upon which the remaining concepts of this chapter can be built.

The Conductive Mechanism

The conductive (mechanical) mechanism anatomically consists of the outer ear and the middle ear. As a whole, the outer and middle ear has the job of gathering the acoustic sound energy from the environment, converting it into mechanical energy, and then delivering this energy to the inner ear (sensorineural mechanism).

The two main portions of the outer ear are the pinna (or auricle) and the external auditory canal (or meatus, also known as the ear canal). The pinna (**FIGURE 3-1**) is the anatomical portion that sits on each side of our heads; this structure is made of cartilage and is covered by skin. Some of the major landmarks on the pinna include the helix, antihelix, tragus, antitragus, concha (bowl-shaped portion), and lobule (earlobe).

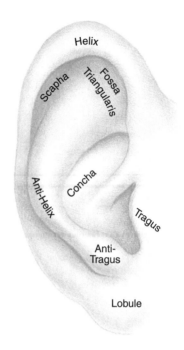

FIGURE 3-1 The pinna (auricle) of the ear.

The external ear canal (**FIGURE 3-2**) is a tube-like structure that is approximately 25 mm (roughly 1 inch) in length and approximately 7 mm in diameter. It starts at the pinna and extends all the way down to the *tympanic membrane* (eardrum). The outer one-third of the ear canal is cartilaginous and is a continuation of the cartilage of the pinna; the inner two-thirds of the canal are bony. The entire ear canal is covered with skin, which continues and forms the outermost of the eardrum's three layers.

The outer ear has several functions—some acoustic (sound-related) and some nonacoustic (Yost, 2007). First, the pinna acts as a collector and director of sound. The "collector" function is accomplished by the cupped shape of the concha; it collects the sound and then directs it down toward the eardrum. In fact, cupping a hand around your ear in an attempt to improve your hearing actually does provide a small loudness boost in the sound level.

The second acoustic function of the pinna is to assist in determining the location of the source of a sound, also known as *localization*. If you look at Figures 3-1 and 3-2 (or, better yet, examine your own or your neighbor's pinna), you may notice that the ear is not a flat surface. Rather, it contains all kinds of nooks and crannies or hills and valleys. The way in which sound bounces off the various curves and grooves of the pinna provides information that the brain can use to determine the direction from which the sound is coming.

Another sound-related function performed by the outer ear is the result of the *resonance properties* of the outer ear structure, which enhance the sound in a particular portion of the *frequency* range. In other

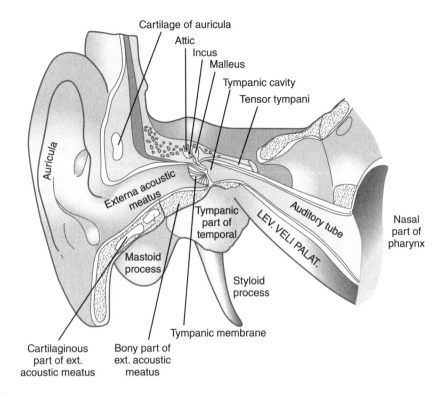

Cartilage of auricula
Attic
Incus
Malleus
Tympanic cavity
Tensor tympani
Auricula
Externa acoustic meatus
Nasal part of pharynx
Auditory tube
LEV. VELI PALAT.
Tympanic part of temporal
Styloid process
Mastoid process
Tympanic membrane
Cartilaginous part of ext. acoustic meatus
Bony part of ext. acoustic meatus

FIGURE 3-2 The ear.

words, some frequencies are given a natural boost, a necessary action if the sound is to eventually reach the fluid-filled inner ear effectively. As a point of interest, both the pinna and the ear canal have a natural design whereby a frequency range of the incoming sounds will be enhanced most effectively (*resonant frequency*). For the pinna, this resonant frequency is approximately 5,000 Hz; for the ear canal, it is approximately 2,000 Hz. In real-life listening situations, this enhancement results in an increase in the frequency range most commonly associated with many of our consonant sounds, thereby providing an ever-so-slight enhancement in receptive speech intelligibility.

In addition to serving these acoustic functions, the outer ear fulfills some nonsound-related roles. Most importantly, it protects the eardrum from direct injury. This is accomplished, at least in part, by the anatomy itself. Examine Figure 3-2 again, noticing that the ear canal does not form a straight horizontal line but rather sits at an angle. Furthermore, it is characterized by curving and bending, and the inner two-thirds of the canal wall is made up of bone. Again, by natural design, the combination of these structural details minimizes injury caused by external sources to the very delicate structure of the tympanic membrane.

Another nonacoustic function of the outer ear relates to cerumen (earwax). This brownish waxy substance found in the ear canal results from secretions of two types of glands (ceruminous and sebaceous), both of which are located in the outer one-third of the ear canal. The secretions act as a protective layer for the skin and tissue underneath, helping to prevent infections by trapping potentially harmful irritants. In addition, the wax serves a self-cleaning function by combining with dirt and sloughed-off (dead) skin cells. This normal process includes the forces of gravity, body heat, and the normal activities of chewing and speaking; collectively, this causes the wax to gradually make its way to the opening of the ear canal. The amount of cerumen produced by an individual varies greatly, and although cerumen production is a natural function of the ear, it can also be the cause of temporary hearing loss (cerumen impaction). Several outer ear disorders, including impacted cerumen, are discussed later in this chapter.

FIGURE 3-3 is a schematic diagram of the middle ear system. The eardrum is the outermost (lateral) border, and the temporal bone (which contains the inner ear, among other structures) makes up the medial wall. Other important structures within the middle ear space include the oval and round windows (on the medial wall), which make up part of the border to the inner ear; the *Eustachian tube* (on the anterior wall that provides a connection to the nasopharynx); and the three smallest bones in the human body—the malleus (hammer), incus (anvil), and stapes (stirrup), which are collectively known as the *ossicular chain*.

The Eustachian tube connects the middle ear space to the nasopharynx (or throat). Its primary functions are to provide circulation of air to the middle ear cavity

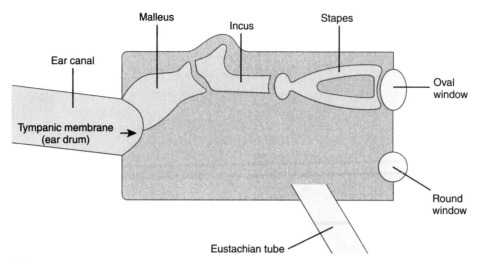

FIGURE 3-3 The middle ear space.

and equalization of the pressure between the middle ear and the outside atmosphere. Rarely is this function more happily appreciated than when a person is going up in an airplane. A brief but pleasing yawn to "pop" one's ears is an excellent example of the function of the Eustachian tube.

The main objective of the middle ear system, however, is to *effectively* deliver sound from the outer ear through the middle ear and to the cochlea in the inner ear. Acoustic energy that is collected by the external ear structures is sent through the ear canal to the eardrum. It is at this point that the acoustic energy is transformed into the mechanical, just like the vibration of a beating drum. This mechanical energy is transmitted through the ossicular chain to the oval window at the entrance of the inner ear. However, since the inner ear is a fluid-filled space as opposed to the air-filled space of the middle ear, this particular function presents a challenge to the middle ear system. The middle ear needs to overcome the resistance of the fluid, and if it does not, the sound energy will not be effectively transmitted through the middle ear to the inner ear and the person will not hear properly. To visualize this difference between the air-filled middle ear cavity and the fluid-filled inner ear cavity, imagine swinging your hand through the air. Now imagine that you are trying to swing your hand through partially set gelatin. Quite obviously, you will use more effort when your hand is going through the gelatin than when it is going through the air. This analogy demonstrates the different in resistance that characterizes the air-filled middle ear versus the fluid-filled inner ear. Overcoming this impedance mismatch is accomplished by the *middle ear transformer function,* which requires a combination of factors.

The first factor affecting the middle ear transformer function is the size mismatch—that is, the comparative size of the eardrum that is much larger—to the size of the stapes footplate at the oval window (where the sound exits the middle ear and enters the inner ear). This size difference alone increases the sound pressure approximately 18-fold by the time it enters the inner ear. The second factor involved is the position of each of the ossicles (refer to Figure 3-3) in relation to the others; this varying placement creates a lever action that also increases the sound pressure. Lastly, the shape of the eardrum and the way it moves adds pressure to the sound energy being transmitted by the ossicular chain. These factors, which are collectively known as the middle transformer function, increase the sound significantly by the time it reaches the inner ear. Without these factors working in unison, the sound energy would not be sufficiently amplified to move through the fluid-filled cochlea. A wide range of factors can throw off this delicate process and result in a hearing loss that is conductive in nature. Conductive hearing losses are discussed in detail later in this chapter.

The Sensorineural Mechanism

The sensorineural mechanism involves both the inner ear and the auditory nerve. The inner ear houses both organs for balance (vestibular labyrinth) and structures concerned with hearing (auditory labyrinth). For this introductory look at the ear, however, we limit our discussion to the anatomy and physiology as they relate to the process of hearing only.

As sound reaches the oval window, it crosses into the inner. The sound is directed toward the auditory labyrinth, which houses the *cochlea.* Inside the cochlea lies the *organ of Corti* (end organ of hearing). FIGURE 3-4a shows the cochlea partially uncoiled; however, in its normal state, the cochlea is coiled up like a conch shell (FIGURE 3-4b). The name "cochlea" itself

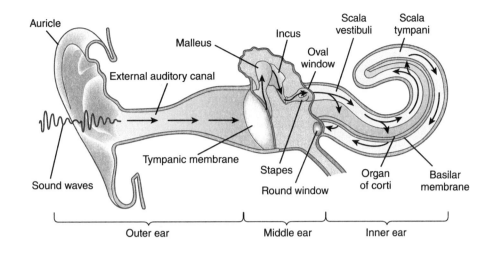

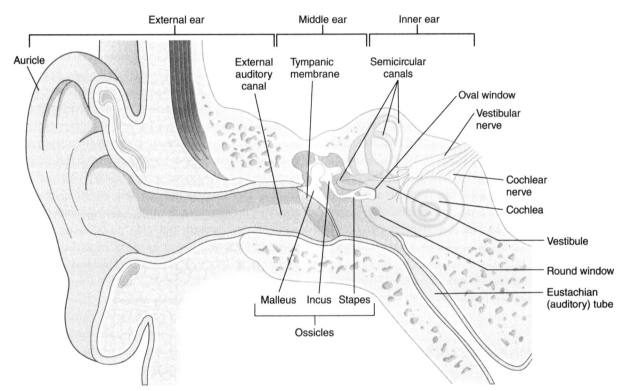

FIGURE 3-4 **(a)** The outer, middle, and inner ear. The cochlea is partially uncoiled. **(b)** The cochlea is coiled (its normal state).

is derived from the Greek words "kokhlias" (meaning snail screw) and "koklos" (meaning spiral shell). For a better understanding and visualization of this structure, imagine that we unroll the cochlea (**FIGURE 3-5**) to take a look at some of the significant structures, namely the scala media (which houses the organ of Corti), the scala vestibuli above it, and the scala tympani below it. The top boundary of the scala media is Reissner's membrane; the bottom boundary is the basilar membrane. Both the scala vestibuli and the scala tympani are filled with a fluid called perilymph, whereas the scala media is filled with a fluid called endolymph. The endolymph and perilymph are both gelatinous fluids, although each has a unique chemical composition. The endolymph has high potassium content, for example, whereas the

perilymph has high sodium content; this difference plays a significant role in the process of hearing.

Because the cochlea is completely filled with fluid, the sound that entered the inner ear as mechanical energy creates a wave (similar to a pebble hitting water) as it enters the scala vestibuli. This wave (known as the *traveling wave*) proceeds all the way through to the top of the cochlear to the structure called the helicotrema and into the scala tympani. The helicotrema is a passageway that permits communication between the scala vestibuli and the scala tympani.

The traveling wave of sound energy, simultaneously, causes displacement (movement) of the basilar membrane within the scala media, as well as the organ of Corti sitting on top of it (refer to Figure 3-4a). Within

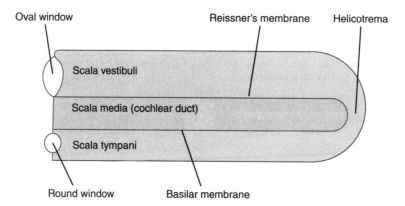

FIGURE 3-5 The cochlea.

the organ of Corti, the wave action sets into motion the structures known as outer hair cells and inner hair cells. The movement causes bending of the tops of these cells, a process referred to as a shearing action. At this point, the mechanical energy (sound) is converted into electrochemical energy. This shearing action causes the mixing of the sodium and potassium ions within the two fluids, which in turn leads to the electrical impulse that causes the auditory nerve to "fire." The resulting electrochemical reaction sends the information along the auditory nerve, which is then delivered to and used by the brain. Any disruption in this process can result in a hearing loss of the sensorineural type. Sensorineural hearing loss is discussed further later in this chapter.

For a more detailed description of this process, you can read *The Auditory System: Anatomy, Physiology, and Clinical Correlates* by Musiek and Baran (2007) or *Fundamentals of Hearing: An Introduction* by Yost (2007).

▶ Normal Auditory Development

The physical properties that make up our auditory mechanism are quite elaborate. Likewise, the natural transmission of sound is a detailed journey through the structures of the ear. However, hearing does not just happen; it is a complex process that itself has developmental milestones. Professionally, a secure understanding of normal auditory development is the precursor to understanding the development of speech and language skills. One should always think "Hearing First" when considering disorders of speech and language in children.

Prenatal Auditory Development

Normal auditory development is a complicated and lengthy process that begins during the gestational period in utero (Holst et al., 2005; Tye-Murray, 2004; Werner, 2003). The physical structures that will form the ear start developing very early in the prenatal period,

beginning roughly during the 3rd week of development (5 weeks gestational age). During the third trimester, the ear begins to function and the fetus starts to respond to sounds that originate from outside of the womb (McMahon, Wintermark, & Lahav, 2012). There is also evidence suggesting that the fetus is capable of more than just the detection of sound. Kisilevsky and her colleagues provide evidence that higher-order auditory perception (more than a mere awareness of sound's presence) begins before birth (Kisilevsky, Hains, Jacquet, Granier-Deferre, & Lecanuet, 2004). Werner (2003) reports that during the last few weeks of pregnancy, the fetus is capable of not only hearing maternal speech while in the womb, but also recognizing after birth some of what was heard in utero. In addition to a fetal response to the mother's voice (Kisilevsky et al., 2004; McMullen & Saffran, 2004), the fetus appears to learn about aspects of linguistic sound such as the prosody, rhythm, and intonation of the mother's native language (McMullen & Saffran, 2004). In fact, some studies have shown that if a mother reads a rhythmic story to her fetus in the last few weeks of pregnancy, her newborn will recognize the story even if another woman reads it (Werner, 2003). This is a clear indication of more than a "mere awareness" of sound's existence and suggests the development of higher-order auditory perceptual ability prior to birth.

Postnatal Auditory Development
Birth Through 6 Months (Stage One)

The gradual development of the auditory system that began during the prenatal period continues well into childhood and adolescence (Werner, 2007a), with the initial postnatal period of sound coding spanning from birth to 6 months of age. This is followed by a stage of development involving greater specificity of acoustic cues that continues through early school years. Finally, as children gain listening experience, they begin developing adult-like sound processing skills.

At birth, the child is thrown into a sea of sound in a nondiscriminatory way. As a matter of fact, a child has the potential at birth to be a native speaker of any language. From this "universe" of sound begins the normal process of language learning, and the child must start on the journey of figuring out what is important to listen to so as to become a competent communicator in their native tongue. The first auditory maturational hurdle for the child to successfully "jump" is that of *sound encoding*. Sound encoding is a basic and essential skill whereby the ear and auditory pathway physically receive and code sound and then send it on its way toward the brain for eventual interpretation. Sound encoding allows, for example, the perception and analysis of the acoustics of speech. In essence, the child learns that sound has meaning and that they can produce sound for the purpose of communication in their environment.

Six Months Through Early Elementary Years (Stage Two)

The maturation of selective listening and discovering new details in sound (Werner, 2007b) begins to develop in this second stage. At 6 months of age, the baby is still listening in a nondiscriminatory way. With the goal of developing normal language and processing skills, it is essential that the infant learn to listen in a selective way. This extended learning process will continue through the preschool and early elementary years. In fact, it continues to be fine-tuned for an extended period after that point as well. During this stage of auditory development, the child becomes more aware of their acoustic environment and begins to listen to more subtle sound cues. This may initially involve the infant selectively focusing on a specific feature of a sound (perhaps the sound made by a favorite toy). As children becomes aware of the auditory world in which they live, they begin to connect sounds with daily events and specific people. It is this bombardment of auditory information that culminates in the momentous occasion of a child's first spoken word at approximately 12 months of age. But one should not think that auditory development ends at the child's first spoken word. The explosion of spoken language noted from 12 to 24 months accompanies the development of the child's ability to listen to complex speech across a wide range of acoustic environments. As the child continues to be exposed to a wide range of auditory experiences, their listening skills become more refined and secure in their native language. Listening to language in both their natural (home) environment and in the educational environment secures their use of both receptive and expressive language skills for the purpose of communication.

School Age Through Adolescence (Stage Three)

At this stage, the maturation of perceptual flexibility (Werner, 2007b) envelops the child's acoustic surroundings. Progressing beyond the early elementary years, listening selectivity involves the development of auditory skills that allow for understanding speech in a background of noise and other acoustically adverse conditions. Although the child is expected to develop selective listening skills by the time they enter grade school, there is evidence that this development continues at least until early adolescence (Putkinen, Tervaniemi, Saarikivi, Ojala, & Houtilainen, 2014), as the child is exposed to unique and challenging listening situations. Clearly then, even normally developing children can and do have more difficulty than adults when it comes to selectively listening, especially when the listening conditions are less than ideal. An example of a "less than ideal" situation that may prove more problematic for a child is one characterized by excessive background noise and/or reverberation that may occur in a typical classroom environment. An abundance of literature documents the negative effects these conditions may have on children and their ability to learn academic materials through audition.

It is important to note that there are nonauditory factors that may prove detrimental to a child's overall ability to hear, perceive, understand, and process the content of speech and language. A common condition is when a speaker's face is not visible to the listener, for example, a child in a noisy classroom not being able to see the teacher's face. Other detrimental nonauditory effects may, for example, include motivational and cognitive issues such as learned helplessness, poor problem-solving skills, low frustration tolerance, and low academic achievement (particularly when it comes to reading) (Bistrop et al., 2002). Each of these conditions presents unique challenges to young children, who must learn to listen with flexibility so that they can communicate effectively when they are thrust into such settings.

What should be obvious at this point is that the accomplishment of normal auditory maturation and associated development of speech and spoken language requires a vast quantity and quality of auditory input and listening practice. **TABLE 3-1** contains a list of aspects related to auditory development and concurrent attainments of speech and spoken language skills (Perigoe & Paterson, 2019).

Hierarchy of Listening Skills Development

Just as neuromaturational changes are observable in auditory behaviors as speech and language skills develop, changes are also seen in the child's

TABLE 3-1 Auditory–Verbal Development in Typically Developing Children with Normal Hearing

	Input: Auditory Development	Output: Speech Production/Spoken Language
Prenatal	*Auditory Experiences in Utero:* A typically developing child has 20 weeks of exposure to auditory stimuli prior to birth Infant emerges literally wired for sound Listens to mother's voice and environmental sounds (both from within and outside of the womb) Born with a preference for mother's voice Born with a preference for songs and stories heard in utero	
Birth to 3 months	*Reactions to Sounds:* Startle reflex, eye blink/eye widening, cessation of activity, limb movement, head turn toward or away, grimacing/crying, sucking, arousal, breathing change *Speech Perception Abilities:* Can identify individual phonemes Capable of detecting virtually every phoneme Prefers vowels *Prosody/Suprasegmentals:* Prefers human voice Attentive to the rise and fall of intonation pattern Attends to patterns of speech Prefers native language to all others *Identification:* Identifies mother's voice Prefers songs heard prenatally	*Reflexive:* Coos, gurgles, reflexive sounds *Physical Response to Sounds:* Stilling, rhythmic movement, searching for sound's source *Vocalization:* Goo sounds, laughter Quasi-resonant nuclei (QRN), immature vowel-like sounds
3–4 months	*Prosody/Suprasegmentals:* Prefers utterances with intonation variation versus flat voice Discriminates high and low sounds	
4–7 months	*Early Auditory Feedback Auditory Tuning In:* Listening to language for longer periods of time Shows awareness of environmental sounds Can be behaviorally pacified by music or song *Speech Perception:* Recognition of mother's voice Reacts to vocal mood differences *Localization:* Localization to sound begins to emerge from eye gaze to head turn to localization to specific sound sources (directly related to motor development) *Auditory Memory:* Beginning of auditory memory (distinguishes between voices of familiar people versus strangers)	*Expanding Vocal Repertoire:* Vocal play Fully resonant nuclei (FRN), vowel-like sounds, consonant-like sounds, consonant-vowel (CV) and vowel-consonant (VC) syllables emerge Plays with streams of sounds, intonation patterns, raspberries, squeals, loudness play Vocal turn-taking exchanges with parent

| **5 months** | *Early Auditory Comprehension:*
Responds to own name | *Vocalization:*
CV syllable and some VC syllable vocalizations
Imitates pitch tone |
| | *Suprasegmentals/Prosody:*
Discriminates own language from others with same prosody | |

6 months

Correlation between achievements and speech perception and later word understanding, word production, and phrase production

Vocalization:
May produce recognizable vowels: /u/a/i/

Speech Perception:
Preference for vowel ends

Early Auditory Feedback:
Listens to self in vocal play

Auditory Identification:
Begins to recognize own name and the names of family members

Reliable Localization:
Begins to respond to directives

Selective Auditory Attention:
Will divert attention from one activity to a more desirable activity based on auditory input.

The Sound with Meaning Connection:
The "melody is the message." Child will interpret parents' intention by listening and reacting to tone of voice change. Happens prior to word comprehension.

8–10 months

Synaptogenesis:
Explosion of synaptic growth may be related to change in perception and production

Vocalization: Canonical "Babble":
Achieves strings of reduplicated and alternated syllable production; timing of syllable production sounds speech-like, stress patterns
Vowels, consonants becoming distinct

Phonotactic Regularities and Prosody:
Sensitive to regularities in word boundaries in infant-directed speech (IDS), even in another language
Begins storing sound patterns for words, although no meaning yet

Increased Vocal Turn-Taking:
Once true babble attained, parents expect more speech-like utterances.

Auditory Comprehension:
Begins to comprehend words

Primitive Speech Acts (PSA):
Expressing intentions nonverbally

8–14 months

Protowords:
Words invented by child, not adult, but have consistent meaning, such as "la-la" for blanket

9 months

Speech Perception:
Prefers nonwords composed of high phonotactic components

Intentionality: "I Know What I Mean":
Child attains cognitive/communication intents
Achieves means–end concept
Uses vocal/verbal means to achieve ends in combination with visual and gestural mechanisms

Auditory Attention:
Sustained auditory attention
Will attend to auditory-based activities for increased periods of time

Vocalization:
Variegated babble: Adjacent and following syllables are not identical

Phonotactic Probabilities:
Predicting likelihood of certain sound sequences, listening preference for nonwords with high phonotactic probability versus those with low probability

(continues)

TABLE 3-1 Auditory–Verbal Development in Typically Developing Children with Normal Hearing   *(continued)*

	Input: Auditory Development	Output: Speech Production/Spoken Language
9–12 months		*9–12 months, Speech to Communicate:* Sound imitation of common household items and animals Distinct word approximations, and in some cases, early single word utterances take the place of crying to fulfill wants and needs Verbal "nicknames" for distinct objects and people develop and remain consistent for that object or person
10 months	*Auditory Tuning In:* Narrows auditory attention and speech perception: tunes in to mother language, loses universal interest in all speech sounds	
10–16 months		*Phonetically Consistent Forms (PCF):* Speech sounds that have sound–meaning relationships, such as "puda" for the family cat *First Words:* Context-bound Following the first word, during the next few months, children add an average of 8–11 words to their vocabularies each month
11 months	*Speech Perception:* Identifies allophones and word boundaries	Variegated babble Word approximations
12 months	*Speech Perception:* Hears word and consonant boundaries	
Ages 12–24 months: Exploring and Expanding	*Listening: Auditory Comprehension*	*Speech Production and Spoken Language*
12–18 months	*Early Auditory Comprehension:* Odd mappings of words Child attends to whole sentence Is able to follow commands Fully aware of the names for familiar objects and family members *Auditory Environment:* Derives obvious pleasure from auditory activities like music, playing with friends, laughing, and being read to *Auditory Experience:* Listening to speech for long periods of time is essential to the ultimate use of even single words	*Overextension and Underextension of Words:* Language develops as a direct correlation of using that developing speech to ultimately gain a desired outcome through a communication interaction between the speaker and the listener *Gradual Decontextualization (to 18 months):* Says first clear, distinct word and assigns that word to a single distinct object or person
16–20 months		*Fast Mapping:* Ability to learn words in one or few exposures

18 months	*Auditory Vocabulary:* Tremendous growth in vocabulary comprehension, 100–200 words understood	*First 50 Words Used: A First Language:* Growth in expressive ability Tremendous growth in one-word usage
18–24 months	*Auditory Localization:* Will independently seek out a sound source in another room *Auditory Comprehension:* Understands and follows verbal directions with two critical elements Begins to respond appropriately to "What, Where" questions	*Word Spurt: Vocabulary Spurt:* "Naming theory" seems to be a basis for noun usage, naming people, objects; occurs for most children when they hit the first 50 words mark Will begin to sing along with songs or mimic the rhythm of a nursery rhyme
Ages 2–3	*Listening*	*Speaking*
24–36 months	*Auditory Identification:* Will identify a sound and share that identification with another person with exuberance Desires to share auditory information with another person *Auditory Memory:* Will share auditory experiences from memory (left brain) Will sing complete or nearly complete songs from memory (right brain)	*Cognitive/Semantic:* Two-word semantic relations, and three-word-plus utterances *Spoken Language and Play:* Will hold a seemingly appropriate conversation with an inanimate object while playing Presyntactic Period
26–32 months		*Phoneme Repetition:* Vocabulary size seems related to ability to repeat phoneme combinations, especially initial position in nonwords
By 36 months		*Early Syntactic:* Recombination of two-plus-two word utterances Early multiple word utterances, correct word order *Early Morphology:* "ing"
Ages 3–4: Peers, Preschool	*Listening*	*Speaking*
3–4 years	*Auditory Memory:* Begins to show listening preferences for favorite stories or music and will follow simple aural commands *Auditory Attention:* Development of sustained auditory attention for increasing periods of time *"Overhearing" or "Incidental" Learning Through Listening:* Does not need to be involved in direct instruction or directly in a conversation to pick up on what is happening; uses words, expressions not directly taught	*Pragmatics:* Able to hold an appropriate turn-taking conversation with a peer; continuing to develop conversational competence Cognitive Semantic *Phonology:* Phonetic repertoire mastered for some phonemes Phonological processes occurring

(continues)

TABLE 3-1 Auditory–Verbal Development in Typically Developing Children with Normal Hearing		_(continued)_
	Input: Auditory Development	**Output: Speech Production/Spoken Language**
	Listening	_Speaking_
	Auditory Feedback Mechanism: Development of auditory feedback mechanism Development of phonemic awareness and temporal processing _Distance Listening:_ Ability to search the auditory environment for information even if engaged in activity	_Preliteracy:_ Recitation by rhyme Rhyme by pattern Alliteration _Early Syntactic Child:_ Increased morphological use, correct sentence word order Begins to produce increasingly complex sentences that adhere to spoken language rules
4–5 years	_Achieves Metalinguistic Ability Through Audition:_ Recognizes and can report when he or she hears someone make an error or slip of the tongue in spoken language Uses auditory cues in conversations to recognize prosodic, pragmatics, semantic and syntactic errors in adult and peer speech	_Pragmatics/Discourse:_ Follows adult conventions for conversation mechanisms; able to take role as "conversational partner" _Preliteracy: Phonologic Awareness:_ Syllable counting (50% of children by age 5)
Ages 5–6: _Preacademic_ _Readiness_	_Auditory Developments_	_Speaking_
5–6 years	_Auditory Attention:_ Development of an attention span for instruction even if the topic is not of high interest _Auditory Memory:_ Stronger development for long-term auditory memory of linguistic information _Internal Auditory Feedback:_ Development of internal auditory feedback (reading voice in head); auditory self-correcting	_Pragmatics/Discourse:_ Oral narrative more developed _Early Literacy: Phonologic Awareness:_ Initial consonant matching Blending 2–3 phonemes Counting phonemes: 70% of children by age 6 Rhyme identification Onset-rime division _Syntax:_ Increasing mastery of complex language forms: relative clauses, coordination, subordination, use of the infinitive verbs Increased mastery of language systems: tense marking, modals and semimodals, pronouns, determiners
Ages 7 and Up: _Refining_ _Auditory Skills_		
7 years	_Assessable Auditory Processing Function:_ Higher level auditory skills are mostly developed and intact: dichotic listening, auditory figure ground, selective auditory attention _Phonemic Awareness:_ Sound blending, sound symbol association _Prosody and Suprasegmentals:_ Ability to sense vocal sarcasm Ability to resist heavy accent and follow conversation (decoding and closure) _Auditory Lexicon:_ 14,000 words (approx.)	_Phonologic Awareness:_ Blending three phonemes Segmentation of three-four phonemes (blends) Phonetic spelling Phoneme deletion _Syntax:_ Expressive vocabulary

	Auditory Developments	Speaking

8 years — *Auditory Processing Overload Strategies:*
Develops compensatory strategies when faced with the challenge of auditory processing overload
Uses volume independently to aid in focus and attention

Auditory Attention for Music:
Begins to have an "ear" for music, auditory attention for musical instruction

Phonologic Awareness:
Consonant cluster segmentation
Deletion with clusters

9 years — *Auditory Input Primary for Instruction:*
Auditory begins to become the primary input system for classroom instruction
Higher-level auditory visual integration skills for organization management like note taking
End of the right ear advantage

Perigoe, C. & Paterson, M. (2019). Understanding auditory development and the child with hearing loss. In Welling, D. R. & Ukstins, C. A. (Eds.), *Fundamentals of Audiology for the Speech-Language Pathologist*, 2nd Edition. Baltimore, MD: Jones & Bartlett.

development of specific listening skills. Not to be confused with the development of auditory system, normal listening skill development involves the acquisition of several individual components leading up to the ultimate and most difficult of the skills, namely comprehension of linguistic and nonlinguistic sounds. The skills discussed in this section are covered in a hierarchical fashion, with the simplest of the levels (detection) being presented first and the most complicated of the levels (comprehension of linguistic and nonlinguistic sounds) being presented last.

Many models have been proposed to describe the normal development of auditory listening skills. On the surface, it might appear that there is considerable variability among these models. A careful investigation, however, reveals that they are actually more similar than not, although some of the models go into more detail than others. The version presented here includes some of the most basic and essential components; it is not intended to be an exhaustive list of all skills necessary to attain the ultimate goal of comprehension.

Detection Level

The *detection level* is the most basic level of sound awareness. In normal hearing individuals, this step in the hierarchical process is simply the answer to the question, "Is sound present?". Determining the existence of auditory information is the most rudimentary level of auditory experience.

Unfortunately, with a hard-of-hearing child, matters become more complex. When a child sustains a hearing loss, the issue of amplification (hearing aid/s

or cochlear implant/s) must be considered first. In order for detection to occur, the device must be in the child's ear/s, turned on, and functioning appropriately. Even with appropriate and adequate amplification, the child's parents and/or caregiver must be diligent in exposing the child to as many different auditory experiences as possible and directing that child's attention to that information ("Oh! Did you hear that?") to complete the first stage in this process.

Discrimination Level

The *discrimination level* is the next higher level of difficulty. In normal hearing individuals, the discrimination level takes on several different forms. One must discriminate between the same sound and a different sound, speech sound versus nonspeech sound, and then move on to the discrimination of speech content.

Within the discrimination level, children first master discrimination of the suprasegmental aspects of language—for example, pitch, prosody, rhythm, stress, and inflection—before they master the segmental aspects. In fact, as described in the section on prenatal development, some evidence suggests that children respond to these suprasegmental aspects of sound before birth. As part of the development of this ability, a young child may be exposed to a parent expressing anger toward a sibling. The child may recognize the anger without needing to understand the entire dialogue that explains what the parent is angry about. Later, children learn to respond to segmental aspects of speech, which include such elements such as phonemes, morphemes, and syllables.

In children with hearing loss, therapeutic intervention is necessary for the development of these skills since incidental language learning is severely impacted. Direct instruction in all aspects of language learning becomes wholly important for the hard-of-hearing child in the development of auditory skills. Since early intervention services typically occur in the home (natural environment) of the child, parents and caregivers work side by side with the professional in a collaborative approach to intervention. One must never assume that the child using hearing aids or cochlear implants, who react to the presence of sound, have achieved this discrimination level. A frequent misconception is that an individual showing awareness of sound has simultaneously discriminated the content.

Identification Level

At the *identification level,* the normal hearing individual is able to identify or label an item; this ability can be shown by naming the item or pointing to it. The identification level is where the child starts to understand and build vocabulary and show an understanding of simple words and phrases (Therres, 2015). Hence, it is at this point that the connection between auditory development and speech and language development becomes strikingly apparent. While each level to this point shows a degree of communicative intent, it is at the identification level in the hierarchy that it becomes an overall indicator of normal childhood development.

In the pediatrician's office, the parent/caregiver is often questioned regarding speech and language development during routine child visits. "How many words does your child use?" is a frequent question. In the rating of normal childhood development, if these milestones are not being met, it may be suspect of hearing loss not identified through the newborn infant hearing screening process and give reason for in-depth follow-up.

In children with hearing loss just learning to use hearing aid/s or cochlear implant/s, these milestone markers may vary significantly from severely delayed to nearing normal depending on the severity of the loss and the extent to which early intervention services have been provided.

Comprehension Level

The *comprehension level*—that is, the comprehension of sound and its meaning—is the ultimate goal of the hierarchical process. Complete comprehension of speech and environmental sounds, in all settings, requires many skills in the areas of listening, language, and learning over a lifetime of experiences. It is the

springboard for spelling, reading, comprehension and writing skills as well as the overall ability to efficiently and effectively communicate in one's everyday environment. In the presence of hearing loss, individuals will certainly struggle with each of these skills without the appropriate diagnosis, instrumentation, and interventions, thus calling for an interdisciplinary team of individuals working with a child with hearing loss.

Other Codeveloping Skills

In conjunction with the hierarchical process, there are other skills that play an important role in the development of higher order listening abilities. *Auditory memory* for later recall is an essential ingredient for an individual to master the overall perception of speech. Another fundamental component of successful speech perception is *auditory attention,* or the intentional ability to focus specifically on the person speaking. *Auditory closure* is yet another necessary skill; it can be defined as the ability to fill in a missing or misspoken part of a word or message.

The hierarchy of listening skills and skill areas related to listening envelop a child's listening learning environment throughout childhood. However, an important issue to be aware of in the development of these skills is that instead of being mastered in the "nice and neat" sequential hierarchy frequently used to describe them, these skills do, in fact, overlap. For example, a child may be mostly at one level yet be able to perform some tasks at the next higher level. This "messiness" occurs because the child is constantly being bombarded with all manners of sound (e.g., speech, environmental) simultaneously. In essence, all speech, whether simple or complex (in addition to environmental sound), is thrown at the child at the same time, and all of the skills are targeted at the same time as well. It would be unreasonable to expect a child to acquire these skills in an orderly, sequential way when the information is being presented in a natural, somewhat random fashion. This interweaving may explain why a child can show abilities at one level while not having completely mastered the level below it. For example, the child may begin to exhibit "discrimination" of simple words, even though they have not fully mastered the "detection" of some types of sound.

Another important issue is the fact that the "natural, somewhat random" language environment to which the child is exposed is not the only way the child can learn the auditory skills necessary for the development of language. A structured approach to enhance language learning may also be employed; in fact, it may be necessary. The issue of the best way for a child to learn language becomes the subject of discussion when a child is not developing speech and language in a normal fashion, for whatever reason, and intervention of some sort is clearly in order.

▶ Hearing Loss

Hearing loss interferes with the foundation necessary for normal speech and language development. It is, therefore, important to understand the types of hearing loss and how hearing loss will impact the development of spoken language skills. With a basic understanding of the anatomy and physiology of the hearing mechanism and how auditory skills develop, we can now discuss the most common types of hearing loss and how each will impact the foundations of language development in children. This section identifies the various types of hearing loss that result from abnormalities in the auditory system, along with some of their more common etiologies and characteristics. The three types of hearing loss are distinguished as follows:

- A *conductive hearing loss* is associated with damage in the outer and/or middle ear.
- A *sensorineural hearing loss* is associated with damage to the inner ear and/or auditory nerve.
- A *mixed hearing loss* is when both a conductive hearing loss and a sensorineural hearing loss are present at the same time.

In many cases, hearing loss occurs in both ears. However, a *unilateral hearing loss* is when one ear has normal hearing and one ear has impaired hearing; the loss in such cases may be conductive, sensorineural, or mixed in nature. In other cases, hearing loss can be asymmetrical. However, for the purpose of this text, we will restrict discussion to the primary types listed previously.

Types of Hearing Loss
Conductive Hearing Loss

When sound is not efficiently conducted through the outer and/or middle ear (i.e., the conductive mechanism), it results in a conductive hearing loss. Examples of conditions that can create a *conductive hearing loss* include a blockage of wax in the outer ear canal, an infection or foreign body in the ear canal, a perforated eardrum, or the all-too-common ear infection. In fact, anything that blocks or stops sound from being effectively transmitted through the outer and/or middle ear will cause a conductive hearing loss.

Conductive hearing loss is usually characterized by a decrease in the loudness of sound (slight, mild, or moderate in degree), but the clarity of speech often remains intact. That is, there is typically no distortion of sound (a characteristic often seen in other types of hearing loss). Conductive hearing loss is often medically and/or surgically treatable. By far, the most common etiology for conductive hearing loss in children is ear infection, also known as *otitis media.*

Otitis media is the nemesis of audiologists and speech-language pathologists alike, not to mention parents, childcare providers, and pediatric healthcare professionals. By the age of 6, nearly all children will have had at least one episode of otitis media, and perhaps as many as two-thirds of children will have had recurring episodes.

The identification of otitis media in the preschool setting is mitigated by the fact that a significant percentage (perhaps one-third, or even more) of otitis media will be asymptomatic. In a study of 302 children younger than 4 years of age, 40% of the children with acute otitis media never complained of, or had symptoms of, an earache. Fever was not present in 31%, and sleep was not disturbed in half of the children with acute otitis media (Pichichero, 2000). Although the specific numbers vary from source to source, recent studies (Ferlito, Paparella, Rinaldo, Schachern, & Cureoglu, 2003; Yildirim-Baylan et al., 2014) continue to demonstrate and discuss the "silent ear infection." The important message here is that if there is no pain, no fever, and no symptoms, there is no cause for a parent to be concerned regarding the child's well-being, and medical follow-up is not pursued. If the child is not verbally sophisticated enough to self-report a change in hearing status (as is frequently the case with young children), the condition will go undetected. To complicate things further, the hearing loss that results from otitis media fluctuates in severity. This ever-changing hearing loss leads to inconsistent responses and behaviors on part of the child; one day, the child may be very responsive, but the next day, they may be quite unresponsive. It is no surprise, then, that otitis media is a major cause of hearing loss and language delay in the preschool population (Roberts & Hunter, 2002; Roberts, Rosenfeld, & Zeisel, 2004; Winskel, 2006).

Sensorineural Hearing Loss

A *sensorineural hearing loss* occurs when damage to a structure within the inner ear and/or auditory nerve pathway (the sensorineural pathway) prevents the transmission of sound to the brain. Such a hearing loss may be the result of an almost unlimited number of causes, such as genetic, prenatal, and postnatal syndromes; diseases; and disorders. Unlike conductive hearing losses, which can respond to medical interventions, sensorineural hearing losses are typically permanent.

According to the American Speech-Language-Hearing Association (ASHA) (2007), genetic (heredity) factors are believed to account for more than half of all cases of sensorineural hearing loss in children. Congenital (present at birth) causes that are common in children include prenatal infection (e.g., rubella or cytomegalovirus), prematurity, anoxia, and Rh-factor complications. The "acquired" category includes etiologies such as meningitis, measles, and mumps, among others.

Sensorineural hearing loss, unlike conductive hearing loss, impairs both loudness (severity ranging from slight to profound in degree) and clarity. It is the aspect of clarity in sensorineural hearing loss that becomes a significant variable in the successful use of amplification and therapeutic outcomes. In many cases of sensorineural hearing loss, there is a distortion of speech that varies not only from one person to the next, but also from one day to the next in the same person. Furthermore, the severity of the loss is not necessarily an indication of what the clarity of the speech signal is likely to be; that is, those with lesser degrees of hearing loss are not necessarily those facing minimal speech understanding problems, and vice versa. The loss of clarity makes the fitting of a hearing aid in some cases a challenging task. Hearing aids amplify sound, making it louder, but they do not necessarily make sounds clearer in an impaired auditory system. Newer hearing aid technologies have made great strides in increasing an individual's ability to understand speech, but the problem as a whole remains. The addition of background noise and/or reverberation, amplified through a hearing aid can also present a listening challenge. This scenario is often present in the average classroom and can present even greater challenges to listening and understanding for the hard-of-hearing child under these circumstances (Anderson & Goldstein, 2004; George, Goverts, Festen, & Houtgast, 2010).

Mixed Hearing Loss

A mixed hearing loss exists when there is simultaneous damage to both the conductive and sensorineural mechanisms. An example of this type of hearing loss is a child who has a sensorineural hearing loss and gets an ear infection. The sensorineural hearing loss *plus* the conductive hearing loss (from the ear infection) *equals* a mixed hearing loss. When we consider the numerous conditions that may result in a conductive or sensorineural hearing loss, we begin to realize the nearly limitless possible combinations of conditions that can create a mixed hearing loss. In light of the almost unlimited supply of etiologies of mixed hearing loss, presenting a discussion of "typical" etiologies and "classic" characteristics becomes nothing less than a daunting task and exceeds the scope of this text.

Unilateral Hearing Loss

A unilateral hearing loss (UHL) is simply a hearing loss that affects one ear only. It may be the result of conductive, sensorineural, or mixed pathologies. The more severe the loss, the more difficulty the child is likely to have. However, the precise outcome depends on other factors as well.

Several characteristic areas of concern arise for an individual with a UHL, including difficulty in the localization of a sound source, which may be the cause for safety concerns for the young child (Augustine, Chrysolyte, Thenmozhi, Rupa, & 2013) and difficulty in hearing and/or understanding if the speaker is facing an impaired ear. The factor that will likely be most damaging for all areas of learning and development is a background filled with noise or reverberant (echoic) conditions (Anderson, 2004; Reeder, Cadieux, & Firszt, 2015). Thus, a child with a UHL may perform as well as a normal-hearing child or as poorly as a severely impaired child depending on the particular conditions and circumstances (Lewis et al., 2016).

Asymmetrical Hearing Loss

As with the case of mixed hearing loss, *asymmetrical hearing loss* can also result from an innumerable combination of disorders involving both the conductive and sensory mechanisms of the ear, the result of a great number of etiological combinations and varying degrees. When the right and left ears differ in degree and (sometime) type of hearing loss, even amplification options become quite elaborate. Interventions can be very complex and planning for such cases should involve a number of individuals from both the medical and educational communities.

▶ Interventions for Hearing Loss

Given that the vast majority of all knowledge and learning (perhaps as much as 90%) occurs incidentally, applying the appropriate intervention for hearing loss becomes imperative. This section considers hearing aids, cochlear implants, hearing assistance technology, and aural rehabilitation. While interventions for hearing loss, hearing assistance technology, and the like are the subjects themselves of textbooks, what follows is merely a brief and general overview of this topic.

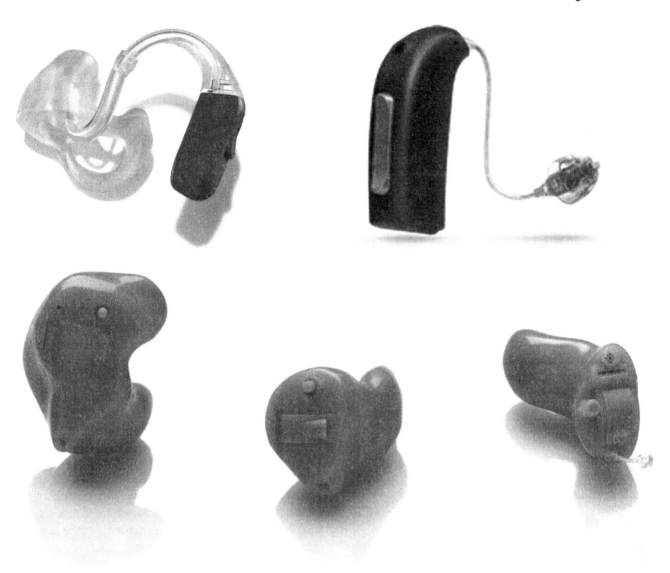

FIGURE 3-6 Hearing aids. **(a)** "Behind the ear" model with earmold. **(b)** "Behind the ear" model with RITE. **(c)** "In the ear" model. **(d)** "In the canal" model. **(e)** "Completely in the canal" model.

Source: Courtesy of Sonic Innovations Inc.

Hearing Aids

A hearing aid is a device that provides acoustic amplification to an individual with hearing loss. It consists of a microphone, amplifier, battery source, and a receiver housed in a small case. The device can be connected to a custom-made portion called an earmold, which channels the amplified sound into the ear canal, or be completely housed in a custom case that fits into the conch a portion of the outer ear or completely in the ear canal. (**FIGURE 3-6a**).The primary hearing aid style used in the pediatric population is the "behind-the-ear" (BTE)-style hearing aid (Figure 3-6a). With the BTE-style hearing aid, when the child has a growth spurt, only the custom earmold portion needs to be remade. Newer technology removes the receiver from the electrical components of the hearing aid itself and places it in a dome that fits into the ear canal.

(**FIGURE 3-6b**) This dome is not custom-made for the individual but rather comes in a number of standard sizes that can accommodate most ears. Other styles of hearing aids are also commercially available, albeit not for the pediatric population. The "in the ear" (ITE) style (**FIGURE 3-6c**) may be used for the older child, perhaps in the pre-teen or teenaged years after the ear itself stops or slows in the growing process, since the custom portion of the device also houses the technical portion. Such hearing aids may be more cosmetically appealing to those in this age group as well. "In the canal" (ITC) hearing aids (**FIGURE 3-6d**) and "completely in the canal" (CIC) hearing aids (**FIGURE 3-6e**) are rarely used for children due to expense and size. It is safe to say that the smaller the hearing aid, the larger the price tag. In children, the smaller the object, the easier it is to lose.

Regardless of style, the basic components of a hearing aid remain the same. The amount of power and other electro-acoustic requirements are based on the hearing loss and are determined by the audiologist for each child individually.

A question that is commonly asked about hearing aids is "Which is better—getting one hearing aid or two?" The answer to this question is not a simple one. The issue of one versus two hearing aids has very little, if anything, to do with the degree of hearing loss (e.g., mild versus severe). Instead, having two hearing aids is the preferred choice whenever possible and regardless of the degree of loss because two hearing aids allow for balanced or stereo listening. This skill is crucial in being able to understand speech in noisy settings. However, there are also many reasons why using two hearing aids might not be advisable (e.g., the existence of physical anomalies or medical pathology). This decision will be made by the audiologist on a case-by-case basis.

The primary goal in selecting the most appropriate and effective intervention technique is always to maximize the auditory input that the child receives. Remember, the vast majority of learning occurs incidentally. Unfortunately, some children receive either no benefit or very minimal benefit from hearing aids, even with the most powerful devices. For these children, cochlear implantation might be a consideration.

Cochlear Implants

Cochlear implant technology was inspired by the desire to help those severely and profoundly hard-of-hearing individuals who were unable to obtain any substantial benefit from conventional hearing aids. Research on cochlear implants began approximately 50 years ago (in adults). The devices did not receive Food and Drug Administration (FDA) approval in the United States for children 2 years of age until 1990 and for children 12 months of age until 2002.

A cochlear implant differs from a hearing aid in that it is not simply another form of acoustic amplification. Rather, this device involves surgically implanting electrodes within the cochlea that in turn provide the sensation of sound by electrically stimulating the auditory nerve.

The cochlear implant contains an external microphone that may look like a BTE hearing aid or a small off-the-ear device that magnetically connects to the internal portion of the implant just above the back of the pinna. This microphone of the cochlear implant collects acoustic energy from the environment (**FIGURE 3-7**). The speech processor portion of the cochlear implant then analyzes the sound and converts it into a digital sound signal, which in turn is sent to the

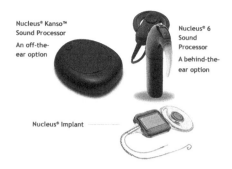

FIGURE 3-7 Cochlear implants. Cochlear implant components. Clockwise from top left: Nucleus Kanso off the ear sound processor, Nucleus 6 behind the ear sound processor, and Nucleus (internal) implant.
© 2018 Cochlear Ltd.

transmitter. Internally, the implant includes a receiver/stimulator and an electrode array. The sound is sent from the transmitter to the receiver, where the sound is converted into an electric impulse. This impulse is transmitted to the electrode array, which then stimulates the auditory nerve.

Cochlear implant candidacy guidelines have changed along with improvements in device technology, and this has resulted in individuals (adults as well as children) with lesser degrees of hearing loss being eligible candidates, while previously their degree of hearing loss made them ineligible for implantation. In addition to having specified audiologic test results, a child must meet other requirements to be considered a candidate for a cochlear implant. Some of these include (but are not limited to) having a functional auditory nerve; having no medical contraindications; having a family with realistic expectations; being willing to work closely with the audiologist, speech-language pathologist, physician, and other professionals; and meeting a stringent auditory-verbal therapy regimen following implantation.

After all of the necessary assessments have been completed, the candidacy approved, and the implantation surgery performed, the process of (re)habilitation for the child can begin. (Re)habilitation starts 3–4 weeks post-surgery, when the child is fit with the microphone and processor, the unit is activated, and programming the implant begins for the individual child. The programming of the unit (referred to as mapping) is an ongoing process because adjustments and reprogramming are frequently necessary, particularly with young children. Simultaneously with the ongoing mapping of the cochlear implant device, the child will undergo speech-language therapy, auditory (skills) training, counseling, and other interventions. Clearly, there is an extensive amount and variety of intervention with children who receive cochlear implants.

Hearing Assistance Technology

One of the most important facts to understand about hearing aids and/or cochlear implants is that they are not a panacea for all hearing problems. They do not restore hearing to "normal," and in some cases, other technology must be employed in order to help an individual with hearing loss navigate their auditory environment. For example, classroom settings (and other poor acoustic environments) are especially problematic for children with a hearing loss due to the presence of background noise and/or *reverberation* (sound bouncing off of hard surfaces, creating an echo-like effect that is then amplified through the device, causing a smearing of sound). In fact, these problems with classroom acoustics may be difficult for normal-hearing children as well. In these cases, devices known as hearing assistance technology (HAT) can be used. An auditory training device can connect to the individual's personal amplification and link wirelessly to a microphone worn by the primary speaker. In essence, this technology allows the teacher's voice to be directly sent to the child's ears, as if they were speaking 6–8 inches away from the child, regardless of where the teacher may be in the classroom. Technologically, this minimizes background noise and the deleterious effects of reverberation for a child with hearing aids or cochlear implants in the typical classroom setting. Similarly, assistive listening devices also equip a teacher with a microphone to amplify his/her voice. However, rather than transmitting to a hearing aid or a cochlear implant, the resulting signal is transmitted to a speaker or similar device that is placed strategically in the classroom. These devices, known as classroom audio distribution systems (CADS), are similar to "surround sound" and are typically used for lesser degrees of hearing loss or to address auditory attention issues within the educational setting.

There is also a wide variety of hearing assistance technology commercially available to assist deaf and hard-of-hearing individuals with daily acoustic events in their personal environments. These may include, but are not limited to, doorbell lights, baby cry alarms, accessibility options for smartphones, fire alarms, and the like. Interested individuals need not look farther than the Internet for resources regarding the most up-to-date technologies.

Aural (Re)habilitation

As we discuss the role that normal hearing has on the development of speech and language skills and the impact a hearing loss will have on the acquisition of normal skills, the purpose of aural (re)habilitation cannot be overlooked. While 21st-century technology provides deaf and hard-of-hearing individuals with the opportunity to optimize their residual hearing, it cannot be done without appropriate professional intervention. A comprehensive aural rehabilitation plan must be put into place any time a child is identified with hearing loss. This plan will involve interprofessional collaboration among the audiologist, speech-language pathologist, educators, and medical professionals, and it should consider each of the following areas for inclusion, which is based, in part, on the preferred practice patterns outlined by ASHA (2006):

- Ongoing audiologic evaluations to monitor the child's hearing status
- Selection, fitting, and ongoing monitoring of and follow-up with the appropriate device (i.e., hearing aids, cochlear implant, HATs, and the like) with consideration for the child's functional ability while using it in different settings
- Parental education about the child's hearing loss; the care, use, and maintenance of the selected device; and educational choices for the child
- Parental counseling regarding the ramifications of the auditory, speech-language, and cognitive effects of the hearing loss on the child and the social-emotional effects on the child *and* other family members
- Referral to the local board of education for child study team (educational) evaluation and determination of the appropriate preschool or educational setting (if appropriate)
- Referral to and ongoing communication with a speech-language pathologist for evaluation and intervention
- Referral to and ongoing communication with other professionals as necessary
- Planning and implementation of an auditory training program to assist the development of essential listening skills (i.e., the developmental skill levels of detection, discrimination, identification, and comprehension)
- Consideration of additional ancillary services as necessary and appropriate

Training for the development of auditory listening skills is an essential element of the aural rehabilitation program. Hard of hearing children will move through the same stages of detection, discrimination, identification, and comprehension observed in normal-hearing children, but they typically need more assistance and perhaps more time to accomplish this development.

▶ Case Studies

🔍 CASE STUDY: JOHNATHON (TD)

Johnathon, a 25-month-old boy, is an example of a typically developing child. In terms of his auditory maturational level, Johnathan's responses to environmental sounds, his name, and attention to verbal requests demonstrate sound encoding and selective listening, as evidenced by his interpretation of the incoming sound and gleaning meaning from the ongoing speech.

Johnathon's development of auditory skill levels and his tendency to develop them in an overlapping manner—an approach typical of a normal-hearing child in a naturalistic environment—are also apparent. This child demonstrates evidence of (age-appropriate) detection, discrimination, identification, and even comprehension of linguistic and nonlinguistic sound, each in varying degrees (as is expected in a normally developing child). Specifically, Johnathon's report notes that his receptive and expressive language skills were demonstrated to be "most typical of a 21- to 24-month-old toddler, with a scatter of skills up to 24- to 27-month age levels."

In conclusion, Johnathon appears to be a classic example of a child developing normal speech, language, and hearing skills. Based on his overall level of achievement and lack of significant history for recurring ear infections, there would be no audiologic or auditory recommendations for this child.

🔍 CASE STUDY: JOSEPHINE (LB)

Josephine is a 22-month-old girl who has been found to have a mild to moderate delay in expressive language development and a moderate delay in speech sound development. Significantly, she has a history of two known episodes of ear infections. Given that approximately one-third (or more) of all cases of otitis media are asymptomatic, it is quite likely that this child has actually had more than two episodes of ear infection or that the episodes were longer in duration than identified by a caregiver or physician.

Josephine's expressive language development, not surprisingly, is significantly delayed, as is her speech sound (phonological) development—also not a surprising finding in light of her history. Remember that the vast majority of learning occurs incidentally; if Josephine's input is inconsistent, her output will be inconsistent as well. Phonological development, vocabulary, and discourse are some of the areas that have been observed to be adversely affected by episodes of otitis media. It appears that Josephine's current level of functioning is in agreement with what has been observed in children who have a history of ear infections.

In terms of Josephine's auditory behavior and skills development, her nonverbal and receptive language skills demonstrate that she has an understanding of encoding, is developing selective listening, and has reached age-appropriate levels in terms of detection, discrimination, identification, and comprehension. Given her prelinguistic skills, strong play and receptive abilities, and the fact that her recent hearing evaluation was within normal limits, her prognosis for overcoming this delay with early intervention is quite good.

🔍 CASE STUDY: ROBERT (LT)

Robert, a 27-month-old developmentally delayed child, has been enrolled in an early intervention program and is receiving physical, occupational, and speech-language therapies. An additional part of his history that is of great significance is a left unilateral hearing loss. This type of impairment puts Robert at risk of further delays in auditory, language, cognitive, and academic development. To have a better assessment of the impact that this hearing loss has already had and may potentially continue to have on his overall development, an audiologic reevaluation must be performed as soon as possible to determine the severity of the hearing loss in the left ear. Additionally, audiologic evaluations must be routinely in place in order to monitor the possibility of progression.

Robert's receptive and expressive language abilities are both delayed and are reported to be most typical of a 9- to 12-month-old child. Likewise, his nonverbal communication is judged to be typical of a 9- to 12-month-old child. While it seems highly unlikely that this delayed development is solely (or in major part) related to a unilateral hearing loss of any degree, its presence, coupled with Robert's already delayed development, might possibly have a synergistic effect. In other words, the resulting deficits that he may experience will very likely be greater than the deficits from a UHL alone or a speech/language delay alone.

Robert's hearing sensitivity and auditory level of functioning must be assessed and regularly monitored, and a program of aural/auditory rehabilitation needs to be carefully planned. Further, Robert may be a candidate for some form of hearing assistance technology (e.g., an assistive listening device); this issue needs to be assessed during the rehabilitation planning process.

Summary

The ability to hear and understand an acoustic signal is the precursor to our ability as humans to develop speech and language skills. It is only when we understand this continuum that we can understand the impact a hearing loss will have on normal speech and language development. Damage to the conductive and/or sensorineural hearing mechanisms can occur at any time, from conception through birth and beyond. While 21st-century technology gives us the ability to maximize an individual's residual hearing, assistive technology provides further assistance when personal devices are not enough to overcome hostile listening environments. Understanding the role that the speech language pathologist has in the process of (re)habilitation is paramount for a child with hearing loss in order to meet therapeutic success and become an effective communicator.

Study Questions

- List and briefly describe both acoustic and nonacoustic functions of the outer ear.
- Describe the middle ear transfer function and state why it is important to the process of hearing.
- List and briefly describe each of the areas in the hierarchy of auditory skill levels presented in this chapter.
- Identify and define the categories of hearing loss described in this chapter.
- Briefly describe some of the typical characteristics of someone with a conductive hearing loss.
- Briefly describe some of the typical characteristics of someone with a sensorineural hearing loss.
- Identify and describe the different styles of hearing aids. How are they the same and how are they different? Which style would be more appropriate for children under the age of 3 years, and why? Which might be appropriate for a child of secondary school age, and why?
- What is hearing assistance technology (HAT) and what does it accomplish for the hard-of-hearing child in a classroom? What can it accomplish for a normal hearing child in a classroom?

References

American Speech-Language-Hearing Association (ASHA). (2006). Preferred practice patterns for the profession of audiology. Retrieved from www.asha.org/policy

American Speech-Language-Hearing Association (ASHA). (2007). JCIH year 2007 position statement: Principles and guidelines for early hearing detection and intervention programs [position statement]. Retrieved from www.asha.org/docs/html/PS2007-00281.html

Anderson, K. L., & Goldstein, H. (2004). Speech perception benefits of FM and infrared devices to children with hearing aids in a typical classroom. *Language, Speech and Hearing in the Schools, 35*, 169–184.

Augustine, A. M., Chrysolyte, S. B, Thenmozhi, K., & Rupa, V. (2013). Assessment of auditory and psychosocial handicap associated with unilateral hearing loss in Indian patients. *Indian Journal of Otolaryngology Head Neck Surgery, 65*(2), 120–125.

Bistrop, M. L., Haines, M., Hygge, S., MacKenzie, D. J., Neyen, S., & Petersen, C. M. (2002). *Children and noise: Prevention of adverse effects.* Denmark, Copenhagen: National Institute of Public Health, Denmark. Retrieved from www.si-folkesundhed.dk/upload/noiseprevention.pdf

Cole, E. B., & Flexer, C. (2011). *Children with hearing loss: Developing listening and talking* (2nd ed.). San Diego, CA: Plural.

Ferlito, A., Paparella, M., Rinaldo, A., Schachern, A., & Cureoglu, S. (2003). The entity known as chronic silent (subclinical) otitis media: A common lesion and a forgotten diagnosis. *Acta Otolaryngologica, 123*, 749–751.

George, E. L. J., Goverts, S. T., Festen, J. M., & Houtgast, T. (2010). Measuring the effects of reverberation and noise on sentence intelligibility for hearing-impaired listener. *Journal of Speech, Language and Hearing Research, 53*, 29–39.

Holst, M., Eswaran, H., Lowery, C., Murphy, P., Norton, J., & Preissl, H. (2005). Development of auditory evoked fields in human fetuses and newborns: A longitudinal MEG study. *Clinical Neurophysiology, 116*(8), 1949–1955.

Kisilevsky, B. S., Hains, S. M. J., Jacquet, A. Y., Granier-Deferre, C., & Lecanuet, J. P. (2004). Maturation of fetal responses to music. *Developmental Science, 7*(5), 550–559.

Lewis, D., Schmid, K., O'Leary, S., Spalding, J., Heinrichs-Graham, E., & High, R. (2016). Effects of noise on speech recognition and listening effort in children with normal hearing and children with mild bilateral or unilateral hearing loss. *Journal of Speech-Language-Hearing Research, 59*, 1218–1232.

McMahon, E., Wintermark, P., & Lahav, A. (2012). Auditory brain development in premature infants: The importance of early experience. *Annals of the New York Academy of Sciences, 1252*, 17–24.

McMullen, E., & Saffran, J. (2004). Music and language: A developmental comparison. *Music Perception, 21*(3), 289–311.

Musiek, F. E., & Baran, J. A. (2007). *The auditory system: Anatomy, physiology, and clinical correlates.* Boston, MA: Pearson Education.

Oller, D. K. (1986). Metaphonology and infant vocalizations. In B. Linkblom & R. Zetterstrom (Eds.), *Precursors of early speech* (pp. 21–35). New York, NY: Stockton Press.

Owens, R. E. (2012). *Language Development: An introduction* (8th ed.). Needham Heights, MA: Allyn and Bacon.

Perigoe, C., & Paterson, M. (2018). Understanding auditory development and the child with hearing loss. In D. R. Welling, & C. A. Ukstins (Eds.), *Fundamentals of audiology for the speech-language pathologist* (2nd ed.). Baltimore, MD: Jones & Bartlett Learning.

Pichichero, M. E. (2000). Acute otitis media: Part 1. Improving diagnostic accuracy. *American Family Physician, 61*(7), 2051–2056.

Putkinen, V., Tervaniemi, M., Saarikivi, K., Ojala, P., & Houtilainen, M. (2014). Enhanced development of auditory change detection in musically trained school-aged children: A longitudinal event-related potential study. *Developmental Science, 17*(2), 282–297.

Reeder, R. M., Cadieuz, J., & Firszt, J. B. (2015). Quantification of speech-in-noise and localization ability in children with unilateral hearing loss and comparison to normal hearing peers. *Audiology and Neurology, 20*(suppl 1), 31–37.

Roberts, J., & Hunter, L. (2002, October 8). Otitis media and children's language and learning. *The ASHA Leader*. Retrieved from http://www.asha.org/Publications/leader/2002/021008/f021008.htm

Roberts, J. E., Rosenfeld, R. M., & Zeisel, S. A. (2004). Otitis media and speech and language: A meta-analysis of prospective studies. *Pediatrics, 113*, e238–e248.

Therres, M. (2015, October). Auditory development series: Auditory development hierarchy. *AudiologyOnline*, Article 15458. Retrieved from http://www.audiologyonline.com

Tye-Murray, N. (2004). *Foundations of aural rehabilitation: Children, adults, and their family members* (2nd ed.). Clifton, NJ: Delmar Learning.

Werner, L. (2003). Prenatal auditory stimuli: Truth, fiction or moot point? *Hearing Health, 19*, 2. Retrieved from http://drf.org/hearing_health/archive/2003/sum03_prenatalaudi_ex.htm

Werner, L. (2007a). Issues in human auditory development. *Journal of Communication Disorders, 40*, 275–283.

Werner, L. (2007b). What do children hear? How auditory maturation affects speech perception. *The ASHA Leader, 12*, 6–7, 32–33.

Winskel, H. (2006). The effects of an early history of otitis media on children's language and literacy skill development. *British Journal of Educational Psychology, 76*, 727–744.

Yildirim-Baylan, M., Schachern, P., Tsuprun, V., Shiabata, D., Paparella, M., & Cureoglu, S. (2014). The pathology of silent otitis media: A predecessor to tympanogenic meningitis in infants. *International Journal of Pediatric Otorhinolaryngology, 78*(2014), 451–454.

Yost, W. A. (2007). *Fundamentals of hearing: An introduction* (5th ed.). San Diego, CA: Elsevier.

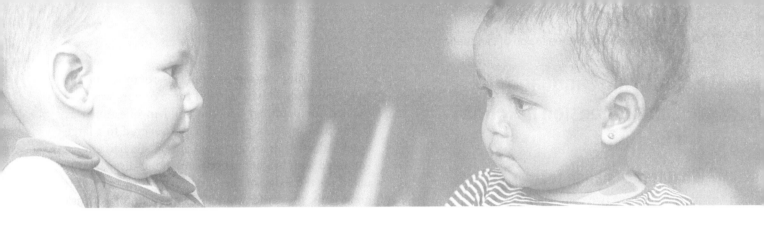

CHAPTER 4

Comprehension of Language

Amy L. Weiss, PhD, CCC-SLP

OBJECTIVES

- Identify developmental principles of children's language comprehension and list several developmental milestones
- Explain why the comprehension competencies of young children are more difficult to measure than their expressive language competencies and provide several solutions for this problem
- Become familiar with several techniques for standardized assessment of language comprehension

KEY TERMS

Assessment   Development
Comprehension   Language

▶ Introduction

A careful perusal of the available textbooks focusing on the scope of children's language development yields much less information about language comprehension than language production. This omission is surprising because language comprehension represents one of the two major processes of language acquisition that young children are learning (Miller & Paul, 1995). The dearth of information in this area may stem from the inherent difficulty of studying language comprehension rather than because the topic is viewed as a trivial matter.

This chapter explores several principles that appear to hold true for children's development of language comprehension, describes what we know about the specific developmental milestones achieved by children during the preschool years, and introduces several different methods for evaluating that development. Several suggestions about how to best incorporate this information into clinical work are also provided.

► Studying Language Comprehension in Young Children

What Is the Challenge?

There are at least two compelling reasons for clinicians and researchers to carefully study and consider the development of young children's language comprehension. The first has to do with the important role that language comprehension plays in young children's understanding of their world, including how it works and how to participate in its workings. The second has to do with the difficulties inherent in accurately evaluating language comprehension. Unlike the study of expressive syntax, phonology, morphology, and sometimes pragmatics, comprehension is not right "out there," but rather has to be inferred from the context (both linguistic and nonlinguistic) as well as the linguistic units provided. Therein resides a daily challenge for both clinicians and family members with young children who are developing language: how do we accurately evaluate children's language comprehension?

Because the evaluation of comprehension is largely inferred from children's nonverbal responses to tasks often conveyed verbally, it is relatively easy to overestimate their language comprehension competencies. Language comprehension competencies are also easy to overestimate because young children who are developing language tend to make guesses about the language they hear around them that they cannot fully understand. Sometimes, these guesses are correct or appear correct; as a consequence, we give credit for a correct response based on what was actually the result of a child's incorrect or incomplete decoding process. For speech-language pathologists, these errors can be useful because we often derive the most insight about language learning by analyzing the mistakes that young children make in their attempts to understand.

An Example

To illustrate how mistakes can yield important information, consider this example of a 5-year-old with age-appropriate language abilities who revealed where the limits of her language understanding were. Notice how important nonverbal context is in this case for interpreting what is going on comprehension-wise. Careful consideration of nonverbal or nonlinguistic context is a crucial clinical tool that we should routinely apply.

The setting was a preschool classroom with multiple centers of activity. One of these centers was designated for painting, and the child in question was busily painting on a piece of paper secured to a large easel. Adorned in an oversized apron, she had a juice can filled with bright orange paint at her disposal, situated on the ledge of the easel in front of her. With great care, the child would dip her paintbrush into the can and, without much dripping, stroke the brush across the paper. She appeared to be more engrossed in the brush and paint process than in creating anything recognizable. Absorbed in her work, the child did not even look up when one of the undergraduate students who volunteered in the classroom walked by the easel. Seeing the child's painting efforts, the student said, "Modern art, huh?" To this comment (and without making eye content with the speaker), the child replied, "Yeah. Orange."

I frequently use this example with my students to gauge their insights into language learning and especially comprehension. This vignette provides a nice illustration of a preschool-age child who understands her role in a conversation, although she does not understand the specific allusion the speaker has made to modern art. In a pragmatic sense, the child has recognized that a door was opened for her to respond (i.e., a tag question, "Huh?," includes a request for a response, thus relating both syntax and semantics as well as pragmatic competencies), and the response she provided had something to do with her painting (i.e., she provided the color of her paint). Clearly, though, this 5-year-old was not able to relate to the more abstract meaning of the student's comment. When evaluating the child's response, you should give her credit for understanding that she has been asked to comment on the statement made by the older, more competent speaker (pragmatics), but acknowledge that her conceptual development has not yet extended to understanding different genres of art (lexical/ semantics) or recognizing that the student was probably being just a little bit sarcastic and has actually made a rhetorical comment that needs no response (pragmatics).

Rather than view the older participant's comment as a disingenuous attempt at communication, I look at it as fortuitous as a clinician. It provided me with an opportunity to achieve some insight into this young child's ability to understand the words spoken, the world around her, and her role in the communication process. We do not expect a 5-year old to understand the abstract term *modern art* or recognize a rhetorical comment when she hears one; thus, her response does not raise any developmental concerns about the young artist's comprehension competencies based on this particular interaction. Nevertheless, analysis of the vignette does provide us with some insight into how context—in this case, the use of orange paint and painting—influenced the manner in which the child revealed her level of comprehension for the language used in this adult-child conversation.

Another important point is brought to light through analysis of this brief interaction. Note how different components of language work together in the child's attempt to make sense of the language input: The child's pragmatics, semantics, and syntax knowledge are all being called upon to resolve the matter of language comprehension. This is a commonly observed phenomenon. That is, demonstration of language comprehension involves much more than simply knowing what individual words mean. Language comprehension is much more than receptive vocabulary. Everything the child understands about language in its broadest sense, including pragmatics, semantics, syntax, morphology, and especially phonology, must become part of the processing of language input for an accurate response to result. Just as it is quite artificial to say that we can study the development of syntax without considering semantics and phonology, we cannot fully evaluate a child's language comprehension without considering the rest of the child's breadth of knowledge about the language.

▶ What Is Language Comprehension?

Speech-language pathologists (SLPs), developmental psychologists, linguists, and others involved in studying language development use a number of different terms to refer to the acquisition of language comprehension. Most often, in addition to language comprehension, the terms *receptive language (learning)* or *the understanding of language* may be used. In all cases, the terminology refers to decoding the language input present in the child's environment as opposed to the production of language. Bishop (1997) refers to language comprehension as "a process whereby information is successfully transformed from one kind of representation to another" (p. 2). Skarakis-Doyle and Dempsey (2008) note that "to comprehend is to construct the meaning of a message or text" (p. 1228). Said another way, language comprehension relates to the process of turning a highly complicated set of acoustic signals into a meaningful message.

In this chapter, we consider young children's understanding of a spoken language. To be sure, much can be gained by studying the development of

comprehension when the input is visual rather than spoken, as in American Sign Language, or written, as when we study reading comprehension. With regard to reading comprehension, the relationship between children's development of oral language comprehension and its necessity as a foundation for reading comprehension monitoring is a particularly critical one (Skarakis-Doyle, 2002; Skarakis-Doyle & Dempsey, 2008). Both of these topics, however, are beyond the scope of this chapter.

Understanding the Role of Context

Language comprehension refers to an individual's ability to understand the linguistic information contained in a message, which is almost always augmented by the message's specific nonlinguistic context (e.g., what is going on at the same time, who is speaking, what was previously said, what visual information is available) and by the listener's knowledge of the world (i.e., how the course of typical events as they occur in the world affects the interpretation of this linguistic message). Milosky (1992) provides a comprehensive discussion of the role of world knowledge in facilitating comprehension.

The balance enforced among these information sources is not always predictable. When children are in the process of acquiring language comprehension, the relative contributions of these information sources are determined by where the child is in development. That is, if complete linguistic knowledge is unavailable, more reliance will probably be placed on the nonlinguistic information available and context becomes more critical for understanding. Miller and Paul (1995) list a number of areas of knowledge that are crucial to successful language comprehension, including but not limited to social knowledge and the understanding of intentionality, inferencing, and scriptal knowledge. These authors note, as does Bishop (1997), that the necessity for such a holistic approach to understanding the process of language comprehension likely explains the difficulties computer programs have in making translations between languages. Put simply, translation is more than a word-by-word transformation from one language to another.

The following example demonstrates the interplay between linguistic and nonlinguistic information. Note the role played by nonlinguistic information (context):

Setting: A mother is busy getting ready for work. Her young child, age 18 months, is watching her mother quickly move around the bedroom, lifting up papers and the bed linens, obviously searching for something. The mother repeatedly mutters to herself but loud enough for the child to hear, "My shoes. Where are my shoes?" The child glances down at her own shoes, reaches forward to touch her right shoe, and chortles, "Mine," as she grasps the shoe. The child then looks up to her mother for approval.

Interpretation: The child probably just understands the word "shoes" (although probably not the plural morpheme). A veteran of many turn-taking exchanges that are prompted by being asked, "Where is your X?", this child provides a response relative to herself and not to her mother. Thus the child has incorporated world knowledge into an attempt to understand the situation unfolding around her in the bedroom. The usual course of events from the child's perspective is that "My mother often asks me where my body parts are and where different items of my clothing are, so that is probably what is happening now." Although she is not specifically being asked a question requiring a response, the child has personalized the exchange by referencing her own shoe.

Does this child have complete understanding of her mother's comment and question? No, it is highly unlikely that she could understand all of the nuances of this communication. In the same situation, an adult might respond with the question, "Which pair of shoes are you looking for?" Another possible adult rejoinder could be, "Where did you last see them?" In both instances, an adult would know that to understand the intended message, one would have to recognize that the mother's shoes are at issue, not her own. Additional world knowledge would reveal that when we are in a hurry, we often cannot find the things we need most, and that comments of encouragement, clarification, and assistance are what are needed. In the example, the child demonstrated incomplete knowledge, both linguistic and nonlinguistic, but still provided a turn in the form of a response to the hypothesized "Where?" question. In the absence of complete information, just as in the example of our 5-year-old artist, this young child attempted to use the information that was at her disposal to participate in the communication exchange.

Interactions Between Context and Comprehension of Meaning

Given the close association between linguistic and nonlinguistic information, a confound may potentially arise from the latter information if we believe we are exclusively looking at linguistic comprehension competencies without making special provisions. Clinicians and researchers who are concerned with the confounding of linguistic and nonlinguistic comprehension make sure to eliminate as much nonlinguistic information as possible when testing young children, for example. Asking questions or making requests in a manner where all gestures are eliminated reduces the possibility that nonlinguistic cues have been relied on for comprehension. Similarly, objects that might serve to cue the child are placed out of sight. Another strategy used by some has been to make requests that run counter to real-world expectations so that linguistic information must be relied on. More information about the elimination of nonlinguistic cues will be provided later in this chapter, when we address the measurement of children's language comprehension.

Why do clinicians and caregivers often disagree about young children's language comprehension? The use of, and perhaps reliance on, nonlinguistic information by young children may lead many caregivers to state with certainty that their toddlers understand everything that is said to them. This expression has been a common occurrence in my clinical experience. What leads to caregivers' strong beliefs that their children, at approximately 2 years of age, understand everything said to them? This is an especially important question because comprehension data collected with tasks that carefully control extraneous cuing have shown that children younger than age 2 understand a corpus of single words, some two-word combinations, and possibly an occasional three-word combination—but they certainly do not understand everything said to them (Miller, Chapman, Branston, & Reichle, 1980).

Given that we empirically know that toddlers cannot understand everything said to them, Chapman, Klee, and Miller (1980) sought to determine why caregivers so often report that their 2-year-olds understand everything said to them. They reported the findings of a preliminary investigation focused on this clinical quandary: why do researchers and caregivers disagree in their perception of young children's comprehension abilities? These researchers looked at half-hour videotaped samples collected from young children, ranging in age from approximately 8 to 21 months, who were engaged in play with their mothers. The investigators carefully analyzed all of the instances where the mothers had made either requests for objects (e.g., *Give me the block*) or requests for action (e.g., *Come over here*) and all of the children's responses. The investigators catalogued use of gestures made on the part of the mothers that may have cued the children to the mothers' linguistic message as well as the use of the children's names to get their attention. In addition, Chapman and her colleagues considered the timing of the requests relative to the children's responses.

A summary of the study's findings demonstrated that not only did the mothers frequently use gesture to gain and direct their children's attention, but they also timed their requests to match the production of their children's responses. This timing sequence had the effect of making the children's responses appear to be correct. Because these responses were actually under way before the request was made, Chapman et al. (1980) called these events *pseudo-successes*. This term derives from the decision by the researchers that credit for a successful response could not be given, although the caregivers may have concluded from the interactions they had observed in real time that their children had understood them based on linguistic information alone.

Here is an example of how such an interaction might look. A mother might say, "Give me the cup," when the child is, in fact, already in the act of handing the mother the cup. In another example, the child might turn their gaze to the mother, and the mother almost simultaneously says, "Look at me." In both instances, the mother's requests are made after the child begins the requested action. In the majority of western culture, middle-class mothers have been observed to shape their utterances to create turn-taking conversation frameworks with their young, language-immature children; the mothers in the Chapman et al. (1980) study may have had the same goal. The effect of their timing, however, was to render the children's participation as looking like linguistic comprehension when it was not.

Chapman et al. (1980) concluded that many mothers who have observed this enhanced connection between their own requests for action, requests for objects, and their children's apparent compliance over many instances have assumed this relationship was evidence of their children's genuine language comprehension. We cannot discount the perspective that parents enjoy seeing their young children's compliant behavior and may not question whether the compliance can be attributed to genuine linguistic comprehension or something else. Morford and Goldin-Meadow (1992) reported that the 41 typically developing children they studied who were producing one word at a time all used gesture when producing their words. Similarly, all of their participants understood gesture when it was presented along with a single spoken word or in place of the spoken word.

My own anecdotal observation has been that parents of children with bona fide expressive language

deficits appear to be even more likely to comment on the strength of their children's language understanding. Part of this perception may derive from the *relative* strength of language understanding when compared with language expression for these children. Also, in lieu of age-appropriate language production skills, anything these parents perceive their children to have mastered—in this case, language comprehension—is viewed with great relief! Experience shows that caregivers who are pleased with their children's apparent skill at language comprehension are less than pleased when told that their perspective is not shared by the SLP who has examined language comprehension in a more controlled environment.

How Do We Incorporate This Information into Our Clinical Work?

The findings of the Chapman et al. (1980) study raise two important issues. First, SLPs need to do more than just take parents' opinion of their children's language comprehension as the final word in language comprehension assessment. This need for further study reflects the difficulty we all experience in getting a pure sample of language comprehension behavior and accurately interpreting what we have. This point is not meant to be dismissive of the important role caregivers play in evaluating their children's language. Second, SLPs have to be sure that when assessing language comprehension skills in young children, they provide tasks that are not confounded by nonlinguistic cues that provide children with the opportunity to look more savvy in terms of their linguistic language comprehension than they actually are.

What Do We Know About the Development of Language Comprehension?

A child setting out to understand their first language face an extraordinary task. If you have attempted to learn a second language (or third or fourth) later in life, you probably remember how difficult it was at first to parse the stream of language that assaulted your ears to determine where one sentence ended and another began. Even more difficult was to determine where one word ended and another began. Infants and toddlers encounter many of the same challenges in making sense of language input and learning language: They have to determine where to segment the stream of sounds they hear. After the stream is segmented, the job of making sense of the phonological information is still left to accomplish.

Anecdotes about young children's early attempts to understand language provide an insight into the difficulties inherent in the parsing process that are fairly common. For example, when I was a doctoral student, I sometimes babysat for my professor's young son. As I was tucking him into bed on one of these occasions, I noticed that his sheets and pillowcases were covered with depictions of a famous cartoon dog both dressed in attire and engaging in activities representing different states in the United States. For example, in Hawaii, the cartoon dog was surfing; in Florida, the dog was sunbathing complete with sunglasses. Remembering that my young friend's parents had lived in Florida before moving to Indiana and, in fact, that this child was born in Miami, I mused out loud, "I wonder whether that's Miami", as I pointed to the sunbathing dog. The child's response was immediate: "No, that's Mommy's ami." We may conclude that whenever this youngster heard his mother say, "Miami" he recognized a word he knew inside it, specifically, "my" (a pretty sophisticated observation on its own). Because he recognized a possessive pronoun, he treated it as such and assumed that whatever an "ami" was, it belonged to his mother. Once again, we see that children use what they understand to figure out what they do not.

For similar reasons, we often see children substitute words they have in their vocabulary for unfamiliar words that have some phonological similarity but are not identical. A number of years ago, a friend's young daughter who had recently arrived in the Midwest with her family from an eastern state explained that she had been told in preschool by her teacher that when the sky became dark and a strong wind blew, hiding in the basement from tomatoes was the appropriate next step. When queried about her statement suggesting that tomatoes could fly and be dangerous to one's life and possessions, the child insisted that that was exactly what her teacher had said: tomatoes were the culprit. My interpretation is that the word "tornado" had been used by the teacher. Not having that word in her receptive lexicon, but having one that sounded somewhat like it, the child substituted the recognized word for the new lexical item.

Which Types of Competencies Are Being Developed to Cope with the Acoustic Information of Speech?

For children to effectively use phonological information from the speech stream they hear, they must be able to detect, discriminate, and classify sounds. First, at the most rudimentary level, children must detect the sounds in the speech stream. That is, can they be heard? Second, children must be able to discriminate between sounds in their input so that they recognize when a /b/ versus a /p/ is produced, although the relevance of that discrimination for their first language is not yet understood. Third, and much more central to specific language learning, is the ability to classify sounds into meaningful categories such as the phonemes in a given language (i.e., /b/ and /p/ are phonemes in English because when used as the initial sound in words formed with the template ____ at, there is a meaningful lexical difference).

Bishop (1997, p. 51) refers to a fourth competency, known as "phonological constancy," as being critical to the ability to utilize the speech signal. This last consideration is related to classification—children have to develop a set of boundaries within which sound productions reflect the same intended sound. In essence, because not every /b/ will sound identical to every other /b/ heard, the child has to set parameters that are forgiving enough so that it will be rare that sounds are confused for others or ignored when they carry meaning.

Assistance from the Environment

Most of word learning is probably associative in nature. Thus, children who are developing language in a typical fashion look to nonlinguistic information to help them map meaning to the consistent sound strings they hear. The strategy of relying on nonlinguistic context to map meaning to sound strings is similar to what adults experience when trying to learn a second language. You may have had the experience of being in a situation where you can understand very little of the language spoken by the people around you. I remember grabbing hold of one word I could understand—like a lifesaver—in a stream of words that I largely could not understand and attempting to figure out the rest of the message from that one word.

Not long ago, the following experience happened to me when I was in a Spanish-speaking country. It was lunchtime, so the fact that I had understood the word for "lunch" made sense when I heard it in conversation. Yes, of course, I would like to join a group of acquaintances who were local to the area for lunch. As it turned out, I had actually been asked if I knew which dining room was serving lunch that day; I had not received an invitation from the group to join them. I was embarrassed for sure, but the experience was a helpful one because it reflected a problem not all that dissimilar from that of language-learning children. The more we can appreciate the disadvantages faced by young children learning language in their attempts to understand the language they hear around them, along with the immense resourcefulness they demonstrate in this situation, the better our position for accurately evaluating their comprehension efforts.

Quality of Input and Context: Helping Children "Map" Language

The study of caregivers' speech and language to young children has provided us with evidence that the input young children receive—at least in majority, middle-class households—is not identical in quantity or quality to the input produced in adult-adult conversation. Specifically, adult-infant/toddler speech and language typically includes more repetition, especially of content words (e.g., *apple, hungry*); longer pauses at grammatical junctures; emphasis on content words; more dramatic shifts of prosody and intonation contours; and longer turn-taking transitions than would be found in adult-adult conversation in the same cultural milieu (Fernald & Kuhl, 1987; Shady & Gerken, 1999). It has been speculated that these differences serve to focus a young child's attention on the stream of speech, specifically on those parts that are most relevant to understanding the message communicated by the adult (Fernald et al., 1989).

More recently, with the use of the Language Environment Analysis (LENA) System, Gilkerson et al. (2017) have provided a compelling corpus of data that demonstrated that on average, the opportunities to engage in child-adult interaction and be exposed to adult word input are significantly fewer for children from lower socioeconomic status (SES) households. Although variability within groups was appreciable, these results point to fewer opportunities for many children to be exposed to input that has been custom-made for language learning as well as fewer vocabulary words. Thus, for many children, the advantages of child-directed speech may not be reaching the intended audience.

Many adults also utilize specific gestures to facilitate communication with young children (Bruner, 1978). For example, it is not unusual for a caregiver to accompany use of the word *here* with a gesture that makes it obvious to the young child where *here* is intended to be, as in "Put your cup *here*." The use of the same strategy with another adult could be viewed as insulting by the adult on the receiving end. The implied message in the latter case would be, "I do not believe you can understand me with my words alone."

We assume that the goal of any child learning language is to determine how to connect or map language input to the context or event that is occurring. Consider the following example of an infant's incorporation into a farewell routine. When the grandmother has put on her coat and headed for the door after giving daddy and infant a substantial hug and kiss, and then daddy says to the infant, "Grandma is going home now," the infant has been provided with an opportunity to more easily connect the language to the event than if the language occurred without the context. The more assistance that an adult (or more sophisticated language user) provides to draw the infant's attention to the symmetry between language and context, the more transparent the mapping task will be for the language-learning child. We can call this symmetry *mapping*, meaning the direct connection of language to event or person or object.

Consider this example of facilitation of mapping that occurred when a friend's son was approximately 8-months old. The infant's 6-year-old sister held out his pacifier (referred to in the family as a "passy") so that it was right in front of him, within easy grasp, as she slowly intoned, "Want passy? Want passy, Joe?" It is not clear whether the child's subsequent grab for his "passy" was prompted by the linguistic information or by the presence of the very attractive pacifier in close proximity to his person. The important information may be that the nonlinguistic context—the presence of the pacifier held by his sister within his reach—was coupled with the production of a linguistic message that fit the scenario. Joe was incorporated into a turn-taking set because his sister asked a question and paused, waiting for her brother to reach for the accessible pacifier. Down the road, multiple instances of this or similar linguistic messages paired with symmetrical nonlinguistic contexts may serve to assist a young child in mapping the likely meaning of *passy* and other words.

Can we credit Joe with understanding the words *want* and *passy*, either singly or in combination? The evidence we have would not allow us to conclude that we can or cannot. Our indecision rests on the remarkable use of comprehension strategies by young children who make the most of nonlinguistic information and/or partial linguistic information in the absence of complete linguistic knowledge.

Development and Use of Comprehension Strategies

Chapman (1978; see also Edmonston & Thane, 1992; Miller & Paul, 1995; Paul, 1990) has written extensively about the existence of language comprehension strategies in the normal development of children's understanding of spoken language. Her conceptualization is a helpful one because it incorporates what young children are doing in terms of cognitive development with their use of what Chapman refers to as formulas for getting around a lack of complete information. Young children learning language in a typical fashion will be much more reliant on nonlinguistic or context information than the more linguistically sophisticated, older child.

For the unsophisticated language user, gesture, proximity to the speaker, attention to what the speaker is attending to, and previous situation experience or world knowledge take on extraordinary importance in decoding language input. Young children are focused on the here and now. Whatever is physically present will significantly figure into the child's attempts to understand any linguistic message.

Examples of "Comprehension" When Little Linguistic Knowledge Has Been Acquired

The example of Joe and his pacifier presented earlier could illustrate one of the comprehension strategies described by Chapman (1978): "Act on objects at hand." That is, when an attractive object is placed in front of Joe, he will try to grasp it. It probably does not matter what his sister said. It does not matter that her utterances are an attempt to help him map language onto context. If Joe is physically able and the pacifier is something he wants, in the absence of linguistic knowledge, you could probably say, "Want hedge trimmer?" and Joe would reach for the pacifier anyway. At 8 months of age, asking Joe whether he wants anything that is not physically present would probably be less successful. Given his 8-month-old motor skills, reaching for something he wants is his response to seeing the pacifier because he can.

An example of another early developing comprehension strategy described by Chapman (1978) has likely been observed by most readers of this text. A 9-month-old child is held in her parents' arms and incorporated into a leave-taking routine by the caregiver. The caregiver starts to wave goodbye to a visitor and tells the baby, "Wave bye-bye." Soon after, the baby begins to wave at the departing visitor. The caregiver is convinced that this movement is occurring in response to the request for action, specifically to wave. According to Chapman's taxonomy, however, the baby is much more likely following a comprehension strategy called "imitate ongoing actions." That is, the caregiver is waving and, regardless of what has actually been said, the child begins to wave too. This situation could be considered a case of actions speaking louder than words.

Why does this response occur? The imitation occurs because at the baby's age, imitation of what caregivers do constitutes a frequent activity on the part of many typically developing children. According to Tomasello

(1995), young children learn early on that there is a benefit to attending to what the speaker attends to for mapping clues. The adult waves, the baby notices, and so the baby waves. If you want your baby to look really smart at this age, just keep saying, "Do what I do;" perform actions your toddler can do; and let cognition take its course! The key is to remember that the ensuing activity by the child is not necessarily the result of linguistic comprehension, but rather a response likely to have occurred regardless of what was said.

Here is another example that meshes well with clinical attempts to estimate young children's language comprehension abilities. Two prepositions that emerge and are mastered quite early in children's expressive and receptive repertoires are the morphemes "in" and "on." Both are part of Brown's (1973) set of 14 grammatical morphemes used to chart the development of morphology in preschool-age children. SLPs often attempt to determine whether 2-year-olds can understand these prepositions, but the nonlinguistic context for assessment must be carefully controlled for test results to have any validity. For example, if children are presented with a bucket and asked to "Put the blocks in the bucket," it is very likely that young children, whether or not they understand the linguistic request, will place the blocks into the bucket. Buckets are receptacles: In "doing what you usually do with objects at hand" (Chapman, 1978), you place smaller things inside something with a natural and clearly visible inside. Similarly, if the SLP tells a child to "put the book on the box" (and supplies the child with a closed cardboard box), it is very likely that the child will place the book on top of the box, not underneath it or next to it. The box has a natural top, so even a child who does not understand more than the words *book* and *box* (and may know quite a bit less) will do what is usually done—that is, place one object on top of another where the top is clearly demarcated.

Comprehension Strategy Use Continues into the Linguistic Period

Chapman (1978) follows the use of comprehension strategies through the young child's early vocabulary acquisition and semantic/syntactic development. The process of making best guesses given knowledge of only part of the linguistic message is related to a phenomenon called *bootstrapping*. That is, children learning language tend to use what they already know to extend their understanding into realms of language where their knowledge is sketchy (Owens, 2012).

For example, children quickly become familiar with the high-frequency occurrence of subject-verb-object

(S-V-O; see the following examples) sentence productions. But what happens when they are presented with a less familiar sentence type, such as a passive construction where the subject and object have exchanged locations in the sentence? Consider the following two sentences, the first in the active voice and the second expressed in the passive voice: (1) The *dog* chased the *cat* and (2) The *cat* was chased by the *dog*. If you provide preschool-age children with a toy dog and cat, and ask them to act out these two sentences one at a time, they are likely to indicate that the first noun is the actor and the second noun is the recipient of the action in both sentences. Mature English-language users know that in both cases the actor and the recipient are the same; it is only the grammatical structure that varies between the two sentences.

In this scenario, the child has used a strategy that can be likened to "playing the percentages." If you are a baseball aficionado and understand why left-hand pitchers and not right-hand pitchers are much more often brought out of the bullpen to pitch to left-handed hitters, you will more easily understand this term. Given the high frequency of S-V-O sentences, a child will impose that template on new, unknown grammatical structures such as the passive construction and, most of the time, be incorrect. Thus, in the first sentence, the child correctly understands that the dog (S) chases (V) the cat (O); in the second sentence, the child erroneously assumes that the cat (S) chases (V) the dog (O). A child who relies on application of the S-V-O rule to unknown sentence constructions may be following a *word-order strategy*. Remember that because the child had mastered the template in which the first noun is always the subject and the second noun is the object/patient, passive-voice sentences will be misinterpreted if the word-order strategy is applied.

Another, more sophisticated, example of a comprehension strategy is application of the *order of mention strategy*, which may occur when children are asked to comprehend sentences with multiple clauses. An example of a situation where this comprehension dilemma could occur is when the adverbs *before* and *after* are used. If the child does not understand the adverbs, a mistake may happen. Look at the four sentences that follow and determine which action would occur first and which action would occur second when children are asked to order two pictures according to the information provided by each sentence:

1. "Show me: 'Before he took a bath, he worked on his homework.'"
2. "Show me: 'He took a bath after he worked on his homework.'"
3. "Show me: 'After he took a bath, he worked on his homework.'"
4. "Show me: 'He took a bath before he worked on his homework.'"

Relying on linguistic knowledge only, you would understand that in the first two sentences, homework was worked on before taking a bath. In the final two sentences, the bath was taken before homework was worked on. For the child applying the order of mention strategy, each of the four sentences would be acted out in the same way. Specifically, the bath occurred first and the homework was worked on second because the first clause includes the word *bath* and the second includes *homework*. The adverbs *before* and *after* are inconsequential to a child who has no knowledge of their role in lending meaning to sequenced actions. Therefore, if a child is presented with only statements such as those in examples 3 and 4, "correct" responses would not necessarily mean that the child understood the adverbs.

SLPs must carefully develop probe test items that will determine whether comprehension strategies are being used and whether the child has true linguistic comprehension of the structure in question. More information about the development of nonstandardized probe items is provided later in this chapter.

One final example of comprehension strategies warrants mention because it represents a crucial portion of the information that children bring to the table in attempting to decipher language input. This piece is referred to as *world knowledge*, and the strategy is referred to as the *probable relation of events strategy* by Chapman (1978); see also Miller and Paul (1995). Using the sample sentences given earlier for *before* and *after* comprehension, consider the case of young children who use world knowledge to figure out sentences that are beyond their competence level. When they are less sophisticated in a linguistic sense, younger children use a "do what you usually do" strategy—for example, when given a brush, they brush hair. When they become more sophisticated in the ways of the world, they interpret what they do not know by thinking about what would make the most sense in that situation based on past experience or how the world typically operates for them. For example, if a child lives in a household where the bedtime routine always includes homework first and then a bath, the use of adverbs the child cannot understand will not hinder them from attempting to understand the four sentences. The answer to the question of which activity occurred first would also be "first homework, then a bath" when a probable relation of events strategy was used because that's how the child's world works regardless of adverbs that might dictate otherwise.

CLINICAL APPLICATION EXERCISE

1. As discussed in this chapter, toddlers often rely on what they know about the world around them in terms of relationships between actions and objects and predictable daily routines to make sense of the world around them in the absence of much receptive vocabulary and syntax knowledge. That is, they are highly dependent on context to help them understand when someone engages them in conversation. This substitution of nonlinguistic knowledge for linguistic knowledge sometimes yields what appears to be a correct response or at least a response that is accepted as evidence of linguistic knowledge. It is easy to forget that even as linguistically sophisticated adults, sometimes, we have to rely on context ourselves because linguistic information is denied to us or at least not fully provided. See whether you can set yourself up for a dose of context dependence and experience an analogous situation to the toddler's face. Here are two suggestions:

   a. Pick up a classic work of literature written in the 19th century and read a random page. Stop when you read a word that you have never seen before. Try to figure out the meaning from the sentence context. Do you now have a general idea of the word's meaning and how it adds to the gist of the sentence? If that does not work, try reading over the paragraph containing the word. Better? If not, try reading the preceding paragraph. If you need even more help from the text, retrieve the chapter title and see if that helps you to predict the meaning of your new word. If you are still not able to figure out the meaning of the word, use a dictionary as your vocabulary resource.

   b. If you are fortunate, you are enrolled in an education setting with a student body representing speakers of different languages and/or different dialects of English. Find a willing conversation partner (perhaps in your class) who speaks a language you do not. Ask that individual to have a brief conversation with you about things in your conversations here and now. Suggest that your partner use simple sentences, a slower than typical speaking rate, as well as gestures to try to help you understand. Using all the nonlinguistic information at your disposal, write down what you believe your partner said and then have the speaker correct your guesses. How close did you come to an accurate translation?

2. Idioms represent a type of figurative language that has to be explicitly learned because an idiom cannot be analyzed word for word. For example, the English idiomatic expressions "rule of thumb" or "throwing a party" express intended meanings that have little to do with thumbs or actually throwing anything. Often, persons who are non-native speakers of English have a difficult time interpreting English idioms just as non-native speakers of any language will have difficulties understanding idioms in that language. Use a search engine to generate a list of idiomatic expressions in English if that is your first language. Determine whether you can accurately interpret each idiom. If not, find an explanation for the origin of the idioms. These are often interesting as well as informative! How would you explain three of the idioms you found to a non-native speaker?

Guessing May Be a Good Strategy for Learning

Children can facilitate adults' miscalculations of their language comprehension because they often make a guess at what is being said when they have understood only a portion of the input. This kind of guessing can be a good thing. Unlike some of the standardized tests we have taken as adults (or nearly adults), where the directions specify that we are not to guess if we do not feel sure of an answer, children's use of partial information, as in the examples of children who have used comprehension strategies to attempt to answer a question, is not without its benefits.

In language-learning contexts, an incorrect response often prompts feedback from a more language-competent person (Demetras, Post, &

Snow, 1986; Farrar, 1990). To see how this works, suppose a child makes what could be called a "best guess" using the information they has available, but the response is wrong. That response may prompt a correction, a model, or a clarification by a caregiver. If they pay attention, the child can use this feedback to determine why the answer was wrong and then generalize this information to another, similar situation in the future. If the response is accepted by the caregiver and the conversation continues, this is also feedback for the child. In this second case, the response produced was probably correct or at least acceptable.

Here is an example of this type of exchange between a caregiver and a 22-month-old child. Notice how the conversation framework plays a vital role.

ADULT: You found the brush for the dolly's hair.
CHILD: (Vigorously shakes her head in affirmation and begins to style the doll's hair with the brush.)
ADULT: Well, okay; if you want to brush the dolly's hair, that's fine. Brush the doll's hair. (Child continues to brush the doll's hair.)

In this example, the child identified the brush as belonging to the doll or being appropriate for the brushing of the doll's hair: brush-doll-hair. These three words, or some combination thereof, were likely understood by the child. The intention of the adult, which was probably just to comment on the child's finding of the brush, was incorrectly interpreted to mean that a request for action had been made. Note how the caregiver has shaped her response to the child's action to fit the conversation flow despite the child's misunderstanding of the adult's original intent. By adding the imperative form, "Brush the doll's hair," the adult has modeled for the child what she would have likely said if the response she had been looking for was the action produced by the child.

Comprehension of Single Words

A number of studies have demonstrated that the vocabularies of young children who are developing normally appear to be somewhat similar in several respects. One feature that appears common to most children is that their *receptive vocabularies*—that is, the single words they understand but do not necessarily produce—begin their development prior to the emergence of their *expressive vocabularies;* early on, receptive vocabularies are typically larger than the child's corresponding expressive vocabulary. Both Nelson (1973) and Benedict (1979) found that children often have receptive vocabularies of approximately 50 different words by the time they have acquired their first 10 expressive vocabulary words. The size differential between receptive and expressive vocabulary appears to diminish as the child moves through the preschool years. In fact, Harris, Yeeles, Chasin, and Oakley (1995) studied a group of six children over an 18-month period and found marked individual differences in the acquisition rate of word comprehension, including differences in the degree to which word comprehension lagged behind word production. Fenson et al. (1994) have demonstrated that by 10 months of age, children may have as many as 10 words in their receptive vocabularies. In fact, thanks to advances in computer technology, Tincoff and Jusczyk (1999) demonstrated that 6-month-old infants will reliably attend to video images of their own mothers when the word *mommy* is presented. Reznick (1990) and others have also demonstrated that infants as young as

6 months can reliably demonstrate visual preference for words they comprehend.

Clinicians should note that a child's early comprehension (or production) of a word does not mean that we can expect the child to have the same sophisticated conceptual understanding for a word that an adult or a much older child might have. To a young child who has just learned to reliably pick out the picture of "*apple*" from a set of four pictures, each depicting something to eat, the actual prototypicality of the apple picture matters. That is, to the child, an apple may have a specific set of features (e.g., is red, can be rolled, has a stem) that describes a very narrowly defined apple by adult standards. Adults know that any trip to a grocery store will likely provide the opportunity to see fruits that do not share these three characteristics yet are considered apples nonetheless.

Over time, and with repeated exposures, we can expect a child's own boundaries of the word to gradually take shape where the adult semantic boundaries lie until, for both child and adult, an apple is an apple. If the boundaries are too narrow, underextension occurs (e.g., *doggy* refers only to my dog); if they are too broadly spaced, overextension occurs (e.g., *doggy* refers to any four-legged animal) (MacWhinney, 1989; Thomson & Chapman, 1977). For young children, overextensions and underextensions appear in both their receptive and expressive vocabularies. Caregiver feedback is often useful in assisting children to revise their word meaning boundaries (Chapman, Leonard, & Mervis, 1986).

Another aspect of vocabulary learning is the development of word category hierarchies from general terms, such as *vehicle*, to more specific terms, such as *car* or *Toyota*. When children develop their first vocabularies, words characterizing mid-level generalities (Owens, 2012), such as *car*, predominate. The internalized organization of these hierarchies likely facilitates word recall and the eventual ability to associate words across abstract domains such as opposites or synonyms. The ability to develop a complex system of semantic linkages is related to both general cognitive development and an increased vocabulary size. The strategy of creating semantic maps helps students consider related words and concepts prior to writing a story, for example. The ability to utilize semantic mapping relies on a foundation of semantic linkages.

Word Learning Mechanisms: Links Between Phonology and Semantics

Vocabulary learning is an activity that extends over one's lifetime but is particularly prodigious during the infant/toddler period. In the last 30 years, researchers have adopted an information-processing paradigm to study vocabulary acquisition. For example, researchers have realized for some time that for children to learn words, they must be able to recognize repeated strings of phonological information and somehow accurately determine what that phonological string references. At the same time, children are increasing their understanding of the world and the things, people, and events in it. They parlay what they have learned about things, people, and events when they were in the preverbal stage into conceptual units, adding information as they go about experiencing their world.

To be successful word learners, children must develop robust phonological representations for words in short-term memory (Gathercole & Baddeley, 1989). This ability provides them with the opportunity to connect specific phonological strings with specific conceptual constructs. It is hypothesized that not only do children have to create phonological representations for short-term memory store, but they also have to be able to retain those representations long enough for the connections to be made. Investigators have also shown that strong nonword repetition skills are related to successful vocabulary learning. That is, children who have formed templates of potential phonological combinations are more likely to draw upon these templates for task repetition purposes than children who lack this type of internalized phonological knowledge.

Bishop's (1997) model of language comprehension focuses on the bridge between phonological representation and meaning. She takes the perspective that determining meaning is a function of all that the young child understands about how language works from the components of the language input message code itself as well as its relationship to the context in which the message has occurred. As Bishop (1997) notes, "[T]he segmentation of a speech stream cannot be a simple bottom-up process, driven solely by perceptual input; the listener uses prior knowledge, context, and expectations to achieve this task and select a meaning from a range of possibilities" (p. 13). Instead, she argues, comprehension probably involves both bottom-up (e.g., phonological representation) and top-down (e.g., world knowledge) processes. Top-down influences on word learning also include what the child knows about the semantic and syntactic neighborhoods in which a novel word appears.

Fast Mapping

Fast mapping refers to the degree of word learning that can occur the first few times a child is exposed to a novel word but not provided with any explicit information about the word (Carey & Bartlett, 1978). To accurately

understand a word presented only once or twice, a child must rely heavily on context to provide salient cues to the word's meaning. Children who are successful "fast mappers" have an advantage in vocabulary learning because fewer exposures to a word are needed before they begin to use the new word. It is likely that some of the context information inferred by the child to be related to the new word is not needed or is incorrectly linked to the new word. This differentiation between what is essential to the new word's meaning and what can be discarded will be refined over multiple exposures to the word (Harris, Barrett, Jones, & Brookes, 1988).

Comprehension of Semantic Relationships and Syntax

Usually, after young children have acquired 50 different words in their expressive vocabularies, they begin to produce two-word combinations. For most children, this language production milestone occurs between 18 and 24 months of age. In fact, many children experience a substantive vocabulary growth spurt once their productive vocabulary includes approximately 100 words (Bates & Carnevale, 1993). This vocabulary spurt may be related to greater ease in the combining of phonological representations and mapped meanings.

For most children, the understanding of two-word combinations begins somewhat before the time those combinations appear in production (Miller et al., 1980). Combining two words together requires that children understand more about the meaning of individual words than the characteristics that define them. In addition, children must learn something about the roles that words serve.

To see how this process works, we will return to learning about the word *apple*, as already discussed. Not only are children learning the characteristics that define the group of items that can be called *apple* and not *peach*, for example, but they are also learning how *apple* can be linked with other words, such as *eat, bake,* and *pick*. With each of these three action words, *apple* can be the recipient of the specified action. Thus, we can talk about *eat apple, bake apple,* and *pick apple*. Children probably hear these combinations as parts of larger, more complex sentences or in sentence fragments directed at their less mature receptive language competencies. As a result, they add to their internal database the information that *apple* not only has distinguishable perceptual characteristics, but, also plays a definite part when linked with certain other words.

Apple can also be described as *red apple* or *wormy apple*. Here, the initial word in the two-word utterance is not an action but a descriptor. The descriptor and what it describes can be linked together to achieve more clarity when indicating which apple is referenced.

As emphasized later in this chapter, when assessing semantic relationships, clinicians must take into consideration how routine the two-word combinations are. If the clinician's goal is to determine when comprehension strategies are being used, it will be important to select combinations of words that are not transparent or rote-learned but require true linguistic comprehension.

Generally, between 1 and 2 years of age, children begin to demonstrate comprehension when actions are paired with expected, familiar words in three-word commands, such as *eat the apple, throw the ball,* and *kiss the dolly*. If we insert unexpected or unfamiliar nouns into those action + object pairs, such as *kiss the apple, throw the dolly,* or *eat the ball*, we are more likely to elicit confusion than compliance. When confused, children often rely on either context cues or world knowledge to determine how to respond. This brings us a full circle back to a consideration of comprehension strategies.

When children master syntactic development in comprehension, where different types of sentences are understood (e.g., declaratives, interrogatives, imperatives), and when they begin to understand how to decode combined clauses and phrases when they have created lengthier and more complicated grammatical structures (e.g., conjoining and embedding), the use of nonlinguistic cues becomes increasingly less necessary. The use of comprehension strategies diminishes as the child begins to rely on linguistic information more often. Once syntactic information is available, young children have the foundation for making predictions about the meanings of novel words from this more sophisticated type of context cue. That is, it becomes possible for children to recognize when the new word is likely to be a noun versus a verb. As noted by Bishop (1997), "syntactic relationships between an unknown word and the other sentence elements can also give critical cues to meaning" (p. 106). This process is also considered to be a top-down method of word learning.

During their third year, children typically add some prepositions (e.g., *in, on, over*), opposites (e.g., *big* and *little, stop* and *go, big* and *small*), and descriptors (e.g., *happy, yellow, beautiful*) to their productive vocabularies and presumably understand the relationships expressed by these elements. With the addition of these concepts to their receptive lexicon, children will be better equipped to understand (and perhaps comply with) one- and two-stage commands such as

Give me the yellow pen or *Pull the blanket over the pillow and bring me the dolly*. Although preschool-age children use conjunctions to combine clauses and phrases (e.g., *and, because*) into the same sentences, it is not until the early school years—ages 7–9 years, according to Owens (2012)—that children understand and are able to incorporate more sophisticated and subtle adverbial conjunctions, including *before, during,* and *while*.

Does Language Comprehension Always Exceed Production?

Generally speaking, although there are anecdotal examples to the contrary (Paul & Norbury, 2012), children's receptive language competencies exceed their production capabilities. That is, when children are reliably demonstrating an understanding of three- and four-word utterances, they may be consistently producing somewhat less lengthy and less sophisticated expressions. Examples where children appear to be producing language in the absence of comprehension generally occur when they have rote-learned a phrase but have not parsed it into its component parts (e.g., "forever and ever"). There is additional evidence from work by Chapman and Miller (1975) and Paul (2000) that some children have shown production of word-order constraints that cannot be demonstrated in their comprehension. Thus, it is crucial for SLPs not to presume that language comprehension always surpasses production abilities for a given child and to be sure to have ample clinical evidence to back up any statements made about relative language abilities.

There are at least two reasons why differential competencies in language comprehension and production must be considered. First, when making recommendations for intervention-targeted structures that are neither comprehended nor produced by a young child, it is probably a good idea to include both comprehension and production training. This is not to say that comprehension teaching must inevitably precede all production training. Lahey (1988) has argued for simultaneous teaching of targets in comprehension and production targets to reflect the way she believes normal language learners acquire language structure. When addressing a child's language disorder in the clinic, for example, the SLP will focus somewhat differently on the problem of inconsistent correct plural use depending on whether the child has demonstrated an understanding of the plural concept ("Show me: 'The cat chases the mice.'"; "Show me: 'The cat chases the mouse.'").

The second reason for carefully considering whether comprehension deficits exist has to do with the following research findings. The results of studies conducted by Thal, Reilly, Seibert, Jeffries, and Fenson (2004) and Whitehurst and Fischel (1994) with children diagnosed with Language Disorder have demonstrated that children with bona fide language disorders who present with deficiencies in only language production have a better prognosis for catching up with their peers than children with deficiencies in both language comprehension and production. This may sound intuitive to the reader: having problems in two language modalities is a more significant therapeutic challenge to overcome than a problem in one modality—specifically, language production.

Question Comprehension: Accurate, Appropriate, or Both?

Question comprehension is an important topic because questions are frequently used by adults and others to invite children into conversations (requests for participation are implicitly made), and conversations are where language learning often takes place. Accurate comprehension of questions versus nonquestions may rely not only on children's ability to detect a rising intonation at the ends of utterances, but also on the grammatical structure that signals a question. Comprehension of question types has been shown to follow a fairly specific order (Parnell, Patterson, & Harding, 1984; Tyack & Ingram, 1977). At a relatively early age, toddlers have been shown to indicate comprehension of yes/no questions by attending to them versus ignoring of *wh*-questions that are beyond their comprehension. Chapman (1978) has noted that young children will use a strategy called "Supply missing information" in response to *wh*-questions they do not fully understand.

Parnell et al. (1984) found that their subjects, ages three through six, responded to *wh*-questions in the following order of difficulty from easiest to most challenging: Where?, Which?, What + be?, Who?, What + do?, When?, Whose?, Why?, and What happened? Specifically, between ages three and four, most children are able to answer "who," "what," and "where" questions as long as they are well supported by context. It is not surprising that the three question types whose answers require the cognitive underpinnings of time ("when"), manner ("how"), and causality ("why") concepts were among the last four question types acquired. In addition to the underlying and specific cognitive knowledge required to comprehend certain *wh*-questions, Deevy and Leonard (2004) demonstrated that children

with language-learning difficulties can be further challenged by processing demands when the questions asked are longer.

For children to be credited with question comprehension, they must demonstrate their ability to answer questions appropriately, though not necessarily accurately. Parnell et al. (1984) made this distinction when categorizing their results, as illustrated in the following example:

ADULT: When do you go to bed?
CHILD: At 10 o'clock.
ADULT: *When?*
CHILD: At 8 o'clock.
ADULT: That's better!

In both of the child's responses to the adult's "When?" question, the child supplied a mandatory time segment, indicating understanding the constraint of answering a "When?" question. Regardless of the adult's indication that the first response given by the child was incorrect (i.e., the child's bedtime is not at 10 p.m.), the answer was appropriate from a comprehension point of view. Leach (1972) provides a comprehensive taxonomy of the constraints on responses inherent in different question types. Question comprehension will be revisited later in this chapter as the basis of a nonstandardized comprehension probe.

▶ Measuring Children's Language Comprehension

This chapter has attempted to make a compelling argument concerning why SLPs must actually assess children's language comprehension and not simply make assumptions of normalcy. The comment in a diagnostic report to the effect that "The child's comprehension appears to be within normal limits" is one that has been known to elicit a reflexive "How do you know that?" from me, either as a clinical instructor or as a clinician reading a report completed by a colleague.

A number of standardized tests are available to assess aspects of the language comprehension of preschool-age children. On many occasions, however, it is necessary for SLPs to design nonstandardized probes to look more carefully at what preschool-age children actually understand when they need to evaluate the range of comprehension deficit of a particular grammatical type.

Whether employing standardized or nonstandardized testing, the tasks SLPs use to evaluate comprehension typically fall into one of three categories:

identification, acting-out, or judgment tasks (Weiss, Tomblin, & Robin, 1999). These tasks will require pointing to a picture that best fits the word(s) or answers the question asked. Acting-out tasks are less frequently used than identification tasks and involve having three-dimensional materials available to the child to demonstrate the action reflected in a sentence (e.g., "Give me the bottle"; "Show me the baby drives the Jeep.") Judgment tasks typically tap the child's ability to make grammaticality judgments. They may involve asking a child to indicate which sentence sounds "silly" or "okay" to avoid the terms *grammatical* and *ungrammatical*. Regardless of the task type, comprehension tasks tend to be limited in the amount of verbal output needed from the examinee; for this reason, comprehension testing may be the preferred place to start when evaluating reticent children.

It is also important to note that sophisticated technology that allows examiners to rely on measurement of eye gaze behaviors may yield the most precise information about children's early word comprehension. Bergmann, Paulus, and Fikkert (2012) used eye tracking measurements to assess pronoun comprehension in a group of 3- and 4-year-olds learning Dutch and found that when compared with use of a more traditional response-based task, children were more likely to demonstrate comprehension with the eye-tracking task. Their younger participants were more reliable in their responses to an eye tracking task, presumably because of their less mature cognitive and linguistic abilities. Moreover, Goldfield, Gencarella, and Fornari (2016) have suggested that an "intermodal preferential looking" task may be the preferred method for assessing comprehension in children with behavioral deficits. They recently reported their success with using an "intermodal preferential looking" task that measured "looking time to target" (LTT) as well as "longest look" (LL) at a target. Goldfield et al. found that both measures increased from the baseline to the target for the assessment of nouns, verbs, and adjectives, although the results for nouns were higher than the other two word groups. Further, a strong correlation was found between children's performance scores on the *Peabody Picture Vocabulary Test-4* when LTT measurements and traditional picture pointing testing results were compared.

A Summary of Caveats

As mentioned previously, young children learning to understand the spoken language in their environment may depend heavily on the nonlinguistic context in which that language is produced in order to fill in any gaps that may exist in their linguistic understanding. Therefore, *if* the clinician's goal is to determine a child's

competence to understand the linguistic portion of a message, he or she must carefully construct tasks that eliminate the nonlinguistic component as much as possible. To do so in a valid manner, SLPs should eliminate unintended gestures that provide clues to understanding. They should also select examples for testing that do not represent routines. For example, handing a child a dolly and saying "Hug the dolly" is a task more likely to bypass comprehension processing than asking the same child to "Hug the apple." For the clinician, a clear understanding of how comprehension strategies are likely to function in the comprehension development of the young child will save the SLP from many instances of misinterpretation and possibly misdiagnosis or *missed* diagnosis.

When designing comprehension tasks to provide children with multiple examples of a comprehension task type, it is also important to carefully take into account the vocabulary included in the task and watch the timing of any requests to the child so that you do not create the "pseudo-successes" that Chapman et al. (1980) found to be so prevalent in the interactions between caregivers and their children. Using multiple examples will reduce the likelihood that the child's response was the result of some extraneous variable connected to that one item. When clinicians use vocabulary that is unfamiliar to the child in test items, they may find that they are testing vocabulary and not comprehension of sentences, for example.

Perhaps the *most* important advice that can be given to clinicians who question the language abilities of young children, whether or not language comprehension is the primary focus of concern, is to be absolutely certain of the child's hearing status prior to formalized language testing. Fortunately, many states have mandated newborn screenings and follow-up for children suspected of hearing loss. Nevertheless, these measures are not a panacea for catching all losses that might lead to negative academic and social ramifications. Given the propensity of middle ear disease in childhood, including repeated episodes of serous otitis media, often with accompanying hearing loss, it is critical to monitor children's hearing levels and determine whether the language input is in an unaltered condition and available for their consumption as intended (Roberts et al., 1986).

Standardized Assessment

Standardized assessment involves two aspects of test giving. The first aspect is that there is a set procedure for the administration and interpretation of the test as well as a standard set of stimuli provided for the examiner's use. These stimuli could consist of specific tasks using specific materials, or they might comprise a prescribed list of questions that are posed to a caregiver familiar with the child's development. The second aspect of standardization involves the substantiation of the psychometric rigor of the test. In addition to evidence of validity and reliability, normative data gleaned from use of a standardized sample of subjects to whom the test has been administered is typically available. The norms can be applied to the performance of a child (i.e., if appropriate for the test, given the criteria delineated in the test manual), thereby enabling the examiner to determine whether the child falls within the range of age-expected ability. For the purposes of this chapter, this section profiles tests that meet either one or both of these criteria for standardized tests.

Assessing Infants and Toddlers

For the clinical assessment of language comprehension in young children, two standardized tools are frequently employed and appear in the case studies found in this text: the *Rossetti Infant–Toddler Language Scale* (Rossetti, 2006) and the *MacArthur-Bates Communicative Development Inventories (CDIs), Second Edition* (Fenson et al., 2007). Although a number of other assessment tools have been published for use with this young population (refer to Paul & Norbury, 2012, for a more complete list), these two tests will serve as examples of the types of tasks used for comprehension assessment.

Rossetti Infant–Toddler Language Scale. Rossetti's assessment tool, the *Rossetti Infant–Toddler Language Scale* (RITLS; Rossetti, 2006), is appropriate for children from birth through age three and yields an overall developmental age, individual developmental ages for language comprehension or language production, or developmental age equivalents for each of the six language-learning areas. Of course, given the age range specified for its use, prelinguistic behaviors are also evaluated in terms of whether they have emerged at an accepted age.

The RITLS can be used as the basis of a caregiver interview about language development. The SLP can supplement the caregiver's responses to queries about the specific language competencies listed on the test (e.g., report) with observation or elicitation of behaviors.

The specific developmental achievements listed in each age group have been gleaned from other developmental resources; that is, there is no normative data accompanying this test derived from test administration. According to Rossetti, the validity of the test derives from the excellence of the developmental sources used for item selection. The author refers to this test as a criterion-referenced measure, noting that it is useful for following a particular child's progress

over time with reference to norms from the general population at large.

The items have been gleaned from other developmental assessment tools and the author's own experiences evaluating infants, toddlers, and young preschoolers. Examples of items from the language comprehension portion of the test are as follows for infants from birth to 3 months of age:

- Shows awareness of a speaker
- Attends to a speaker's mouth
- Moves in response to a voice

For a child to receive credit for reaching a specific language comprehension age, *all* items at that age level must have been achieved. Note that each of the items is viewed to be equally representative of the age level in question.

MacArthur-Bates Communicative Development Inventories. The *MacArthur-Bates Communicative Development Inventories (CDIs), Second Edition* (Fenson et al., 2007) was first published by Fenson et al. (1993) and consisted of two different test protocols: the Infant form (Words and Gestures), which is appropriate for children ranging in age from 8 to 16 months, and the Toddler form (Words and Sentences), which is appropriate for children ranging in age from 16 to 30 months. The newer version of the test, in addition to it being renamed in honor of the late Dr. Elizabeth Bates, includes the CDI-III, an extension of the existing inventories appropriate for children 30–37 months of age. This three-part addition focuses on expressive vocabulary through a checklist, word combinations from a set of 13 questions, and a list of 12 yes/no questions that investigate a child's language comprehension as well as age-appropriate aspects of semantics and syntax.

In terms of language comprehension testing, this test provides a standardized format for collecting information about a young child's early single-word and phrase vocabulary. By providing caregivers with closed sets of options for selecting words and phrases that their children comprehend (and produce), the authors generally find that parents are easily able to complete the checklist in a brief period of time with minimal, if any, assistance from professional examiners. The normative data provided by the authors is extensive (Dale & Fenson, 1996), but comprehension data is available for the Infant form only. This limitation likely reflects the fact that as children's vocabularies grow substantially into their second year, it becomes more difficult to determine, in the absence of production, which words the toddler actually understands and which words are perceived by caregivers as understood due to context confounds. The normative data is also divided between males and females.

A look at the vocabulary comprehension data provided by Fenson et al. (1993) demonstrates the rapid acquisition of single-word vocabulary. For example, girls ranking at the 50th percentile comprehend 14 different words at 8 months of age and 191 at 16 months of age. Vocabulary "stars" functioning at the 99th percentile understand 142 words at 8 months of age and 392 words by 16 months! When we consider these same "stars" in terms of their vocabulary production, they have an average of 7 words at 8 months of age and 281 words at 16 months of age, demonstrating a substantive difference between the size of their comprehension and production vocabularies.

Standardized Testing Procedures for Older Preschool-Age Children

Most often, standardized assessment of children in the 2–5-year age range involves having children identify pictures that are the best referents for the words, phrases, or sentences produced by the examiner. Typically, several foil items appear on the page in addition to the correct answer. Children are encouraged to look at all of the options before selecting the picture that answers the query, and the test administrator should use any sample items provided by the test authors to be sure that the child understands the task. Examiners should be alert to children who appear to persevere in pointing to one location for all pictures because this behavior may mean that they are not considering all of the picture options. Examiners also need to be careful not to accidentally point to the correct picture choice.

Paul & Norbury (2012) list 34 language assessment tools that are appropriate for use with children at the developing language level. Of these, only 14 are identified as focusing on the assessment of comprehension competencies of preschool-age children. Some of these tests provide SLPs with the opportunity to evaluate both comprehension and production. A smaller number evaluates language comprehension only.

Two of the most commonly used tests in this age group are the *Peabody Picture Vocabulary Test-4* (*PPVT-4*; Dunn & Dunn, 2007), a test of hearing vocabulary only, and the *Test for Auditory Comprehension of Language-3* (TACL-3; Carrow-Woolfolk, 1999), an assessment tool that consists of three parts— vocabulary, grammatical morphemes, and elaborated phrases and sentences. Both of these tests use identification tasks to elicit responses from test takers and utilize a basal/ceiling scoring regimen. The pictures that make up the PPVT-4 items are displayed four on a page; the TACL-3 items consist of three pictures located side by side. Because examiners are asked to determine basal and ceiling scores, they are provided with suggestions for where to start in the test given the child's chronological age.

Examiners can derive the following scores from the PPVT-4: standard scores, percentiles, normal curve equivalents, stanine scores, age equivalents, grade equivalents, and growth scale value scores. The TACL-3 provides the SLP with the opportunity to compare the child's performance with normative data to derive percentile ranks, standard scores, and age equivalents.

As psychometrically sound as these standardized tests are, their usefulness—especially when deciding where to begin therapy—can be limited, perhaps due to the small number of items available to test the comprehension of a particular comprehension construct. For that reason, the use of nonstandardized probes to fine-tune the results from diagnostic tests is often recommended (Weiss et al., 1999).

Nonstandardized Comprehension Probes

Sometimes, the standardized tests do not provide SLPs with the opportunity to fully evaluate specific areas of language comprehension. To perform a more complete assessment of a child's comprehension competencies, SLPs may have to devise their own tasks to collect the information we need for clinical decision-making. That is, SLPs may need to develop their own nonstandardized probes.

Here is an example of a nonstandardized comprehension probe that may prove very useful—it was designed to fill a gap in available testing. This tool is meant to account for the fact that standardized tests do not do a particularly good job in providing clinicians with the means to assess children's comprehension of different question forms. For example, the TACL-3 (Carrow-Woolfolk, 1999) contains very few items that directly address *wh*-question comprehension. Specifically, these questions are framed as follows: "When do you sleep?" and "What do you eat?" Children are told to point to the one of three pictures that best represents an answer to the question. Actually, the task is a little less specific than that: examiners tell children to show them the picture that best represents the utterance produced by the examiner. Note how decontextualized the use of the question is in this test-taking situation. Typically, a question turns the speaking floor over to another conversation partner. During test-taking, however, no verbal response is called for. It is no wonder that many children will answer the question when it is produced by the examiner!

Given that question comprehension plays a vital role in children's ability to function in academic and social settings, determining the adequacy of a child's question comprehension is not a simple matter. Relying on the TACL-3 will not achieve this goal. Thus, a nonstandardized assessment tool can be developed to provide more and different examples of questions.

TABLE 4-1 shows one such nonstandardized probe. Note that several examples per question type are used. The question types selected reflect the results of a study that demonstrated the question forms typically understood by children ages 3 through 6 (Parnell et al., 1984). This article serves as the only normative referent. Completion of this nonstandardized test will provide a clinician with the data needed to determine whether question comprehension is

progressing within normal limits or whether it represents an appropriate goal for therapy for a particular child.

An advantage of developing nonstandardized assessment probes is that you can design the tool to fit the specific children you are evaluating. Not only can you be sure to focus attention on the area of language comprehension you may be curious about, but you can also select the type of task that you believe will work best (e.g., identification, acting out, judgment, response to question) for the child. In addition, you can control the vocabulary used so that the performance of the child is not confounded by use of unfamiliar words in the tasks (Weiss, 2001).

TABLE 4-1 A Nonstandardized Probe for *Wh*-Questions	
Question Type and Examples	**Functionally Appropriate**
What + be: e.g., "What is this?"	
What is a banana? etc.	
What is your name? etc.	
Which: e.g., "Which puppy is cuter?"	
Which ball is orange? etc.	
Which boat is a sailboat? etc.	
Where: e.g., "Where do you live?"	
Where are your toys? etc.	
Where do you sleep? etc.	
Who: e.g., "Who takes you to school?"	
Who do you play with? etc.	
Who is your best friend? etc.	
Whose: e.g., "Whose hat is that?"	
Whose toy is that? etc.	
Whose hair is curliest? etc.	
What do: e.g., "What are you doing?"	
Why: e.g., "Why did he fall down?"	
When: e.g., "When is your bedtime?"	
What happened: e.g., "What happened yesterday?"	

▶ Case Studies

Given our discussions about language comprehension in this chapter, how can we relate that information to the following three case studies?

🔍 CASE STUDY: JOHNATHON (TD)

A Typically Developing Child at Age 25 Months

The speech-language evaluation report provided for the typically developing 2-year old, Johnathon, includes some information in the history paragraph about the child's receptive language abilities. As noted in the report, Johnathon was able to follow age-appropriate directions provided without contextual support. Although there might be a problem with the example used (i.e., "Bring me your bottle" is fairly stereotypical of what one would be asked to do with a bottle), at least the clinician viewed comprehension as important enough to inquire about it on the front end of the evaluation. The section chronicling Johnathon's receptive language could have been supplemented with nonstandardized tasks that would determine the extent to which the child used comprehension strategies in response to requests for actions or objects.

The comment that Johnathon understands new words rapidly should be clarified. An example or two would be helpful here. Does this comment refer to Johnathon penchant for fast mapping? That is, is he likely to use a word correctly after being exposed to it only one or two times? We know that children who are considered good at fast mapping typically show accelerated word learning. These children are risk-takers in terms of language learning. Their ability to observe how a word is used is keen, which means they can pick out salient features of the verbal and nonverbal context to generalize the word to future circumstances. Also, they do not seem to be shy about trying out new words.

A comparison between the child's receptive and expressive language abilities demonstrated that Johnathon's skills were closely aligned; that is, there was no discrepancy between receptive and expressive competencies, as indicated by the RITLS (Rossetti, 1990). We have already discussed the importance of not making assumptions about expressive language skills based on receptive skills and vice versa.

🔍 CASE STUDY: JOSEPHINE (LB)

A Late Talker at Age 22 Months

Josephine's significant history included the observation that her receptive language was a relative strength. Although Josephine did not produce her first word until the age of 15 months, and her mother's perception was that her daughter had a smaller expressive vocabulary than would be expected for her age, the child was reported to be following two-step commands. Note that the example given by the mother could be reflective of an overestimation of Josephine's language comprehension: "Go to the family room and get your diaper." If Josephine recognizes the word "diaper" and, as most children do, knows where they are kept, the first portion of the command is unnecessary. That is, when retrieving a diaper, Josephine will go to the family room whether told to or not. Thus, Josephine's response to this particular two-step command may mean as little as comprehension of the word "diaper" and "locate the objects mentioned," one of Chapman's comprehension strategies.

According to her performance on the RITLS, Josephine's receptive language abilities slightly exceeded those expected for her chronological age. This estimate included successful completion of tasks requiring responses to two-step commands. When comparing Josephine's expressive and receptive test results, it is clear that her language comprehension abilities significantly exceed her language production abilities. This is a child whose caregivers may believe "she understands everything" partly because of the discrepancy between receptive and expressive language and partly because of the facility with which her comprehension strategies are used. Clinicians should take care to explain to the parents that Josephine's strength is certainly her understanding of language and that this strength will be used in therapy to help increase her expressive language abilities. Under no circumstances, however, should the parents be encouraged to believe that their child understands everything that is said to her: no 2-year-old does.

Research has demonstrated that children whose problems are confined to expressive language tend to make swifter language development gains than those with both receptive and expressive language needs (Thal et al., 2004). Because Josephine's receptive language or language comprehension is a relative strength for her, this child's ability to catch up to her same-age peers in terms of language development is more likely than that of another child who demonstrated both comprehension and expressive language deficits.

🔍 *CASE STUDY: ROBERT (LT)*

A Child with Bona Fide Language Impairment at Age 27 Months

Robert has displayed a number of developmental concerns, only one of which is language learning. Diagnosed with developmental delay by a physician in his first-year examination, Robert's language comprehension development was not addressed in his history other than the mention of his ability to follow simple directions. Of some concern is the lack of definitive information provided regarding Robert's hearing levels. Accurate/adequate hearing will supply Robert with not only the verbal information necessary to understand language, but also the context information necessary for understanding the more subtle nuances of communicated messages.

Standardized testing on the CDI: Words and Gestures form (normally used for children somewhat younger than Robert) revealed that Robert's receptive vocabulary was typical of an 18- to 24-month-old child. Results from the RITLS revealed a less mature picture, with his receptive language developmental age being closer to 1 year, although the report did note a scattering of skills up to the 21- to 24-month-old level. Because both receptive and expressive language competencies appear to be slow to develop, and given the pervasive delays observed in Robert's other developmental areas, the prognosis for Robert to make significant gains without continued provision of dedicated, intensive speech-language therapy is not very positive.

▶ Summary

Language comprehension, though an important aspect of language development, does not always receive the attention it deserves. Whether our interest is in normally developing or clinical populations, focusing on language comprehension competencies allows us to forge a more holistic picture of a child's language competencies, provide some hypotheses about how the child learns best, or, in the case of children with language deficits, give some insight into how to approach their language problems in the clinic. Further more, the study of language comprehension provides a wealth of evidence, indicating that children's learning of language necessitates the interweaving of knowledge not only about specific linguistic parameters, but also about how their world operates.

Study Questions

■ You have received a catalogue from a publisher of speech and language tests. While perusing its pages, you notice that one of the products highlighted is a brand-new comprehension test advertised as appropriate for children 2–5 years of age. Before purchasing this test for use in your work setting, you think about your practice. Which specific information about language comprehension

in children will assist you in evaluating the benefit of owning this new test instrument?

■ Using a university library's research engine, find an issue of a journal that publishes information about language learning in either normal or atypical children (e.g., *First Language; Journal of Child Language; Journal of Speech, Language, and Hearing Research*), including an article chronicling some aspect of children's developing language comprehension. Determine which types of tasks were used to assess comprehension. Were the procedures used for data collection valid? That is, did the tasks account for the possibility of an overestimation of children's comprehension abilities?

■ Go to the YouTube website and search for video clips under the term "babies waving." Look for a video starring a toddler who is being coaxed to wave by a caregiver, who asks him or her to wave "bye-bye." Watch the segment carefully. Given what you know about children's early language comprehension and the appearance of early language, would you or would you not give this child credit for understanding the command "Wave bye-bye"? Be sure that there is a caregiver involved in the clip as well so that you can determine how much, if any, nonverbal cuing was provided.

References

Bates, E., & Carnevale, G. (1993). New directions in research on language development. *Developmental Review, 13*, 436–470.

Benedict, H. (1979). Early lexical development: Comprehension and production. *Journal of Child Language, 6*(2), 183–200.

Bergmann, C., Paulus, M., & Fikkert, P. (2012). Preschoolers' comprehension of pronouns and reflexives: The impact of the task. *Journal of Child Language, 39*, 777–803.

Bishop, D. (1997). *Uncommon understanding: Development and disorders of language comprehension in children*. East Essex, UK: Psychology Press.

Brown, R. (1973). *A first language: The early stages*. Cambridge, MA: Harvard University Press.

Bruner, J. (1978). The role of dialogue in language acquisition. In A. Sinclair, R. Jarvella, & W. Levelt (Eds.), *The child's conception of language* (pp. 241–256). New York, NY: Springer-Verlag.

Carey, S., & Bartlett, E. (1978). Acquiring a single new word. *Papers and Reports on Child Language Development, 15,* 17–29.

Carrow-Woolfolk, E. (1999). *Test for auditory comprehension of language* (3rd ed.). Austin, TX: Pro-Ed.

Chapman, K., Leonard, L., & Mervis, C. (1986). The effect of feedback on children's inappropriate word use. *Journal of Child Language, 13,* 101–117.

Chapman, R. (1978). Comprehension strategies in children. In J. Kavanaugh & W. Strange (Eds.), *Speech and language in the laboratory, school and clinic* (pp. 308–327). Cambridge, MA: MIT Press.

Chapman, R., Klee, T., & Miller, J. (1980, November). *Pragmatic comprehension skills: How mothers get some action.* Presented at the annual meeting of the American Speech and Hearing Association (Detroit, MI).

Chapman, R., & Miller, J. (1975). Word order in early two- and three-word utterances: Does production precede comprehension? *Journal of Speech and Hearing Research, 18,* 355–371.

Dale, P. S., & Fenson, L. (1996). Lexical development norms for young children. *Behavior Research Methods, Instruments, & Computers, 28,* 125–127.

Deevy, P., & Leonard, L. (2004). The comprehension of *Wh*-questions in children with specific language impairment. *Journal of Speech, Language, and Hearing Research, 47*(4), 802–815.

Demetras, M., Post, K., & Snow, C. (1986). Feedback to first language learners: The role of repetitions and clarification questions. *Journal of Child Language, 13,* 275–292.

Dunn, L., & Dunn, L. (2007). *Peabody picture vocabulary test—IV* (4th ed.). Circle Pines, MN: American Guidance Service.

Edmonston, N., & Thane, N. (1992). Children's use of comprehension strategies in response to relational words: Implications for assessment. *American Journal of Speech-Language Pathology, 1,* 30–35.

Farrar, M. (1990). Discourse and the acquisition of grammatical morphemes. *Journal of Child Language, 17*(3), 607–624.

Fenson, L., Dale, P., Reznick, S., Bates, E., Thal, D., & Pethick, S. (1994). Variability in early communicative development. *Monographs of the Society for Research in Child Development, 59* (Serial No. 242).

Fenson, L., Dale, P., Reznick, S., Thal, D., Bates, E., Hartung, J. P., & Reilly, J. S. (1993). *The MacArthur communicative development inventories.* San Diego, CA: Singular Publishing.

Fenson, L., Marchman, V., Thal, D., Dale, P., Reznick, S., & Bates, E. (2007). *MacArthur-Bates communicative development inventories (CDIs)* (2nd ed.). Baltimore, MD: Paul H. Brookes Publishing Co.

Fernald, A., & Kuhl, P. (1987). Acoustic determinants of infant preference for motherese speech. *Infant Behavior and Development, 10,* 279–293.

Fernald, A., Taeschner, T., Dunn, J., Papousek, M., deBoysson-Bardies, B., & Fukui, I. (1989). A cross-language study of prosody modifications in mothers' and fathers' speech to preverbal infants. *Journal of Child Language, 16*(3), 477–501.

Gathercole, S., & Baddeley, A. (1989). Evaluation of the role of phonological STM in the development of vocabulary in children: A longitudinal study. *Journal of Memory and Language, 28*(2), 200–213.

Gilkerson, J., Richards, J., Warren, S., Montgomery, J., Greenwood, C., Oller, D., … Paul, T. (2017). Mapping the early language environment using all-day recordings and automated analysis. *American Journal of Speech-Language Pathology, 26,* 248–265.

Goldfield, B., Gencarella, C., & Fornari, K. (2016). Understanding and assessing word comprehension. *Applied Psycholinguistics, 37,* 529–549.

Harris, M., Barrett, M., Jones, D., & Brookes, S. (1988). Linguistic input and early word meanings. *Journal of Child Language, 15*(1), 77–94.

Harris, M., Yeeles, C., Chasin, J., & Oakley, Y. (1995). Symmetries and asymmetries in early lexical comprehension and production. *Journal of Child Language, 22,* 1–18.

Lahey, M. (1988). *Language development and language disorders.* New York, NY: MacMillan.

Leach, E. (1972). Interrogation: A model and some implications. *Journal of Speech and Hearing Disorders, 37*(1), 33–46.

MacWhinney, B. (1989). Competition and lexical categorization. In R. Corrigan, F. Eckman, & M. Noonan (Eds.), *Linguistic categorization* (pp. 195–242). New York, NY: John Benjamins.

Miller, J., Chapman, R., Branston, M., & Reichle, J. (1980). Language comprehension in sensory motor stages 5 and 6. *Journal of Speech and Hearing Research, 23,* 1–12.

Miller, J., & Paul, R. (1995). *The clinical assessment of language comprehension.* Baltimore, MD: Paul H. Brookes.

Milosky, L. (1992). Children listening: The role of world knowledge in comprehension. In R. Chapman (Ed.), *Processes in language acquisition and disorders* (pp. 20–44). St. Louis, MO: Mosby Year Book.

Morford, M., & Goldin-Meadow, S. (1992). Comprehension and production of gesture in combination with speech in one-word speakers. *Journal of Child Language, 19,* 559–580.

Nelson, K. (1973). Structure and strategy in learning to talk. *Monographs of the Society for Research in Child Development, 38*(1/2), 1–135.

Owens, R. (2012). *Language development: An introduction* (8th ed.). Boston, MA: Pearson.

Parnell, M., Patterson, S., & Harding, M. (1984). Answers to *wh*-questions: A developmental study. *Journal of Speech and Hearing Research, 27,* 297–305.

Paul, R. (1990). Comprehension strategies: Interactions between world knowledge and the development of sentence comprehension. *Topics in Language Disorders, 10*(3), 63–75.

Paul, R. (2000). Understanding the "whole" of it: Comprehension assessment. *Seminars in Speech and Language, 21*(3), 10–17.

Paul, R., & Norbury, C. (2012). *Language disorders from infancy through adolescence: Listening, speaking, reading, writing, and communicating* (4th ed.). St. Louis, MO: Mosby Elsevier.

Reznick, J. (1990). Visual preference as a test of infant word comprehension. *Applied Psycholinguistics, 11*(2), 145–166.

Roberts, J., Sanyal, M., Burchini, M., Collier, A., Ramey, C., & Henderson, F. (1986). Otitis media in early childhood and its relationship to later verbal and academic performance. *Pediatrics, 78,* 423–430.

Rossetti, L. (1990). *The Rossetti Infant-Toddler Language Scale.* East Moline, IL: LinguiSystems, Inc.

Rossetti, L. (2006). *The Rossetti Infant-Toddler Language Scale: A measure of communication and interaction.* East Moline, IL: Linguisystems.

Shady, M., & Gerken, L. (1999). Grammatical and caregiver cues in early sentence comprehension. *Journal of Child Language, 26,* 163–175.

Skarakis-Doyle, E. (2002). Young children's detections of violations in familiar stories and emerging comprehension monitoring. *Discourse Processes, 33,* 175–197.

Skarakis-Doyle, E., & Dempsey, L. (2008). The detection and monitoring of comprehension errors by preschool children with and without language impairment. *Journal of Speech, Language, and Hearing Research, 51*(5), 1227–1243.

Thal, D., Reilly, J., Seibert, L., Jeffries, R., & Fenson, J. (2004). Language development in children at risk for language impairment: Cross-population comparisons. *Brain & Language, 88*(2), 167–179.

Thomson, J., & Chapman, R. (1977). Who is "Daddy" revisited: The status of two year olds' over-extended words in use and comprehension. *Journal of Child Language, 4*, 359–375.

Tincoff, R., & Jusczyk, P. (1999). Some beginning of word comprehension in 6 month olds. *Psychological Science, 10*(2), 172–175.

Tomasello, M. (1995). Pragmatic contexts for early verb learning. In M. Tomasello & W. Merriman (Eds.), *Beyond names for things: Young children's acquisition of verbs* (pp. 115–146). Hillsdale, NJ: Erlbaum.

Tyack, D., & Ingram, D. (1977). Children's production and comprehension of questions. *Journal of Child Language, 4*(2), 211–224.

Weiss, A. (2001). *Preschool language disorders: Resource guide.* San Diego, CA: Singular Publishing/Thomson Learning.

Weiss, A., Tomblin, J., & Robin, D. (1999). Language disorders. In J. Tomblin, H. Morris, & D. Spriestersbach (Eds.), *Diagnosis in speech-language pathology* (2nd ed., pp. 129–173). Chicago, IL: University of Chicago Press.

Whitehurst, G., & Fischel, J. (1994). Early developmental delay: What, if anything, should the clinician do about it? *Journal of Child Psychology and Psychiatry, 35*, 613–648.

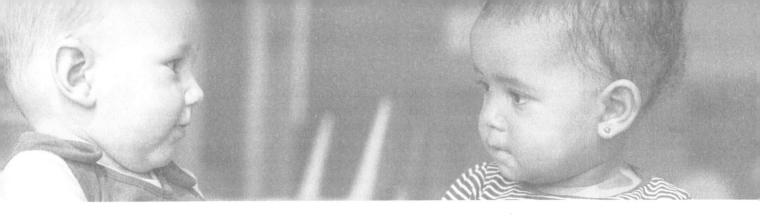

CHAPTER 5

Gesture Development: Setting the Stage for Language Development

Nina Capone Singleton, PhD, CCC-SLP

▶ Introduction

This chapter gives an overview of gesture development and its relationship with language. *Gestures* are manual, facial, or other bodily movements. These movements can communicate meaning or simply accompany the forward flow of speech.

The act of gesturing is inherent to the act of speaking (Goldin-Meadow, Butcher, Mylander, & Dodge, 1994; Iverson & Goldin-Meadow, 2001). For example, children gesture regardless of their cultural background or the language that they speak. Further, blind speakers gesture to blind listeners, and deaf children create their own representational gestures to communicate even though their parents have not signed or modeled these gestures.

Gestures are not random movements. Indeed, many gestures convey meaning such that a child's gesture reflects what they know (Capone, 2007; Evans, Alibali, & McNeil, 2001; Goldin-Meadow, 2003; Goldin-Meadow & Wagner, 2005). Gesturing becomes fully integrated with spoken language. School-age children are rarely observed to gesture in isolation, without speaking (Church & Goldin-Meadow, 1986).

When the child's gesture and spoken language are examined for the meaning each expresses, we see that the information conveyed by gesture may be the same or different from what they are saying. Thus, gesture can express knowledge that the child has represented in memory, but that information may or may not be expressed with spoken language. When the child conveys some information in gesture and different information in spoken language, it reflects how richly the child has knowledge represented in memory. For example, as the child learns new information, they may not yet have consolidated it well enough in memory to formulate the language to talk about it. Instead, they express new information via gesture. The child also pays attention to and uses the *adult's* gesturing to expand their own gesture repertoire and learn spoken language. In this way, gesture is a rich source of information for the child as a speaker and a listener.

This chapter first defines types of gestures and delineates the developmental course of gesturing. The remainder of the chapter discusses the relationship between gesture and spoken language development.

▶ Defining Gesture Types

The first gestures to emerge in development are *deictic gestures*. Deictic gestures, which include *showing*, *giving*, *pointing*, and *ritual request* gestures, are also referred to as prelinguistic gestures because they emerge before the child speaks their first word. Deictic gestures make a reference to something in the environment and rely on that context to convey meaning. For example, a speaker may announce, "I can't find my book," while extending a hand toward the table. The gesture conveys the location that the book was last found even though the speaker has not said this explicitly.

Deictic gestures have the pragmatic function (i.e., communicative intention) to gain or maintain adult interaction or request or draw attention to a referent. Infants may point to their cup before they have the word *cup* in their vocabulary. The infant's intention may be to draw attention to the cup or to request it, much like labeling it would. Other early communicative gestures are taught through social routines. These gestures include hand waving to signal greeting; shaking or nodding the head for *no* and *yes*, respectively; blowing kisses; shrugging to indicate an inability to answer the question *Where did it go?*; and placing a finger to the lips to indicate a *hush* (Fenson et al., 2007).

A student of language would be wise to understand that gesture is central to language development. Much research has been dedicated to the relationship between gesture and language, and several tests used by speech-language pathologists include items and questions about gestures as part of the language assessment protocol (e.g., *MacArthur-Bates Communicative Development Inventories, Rossetti Infant-Toddler Language Scale or RITLS*). **TABLE 5-1** presents some recent research on the relationship between pointing, language development, and early indicators of language delay.

The second gesture type children develop is the *representational gesture*. Representational gestures

TABLE 5-1 Relationships Between Pointing and Early Language Development

Lüke, Ritterfeld, Grimminger, Liszkowski, and Rohlfing (2017)	▪ Typical infants point often by 12 months ▪ Delay to point until 21–24 months is associated with delayed language acquisition ▪ Indicating with an open-hand point (versus index finger) precedes the index finger point ▪ At 18 months of age, children showing signs of language delay are still relying on more open-hand points than toddlers with typical language development
Esseily, Jacquet, and Fagard (2011)	▪ By 14 months, pointing is largely one-handed and lateralized (showing a preference to right or left) ▪ Pointing is often lateralized to the right hand ▪ Right-handed pointing in 14-month-olds is associated with stronger vocabulary skills

are iconic. They convey some aspect of the referent's meaning, so they can be understood even when they are produced without the referent in sight. The meaning conveyed by representational gestures might be the form of an object, the function of an object, the path or quality of an action, or the spatial relationship between two objects expressed by a preposition. For example, Goldin-Meadow and Butcher (2003) reported a child in their study who said the word *bear* while also producing scratching hand movements. From this clawing motion, we see that the child has some knowledge of what bears do as well as how we label them. As another example, the young child might extend their tongue in reference to a *frog* because this action is often characteristic of our idea of what frogs do. Similarly, the child may extend two fingers in a V to signal *bunny*. Here, the gesture represents the form of the bunny's ears. In another example, the child may extend an index finger upward toward a ceiling fan and use a quick circling motion. The child is commenting through gesture on the trajectory and quality of the fan's movement.

Representational gestures are also referred to as *iconic gestures* and *baby signs* (Acredolo & Goodwyn, 1996). Acredolo and Goodwyn (1996) published a popular press book for parents about baby signs. It included a glossary of representational gestures that were created by infants. The term *baby signs* should not be confused with sign language, such as *American Sign Language* (ASL). ASL signs are symbols, in the same way that spoken language is a symbol. That is, ASL signs convey meaning, but many ASL signs are not iconic in the way that representational gestures are iconic. They do not convey semantic content in the form they take (i.e., in the actual form of the sign itself). Signed languages are further differentiated from representational gesturing in that the child needs exposure to signed language to learn it in the same way that spoken language must be taught. Another difference between gesturing and signing is that signed language encompasses more than single vocabulary items. Like spoken language, it adheres to a grammatical rule system.

Another symbolic gesture added later to the repertoire is the emblem gesture. *Emblems* are conventional symbols such as the *high-five* to convey camaraderie, *okay* or *thumbs up* gestures to signal agreement, and the *hand across the throat* to signal stop. These gestures are language-like in that they are abstract symbols. Like spoken language symbols, they do not change referents. Each emblem conveys a particular meaning consistently, and each gesture-referent pairing is agreed upon by the communication partners. This is

also the case with representational gestures, although often, the representational gesture is dependent upon the spoken language or context that accompanies it. Also, the community that understands the child's representational gesture may be their immediate caregivers, whereas other early communicative and emblem gestures are shared by the larger community of the culture (Goldin-Meadow, 2003). Note that in some cases, an emblem gesture can be considered benign in one culture but offensive in another culture.

Another gesture to emerge in development is the *beat gesture.* These gestures follow the rhythm of speech and may provide emphasis on a particular idea, but they do not convey semantic information. For example, you may notice that while your professor is lecturing, their hands move up and down but then stop when they pause. These movements are paced with the forward flow of speech.

The remainder of this chapter reviews the course of gesture development and the relationship between gesture and spoken language for the child as a speaker and a listener.

▶ The Emergence of Gesture

Gesture development is predictable in terms of the sequence of gestures as they appear in the child's repertoire and the timeline of each gesture's emergence. This predictability provides the clinician with expectations regarding where the child falls along the continuum of communication development. The emergence of gestures predicts and parallels spoken language development. The *First Words Project* (http://firstwordsproject.com) through Florida State University offers several 16 by 16 series™ Lookbooks. The series offers the 16 Gestures by 16 Months Lookbook, which provides caregivers the types of gestures that children use and the timeline of gesture emergence. In essence, the Lookbook shows that children should be developing around one or two gestures each month from 8 months onward.

Children first communicate intentionally during the illocutionary stage of communication development by using deictic gestures. At approximately 8–10 months of age, the infant begins to show objects to engage the adult partner in an interaction, though the infant will not hand over the object. Within weeks, however, the infant will give the object to their partner to communicate. During the 10–12 month age range, infants also produce ritual request gestures. Ritual request gestures convey the infant's want or need for something by reaching with an open hand or moving an adult's hand to the referent of interest. For example, an infant may take the adult's hand and move it to a bottle of bubbles, indicating that they want the mother to engage in this activity.

Once ritual request, showing, and then giving gestures are in the infant's repertoire, but just before first words emerge, the infant begins pointing. Pointing is particularly important in communication development because it predicts the emergence of language symbols. This prenaming behavior predicts the child's ability to use symbols. Specifically, the hearing child begins to point just before speaking their first word, and the hearing-impaired child points before their first signs (Folven & Bonvillian, 1991). Pointing may in part grow out of the child's use of his or their index finger exploring objects (Locke, Young, Service, & Chandler, 1990). The child explores objects with the index finger while they are alone or with others, but they do not search for adult attention. Later, the index finger is extended and is not in contact with the object. A full-hand point is observed around the same time that the extended index finger is used to point (Lüke et al., 2017). The pointing gesture is now coordinated with social interaction (e.g., eye contact with the caregiver). Other early communicative gestures are also learned starting early in the second year (Fenson et al., 2007).

The emergence of representational gestures coincides with first words, at approximately 12 months of age. However, Goodwyn and Acredolo (1993) found that infants had an advantage in expressing themselves via representational gestures when compared to spoken words. Their first gestured symbol was documented 1 month before their first word. This is the first piece of evidence that children will use gesture to express what they know before they have the spoken language to do so. Put another way, children know more than they say; if we pay attention to the child's gesture, we are observing the knowledge they have represented in memory. This information could be missed if we attended to only spoken language.

On average, infants can have 3–5 representational gestures in their repertoire and as many as 17 gestures by toddlerhood (Acredolo & Goodwyn, 1988). Between 12 and approximately 16 months of age, infants communicate with gestures or words, used individually. Their gesture repertoires, although small, tend to complement or supplement their spoken vocabulary. That is, children in this age group do not have a word *and* a gesture for the same referent but rather have a word *or* a gesture for a referent. When symbols (lexical and gestured) are combined, the sum is referred to as a conceptual vocabulary. Bilingual children (i.e., children learning two languages) also show a larger conceptual vocabulary than would be documented if the clinician only tallied lexical items from one language (Genesee, Paradis, & Crago, 2004).

As children's spoken vocabulary grows, they integrate gesturing with speech. The toddler starts to combine words between 18 and 24 months of age. Just before the emergence of two-word utterances, the child starts putting gestures and words together into gesture-word combinations (Capirici, Iverson, Pizzuto, & Volterra, 1996; Goldin-Meadow & Butcher, 2003; Iverson & Goldin-Meadow, 2005; Morford & Goldin-Meadow, 1992; Özçalışkan & Goldin-Meadow, 2005). These gestures are predominately pointing gestures. The semantic relations expressed in spontaneous gesture-word combinations (e.g., *mommy* + POINT to chair) have been found in the first spoken word combinations (e.g., *mommy chair*) that toddlers produce (Iverson & Goldin-Meadow, 2005; Özçalışkan & Goldin-Meadow, 2005). Findings such as these provide a second piece of evidence that the child has more complex language represented in the mind than spoken language alone would indicate. It is, therefore, important for the clinician to observe gesture as a valid modality of expression.

Emblem gestures seem to appear in early toddlerhood and are most likely routine-based gestures at this point in children's development. For example, the *Rossetti Infant-Toddler Language Scale* (RITLS; Rossetti, 2006)—an assessment of children's language, social–emotional, play, and gesture development from birth to 36 months—first surveys children for emblem gesture (*give me five*) at the 24- to 27-month age interval. They are the last type to emerge. They have been reported for the child as they move toward advancing morphological and syntactic domains of language development (Nicoladis, Mayberry, & Genesee, 1999). Nicoladis et al. (1999) studied bilingual preschoolers who were learning French and English. These children varied in their proficiency with each language. More beat (and representational) gestures were produced for utterances in the child's more proficient language.

As the child's vocabulary expands to include a variety of word classes, gesture will accompany not only nouns, but also verbs, adjectives, and adverbs (Nicoladis et al., 1999).

In summary, gesturing emerges as a natural course of development. Gestures include deictic gestures (ritual request, show, give, point), representational gestures, early communicative and emblem gestures, and beat gestures. Deictic gestures emerge during the prelinguistic period (before age 12 months), and pointing predicts first words. Representational and other early communicative gestures appear with first words and act to complement or supplement spoken vocabulary. Soon after, gesture-spoken language combinations predict two-word utterances. Beat gestures are observed once morpho-syntax begins developing.

Case Study

Given the expectations of development, the clinician knows that the child who points may be closer to first words than the child who is not yet pointing. If we examine the three case studies presented (25-month-old Johnathon, 22-month-old Josephine, and 27-month-old Robert), we see that all three children are using prelinguistic gestures. This places each *at least* at the 12-month-old milestone for gesture development. Each child has the gestural precursor to the single-word stage of development. However, there are children evaluated by the speech-language pathologist who do not yet point. In planning treatment goals for those children, the clinician will work on teaching gestures, particularly pointing, to indicate people, places, and things in the environment (much like initial words do!).

Next, we have an expectation that the child who combines gestures and words is developmentally approaching the 18 to 24 month age range and is closer to two-word utterances than the child who is not yet producing cross-modal communications. All three children should be producing words in combination and gesture in combinations with words. Here, only Johnathon is combining gesture and words and two words in utterances. This places Johnathon within normal limits for expressive language and gesture for his age. Josephine is not yet producing words, words in combinations, or words in combination with gestures. This represents a delay for Josephine in expressive language development. However, she demonstrates two strengths in gesture: (1) She combines gesture and vocalizations, and (2) she produces representational (iconic) gestures to communicate. These behaviors fall within the 12- to 18-month-old developmental range. Robert demonstrates the greatest delay. He is the oldest of the three children, yet he is using only prelinguistic gestures and some social gestures (e.g., shaking head *no*) for basic needs. He is not yet using words, representational gestures, or gesturing in combination with vocals. Therefore, he is delayed in expressive language as well as gesture development.

A strength for both Robert and Josephine is that although their gesture repertoire differentiates their delays, they both used the gestures they had to communicate. Therefore, an initial intervention goal for Robert would be to expand his gesture repertoire to include representational gestures. This would provide him with more communication opportunities and establish semantic representations (meanings or concepts) of the words that he will eventually learn. The next section discusses the relationship between spoken language and deictic and representational gestures.

▶ Gesture Reflects the Child's Mental Representations

Gesture and spoken language tap the same mental representations in memory, particularly semantic representations. The term *mental representation* can be thought of as knowledge that is stored, or represented, in memory. For example, we have mental representations for the meaning of a word (i.e., semantic representation), for our understanding of how gears work, and for problem-solving procedures such as those for the Tower of Hanoi puzzle, conservation problems, or mathematical equivalence. We can, on some level, equate mental representation with knowledge, concept, or meaning. Something else we know is that mental representations evolve through experience (e.g., Barsalou, 1999). That is, learning is not an all-or-nothing phenomenon. Rather, learning is gradual and there is a process of trial and error to update our existing ideas, reorganize incorrect information, and establish accurate and rich mental representations of concepts. Gesture reflects not only the content of a mental representation (remember the *bear* example earlier), but also the richness or stability of that mental representation (Capone, 2007; Church & Goldin-Meadow, 1986).

One underlying cognitive skill that gesture and spoken language share is the symbolic ability to decontextualize a mental representation. Decontextualization refers to the gradual distancing of a symbol from the original referent or learning context (Werner & Kaplan, 1963). It is a skill that's needed to use more complex and abstract spoken language, and later, written language. When children first learn words, their use tends to be contextualized or tied to the original context of learning. For example, a child may use the word *cup* to label only their cup. The context of their cup (i.e., their red sipper cup) is the original context of learning the spoken symbol *cup*. Children gradually begin to decontextualize spoken language by using the word *cup* to refer to all cups that are similar in appearance (i.e., shape) and to request a cup without the object being present. Children extend known words to novel exemplars, even though no one has explicitly taught them each word-new-referent pairing (e.g., *cup* refers to the mother's cup too).

Before children do this with words, this ability to decontextualize, or distance the word from its referent or themselves from a referent, is observed in the deictic gesture sequence. As the child progresses from showing an object to giving an object to pointing to an object, this evolution reflects the child's early ability to see objects as separate from themselves or distance themselves from an object when referring to it. As a second example, representational gestures can meet the same criteria of symbolic use that words satisfy (Goodwyn & Acredolo, 1993; McGregor & Capone, 2004). For example, in Goodwyn and Acredolo's work (1993), representational gestures met symbolic criteria that are applied to words as symbols (p. 695; see also McGregor & Capone, 2004). Specifically, the representational gestures that infant-toddlers produced:

1. Referred to multiple exemplars (e.g., objects and pictures).
2. Were used in the absence of the referent.
3. Were produced spontaneously, without models.
4. Were not part of a well-rehearsed routine (e.g., *eensy-weensy-spider*).

An interesting parallel between the gesture lexicon and the spoken lexicon is found in their relationship to other developing language skills. Early in development, children tend to have many object words in their lexicon when compared to other word classes, such as social words, verbs, and adjectives. Children with more objects in their spoken lexicons tend to have larger vocabularies overall and meet semantic and early grammar milestones earlier than children who have fewer object labels in their spoken lexicons (Bates, Bretherton, & Snyder, 1988; Nelson, 1973). The early gesture lexicon parallels the infant's spoken vocabulary in this relationship. The early gesture lexicon also tends to have a high proportion of object gestures when compared to other word classes. Like children with a high proportion of spoken object labels in their vocabulary, children with more object gestures in their repertoire tend to have larger spoken vocabularies than children with fewer object gestures do.

Gesture Reflects the Child's Readiness to Learn

As gesture and spoken language become integrated and the child begins developing a variety of complex concepts, gesture continues to be a window into the child's developing mental representations. The relationship between what is expressed via gesture and spoken language in an utterance becomes a marker of where the child is in acquiring a particular mental representation (Alibali & Goldin-Meadow, 1993; Capone, 2007; Church & Goldin-Meadow, 1986; Garber, Alibali, & Goldin-Meadow, 1998; Garber & Goldin-Meadow, 2002; Goldin-Meadow, 2000; Goldin-Meadow, Alibali, & Church, 1993; Kelly & Church, 1998; Perry, Church, & Goldin-Meadow, 1988; Pine, Lufkin, & Messer, 2004). To reiterate, we have mental representations of a word, an understanding of how gears work, and solutions to conservation problems, mathematical equivalence problems, or the Tower of Hanoi puzzle, and many others. Because learning is gradual, children move from an inaccurate or incomplete understanding of a concept to an accurate and stable state of concept acquisition over time. Gesture-spoken language combinations change and reflect where the child is in the process of acquiring concepts.

To understand the literature that deals with this issue, it is important to be clear on the methods used to document the phenomenon. Across many of these studies, participants are presented with a task that requires problem-solving, and then participants are asked to explain its solution. Consider the concept of conservation of quantity as tested by Church and Goldin-Meadow (1986). In their study, 5- to 8-year-old children were shown two equivalent glasses of liquid. The liquid from one glass was then poured into a dish. Children were first asked whether the amount of liquid in the dish was equivalent to the liquid that was in the glass. This task tests whether children understand that liquid quantity is conserved (i.e., stays the same) even when the shape of the container holding it changes. The children's task solutions were analyzed for accuracy. Their accuracy in solving the problems served to classify them as having an inaccurate representation of the problem, a transitional representation of the problem, or a stable and accurate representation of the problem. The correct answer is that liquid quantity does not change simply because the shape of the container that holds it changes.

Second, children were asked to explain their response (e.g., "Why?", "How can you tell?"; p. 47). The children's explanations were analyzed for several variables, including the following:

- The modality of the child's response (spoken language, gesture-spoken language combination)
- The information expressed in gesture and the information expressed in their spoken language
- Whether gestured information was the same (matched) or different from (mismatched) the spoken information
- The accuracy of the information expressed in each modality

Three types of gesture-spoken language combinations were analyzed:

- Inaccurate match combination: gesture and spoken language match but express an inaccurate explanation (i.e., inaccurate or incomplete understanding)
- Mismatch combination: gesture and spoken language mismatch and may contain at least one piece of accurate explanation (i.e., transitional understanding)
- Accurate match combination: gesture and spoken language match and express the accurate explanation (i.e., stable and acquired understanding)

For example, a child who understands that liquid quantity is conserved may explain that "The glass is tall and skinny" while producing a pouring motion from the *dish* to the *glass* (Church & Goldin-Meadow, 1986, p. 58). Here, the child expresses two beliefs about why liquid quantity conserves: the compensatory features of the container's shape in two dimensions (in spoken language) and the reversibility of the liquid's transformation (in gesture). Now that we understand the method, we can better understand the findings.

Research shows that as children transition from an incomplete understanding to a stable and accurate understanding of a concept, they transition from mismatch combinations to match combinations in their explanations over time with acquisition of the concept (e.g., Alibali & Goldin-Meadow, 1993; Church, 1999; Perry et al., 1988). Put another way, when children produce mismatch combinations in their explanations, it reflects a transitional knowledge state. During this stage of learning, the child is moving from an incomplete or inaccurate understanding of a concept toward a complete and accurate understanding of that concept. But why do these mismatches occur? It has been suggested that a child who is in transition is still considering multiple hypotheses—both accurate and inaccurate—about the solution to the problem. These hypotheses about the task's solution are simultaneously activated in memory as the child engages in thinking about the task. This simultaneous activation leads to some of these hypotheses being expressed via

gesture and others with spoken language (Garber & Goldin-Meadow, 2002; Goldin-Meadow, Nusbaum, Garber, & Church, 1993).

When children's gesture-spoken language combinations are examined, children who produce many mismatch combinations during their explanations are more likely to benefit from instruction than children who produce few to no mismatch combinations (e.g., Alibali & Goldin-Meadow, 1993; Church & Goldin-Meadow, 1986; Perry et al., 1988). Take as an example a study by Alibali and Goldin-Meadow (1993). This study examined school-aged children's understanding of mathematical equivalence. In this study, children were asked to solve equivalence problems of addition and multiplication and then explain their solutions. All children were provided with instruction on addition equivalence problems, but children who produced mismatch combinations in their explanations were more likely to advance to a correct understanding with this instruction. In addition, children who produced mismatch combinations generalized learning from trained items to untrained exemplars that also tested the concept. Children who did not produce mismatches were also provided with instruction but were less likely to generalize their knowledge to untrained exemplars. This result suggests that learning was richer for children who were already in a transitional phase of learning and that their mismatch combinations reflected their readiness to learn.

Gesture has access to accurate ideas the child has represented in memory, even though they may not be heard in speech (Capone, 2007; Evans et al., 2001; Garber et al., 1998; Goldin-Meadow et al., 1993; Pine et al., 2004). Goldin-Meadow et al. (1993) also found that children expressed more accurate explanations in gesture than in speech. That is, children had beliefs represented about the task's solution, but this knowledge would have gone unnoticed had only speech been assessed. In the study carried out by Alibali and DiRusso (1999), undergraduates explained solutions to algebra word problems. In mismatch combinations, gesture was just as likely as speech to convey the strategy that the participant actually used to solve problems.

Transitional Knowledge in Word Learning

Capone (2007) examined gesturing in a developing language task reported on by Capone and McGregor (2005). This study extended the work of Goldin-Meadow and colleagues in two ways. First, a younger group of children (30-month-old toddlers) was the focus of study. Second, a new task—learning new words—was examined. Toddlers were placed in a transitional learning state by teaching them the names of new object words under three different conditions. In two learning conditions, semantic enrichment was provided by the adult. Semantic enrichment highlighted the shape or function of the trained objects. The third learning condition was a control condition, so no semantic enrichment was provided beyond what experience with the object itself provided for the child. Learning was measured via naming of the objects at the end of the study. In this study, toddlers learned more names for objects taught in the semantic enrichment conditions than in the control condition.

Of importance to our discussion on gesture is an analysis of toddlers' gesture-spoken language combinations during this time of learning. Gesturing was analyzed at the beginning and end of instruction in a separate task that required children to state the functions of objects (*What do we do with this one?*). Several parallels were observed between these toddlers' gesturing and the older children's gesturing from previous studies. First, toddlers responded to these function probes with gestures and spoken language. Second, a transition from mismatched combinations at the beginning of training to accurate match combinations at the end of training was observed only under conditions where naming of the trained objects also occurred (i.e., stability in learning). Also consistent with other studies, accurate knowledge tended to be expressed in gesture before spoken language in mismatched combinations.

It seems then that from the time that gesture and spoken language have started becoming integrated, the relationship between gesture and spoken language serves as an index of the child's readiness to learn a variety of concepts, including new words.

Can caregivers and clinicians see a child gesturing and identify that child's readiness to learn new words? You bet! A study by DiMitrova, Özçalışkan, and Adamson (2016) examined three groups of toddlers—typically developing toddlers, toddlers with autism, and toddlers with Down syndrome. The researchers were interested to know:

1. Are parents in each group aware of their children's gestures?
2. Do parents offer spoken word translations of the gestured referents? For example, if the child gestured by pointing to the bottle but did not have *bottle* in their expressive vocabulary, the parent could translate by saying "that is a bottle" or could opt not to translate by simply handing the child the bottle.
3. If parents translate the gesture by offering the spoken word, will the child learn that word before other words not translated by the parent?

DiMitrova et al. found exciting answers to these questions. First, all three groups of children—including children with autism and children with Down syndrome—gestured before using words. Parents of all three toddler groups translated those gestures into words by labeling what the children were referring to. Finally, children acquired those spoken words that parents had translated from gestures. Children—typically developing, those with autism and those with Down syndrome—more often added the words parents labeled than the words they had not translated from gestures. Gestures that parents did not label were not words that tended to be acquired by the children.

In summary, a child's gesture provides a lens into their readiness to link a new spoken word with an already established representation in memory. As a caregiver—whether parent, teacher, or clinician—be sure to pay attention to the child's interest. Each gesture has the potential to be a stimulus for expressive vocabulary teaching.

▶ Gesture Input for the Child

Although gesture emerges as a natural course of development, the adult's gesture input for the child can be quite influential in shaping the child's gesture expression (Capone, 2007; Goodwyn, Acredolo, & Brown, 2000; Iverson, Capirici, Longobardi, & Caselli, 1999; Iverson, Capirici, Volterra, & Goldin-Meadow, 2008). Iverson et al. (1999) found a gestural analogue to the motherese of speech directed to 16- and 20-month-old children. That is, mothers' gestures co-occurred with speech—approximately 15% of maternal utterances were supported by gesture. Gestures were conceptually simple, referred to the immediate context, and reinforced spoken messages (p. 70).

A cross-cultural study by Iverson et al. (2008) compared American toddlers to Italian youngsters. The Italian infants were part of a culture that is rich in its use of representational gesturing. This rich gesture input was reflected in Italian infants' repertoires of early symbols. When compared to their American counterparts, Italian infants had a larger repertoire of representational gestures and fewer spoken words. When gesture and spoken symbols were combined, Italian infants demonstrated total vocabulary sizes that were comparable to the size of the American infants' vocabularies.

Goodwyn et al. (2000) manipulated the representational gesture input to young toddlers and observed changes in their gesture repertoire. One group of parents was trained to use gestures and spoken words in combination while interacting with their children; two other groups of parents were either trained to increase spoken labeling or received no training. Children of parents who were trained to model gestures and words had larger gesture repertoires at the study's end than the children in the other two groups did. In addition, these children performed better than the other groups on measures of spoken language development. Thus, gesturing by adults produced a benefit not only on the children's own gesture communication but also on their language development more generally.

In the study described earlier, Capone and McGregor (2005) provided semantic enrichment during word learning via the experimenter's gesture cues to the shape or function of the objects. These representational gestures took either the shape of the object being trained or the function of the object being trained. Capone (2007) observed that toddlers from Capone and McGregor's (2005) study produced more representational gestures in isolation when explaining object functions than is typically reported in studies of non-enriched environments. This outcome was partially attributed to the rich gesture environment that the children were provided during instruction by the experimenter.

Gesture input by adults for the child can also influence spoken language development. This type of gesture input can serve as a visual cue or scaffold to the spoken language of the adult. For example, gesturing the function of an object while labeling it highlights important semantic information via the gesture and lexical information via the word model. Capone and McGregor (2005) found that gesture cues to salient object features (object shape or object function) enriched semantic knowledge of the objects and had an effect on word retrieval for naming the objects after instruction was provided (over a no gesture input condition). This effect on word retrieval was replicated in a follow-up study (Capone Singleton, 2012). Capone Singleton (2012) found that teaching an object name paired with an iconic gesture that highlighted its shape was more effective than pointing to the object while naming it. In addition to naming more taught objects, children extended the names learned with shape gestures to novel exemplars of the object category.

McNeil, Alibali, and Evans (2001) compared preschoolers' performance in the following directions when provided gesture cues versus no gesture cues. Results showed that gesture cues were particularly helpful relative to no gesture cues when preschoolers were asked to follow complex directions versus simple directions. Grimminger, Rohlfing, and Stenneken (2010) studied direction following by toddlers with and without language delay. Mothers were asked to have the toddlers follow directions of varying difficulty. Grimminger et al. found that mothers gestured more with spoken directions and held the gestures longer for the toddlers with language delay when directions were more challenging. In turn, the toddlers with language delay performed comparably to their typical peers. Results such as these tell us that when spoken language outpaces a child's level of understanding, the child will access gesture as a visual scaffold to success.

Weismer and Hesketh (1993) examined the effect of gesture cues on learning words that conveyed spatial relations (e.g., *away from, on top of, beside*). These are words that are often found in spoken directions. They compared gesture and no-gesture conditions, but they also compared the effectiveness of this scaffold to other modalities of scaffolding, such as rate of speech in teaching the words and prosodic stress in saying the words (emphatic, neutral). These authors reported that children (with and without language delay) comprehended more words when they were taught with gesture cues than without gesture cues.

A recent study with adults showed that when a speaker uses gesture and spoken language in combination, the listener is sensitive to both (Wu & Coulson, 2007). Brain activation changes as a function of the speaker's use of gesture and spoken language together versus spoken language alone. In their work, Wu and Coulson (2007) measured evoked related potentials (ERP) while adults listened to and saw a speaker in discourse. Greater activation was observed for gesture-spoken language than for spoken language alone at the N400 mark. The N400 mark is a measure of semantic processing and integration in milliseconds after a stimulus is given. Wu and Coulson suggest that gesture activates visual-spatial representations that include shape, functions, and locations of entities.

In summary, gesture input for the child can influence both the child's own gesture repertoire and the child's performance on language tasks. Gesture appears to serve as a scaffold for the child's transition to more advanced language development. This makes gesture a very useful tool in teaching children with and without language impairments to use and understand language.

If we, again, examine the three children from the case study, we see that Johnathon readily uses gesture cues by the adult to understand more complex directions and that Josephine readily imitates adults' gestures. These gesture cues are useful scaffolds for continued language development. In contrast, Robert does not consistently use gesture cues to scaffold his understanding of language, which puts him at a disadvantage in language learning. Improving Robert's attention to gesture cues by the adult, which will provide him with a scaffold for additional language learning, would be a prudent first goal of language intervention.

The next section reviews why gesturing may be useful for the child as both a speaker and a listener.

The Function of Gesturing

When linguistic or metalinguistic skills are immature, all that a child knows may be missed if only their spoken language is assessed. Infants, toddlers, and other children with limited spoken language abilities use gesture to compensate for limitations or immaturities in articulatory or language skills (Acredolo & Goodwyn, 1988; Iverson & Thelen, 1999). In addition, the retrieval and formulation of spoken language to convey what the child knows seems to rely on a rich mental representation, whereas gesture taps into the still evolving or weak mental representation (Alibali & Goldin-Meadow, 1993; Capone, 2007; Capone & McGregor, 2005; Church & Goldin-Meadow, 1986). Gesture allows the child to express ideas that are still forming (the immature, weak, and still evolving mental representation). This may be the case because gestures represent knowledge visually without the demand of formulating a verbal description (Goldin-Meadow, 2003). Speaking places greater demands on memory compared to gesture because speech is encoded sequentially, one piece of information at a time, over time, whereas gesture expresses information holistically, in a chunk.

Gesturing may also ease the child's thinking process. The brain has a limited set of processing resources (Baddeley, 2000). To use an analogy, we can think about neural processing resources as being akin to scholarship money. We have a limited set of resources, or scholarship money. The brain (university administration) can divide the processing resources among several aspects of a task (several students get a little bit of money toward tuition) or, alternatively, those resources can be redirected to one or fewer tasks (funding the entire tuition of one or two students). As with the supply of scholarship money, we cannot increase processing resources. Therefore, we must make the most efficient use of our resources to benefit learning or explaining the task at hand.

How might the child maximize this limited set of brain resources? When the child gestures, they externalize a mental representation. Put another way, when the child gestures, the information that is gestured no longer needs to be remembered and kept track of in the mind because it is expressed externally, by the hands. Externalizing the thought process this way may free the brain's resources so that there are more resources for processing other aspects of a task (Alibali & DiRusso, 1999; Goldin-Meadow, Nusbaum, Kelly, & Wagner, 2001). In summary, gesturing may

make the child's thought process more efficient for learning or performing.

The child's gesture can have an indirect effect on their learning as well because adults can interpret the child's gestural communication. Researchers have shown that adults both with and without training in recognizing gesture communication can glean information from the child's gesture. These adults will subsequently tailor their instruction to the child according to what they understand the child to know (Goldin-Meadow & Singer, 2003; Kelly & Church, 1998; Kelly, Singer, Hicks, & Goldin-Meadow, 2002). In the same vein, the child's gesturing sets up opportunities for the adult to model the spoken language that labels what the child is gesturing. For example, a child may touch their lip with an index finger and round their lips in a blowing motion. This representational gesture conveys a request that the mother blow bubbles. The adult can then model the spoken language used to make this request—for example, "Mommy, blow more bubbles." The child now has an opportunity to imitate and learn the spoken language to request an activity.

The functions that gesturing serve for a child who is typically developing also can serve a child who has difficulty learning spoken language. For example, two of the three children in our case studies are delayed in spoken language. Their gesturing can serve as a focus of language modeling during the language intervention process. The next section briefly gives examples of gesture development in children with language impairments.

Children with Language Learning Impairments

The tight coupling of gesture and spoken language in development is illustrated by children with delays in learning language. Gesture development is a robust phenomenon. Even in the face of sensory, cognitive, and/or language impairments, gesturing emerges in children. Several characteristics of gesture development in typically developing children are also observed in children who are delayed in learning language. Children with language delays are limited in communication and verbal language.

Upon review of the developmental course and the functions of gesturing in typical development, we can see that gesture could serve the clinician in assessment and treatment of children with language delays. The speech-language pathologist encounters a variety of children with language delay, including those with early language delay (ELD) (also referred to as late talkers), specific language impairment (SLI), Down syndrome, autism, and delays caused by multiple-birth pregnancy, to name a few. Gesture provides the speech-language clinician a modality of communication with which to better assess the child. Children with delays in learning language may show a delay in gesture development but like younger, typically developing children, they also use gesture to compensate for limited spoken language in communication.

The robust relationship between the prelinguistic gesture sequence (showing, then giving, then pointing) and first words has been observed in children who demonstrate language delays due to multiple-birth risk factors. McGregor and Capone (2004) studied a set of quadruplets who were at risk of language delay as a result of biological (e.g., prematurity) and environmental (e.g., shared caregiver) factors. Although delayed in language development, the quadruplets were observed to progress from showing to giving to pointing before speaking their first words, albeit at a later age milestone.

Combinations of gesture and spoken language in an utterance were also observed in the set of at-risk quadruplets studied by McGregor and Capone (2004). As part of their study, these authors trained the quadruplets on a small vocabulary set by modeling words paired with representational gestures. These infants showed the developmental sequence of communicating these referents initially via gestures and then later with spoken words, just as observed in typical development. Further, the identical-twins pair of the four children showed a preference for combining gesture and spoken combinations as they transitioned to spoken naming.

Gesture serves a compensatory function for children who demonstrate a delay in language development (Evans et al., 2001; Mainela-Arnold, Evans, & Alibali, 2006; Thal & Tobias, 1992). For example, Thal and Tobias (1992) reported that late talkers gestured more than language-mates but on par with age-mates. Rescorla and Merrin (1998) found that late talkers relied more on several types of nonverbal communication, including gestures as well as gesture-spoken language combinations, to communicate when compared to their normally developing peers.

Capone Singleton and Saks (2015) reviewed the evidence on co-speech gestures as a support for word learning in children with and without language delay. In a pilot study of toddlers with ELD, the authors showed that toddlers learned words presented with shape gestures over no gesture or point gestures. In a follow-up study, Capone Singleton and Anderson (2016) implemented two simultaneous word-learning treatments. In one learning treatment, toddlers heard words paired with shape gestures; in the other learning treatment, the words were paired with other indicators, such as showing or touching gestures. Consistent with other studies, three of the four toddlers with ELD learned more taught words when word models were paired with shape gestures rather than other indicator gestures. In addition, they extended those learned words to novel objects in the learned object categories.

Evans et al. (2001) and Mainela et al. (2006) studied school-aged children with SLI and children who were matched for their ability to solve conservation problems like the ones discussed earlier. Even though the younger children were just as accurate in solving the problems, the children with SLI conveyed more advanced explanations in their gestures in both studies. In particular, children with SLI expressed more information in gesture that was not heard in spoken language and expressed more advanced knowledge when gesture was combined with spoken language than when spoken language was used alone. If only spoken language was assessed, the child with SLI would be penalized for not knowing these concepts when in fact they do understand them.

Gesture production is a strength for children with Down syndrome relative to their development in receptive and expressive language. When compared to typically developing children matched for vocabulary size, children with Down syndrome show greater gesture use (Caselli et al., 1998; Singer Harris, Bellugi, Bates, Jones, & Rossen, 1997). A systematic review of the research that examined gesture development relative to spoken language development in children with Down syndrome confirmed several findings reported over time (Te Kaat-van den Os, Jongmans, Volman, & Lauteslager, 2015). The main findings are summarized as follows:

- Children with Down syndrome use deictic gestures with the exception of a specific deficit in ritual requesting gestures. This has been referred to as a nonverbal requesting deficit in children with Down syndrome (Mundy, Kasari, Sigman, & Ruskin, 1995).
- Early in vocabulary development, children with Down syndrome gesture more frequently than typically developing children who are matched for mental age (and are, therefore, younger). In this case too, they rely on gestures over words.
- Children with Down syndrome use co-speech gestures (e.g., wave bye + say "bye"), but these are not two-concept combinations; they rarely use complementary and supplementary co-speech gesture combinations that convey two concepts (e.g., point to bird + say "fly").

Te Kaat-van den Os et al. (2015) suggest that this is a deficit that children with Down syndrome present in supplementary and complementary co-speech gesture combinations. Further more, this deficit may be a window onto a specific grammatical deficit we see in their spoken language as they age.

Children with autism show impairments in pointing. They have been shown to use pointing to refer as a prenaming activity while looking at a picture book. However, pointing in this kind of context is often accompanied by eye contact in a typically developing child. Children with autism do not point concurrent with eye contact with a communicative partner. Therefore, their atypical gesture development here appears to be related to their social-emotional development rather than their referential development (Charman, 1998; Goodhart & Baron-Cohen, 1993). Some very promising findings in this regard were reported by Capps, Kehres, and Sigman (1998). These authors found that older children with autism use representational gestures in conversational contexts. Because children with autism tend to show great heterogeneity in their profiles, including behavioral, cognitive, and language profiles, greater attention needs to be paid to how gesture development relates to their development in other areas of language and cognition.

▶ Final Thoughts for the Clinician

More research on gesture development in children with a variety of language impairments is still needed. Nevertheless, a clinician who is armed with the knowledge of the typical course of gesture development can begin to use this knowledge in the assessment and intervention of children. They can observe when children are not using gesture to communicate at expected age milestones and can identify this absence as indicative of a delay in development. At the same time, it is important to acknowledge the child who uses gesture to compensate for limited spoken language. It will be important for clinicians to also train parents and other caregivers to recognize gesture as a valid modality of communication.

Study Questions

- List the types of gestures discussed in this chapter and create a timeline indicating when they emerge in development.
- Compare and contrast the types of gestures. How does gesture differ from a signed language such as ASL?

As an intervention tool, the clinician can take the opportunity to observe what the child has already represented (and expressed via gesture) and provide language models for that knowledge. Modeling language, so that the child can hear and imitate it, is a useful scaffold that clinicians use to expand children's language learning. Gesture provides children with a means of expressing what they know and provides the clinician with a jumping-off point in language therapy. Finally, gesture cues can be useful as a visual scaffold for communication attempts as well as for enriching the mental representations of spoken language.

▶ Summary

The act of gesturing is a robust phenomenon. Children begin to gesture within the first 12 months of their lives. Gesturing never disappears—in fact, it becomes integrated with spoken language early on, by 24 months of age. Gesture development is predictable in its own developmental course and in relation to spoken language development. The clinician can use this predictability to their advantage in the clinical process.

Gesture serves many functions for children. Because it reflects what children know, it allows children to communicate before they have the spoken language to do so. Gesture reveals children's learning status through their use of gesture and spoken language in combination, as well as their readiness to learn. Evidence indicates that gesturing eases children's thinking processes, both directly and indirectly (through adult interaction). In addition, adult gestures provide children with a rich source of information. Adults' gesturing positively influences children's gesturing and subsequently their spoken language.

Gesture development in children with language impairments proceeds in much the same way as it does in typically developing children. The exception is that the emergence of gesture may be delayed in children with language impairment, though such children may then use gesture longer to compensate for their difficulties related to spoken language. A clinician who is knowledgeable about gesture development can use this knowledge in the assessment and intervention process for children with language impairments.

- How does the clinician use the predictability of gesture development in clinical assessment of children?
- What is one piece of information the adult can gain by paying attention to the child's gesture? More specifically, state the relationship between gesture and the child's mental representation.

References

Acredolo, L., & Goodwyn, S. (1988). Symbolic gesturing in normal infants. *Child Development, 59*(2), 450–466.

Acredolo, L., & Goodwyn, S. (1996). *Baby signs: How to talk to your baby before your baby can talk.* Chicago, IL: NTB/Contemporary.

Alibali, M. W., & DiRusso, A. A. (1999). The function of gesture in learning to count: More than keeping track. *Cognitive Development, 14*(1), 37–56.

Alibali, M. W., & Goldin-Meadow, S. (1993). Gesture speech mismatch and mechanisms of learning: What the hands reveal about a child's state of mind. *Cognitive Psychology, 25,* 468–523.

Baddeley, A. (2000). The episodic buffer: A new component of working memory? *Trends in Cognitive Science, 4*(11), 417–423.

Barsalou, L. W. (1999). Perceptual symbol systems. *Behavioral and Brain Sciences, 22*(4), 577–660.

Bates, E., Bretherton, I., & Snyder, L. (1988). *From first words to grammar: Individual differences and dissociable mechanisms.* New York, NY: Cambridge University Press.

Capirici, O., Iverson, J., Pizzuto, E., & Volterra, V. (1996). Gestures and words during the transition to two-word speech. *Journal of Child Language, 23,* 645–673.

Capone, N. C. (2007). Tapping toddlers' evolving semantic representation via gesture. *Journal of Speech, Language, and Hearing Research, 50*(3), 732–745.

Capone, N. C., & McGregor, K. K. (2005). The effect of semantic representation on toddlers' word retrieval. *Journal of Speech, Language, Hearing Research, 48*(6), 1468–1480.

Capone Singleton, N. (2012). Can semantic enrichment lead to naming in a word extension task? *American Journal of Speech-Language Pathology, 21,* 279–292

Capone Singleton, N. C., & Anderson, L. (2016). *Co-speech gesture to support word learning in toddlers with small vocabularies.* Poster presented at the annual conference of the American Speech-Language-Hearing Association, Philadelphia, PA.

Capone Singleton, N. C., & Saks, J. (2015). Co-speech gesture input as a support for language learning in children with and without early language delay. *Perspectives on Language Learning and Education, 22,* 61–71.

Capps, L., Kehres, J., & Sigman, M. (1998). Conversational abilities among children with autism and children with developmental delays. *Autism, 2*(4), 325–344.

Caselli, M. C., Vicari, S., Longobardi, E., Lami, L., Pizzoli, C., & Stella, G. (1998). Gestures and words in early development of children with Down syndrome. *Journal of Speech-Language-Hearing Research, 41,* 1125–1135.

Charman, T. (1998). Specifying the nature and course of the joint attention impairment in autism in the preschool years: Implications for diagnosis and intervention. *Autism, 2*(1), 61–79.

Church, R. B. (1999). Using gesture and speech to capture transitions in learning. *Cognitive Development, 14,* 313–342.

Church, R. B., & Goldin-Meadow, S. (1986). The mismatch between gesture and speech as an index of transitional knowledge. *Cognition, 23,* 43–71.

DiMitrova, N., Özçalışkan, S., & Adamson, R. B. (2016). Parents' translations of child gestures facilitate word learning in children with autism, Down syndrome, and typical development. *Journal of Autism and Developmental Disorders, 46,* 221–231.

Esseily, R., Jacquet, A., & Fagard, J. (2011). Handedness for grasping objects and pointing and the development of language in 14-month old infants. *Laterality, 16*(5), 565–585.

Evans, J. A., Alibali, M. W., & McNeil, N. M. (2001). Divergence of verbal expression and embodied knowledge: Evidence from

speech and gesture in children with specific language impairment. *Language and Cognitive Processes, 16*(2/3), 309–331.

Fenson, L., Marchman, V. A., Thal, D. J., Dale, P. S., Reznick, S., & Bates, E. (2007). *Macarthur-bates communicative development inventories* (2nd ed.). Baltimore, MD: Brookes.

Folven, R., & Bonvillian, J. D. (1991). The transition from nonreferential to referential language in children acquiring American Sign Language. *Developmental Psychology, 27*(5), 806–816.

Garber, P., Alibali, M. W., & Goldin-Meadow, S. (1998). Knowledge conveyed in gesture is not tied to the hands. *Child Development, 69*(1), 75–84.

Garber, P., & Goldin-Meadow, S. (2002). Gesture offers insight into problem-solving in adults and children. *Cognitive Science, 26,* 817–831.

Genesee, F., Paradis, J., & Crago, M. B. (2004). *Dual language development and disorders: A handbook on bilingualism and second language learning.* Baltimore, MD: Paul H. Brookes.

Goldin-Meadow, S. (2000). Beyond words: The importance of gesture to researchers and learners. *Child Development, 71*(1), 231–239.

Goldin-Meadow, S. (2003). *Hearing gesture: How our hands help us think.* Cambridge, MA: Harvard University Press.

Goldin-Meadow, S., Alibali, M. W., & Church, R. B. (1993). Transitions in concept acquisition: Using the hand to read the mind. *Psychological Review, 100*(2), 279–297.

Goldin-Meadow, S., & Butcher, C. (2003). Pointing toward two-word speech in young children. In S. Kita (Ed.), *Pointing: Where language, culture, and cognition meet* (pp. 85–107). Mahway, NJ: Lawrence Erlbaum Associates.

Goldin-Meadow, S., Butcher, C., Mylander, C., & Dodge, M. (1994). Nouns and verbs in a self-styled gesture system: What's in a name? *Cognitive Psychology, 27*(3), 259–319.

Goldin-Meadow, S., Nusbaum, H., Garber, P., & Church, R. B. (1993). Transitions in learning: Evidence for simultaneously activated strategies. *Journal of Experimental Psychology: Human Perception and Performance, 19*(1), 92–107.

Goldin-Meadow, S., Nusbaum, H., Kelly, S. D., & Wagner, S. (2001). Explaining math: Gesturing lightens the load. *Psychological Science, 12*(6), 516–522.

Goldin-Meadow, S., & Singer, M. A. (2003). From children's hands to adults' ears: Gesture's role in the learning process. *Developmental Psychology, 39*(3), 509–520.

Goldin-Meadow, S., & Wagner, S. M. (2005). How our hands help us learn. *Trends in Cognitive Sciences, 9*(5), 234–241.

Goodhart, F., & Baron-Cohen, S. (1993). How many ways can the point be made? Evidence from children with and without autism. *First Language, 13*(3), 225–233.

Goodwyn, S., & Acredolo, L. (1993). Symbolic gesture versus word: Is there a modality advantage for onset of symbol use? *Child Development, 64,* 688–701.

Goodwyn, S. W., Acredolo, L. P., & Brown, C. A. (2000). Impact on symbolic gesturing on early language development. *Journal of Nonverbal Behavior, 24*(2), 81–103.

Grimminger, A., Rohlfing, K. J., & Stenneken, P. (2010). Children's lexical skills and task demands affect gestural behavior in mothers of late-talking children and children with typical language development. *Gesture, 10*(2–3), 251–278.

Iverson, J. M., Capirici, O., Longobardi, E., & Caselli, M. C. (1999). Gesturing in mother-child interactions. *Cognitive Development, 14,* 57–75.

Iverson, J. M., Capirici, O., Volterra, V., & Goldin-Meadow S. G. (2008). Learning to talk in a gesture-rich world: Early communication in Italian vs. American children. *First Language, 28*(2), 164–181

Iverson, J. M., & Goldin-Meadow, S. (2001). The resilience of gesture in talk: Gestures in blind speakers and listeners. *Developmental Science, 4*(4), 416–422.

Iverson, J. M., & Goldin-Meadow, S. (2005). Gesture paves the way for language development. *Psychological Science, 16*(5), 368–371.

Iverson, J. M., & Thelen, E. (1999). Hand, mouth, and brain: The dynamic emergence of speech and gesture. *Journal of Consciousness Studies, 6*(11–12), 19–40.

Kelly, S. D., & Church, R. B. (1998). A comparison between children's and adult's ability to detect conceptual information conveyed through representational gesture. *Child Development, 69*(1), 85–93.

Kelly, S. D., Singer, M., Hicks, J., & Goldin-Meadow, S. (2002). A helping hand in assessing children's knowledge: Instructing adults to attend to gesture. *Cognition and Instruction, 20*(1), 1–26.

Locke, A., Young, A., Service, B., & Chandler, P. (1990). Some observations on the origins of the pointing gesture. In V. Volterra and C. J. Erting (Eds.), *From gesture to language in hearing and deaf children* (pp. 42–55). New York, NY: Springer-Verlag.

Lüke, C., Ritterfeld, U., Grimminger, A., Liszkowski, U., & Rohlfing, K. J. (2017). Development of pointing gestures in children with typical and delayed language acquisition. *Journal of Speech, Language, and Hearing Research, 60*, 3185–3197.

Mainela-Arnold, E., Evans, J. L., & Alibali, M. W. (2006). Understanding conservation delays in children with language impairment: Task representations revealed in speech and gesture. *Journal of Speech, Language, and Hearing Research, 49*, 1267–1279.

McGregor, K. K., & Capone, N. C. (2004). Genetic and environmental interactions in determining the early lexicon: Evidence from a set of tri-zygotic quadruplets. *Journal of Child Language, 31*(2), 311–337.

McNeil, N. M., Alibali, M. W., & Evans, J. (2001). The role of gesture in children's comprehension of spoken language: Now they need it, now they don't. *Journal of Nonverbal Behavior, 24*(2), 131–149.

Morford, M., & Goldin-Meadow, S. (1992). Comprehension and production of gesture in combination with speech in one-word speakers. *Journal of Child Language, 19*(3), 559–580.

Mundy, P., Kasari, C., Sigman, M., & Ruskin, E. (1995). Nonverbal communication and early language acquisition in children with Down syndrome and in normally developing children. *Journal of Speech, Language and Hearing Research, 38*, 157–167.

Nelson, K. (1973). Structure and strategy in learning to talk. *Monographs of the Society for Research in Child Development, 143*(38).

Nicoladis, E., Mayberry, R., & Genesee, F. (1999). Gesture and early bilingual development. *Developmental Psychology, 35*(2), 514–526.

Özçalışkan, S., & Goldin-Meadow, S. (2005). Gesture is at the cutting edge of early language development. *Cognition, 96*(3), B101–B113.

Perry, M., Church, R. B., & Goldin-Meadow, S. (1988). Transitional knowledge in the acquisition of concepts. *Cognitive Development, 3*(4), 359–400.

Pine, K. J., Lufkin, N., & Messer, D. (2004). More gestures than answers: Children learning about balance. *Developmental Psychology, 40*(6), 1059–1067.

Rescorla, L., & Merrin, L. (1998). Communicative intent in late-talking toddlers. *Applied Psycholinguistics, 19*(3), 393–414.

Rossetti, L. (2006). *The Rossetti Infant-Toddler Language Scale.* East Moline, IL: LinguiSystems, Inc.

Singer Harris, N. G., Bellugi, U., Bates, E., Jones, W., & Rossen, M. (1997). Contrasting profiles of language development in children with Williams and Down syndromes. *Developmental Neuropsychology, 13*(3), 345–370.

te Kaat-van den Os, D. J. A., Jongmans, M. J., Volman, M. J. M., & Lauteslager, P. E. M. (2015). Do gestures pave the way? A systematic review of the transitional role of gesture during the acquisition of early lexical and syntactic milestones in young children with Down syndrome. *Child Language Teaching and Therapy, 31*(1),71–84.

Thal, D., & Tobias, S. (1992). Communicative gestures in children with delayed onset of oral expressive vocabulary. *Journal of Speech and Hearing Research, 35*(6), 1281–1289.

Weismer, S. E., & Hesketh, L. J. (1993). The influence of prosodic and gestural cues on novel word acquisition by children with specific language impairment. *Journal of Speech and Hearing Research, 36*, 1013–1025.

Werner, H., & Kaplan, B. (1963). *Symbol formation.* New York, NY: John Wiley & Sons.

Wu, Y. C., & Coulson, S. (2007). How iconic gestures enhance communication: An ERP study. *Brain and Language, 101*(3), 234–245.

SECTION II
The Domains of Language

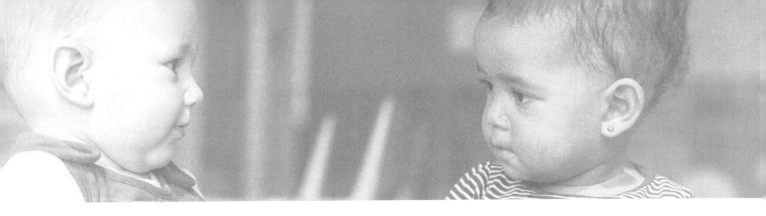

CHAPTER 6

Social-Emotional Bases of Pragmatic and Communication Development

Carol E. Westby, PhD, CCC-SLP

OBJECTIVES

- Describe the social/cognitive underpinnings of language and communicative competence
- Explain the ways in which child characteristics, disabilities, and environmental factors influence the development of social and communicative competence and pragmatic language skills
- Assess children's social-emotional and language bases for communicative competence
- Describe a philosophy of intervention for social-communicative pragmatic deficits

KEY TERMS

Attachment
Attunement
Autobiographical memory
Communicative competence
Coordination/coregulation
Emotions
Endogenous/intrinsic factors
Episodic memory
Epigenetics/epigenesist

Exogenous/extrinsic factors
Horizontal development
Independent/individualist
Initiating behavior request (IBR)
Initiating joint attention (IJA)
Intentionality
Interdependent/collectivist
Joint attention (JA)
Pragmatics

Primary intersubjectivity
Referencing
Responding to joint
 attention (RJA)
Secondary intersubjectivity
Temperament
Theory of mind (ToM)
Vertical development

▸ Introduction

Language acquisition involves three components: (1) the learning of well-formedness—that is, the rules of grammar (syntax); (2) the capacity to refer and to mean (semantics); and (3) communicative function or intent—that is, the ability to get things done with gestures and words (pragmatics). Without communicative intent, other aspects of language are meaningless. Some children appear to master syntax and semantics but fail to use them for interactive communication. True language is a social activity, and a primary function of language is to sustain and maintain emotional attachments.

Each of these components of language is addressed in the three case studies discussed in the chapter. For all three children, the evaluator claims that aspects of pragmatics are the children's communicative strengths. The evaluator notes that all three children engage in joint attention, turn-taking, and prelinguistic gestures; furthermore, the evaluator also suggests that Josephine (the late bloomer) and Robert (the late talker) show strengths in these areas. Some children with developmental delays or language impairments, however, exhibit delays or disorders in these early pragmatic elements; in some cases, deficits in pragmatic aspects of communication are most delayed or different. Also, many children who initially appear to exhibit fairly typical pragmatic skills, despite delays or deficits primarily in syntax and semantics, later exhibit difficulties with social-emotional/pragmatic aspects of communication. Today, increasing attention is being given to the early precursors of communicative intent and pragmatic communication skills as well as the long-term influences of both early and later differences in social-emotional development.

This chapter discusses the nature and development of social competence—the foundations for pragmatic language skills—including precursors to a theory of mind and the affective and social bases of communication. It also explores the development of communicative intent and social uses of language, factors affecting social-emotional aspects of communication, and methods for assessing and facilitating the social-emotional bases of communication and communicative competence.

▸ Underpinnings of Social Competence and Language

Beauchamp and Anderson (2010) presented a conceptualization of social skills development they termed SOCIAL for "socio-cognitive integration of abilities." SOCIAL defines and integrates the core dimensions of social skills: biological, psychological, and social. Social competence has underlying neurological foundations (the biological dimension); it requires cognitive-executive and social-affective processes (the psychological dimension) and social experiences that influence the ways social skills develop and their specific manifestation (the social dimension). SOCIAL addresses both what the child brings to the process of social-emotional development and what and how the environment influences this development.

SOCIAL proposes a set of relationships between *cognitive functions* (e.g., attention/executive functioning, communication, socioemotional skills), *mediators* (e.g., intrinsic/extrinsic factors) that influence the cognitive functioning, and resulting *social competence* (i.e., appropriate, effective, skillful functioning in social situations).

Social competence in social situations requires the following steps:

- Observe/encode social cues
- Interpret social cues
- Form an intent/goal to respond to the social cues
- Have access to generating a vocal/verbal/behavioral response
- Carry out the social response
- Evaluate the response/repair response when necessary

These steps are developmental, but even by the preschool years, children have some ability to evaluate the effectiveness of their communicative responses and repair or modify them. Refer to **FIGURE 6-1**. The SOCIAL model can be used to explain why and where breakdowns in social competence may occur.

Cognitive Functions

Social competence requires underlying cognitive functions. Children must attend to their environments, be motivated to interact, use their executive functions to regulate their interactions, and process cognitive/linguistic information and social cues. Children communicate to maintain social contact, often for no other reason than to share an experience, feeling, or thought with another person (Bates, Bretherton, Beeghly-Smith, & McNew, 1982). This motivation for sharing reflects the need infants have to sustain *intersubjectivity*—that is, an interfacing of mind with other persons—the earliest aspect of social-emotional development. *Intentionality* drives language acquisition, and intersubjectivity drives intentionality. Initially, this intersubjectivity reflects

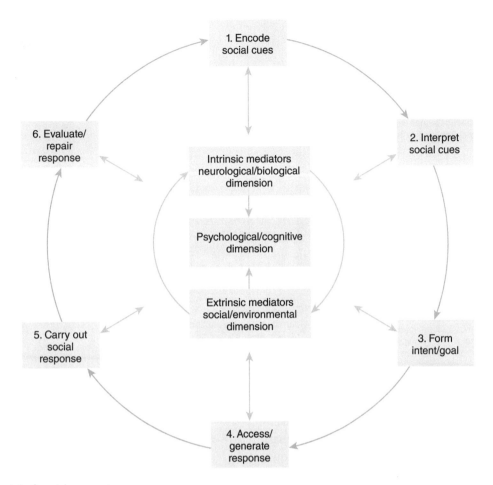

FIGURE 6-1 Model of social competence.

the child's experience of emotions. Gradually, however, children come to recognize others' experiences of emotions. Increasingly, this appreciation of inter-subjectivity, or what has been termed a *theory of mind* (ToM), contributes to children's ability to predict behaviors of others and participate in effective social conversation (Bretherton, 1991; Bruner, 1986; Hewitt, 1994; Zlatev, Racine, Sinha, & Itkonen, 2008). Participating in discourse—particularly discourse about past experiences—further promotes ToM and the ability to make appropriate inferences that are essential for appropriate social interactions and text comprehension.

ToM is not a unitary construct; there are several types of ToM, each with differing neurophysiological underpinnings (Abu-Akel & Shamay-Tsoory, 2011; Northoff et al., 2006). **FIGURE 6-2** shows the types of ToM. Cognitive ToM involves the ability to attribute mental states—beliefs, intents, desires, pretending, knowledge, etc.—to oneself and others and to understand that others have mental states that are different from one's own. Affective ToM has two aspects: affective cognitive ToM—the ability to recognize emotions in oneself and others, reflect on one's own emotions, and regulate one's emotions; and affective empathy, which is the ability to share and respond to the feelings

of others. Cognitive and affective ToM can be further differentiated into interpersonal ToM, used to infer mental states and emotions of others, and intrapersonal ToM, used to reflect on one's own mental states and emotions. Each of these types of ToM has different developmental trajectories, and it is possible for persons to have differing strengths and weaknesses in each of these areas. Affective ToM begins to develop during the earliest infant-caregiver interactions and continues to develop into adulthood (Sebastian et al., 2012). Cognitive aspects of ToM develop along with language development. By age 16, adolescents' response to cognitive ToM tasks is similar to that of adults. ToM cannot develop without social interactions, and effective social interactions are not possible without ToM.

ToM, or intersubjectivity, which underlies developing social and language competence, is influenced by endogenous or intrinsic factors within the child and exogenous or extrinsic factors in the environment. Primary intersubjectivity occurs early (when the child is 0–6 months of age) and reflects a system that promotes the infant's tendency to use and respond to eye contact, facial affect, vocal behavior, and body posture in interactions with caregivers. Primary intersubjectivity involves a sharing of emotions between persons.

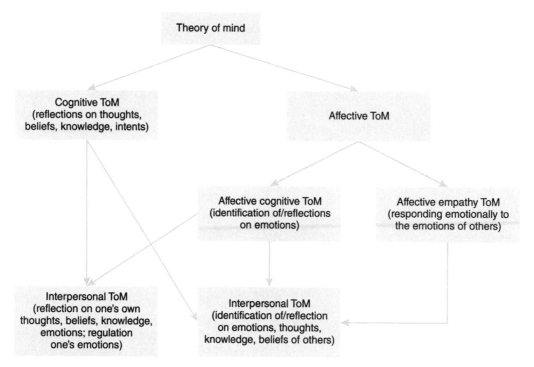

FIGURE 6-2 Theory of mind dimensions.

This primarily dyadic interactive phase of social development provides the information and experience that, in combination with cognitive maturation, allows infants to begin to develop representations of themselves and others as having both distinct and shared affective experiences.

Secondary intersubjectivity requires *joint attention* (JA), which involves conscious awareness of both self and others looking at the same object or as sharing an experience and occurs between 6 and 18 months of age (Tomasello, 1995). In addition to joint attention, secondary intersubjectivity involves *social referencing* or borrowing the perspective of other persons. The child interprets the adult's emotional expression and uses the affective display to regulate their behaviors toward environmental objects, persons, and situations. This enables children to use others' reactions to resolve uncertainty about a situation and determine the effects of their behaviors on others. This type of early engagement is integral to the development of the ability to understand others' thoughts, intentions, and feelings, and it reflects sensitivity to the reward values of sharing with others. The experience of secondary intersubjectivity has positive reinforcement value for the child and, therefore, contributes to ongoing motivation for social interactions. Infant joint attention predicts childhood cognitive and language outcomes, self-regulation, and individual differences in childhood social interactive competence in typically developing children, at-risk children, and children with autism (Mundy, 2016).

Several types of joint attention develop in the 3- to 18-month period of infancy:

- *Responding to joint attention (RJA)*: The infant follows the direction of gaze, head turn, and/or point gesture of another person.
- *Initiating joint attention (IJA)*: The infant uses eye contact and/or deictic gestures (pointing or showing) to spontaneously initiate coordinated attention with a social partner. This communication is a type of protodeclarative. In other words, the infant is seeking interaction with another person simply for the sake of sharing an experience.
- *Initiating behavior requests (IBR)*: The infant uses eye contact and gestures to initiate attention coordination with another person to elicit aid in obtaining an object or event. IBR is a protoimperative; it is used for less social but more instrumental purposes.

RJA is a type of primary intersubjectivity; IJA and IBR reflect secondary subjectivity. RJA and IJA serve social functions. The goals and reinforcement of RJA and IJA behaviors revolve around the sharing of experiences with others and the positive emotions that such early social sharing engender in young children. IJA and RJA are both related to later language development and social outcomes in the second and third years of life and decreased risk of later disruptive behaviors (Mundy & Thorp, 2006). In contrast, high rates of IBR, which may reflect an impulsive and object-driven style of behavior, are associated with greater externalizing or disruptive behaviors in later life (Sheinkopf, Mundy, Claussen, & Willoughby, 2004).

Social-emotional development reflected in joint attention initially triggers or enables language; later, language becomes the medium through which children further develop social-emotional cognition that enables understanding of their social world and acquisition of their culture. It enables them to share and understand emotions, goals, and expectations (Bloom, 1993; Bretherton & Beeghly, 1982; Lewis, 2014; Tronick, 2007). Language acquisition cannot be understood by looking at only the child's cognitive and linguistic abilities because it is the child's emotional development that drives communication. Instead, language acquisition can only be understood by also looking at the social interactions or cultural settings in which language occurs (Bruner, 1983). To acquire language, children must be sensitive to the sound patterns and grammatical constraints of the language, referential requirements, and communicative intentions. Such sensitivity grows in the process of fulfilling certain general nonlinguistic functions—predicting the environment, interacting transactionally, getting to goals with the aid of another, and so on. Bruner has suggested that such functions must first be fulfilled by prelinguistic communicative means; only after these means reach certain levels will children generate linguistic hypotheses.

Because communication depends on effective interactions between infants and adults, we must understand the intrinsic and extrinsic mediators children and adults bring to interactive episodes and the ways in which these interactions are organized.

Intrinsic Mediators the Child Brings to Interactions

The child's neurobiological system influences their cognitive functioning. Infants are born with a motivational system that drives them to attach to their caregivers, and each infant comes with their own unique temperament and response to interactions with caregivers.

Infant Engagement Cues

Infants are born with endogenous processes that enable them to perceive people as being similar to themselves. This awareness is not based on facial features or movement but rather on affective awareness. Legerstee (2005) proposed that infants are born with an affect sharing device (AFS) that has three components:

- Self-referential processes that allow infants an awareness of their own mental states
- Interpersonal awareness that allows infants to recognize the emotions of others
- An innate sense of emotional attunement

The AFS enables infants to recognize whether their own emotions and the emotions of others are similar. Mirror neurons in the cortex may be implicated in this attunement process (Bertenthal & Longo, 2007). Mirror neurons respond similarly both when individuals initiate an action or experience an emotion and when they see the same action performed or the same emotion experienced by someone else (Schulte-Ruther, Markowitsch, Fink, & Piefke, 2007).

At approximately 6 weeks of age, infants can visually fixate on their mothers' eyes, hold the fixation, and widen their own eyes. This fixation results in the mother feeling a greater sense of connection with the infant. With this eye fixation, social play between infant and adult begins in earnest. Infants can not only seek out interaction, but also terminate interaction. They can gaze directly into the adult's eyes, can turn their heads slightly so that they see the adult out of the corner of their eyes, or can lower their heads and turn far enough away to totally avoid visual contact. These engagement-disengagement behaviors enable infants to control the amount of stimulation they desire (Schaffer, 1984; Stern, 1977).

By the end of the third month after birth, infants' mature motor control of gaze direction gives them complete control over what they see. With this ability, they can start or stop face-to-face interaction because these interactions are built around mutual gaze. By looking at the mother, infants can start an encounter because the mother will look back. Children can continue the interaction by smiling or end it by averting their eyes or turning their heads away. Mutual gaze represents the turn-taking that is later seen in verbal conversation. In these early months, babies are learning the nonverbal basis of social interaction upon which language is later built. They are able not only to fixate on an object, but also to pursue it. In the second half of the first year, infants become interested in objects as their increasing motor abilities enable them to reach, grasp, and manipulate the objects in their world. Once this occurs, the mother-infant interaction becomes a triadic affair between the mother, infant, and object.

Infants younger than 1 week old can distinguish and imitate facial expressions such as happy, sad, and surprised (Meltzoff & Moore, 1977). Near the end of the first year, they are able to engage in social referencing—that is, they are able to perceive the link between a person's affect and the eliciting stimulus.

Infants use this social referencing to make judgments about how to respond to a situation. They are particularly alert to a parent's indications of fear. By the end of the first year, child and parent start engaging in ongoing co-referencing, each noting and responding to the emotional sharing of the other. These social-emotional characteristics lead infants to interact with adults in ways that are useful for language development. All neurotypical babies exhibit these gaze and emotional expression behaviors. They do not, however, all respond in the same way to their social and physical environments.

Temperament

Each baby has their own personality or *temperament*. *Temperament* is defined as the behavioral style or the, "how of behavior. Temperament significantly determines the pattern of interactions infants experience with their environments, including what infants respond to and how they respond. Variations in infant temperament involve differences in general mood, activity level, and adaptability to changes in routine. Large differences also exist between babies in terms of the intensity of their responses, their tendency to approach or withdraw from new experiences, their persistence, their distractibility, and their sensitivity to stimulation.

Thomas and Chess (1977) described three temperamental patterns: *easy, slow-to-warm-up,* and *difficult.* Recently, more positive terms have been substituted for Thomas and Chess's original labels: *flexible, fearful,* and *feisty.* Flexible babies have a regular overall pattern. They accept new experiences readily, exhibit mild reactions to discomfort, and make smooth adjustments to changes in routines. Fearful babies share some of the same style of flexible babies, but tend to withdraw from new experiences and are shy around others. They will gradually adapt to new situations but need to be handled sensitively in the process. Such babies generally cannot be pressured into new experiences. Feisty babies are easily distressed. They express their likes—and more often, their dislikes—in no uncertain terms. They react forcefully and negatively to new experiences and even minor changes in routine, and they show little or no consistency in their schedule. It is difficult for caregivers to predict the behaviors of these children. Temperament acts as a modulator of joint attention. Infants with fearful or feisty temperaments engage in less frequent gaze-following or RJA (Todd & Dixon, 2010). This reduced RJA may be the mechanism underlying temperament-language relationships. Toddlers with fearful or feisty temperaments show poorer vocabulary and morphological abilities (Garello, Viterbori, & Usai, 2012).

Infants' intrinsic biological temperaments interact with external environmental factors. Their temperaments influence the ways that caregivers interact with them and the types of interactions they experience can influence their temperaments. Environmental factors can either ameliorate or potentiate genetically based temperamental risks. What is essential for the best development of children is the existence of a "good fit" between infant and caregiver. Flexible babies, who are abundantly adaptable, can be reared by nearly anyone. Raising fearful and feisty infants takes more sensitivity and insight on part of the caregivers. Goodness of fit results when the expectations and demands of the environment are in accord with the child's own capacities, motives, and behavioral style. Poorness of fit occurs when dissonances between the two lead to incompatibility. An active, intense parent may be comfortable with an intense baby who cries vigorously with change. A parent who expects the infant to have a regular time routine and be able to tolerate changes in caregivers may be unnerved by a feisty baby and have no idea how to calm or interact with the child. Children with flexible temperaments adapt to a variety of caregiving styles; in contrast, children with fearful or feisty temperaments require more sensitively attuned caregiving interactions if they are to develop the ability to regulate their social interactions (Bakermans-Kranenburg & van IJzendoorn, 2006). Children's temperaments also influence the ways in which mothers engage in reminiscing or talking about past experiences (Laible, 2004). Mothers are more likely to elaborate when discussing a child's past behavior if they perceive that the child is high in effortful control. Mothers are better able to elaborate in reminiscing with children whose temperaments are easy or flexible because such children are inclined to self-regulation and attention. In contrast, children with feisty temperaments may limit their mother's ability to effectively communicate with them when discussing the past. Laible (2004) noted that children ages 3 to 5 years whose mothers engaged in more elaborated discussion of past experiences displayed more behavioral internalization and higher levels of emotional understanding than children whose mothers did not elaborate in the same way.

Extrinsic Mediators Caregivers Bring to Interactions

Children set the tone for interactions, but caregivers determine what children learn about interactions within a family and culture. Child-caregiver interactions can cause epigenetic changes (modifications of genetic expression) that result in changes in the child's biological/neurological functioning that influence the child's cognitive functioning.

Attunement/Attachment

Parents vary in the degree to which they respond sensitively to their infants' cues. In some instances, parents may be less able to read children's cues, may be less available to engage in interaction with children, or may misinterpret an infant's behavior (Tronick, 2007). Some parents may simply be poor matches with their infants. They may not be able to cope effectively with the temperamental style of their infants, or they may fail to attune to their infants affectively. Affect attunement refers to the ways in which internal emotional states are brought into communication within infant-caregiver interactions. Both the adult and the infant can be active in the attunement (Legerstee, 2005).

Alignment is one component of affect attunement in which an individual alters their state to approximate that of the other member in the dyad. For example, a parent might notice a child's smile and mirror back a smile; an infant may notice a parent's apprehensive or fearful look when watching the child crawl to some steps and mirror the parent's expression. Alignment can be primarily a one-way process in which either the adult's or the infant's state changes to match and anticipate that of the other, or it can be a bilateral process, in which both the parent and the infant modify their states.

When there are high levels of attunement between parents and children, they develop an emotional resonance that influences their sensitivity to other aspects of each other's minds. Some parents, however, do not easily attune to their infants. They may not be sensitive to their infant's states and hence may either overstimulate or understimulate their infants. Adults who overstimulate tend to engage in overcontrolling, intrusive behaviors with infants. Overstimulating adults may fail either to read or respond to infants' efforts to control stimulation. What the baby does matters relatively lesser. Highly attuned or high-affect-monitoring parents spend more time than less attuned or low-affect-monitoring mothers focused on the objects their infants are focused on.

Attunement in secure parent-child interactions is related to later language development. Depressed, emotionally disturbed, or intellectually limited parents are more likely to be low-affect monitors and may understimulate their infants. Infants with understimulating or overstimulating caregivers have fewer opportunities to participate in satisfying social interactions and discover ways in which they can affect their environments through communication.

Children reared in abusive and/or emotionally neglectful circumstances may experience fewer instances of positive social interactions; even when such an interaction is available, the children may be in such a constant state of "fight or flight" that they cannot attend to the communication (Perry, 1997). Such children may suffer long-lasting social-behavioral-communicative deficits. The lack of appropriate affective experiences in early life can result in neurological differences and associated malorganization of attachment capabilities. During development, abused/neglected children spend so much time in a low-level state of fear that they are constantly focusing on nonverbal cues. Such children feel no emotional attachment to other humans, and they fail to develop appropriate social-interactive relationships and communication skills (Alessandri & Lewis, 1996).

Caregivers' alignment/attunement with infants influences the types of attachments children form. Children's attachments to their caregivers are influenced by what the child brings to the interaction, but are highly dependent on their experiences with caregivers. Mothers' communication with their children and the child's attachment to the mother have been shown to be related to the caregiver's own attachment history and their interpretation of that history (Main, 1996). Four types of caregiver-child attachments have been identified based on children's behavior in the "Strange Situation" (Ainsworth, Blehar, Waters, & Wall, 1978). With this assessment method, the caregiver brings the child into a playroom, leaves the room briefly, and then returns. Attachment categories are based on what the child does upon the caregiver's return:

- Children with *secure attachment* protest the mother's departure and quiet down promptly on the mother's return, accepting comfort from her and returning to exploration or play. Children with secure attachment have caregivers who are attuned to their child's emotions.
- Children with *avoidant attachment* show little to no signs of distress at the mother's departure, a willingness to explore the toys, and little to no visible response to the mother's return. The caregivers of children with avoidant attachment are rejecting or unavailable.
- Children with *resistant-ambivalent attachment* show sadness on the mother's departure and on the mother's return; they also show some ambivalence, signs of anger, or reluctance to "warm up" to her, and they fail to return to play. Children with resistant-ambivalent attachment have caregivers who are inconsistent. They may be sensitively

attuned with the child at one time but intrusive, rejecting, and angry at other times.

- Children with *disorganized-disoriented attachment* seem to have no clear strategy for responding to their caregivers. They may at times avoid or resist approaches to the caregiver; they may also seem confused or frightened by them or freeze or still their movements when they approach them. Caregivers of children with disorganized-disoriented attachment ignore the child's needs or may react to the child in frightening/traumatizing ways.

If infants/toddlers experience severe abuse or neglect with a caregiver who seeks an attachment with them (for example, it may happen to children raised in institutions from infancy), they may develop what is term *reactive attachment*. Children with reactive attachment disorder fail to develop a conscience and attachment to anyone. Caregiver-infant attachment has life-long consequences for a person's social emotional and communicative development (Siegel, 2012).

Caregiver-infant attachment patterns influence children's cognitive abilities to encode and interpret social-emotional cues. Mothers of children of securely attached children talk more with their children about emotions. This facilitates children's development of affective ToM. They have greater emotion awareness, the ability to attribute mental states to others, and a greater capacity to regulate their emotions. In contrast, mothers of children in insecure relationships are less comfortable in talking with their children about difficult emotions and are less likely to respond to their children's expressions of emotions. Children who are insecure and avoidant may ignore mental states of others, while those who are insecure and resistant may focus only on their own mental states, avoiding interactions that they find overwhelming (Thompson, 2014).

Mainstream Caregivers' Interaction Style

The majority of information regarding socialization of communication comes from studies of white, middle-class families. Most caregivers use a variety of behaviors to engage and maintain the interest of infants. When caregivers interact with infants, they often exaggerate their facial expressions in space and time. Caregivers may use an expression of mock surprise—opening their eyes wide, raising their eyebrows—and saying something like *oooooh* or *aaaaah* to signal a readiness to interact. They may move their heads from side to side or toward the infant. The facial expressions are slow to form and are then held. Caregivers may play with the speed and rate of these behaviors, speeding up and then slowing down. As the interaction continues,

they may smile to indicate that the interaction is going well or they may use an exaggerated frown or pout when the interaction is running down or in trouble. The repertoire of facial exaggerations is limited, and a few patterns are repeated frequently. These facial exaggerations facilitate infant's abilities to read facial expressions (Lewis, 2014; Stern, 1977).

Mainstream caregivers also tend to engage in baby talk (Snow & Ferguson, 1977). They simplify syntax, use short utterances, use many nonsense sounds, transform words (e.g., *pwitty wabbit* for "pretty rabbit"), raise vocal pitch, and exaggerate loudness and intensity of vocalizations—ranging from a whisper to a loud "pretend scary" voice. Sometimes, the speech is sped up, and other times, it is slowed down, elongating vowels on certain words—for example, *What a goooooooood little baby*. Pause times between utterances are also elongated, as though to allow time for the infant to respond. In essence, the caregiver appears to be shaping the infant's turn-taking behavior to the form necessary when the child becomes verbal. The mother also tends to repeat runs of interactions: You're a pretty baby; *you're such a pretty baby, you're the prettiest baby mommy has ever seen*. Many of these runs involve questions and answers, *Are you hungry? Are you? Huh? I think you are*. During each vocalization, the mother brings her head closer to the infant. Between questions, the mother moves away. Each question is accompanied by a distinct facial expression.

From the infant's birth, mainstream adults look for reasons for infants' behaviors and comment to the infants about possible intentions: *You're so hungry. You don't like beets. You want mommy to pick you up.* When adults view infants as intentional, they attempt to find the object or event (referent) that is triggering the child's behavior: *You're looking at your teddy bear. You want your bottle.* In doing so, adults guide children into referencing (labeling) and requesting behaviors.

As children develop the verbal ability to label and request, adults provide scaffolding questions to assist the children in producing more information. In mainstream homes, this scaffolding especially occurs during storybook reading, as in the following example:

MOTHER: Look!
CHILD: (touches picture)
MOTHER: What are those?
CHILD: (vocalizes a babble string and smiles)
MOTHER: Yes, they are rabbits.
CHILD: (vocalizes, smiles, and looks up at mother)
MOTHER: (laughs) Yes, rabbit.
CHILD: (vocalizes, smiles)
MOTHER: Yes.
(Bruner, 1983, p. 78)

As children acquire the routine and begin to take over their pieces (e.g., labeling the picture), the adult ups the ante by asking a more complex question: *What's the rabbit doing?* After the child labels the object and what it is doing, the caregiver ups the ante again: *Why is the rabbit doing that? How does he feel about what he is doing?* Through these social exchanges, children come to understand how to take turns in conversations, maintain a topic, and provide information in their culture. In addition, they are learning how to structure narratives.

Many caregivers reminisce with children about past events. Those who reminisce in elaborative ways ask open-ended questions that provide information and encourage the child to recall additional information ("What did we do at the zoo today?"); integrate their children's responses into the ongoing narrative ("That's right, we saw the gorillas. What were they doing?"); and refer to thoughts and feelings to evaluate experience ("I don't remember what we ate." "The gorillas looked so silly." "We got scared when the lions roared."). Mothers who reminisce with their young children in elaborated and evaluative ways have children who develop a better self-concept and show more insight into their own and others' thoughts and feelings (inter- and intra-personal cognitive and affective ToM) (Salmon & Reese, 2016; Taumoepeau & Reese, 2013). The children's greater self-awareness is reflected in more detailed, coherent, *autobiographical memory*. Autobiographical memory consists of episodic memory for personally experienced events (times, places, associated emotions, and other contextual who, what, when, where, why knowledge) and semantic memory for general knowledge and facts about the world. Children with better autobiographical memory tell more coherent personal stories (Fivush, 2011; Reese & Sutcliffe, 2006) and children who tell more coherent personal narratives exhibit better self-regulation and social problem-solving (Brown, Dorfman, Marmar, & Bryant, 2012).

Cultural Variations in Caregiver–Child Interactions

Anthropological studies have made it clear that cultures differ in their child-rearing practices. Each culture has its own perspective on infant capabilities and provides cares for infants, the types of interactions between adults and children, and the role of the infant and young child in the family. Because of these variations, people of different cultures respond to and interact with infants and young children in different ways (Chen & Rubin, 2011; Field, Sostek, Vietze, & Leiderman, 1981; Greenfield & Cocking, 1994; Johnston & Wong, 2002;

Lynch & Hansen, 2004; Vigil, 2002). Children's cultural contexts are highly influential in their social-emotional and ToM development (Slaughter & De Rosnay, 2017).

Cultures tend to differ in terms of whether they are socializing children to become independent or to become interdependent. Cultures that socialize children toward *independence* promote *individualism*—that is, a focus on the individual; cultures that socialize children toward *interdependence* promote *collectivism*—that is, a focus on the group. Caregivers in individualistic cultures are more likely to follow the infant's lead in interactions. They follow the child's line of regard when establishing joint attention and are likely to label what they see the child looking at or to interpret what they think are the child's desires. In contrast, caregivers in collective cultures are more likely to expect the child to follow their line of regard and attend to the desire of the caregiver. In these instances, caregivers are more likely to give directives that children are to follow (Vigil & Westby, 2004) and children may have proportionally more action words compared to children in individualistic cultures (Waxman et al., 2016). Individualistic cultures tend to attribute intentional behavior to infants, whereas collectivistic cultures may be less likely to expect infants to exhibit intentional, goal-directed behavior. When adults do not view infants as intentional, they are unlikely to talk with them, provide labels, or ask questions, and they are less likely to support them in their attempts to produce lengthy, topic-maintaining dialogues (Heath, 1983; Whiting & Edwards, 1988).

Families in individualistic and collectivistic cultures reminisce with children in different ways. Mothers in individualistic cultures tend to be highly elaborative when reminiscing. They give voluminous descriptive information about experiences, prompt children to give embellished narratives, and encourage children to focus on the self and feelings about the past. In contrast, mothers in collectivistic cultures tend to talk less about the past, offer fewer details, and emphasize cooperation and accommodation to others. In response to these maternal reminiscing styles, children in collectivistic cultures give a skeletal description of multiple events and show a greater orientation to social engagement, moral correctness, and concern for authority. Children in individualistic cultures elaborate on one or two events when reminiscing, make more references to themselves and more personal evaluations, and indicate little concern for authority (Wang, 2013).

The remainder of this chapter addresses the social-emotional bases of communication in mainstream children. Some principles are applicable to all children, but one must be alert to ways in which culture may affect the structure and functions of children's communications.

▶ Communicating with Others

Children's social communicative abilities develop in two directions. *Vertical development* refers to increasing hierarchical development associated with increasing age and cognitive understanding. *Horizontal development* refers to the range of abilities or communicative functions within a particular developmental level.

Vertical Development

Intentionality

Bates (1976) described three stages in children's emergence of pragmatic or intentional communicative behaviors: perlocutionary, illocutionary, and locutionary. In the *perlocutionary* stage, from birth to approximately 9 months, infants have a systematic effect on adults without intending to. Adults interpret the infant's smiles, cries, and coos as though they were intentional, although they are not. The infant does not intentionally cry or smile to seek a response from an adult, yet adults talk to the infants as though the infant is being intentional: *Oh, you want mommy to sing that again*, or *You don't want any more carrots; mommy will take them away*. Perlocutionary behavior is sometimes referred to as functional communication. The infant's or child's behavior functions as a communication to adults, even though the child's behavior is not intentionally goal-directed.

Around 9 months of age, when infants are able to establish joint attention, they enter the *illocutionary* stage. Infants now use behaviors intentionally to gain the adult's attention. Many of these behaviors become conventionalized; that is, they are gestures that others would use (e.g., reaching, waving bye-bye). If a child wants a toy and the child's mother is not looking at it, he (say) will point at the toy with an arm outstretched and index finger pointed, look toward the toy, shift his gaze to his mother's face, and then shift his attention back and forth. A cry or vocalization is deliberately used to get another's attention. The child may whine and then check whether the adult is attending. If not, the child may escalate the whine to a cry, but again may stop to check whether the adult is attending.

During this stage, one observes what Bates (1976) considered precursors to language: the protoimperative (IBR) and the protodeclarative (IJA). The *protoimperative* is defined as the child's use of a means

to cause the adult to do something. It grows out of their attempts to do something themselves. Hence, the first protoimperatives (IBRs) involve instances of reaching and looking between the desired object and the event. Later, the child may bring an object or toy to an adult, seeking assistance with operating it. For example, the child may recognize a music box, yet be unable to wind it himself/herself. The child brings the box to an adult, hands it to the adult, and then waits expectantly for the adult to wind it. By contrast, a *protodeclarative* (IJA) is defined as a preverbal effort to direct the adult's attention to an event or object in the world. Included here are showing objects and exhibiting oneself for the sole purposes of gaining attention. For example, a child may bring a toy to an adult simply to capture the adult's interest and attention.

Between 13 and 18 months of age, children enter the *locutionary* stage. During this phase of development, they begin to use conventionalized words to make things happen. The child who earlier pointed to the cookie now says, "*cookie;*" the child who simply handed the mother a toy to wind now says, "*help.*"

Referencing and Requesting

To engage in illocutionary and locutionary behavior, children must be able to engage in joint attention with another person—looking at what another person is looking at and knowing that they and the other person are looking at the same thing. Furthermore, they must be able to socially *reference*—use caregivers' expressions to form their responses to events and situations. People use joint attention to manage and direct one another's attention by linguistic means. Initially, the management of joint attention is under the control of the adult. For instance, the caregiver highlights objects by moving them into the infant's view. After the infant's attention can reliably be gained by showing objects, the caregiver begins to prepare the child for the object by calling the child's name or saying, *Oh, look*, or *See what I have*. Between 8 and 12 months of age, infants discover that the adult's speech signals that the adult is looking at something and the infants begin to follow the adults' line of regard. By age 12 months, infants follow the adult's line of regard, search for an object, and, if they find none, they look at the adult's face again, and then again look outward. Shortly after this, the child begins to point. After pointing and consistent words appear, caregivers initiate *what* and *where* games (*What's this? Where did it go?*).

When children can engage in joint attention and social referencing, they can request. This entails not only coordinating one's language with the requirements of action in the real world, but doing so in culturally prescribed ways. Bruner (1983) distinguished three types of early requests:

- Request for an object
- Invitation or request to an adult to share a role relationship in play or in a game
- Request for supportive action in which the child tries to recruit an adult's skill or strength to help the child achieve a desired goal

The caregiver's role is different in each of these requests. In the first type of request, the caregiver must figure out what the child wants; in the second, what the invitation is for; and in the third, what kind of help the child needs. Requests for visible and near objects occur before one year of age. Requests for remote or absent objects and for supportive action or assistance emerge around 18 months, when children develop representational capacity.

After children start using words to request absent objects and supportive actions, caregivers begin to enforce the cultural expectations for requests. Children are expected to really need the object or the assistance and not request something they can get or do for themselves. Requests should not require unreasonable demands from caregivers (e.g., *I can't go upstairs and find your book now—I'm fixing dinner*) and the child must respect the voluntary nature of responses to requests (e.g., the caregiver requires the child to say *thank you* after the request is fulfilled). Certain requests are related to time and can be fulfilled only within a particular time frame (e.g., *You can't have cookies before dinner*).

Verbal requests can be one of three types:

- Direct requests: *Gimme that! More milk. Please pass the butter.*
- Indirect requests: *Could you get that pencil? Why don't you close the door?*
- Hints or nonconventionalized requests: *It's cold in here. I haven't gotten my allowance yet.*

Successful requesting requires that children gain attention, their requests be clear and persuasive, they maintain the desired or expected social relationships, and they have strategies for making repairs when their request is not understood (Ervin-Tripp & Gordon, 1986). In addition, children must produce requests that recognize the following aspects:

- The social status or the relative power of the speaker and the addressee
- The intrusiveness of the request
- Ownership/possession
- Rights and obligations (Gordon & Ervin-Tripp, 1984)

In general, children are sensitive to roles, rights, and possessions by age 2, knowing that they should be more polite when asking for something from someone older, when asking for something that is not their own, and when the person they are asking is not obligated to respond. They have limited awareness of intrusiveness before school age. Lawson (as cited in Ervin-Tripp & Gordon, 1985) reported that a 2-year-old child used different forms of speech to her father, her mother, and children at nursery school depending on whether they were her own age or older. She used direct imperative requests to 2-year-olds, and embedded requests or requests with tags such as *please* or *okay*.

Ervin-Trip and Gordon (1986) reported that 60% of 2- and 3-year-old children's requests to outsiders used politeness markers, whereas only 1% of requests to mothers and 14–24% of requests to other children were polite. These researchers suggested that children assume that mothers must be available for services, whereas older children and visitors do not have to be available. Requests for objects that belonged to others were usually polite even to mothers and siblings.

Two- and three-year-old children seldom provide justifications for their requests. A marked increase in justification of requests occurs around age 4 (e.g., *I need a red crayon 'cause mine is broke*). At this age, children begin to challenge adults' refusals of requests. They later use information gained from adults' reasons for their refusals to persuade adults of their needs, desires, or intents (e.g., *I'll eat all my dinner if I can have a popsicle now*).

As children become sensitive to the social rules underlying requests, they produce more indirect and nonconventualized requests. Between ages 4 and 8 years, children not only use politeness modifications for issues of status and rights, but they also become sensitive to how their requests might intrude the activities of others. Children understand direct and indirect requests during the preschool years but comprehend nonconventualized requests or hints only when they reach approximately 8 years of age. Conventionalized requests (directives and indirectives) can be learned as formulas; that is, caregivers can tell a child what to say in a particular situation. By comparison, nonconventionalized requests require greater cognitive and social knowledge.

Joint attention plus a vocalization or behavior (e.g., touching the caregiver or gesturing) can be sufficient for an initial request for an action or object. But social referencing, or secondary intersubjectivity, is required if the caregiver does not give an initial response or if there is to be further engagement after the request is granted. Children must take the perspective of the caregiver, interpret the caregiver's response, and determine whether the caregiver considers the request acceptable or unacceptable.

Horizontal Development

After children engage in illocutionary and locutionary behavior, they communicate a variety of intentions. A number of taxonomies have been developed to code communicative intents. The categories vary depending on the age of the children studied, the philosophical orientation of the researcher, and the degree to which discourse and social context are considered (Chapman, 1981). Taxonomies may classify gestures or language at the following levels:

- *The utterance level.* Each utterance is coded based on what the speakers are doing at the moment. Are they labeling, requesting, warning, promising, or ordering?
- *The discourse level.* In this taxonomy, the utterance is categorized according to its relationship with other utterances. Does the utterance initiate a conversation, maintain the conversation, acknowledge another speaker, clarify an utterance, or terminate the conversation? Utterances coded at the utterance level can also be coded at the discourse level. An utterance may function as a label at the utterance level and as a topic initiator

at the discourse level. At the discourse level, utterances may also be considered in terms of how they manage the conversation. Does the utterance function to get a turn, hold one's turn, or allow another person to take a turn?

- *The social level.* The utterance can be placed in its social context. Language varies according to the setting and the roles of the participants in these settings. This is particularly true with politeness and argumentative behavior. How does the utterance function to soften or strengthen the communication?

Communication in the illocutionary and early locutionary phases involves efforts to regulate another's behavior for purposes of achieving a goal, seeking social interaction, or establishing joint attention for the purpose of sharing information. **TABLE 6-1** presents communicative intents, coded at the utterance level, that have been reported during the illocutionary and early locutionary stages (Coggins & Carpenter, 1981; Dore, 1975; Halliday, 1975; Wetherby & Prizant, 1989). Communicative intentions in this stage can be gestures or verbal utterances that serve to (1) regulate behavior, (2) engage in social interaction, and (3) establish joint reference. In the table, items marked with an asterisk (*) generally appear only in the locutionary period.

Even during the illocutionary stage, children are likely to use all three major functions. As they move

---

TABLE 6-1 Early Communicative Intents

Behavioral Regulation
- Request for specific object — demands an object
- Rejection of an object — refuses an object
- Request for action — commands someone to perform an action (e.g., raises arms to be picked up)
- Protest of action — refuses an activity by someone

Social Interaction
- Greeting — gains attention, indicates notice of initiation or termination of activity (e.g., *hi, bye*)
- Request for social routine — initiates routines such as peek-a-boo or pat-a-cake
- Showing off — attracts attention
- Calling — gains the attention of someone
- Acknowledging — indicates that the speaker's communication was received
- Requests permission — seeks approval to carry out an activity
- Personal — expresses moods or feelings

Joint Attention
- Transferring — places an object in another's possession
- Comment on an object — directs someone's attention to an object
- Comment on an action or event — directs someone's attention to an event
- Request for information — seeks information, explanations, or clarifications*
- Clarification — utterances used to clarify previous communication*

* Generally appear only in the locutionary period.

TABLE 6-2 Communicative Functions in Preschool Children

Requests	For information	Where's Michael going?
	For action	Get me some more paste.
	For acknowledgment	You know what?
Responses to requests	Providing information	(Why isn't Karen here?) She's sick.
	Expressing acceptance, denial, or acknowledgment	Okay. You can't have it.
Descriptions of past and present facts	Labeling or describing objects and actions	I'm eating my lunch. Anna spilled her milk.
	Describing properties and locations	My candle has lots of red paint on it. I put it in my cubbie.
Statements	Of facts or rules	It's not nice to grab. We have to share the wagon.
	Of explanations, reasons, or causes	Sara can't go swimming 'cause she's got a cold.
Acknowledgments	Recognizing responses	Okay, yes, right
	Evaluating responses	That's not what teacher said.
Organizing devices	Regulating contact and conversation	Hi, bye, my turn, sorry
Performatives	Accomplishing event by speaking (protests, jokes, claims, teases, warnings)	Stop. Don't touch it. Josh is a baby.

Source: Data from Dore, J. (1978). Requestive systems in nursery school conversations: Analysis of talk in its social context. In R. Campbell & P. Smith (Eds), *Recent advances in the psychology of language: Language development and mother-child interaction* (pp. 271–292). New York: Plenium Press.

into the multiword locutionary stage, requests for social routines and showing decrease, whereas calling, requesting permission, acknowledging, requesting information, and requesting clarifications increase. The rate increases substantially between the early illocutionary and multiword locutionary stages. Children display an average of about one act per minute during the prelinguistic stage, two acts per minute in the one-word stage, and five acts per minute by the multiword stage.

During the preschool years, communicative functions become less tied to the concrete environment and more closely related to language referring to language. **TABLE 6-2** presents Dore's schema (1978) for coding communicative functions for preschool-aged children.

Development of Emotional Understanding

Appropriate use of communication in social interactions requires increasing awareness of one's own emotionality, the emotionality of others, and the social rules governing the appropriate display of emotions. At least six emotions are considered primary and universal: happy, sad, mad/angry, afraid, surprised, disgusted. Children's understanding of these emotional terms begins to develop early and follows a regular pattern of emergence (Baron-Cohen, Golan, Wheelright, Granader, & Hill, 2010; Harris, 2008; Harter, 1987; Michalson & Lewis, 1985; Pons, Harris, & de Rosnay, 2004). Between ages 3 and 4 years, approximately 55% of children are able to recognize and name basic emotions (happy, sad, afraid, angry) on the basis of facial expression when presented with pictures. By age 5 years, 75% of children can do so. Moreover, by 5 years of age, a majority of children understand the relationship between emotions and memory, namely they realize that the intensity of the emotion decreases with time and that some elements of a present situation can result in past emotions. More than half of

5-year-olds can also identify external causes of emotions and link a facial expression to a situation (e.g., one feels sad at the loss of a favorite toy or happy when receiving a desired gift). For social emotions, such as embarrassment, guilt, shame, and contempt, children rely more on the situation than facial expression to determine the emotion. Although preschool children may exhibit these social emotions, they are not good at identifying them in others or in story scripts (Widen & Russell, 2010).

By age 7 years, the majority of children understand that a person's beliefs—whether true or false—will determine a person's emotional reaction to a situation. For example, if a child is afraid of snakes and thinks they see a snake, the child will be afraid, even if what the child sees is a garden hose. Seven- to nine-year-olds develop an understanding of situations in which they should hide emotions. For example, if a neighbor gives them a piece of cake that tastes disgusting, they realize that they should smile and say, "Thank you," and not grimace and say, "This is really yukky."

By 9 years of age, the majority of children understand that a person can have multiple, and even ambivalent or contradictory, emotions in a given situation. For example, the child might be both excited and fearful to go on a roller coaster. Furthermore, 9-year-olds understand that negative feelings are typically associated with morally inappropriate actions (lying, stealing) and positive feelings are associated with praiseworthy actions (making a sacrifice, resisting a temptation). By age 11 years, nearly all children understand that failure to confess a misdemeanor provokes sadness.

▶ Neurological/Biological Factors Affecting Social-Emotional Aspects of Communication

The social brain network underpins normal social development and function. Disruptions of this network can occur as a result of genetic disorders, developmental disabilities, infections, traumas, and degenerative processes. A number of developmental disabilities illustrate the bio-psycho-social relationships central to social-emotional development and pragmatic language skills. Disruption in any aspect of neural development sond integration places an individual at increased risk for deficits in social competence. Hence, children with sensory, cognitive, or attention

deficits or syntactic and semantic language impairments are also likely to show delays and differences in social or pragmatic aspects of communication that may result in their being less able to be involved in communicative interactions or in the adult being less able to read the child's involvement. Children who were born prematurely and have significant medical problems or cognitive impairments as a consequence, are less able to engage in the conversational dance during infancy. They are, therefore, at risk of pragmatic deficits beyond what would be expected based on their cognitive abilities alone.

In the *Diagnostic and Statistical Manual of Mental Disorders-5* (DSM-5; American Psychiatric Association, 2013), the American Psychiatric Association added a new diagnostic category—social communication disorder (SCD). SCD is defined as persistent difficulties in pragmatics or the social uses of verbal and nonverbal communication as manifested by all of the following:

- Deficits in communication for social purposes, such as greeting and sharing information, in a manner that is appropriate for the social context.
- Impairment of the ability to change communication to match context or needs of the listener, such as speaking differently in a classroom than on a playground, talking differently to a child than to an adult, and avoiding the use of overly formal language.
- Difficulties following rules for conservation and storytelling, such as taking turns in conversation, rephrasing when misunderstood, and knowing how to use verbal and nonverbal signals to regulate interaction.
- Difficulties understanding what is not explicitly stated (e.g., making inferences) and nonliteral or ambiguous meanings of language (e.g., idioms, humor, metaphors, multiple meanings that depend on the context for interpretation) (pp. 47–48).

A social communication disorder may be a distinct diagnosis or may occur as part of other conditions, such as autism spectrum disorder (ASD), specific language impairment (SLI), learning disabilities (LD), language learning disabilities (LLD), intellectual disabilities (ID), developmental disabilities (DD), attention deficit hyperactivity disorder (ADHD), traumatic brain injury (TBI), hearing loss, or psychological/emotional disorders.

The SCD diagnostic category may have been meant to fill a gap resulting from changes in other diagnostic categories. DSM-5 redefined the criteria for a diagnosis of autism, requiring deficits not only in social communication and social interaction, but also narrow interests and repetitive behavior. Hence, persons with only social communication deficits no longer receive the autism diagnosis. DSM-4 also modified diagnostic categories for what, in some contexts, has been termed specific language impaired. The *Diagnostic and Statistical Manual of Mental Disorders-4* (DSN-4; American Psychiatric Association, 2000) used the diagnostic categories of Expressive Language Disorder and Mixed Receptive-Expressive Language Disorder. DSM-5 placed these categories with the category Language Disorder, which addresses primarily vocabulary and grammar-structural aspects of language rather than pragmatic aspects. The SCD diagnosis may be used for children who do not quite meet the stringent criteria for diagnosing autism or to identify persons who have adequate vocabulary and syntactic language but face problems in using these skills in natural communication.

Some language researchers have been using the diagnostic label pragmatic language impairment (PLI) in a way that is compatible with the SCD diagnosis. The diagnosis of SCD or PLI is somewhat controversial. There is little evidence that SCD is a reliably or validly distinct category independent of autism and language disorder (Ozonoff, 2012). SCD symptoms are comorbid features across a wide range of other disorders and, therefore, many children and adolescents with language and behavioral impairments should be evaluated for social communicative competence. It is possible that pragmatic difficulties or SCD represent residual language problems.

Autism Spectrum Disorder

ASD is probably the condition most commonly associated with deficits in social/emotional aspects of communication. Children with ASD exhibit a fundamental failure in socialization. The social dysfunction observed in children with autism is never observed in neurotypical children of any age and cannot be accounted for on the basis of cognitive impairments alone. Children with ASD show deficits in three areas related to social engagement: sociability and social communication, attachment, and understanding and expressing emotions (Volkmar & Klin, 2005).

Deficits in socialization may be noted early. In fact, many children with ASD exhibit deviant patterns of gaze from early infancy. Young children with autism may avoid eye gaze, while some older children may stare fixedly and inappropriately. Deficits in joint attention and referential pointing readily discriminate toddlers with and without ASD. Communication requires that one be able to perceive

of another's sharing an interest about an object or topic. A key symptom of ASD is the child's inability to enter into joint attention and affective contact with other people.

The majority of children with autism eventually develop RJA and IBR, but they continue to exhibit deficits in IJA (Mundy, Sigman, & Kasari, 1994). Even though they may follow another's line of regard (RJA), they do not necessarily reference the emotional expression of the person they are observing; that is, they do not attempt to interpret the person's reason for looking or response to looking. Children who cannot engage in joint attention, or who avoid it, would have difficulty in grasping early language functions. Without RJA, IJA, and social-emotional referencing, children with ASD continue to exhibit poor skills in emotional sharing; without emotional sharing, they fail to develop higher levels of ToM essential for social understanding, interpersonal relationships, and communicative competence. RJA in young children with autism predicts their nonverbal communication and social skills as adults (Gillespie-Lynch, 2012).

Children with ASD exhibit a sparsity of intentional communicative behaviors. They use fewer communicative acts during interactions, and many of the communicative intentions they do use are not conventionalized. For example, some children with autism use echolalia (repetitions of words and phrases they have heard spoken) to make a request. For example, they may say, *Do you want a drink?* instead of *I want water*. They use a high degree of nonreciprocal speech, fail to listen, make irrelevant comments, and fail to leave a topic of obsessive interest or to look for cues in the listener as to their interest or desire to take a turn (Paul, Orlovski, Marcinko, & Volkmar, 2009). They tend to be poor at initiating conversation, although they may not be unresponsive if another person initiates it (Loveland, Landry, Hughes, Hall, & McEvoy, 1988). When they do bring up a topic, it is often related to their own preoccupations, and their remarks or questions are usually uttered without varied inflection (Rutter & Garmezy, 1983). Children with ASD are also likely to interrupt and respond inappropriately in conversations (Capps, Kehres, & Sigman, 1998). Some engage in persistent and perseverative questioning that does not serve the purpose of requesting information (Hurtig, Ensrud, & Tomblin, 1982). Although some basic intention to communicate exists, children with ASD have little skill in participating in communicative activities involving joint reference of shared topics, particularly in supplying new information relevant to the listener's purposes (Tager-Flusberg, Paul, & Lord, 2005).

Visual Impairment (VI)

Early social interactions, joint attention, gesturing, and the development of referencing are all dependent upon vision. The research literature indicates that even a small amount of form vision leads to better developmental outcomes (Sonksen & Dale, 2002). Hence, it is important to make a distinction between children with a profound VI (PVI, no vision or light perception at best) and severe VI (SVI, severely impaired vision, but the ability to detect form). It is also important to distinguish between peripheral VI (damage to the eye, retina, or optic nerve) and cerebral VI (damage to the posterior optic pathway to visual cortex). (Some children have both peripheral and cerebral impairment.) Children with SVI tend to have better outcomes than children with PVI, and children with peripheral only VI tend to have better outcomes than children with cerebral VI (Greenaway & Dale, 2017).

By 6 months of age, the sighted infant has developed a large repertoire of social interactions. Infants with VI, however, have no way of watching their mothers' facial expressions and, therefore, cannot engage in the face-to-face emotional sharing that is part of early attuned caregiver–infant interactions. Developing joint or shared attention to objects, which is essential for establishing referencing, is particularly challenging for infants with VI. Children with VI may have difficulty determining whether their intended listeners are attending to them or even whether the persons are present. Knowing that the person is present, however, is no guarantee that they are paying attention. Even if the person is present and has been listening, the child has no way of knowing whether the person's attention has shifted to something else. The child must gain the listener's attention. Children with VI do not have the option of establishing mutual gaze or gesturing. Instead, they must either touch the listener or vocalize. For sighted children, vocalizing to gain attention and establishing joint referencing are initially superimposed on earlier gestural strategies. Without vision, children with VI develop few gestural communications. They also may not be certain whether the referent exists in the environment or whether the listener is attending to it.

Absence of eye gaze makes it more difficult for caregivers to interpret the child's communicative intent. In early interactions, infants with VI tend to be less expressively responsive, less likely to initiate social interaction, and less likely to share experiences with toys. Caregivers initiate interactions more frequently than toddlers and are more likely to talk about objects that are not in the child's focus of attention (Moore & McConachie, 1994). These challenges to early joint attention and referencing make it harder for children to learn that experiences can be shared with others, and as a result, they are at risk for delays and deficits in ToM. Children with VI are delayed in passing ToM false belief tasks (Peterson, Peterson, & Webb, 2000; Roch-Levecq, 2006), but their performance typically improves with age. They are, however, likely to exhibit some difficulties with situations that require them to interpret the thoughts, beliefs, and feelings of others (Sak-Wernicka, 2016). Their hearing and language skills do not compensate for all that is lost because of their VI. Surprisingly, adolescents with VI have greater difficulty recognizing emotionality in voice than sighted adolescents (Dyck, Farrigoa, Shochet, & Holmes-Brown, 2004)

Children with VI are generally delayed in acquisition of first words. They repeat words to themselves and fail to produce them to initiate interactions until well into their third year (Urwin, 1984). Later, they may ask many questions, sometimes inappropriately; they may use echolalia; and they may make 'off-the-wall' comments (Mills, 1993). Many of the early referents of children with VI are names of people rather than names of objects. Use of language for requesting purposes appears in sighted children by the end of the first year after birth but emerges closer to the end of the second year in children with VI. Because children with VI's nonverbal behavior so often fails to provide topics for comment, parents frequently adopt a questioning mode of interaction. Although questioning may facilitate an early form of turn-taking between parent and child, because the initiative always remains with the adult, the practice inhibits the child's development of awareness of their own agency—that is, the ability to make things happen in the environment (McGurk, 1983).

Although there is considerable variability among children and adolescents with VI, as a group, they are likely to have more difficulty with pragmatic skills than structural language skills (Greenaway & Dale, 2017). On the CCC-2 (Bishop, 2006), they are likely to exhibit more difficulty on all the pragmatic and social communication behavior scales than on the scales that assess articulation, language structure, vocabulary, and discourse (James & Stojanovik, 2007; Tadic, Pring, & Dale, 2010). Despite these early deficits, children with ocular-only VI, who have no other handicapping conditions and have adult caregivers who are alert to the interaction of VI and language, can develop normal communicative interaction patterns during the preschool years (Begeer et al., 2014; Wilton, 2011). Many, however, show patterns of delays and disorder in pragmatic communicative interactions (James & Stojanovik, 2007; Tadic, Pring, & Dale, 2010).

Deafness/Hearing Loss

The ongoing effects of a hearing loss and the resulting delayed language and disruption of caregiver-child interactions puts children who are deaf or hard of hearing (DHH) at risk of deficits in social competence. Children who are DHH exhibit significantly more challenging, inappropriate social behaviors (Austen, 2010). They exhibit more difficulties in pragmatic skills in conversations and social situations than hearing children, even when they are matched on vocabulary and syntactic skills (Goberis et al, 2012; Toe, Rinaldi, Caselli, Paatsch, & Church, 2016). Some of these pragmatic deficits may be related to ToM delays and deficits. Parents of children who are DHH and late-signing deaf children typically are also quite delayed in cognitive ToM associated with false belief (i.e., recognizing that what someone believes is untrue) (de Villiers & de Villiers, 2012; Peterson, 2009). Deaf children of deaf parents typically pass formal cognitive ToM false-belief tasks at the same age as hearing children; however, they exhibit significant delays in developing higher order aspects of cognitive ToM (O'Reilly, Peterson, & Wellman, 2014). It is possible to pass cognitive ToM false-belief tasks yet not be able to comprehend all the nuances of perspective taking in naturalistic situations. Development of ToM requires not only an intact neurological system, but also experiences with persons who talk about the mind. The hearing loss and associated reduced communicative interactions experienced by deaf children have been used to explain delays in language development, which in turn has been used to explain their delayed ToM development (de Villiers, 2005). Yet language delays cannot explain the ToM deficits exhibited by many children and adolescents with hearing loss.

Children and adolescents who are DHH also exhibit delays and deficits in affective ToM that are not necessarily dependent on language skills. They are less accurate than hearing children in following line of regard (JA) to interpret person's intention. They are not as proficient at sorting faces that express emotion or labeling emotional expressions as hearing children (Ludlow, Heaton, Rosset, Hills, & Deruelle, 2010; Wiefferink, Rieffe, Ketelaar, De Raeve, & Frijns, 2013). They also exhibit greater difficulty in matching emotional expressions to pictures of situations that might trigger than emotion and they tend to give different rationales for the emergence of emotions than their hearing peers (Rieffe, Terwogt, & Smit, 2003). For example, when identifying the emotion that would occur in a situation, deaf children tend to focus on the outcome of a situation in terms of whether a person's desires are fulfilled. As a consequence, they are likely to judge a person's emotional response to a situation in terms of being happy or sad depending on whether the outcome was desired. In contrast, hearing children tend to consider both the controllability of a situation and the final outcome. Hence, if a child cannot go on a picnic because it is raining, they judge that the child will be sad; in contrast, if the child cannot go on a picnic because a parent insists that the child clean their room instead, then they are likely to judge that the child will be angry. Children who are DHH are likely to judge the child to be sad in both instances. Furthermore, they also misinterpret the types and causes of emotions of characters in stories (Gray, Hosie, Russell, Scott, & Hunter, 2007). Failure to distinguish the reasons behind an outcome will result in the latter children having fewer strategies to cope with social situations. These reduced strategies for coping with social situations may contribute to the frequently noted externalizing behavior problems of deaf children (Vostanis, Hayes, Du Feu, & Warren, 1997).

Children who are DHH also score lower in empathy than their hearing peers. On self-rating measures, they report lower levels of empathy and prosocial motivation than hearing children, regardless of their type of hearing device, and they show less supportive behaviors to peers (Netten et al., 2015) and teachers rate them as less empathic (Peterson, 2016). If children have difficulty recognizing emotions, it is not surprising that they are less empathic. Because empathy is of major importance in initiating and maintaining social relationships, this could have ongoing consequences in the social/pragmatic development of DHH children.

Language Disorder/Specific Language Impairment

A strong correlation exists between language skills and social-emotional behavior (Baker & Cantwell, 1987; Brinton & Fujiki, 1993; Giddan, 1991; Hollo, Wehby, & Oliver, 2014). Specific language impairment (SLI) is typically identified initially when children exhibit obvious delays in vocabulary and morphosyntactic skills but no hearing loss or other obvious developmental delays. As children with SLI develop the structure of language, their problems with pragmatic aspects of language become more obvious. (Note: The term SLI has been used in much of the research literature in the United States, yet the term has become controversial because it has become clear that language impairment does not exist in isolation. Children with language impairments are likely to have other comorbid conditions—symbolic play delays, reduced attention, working memory/executive function deficits [Bishop, Snowling, Thompson, Greenhalgh, & CATALISE-2 consortium, 2017]).

Language impairment disrupts the ability of children with SLI to participate effectively in social communication. Negative social consequences of SLI are manifested in the early preschool years when children as young as three years avoid conversing with language-impaired peers. By four years of age, children with SLI are chosen as least liked by their typically developing peers. This reduced popularity continues throughout the school years. Longitudinal studies have shown that social difficulties of children with SLI increase through adolescence and are related to their pragmatic skills (Conti-Ramsden, Moka, Pickles, & Durkin, 2013; St. Clair, Pickles, Durkin, & Conti-Ramsden, 2011; van Agt, Verhoeven, van den Brink, & De Koning, 2010). Adolescents with a history of SLI are more likely than their TD peers to report higher levels of peer problems, emotional symptoms, hyperactivity, and conduct problems. Although there is agreement that, in most instances, language and social impairments are causally linked, there is less agreement about the nature and direction of this relationship. Perhaps a biological or neurophysiological factor underlies both the social-emotional and linguistic difficulties. Caregivers of children with SLI employ a less facilitative conversational style and over time decrease their initiations and responses (van Balkom, Verhoeven, & van Weerdenburg, 2010). As a result, children have less opportunity to learn pragmatic skills. Deficits in one area might drive further deficits in the other area. Research is increasingly showing that children with specific language impairment (SLI) have more difficulties in social interactions than can be explained by their language impairment alone (Adams, Clarke, & Haynes, 2009; Fujiki, Brinton, Isaacson, & Summers, 2001).

Some children with SLI may exhibit early appropriate social-emotional interactions, but later problems in word-finding, constructing requests or comments, repairing communication breakdowns, or comprehending what is said may adversely affect their social skills. Children with language impairments are less willing to engage in conversation, and they are more likely to be ignored or rejected when they do attempt to communicate (Fujiki, Brinton, & Todd, 1996; Rice, 1993). In addition, deficits in social and language skills frequently result in reduced opportunities for social interaction (Rice, 1993). Because social interactions are so critical in driving language and social development, a child with social and language impairments experiences further delays in development.

The language impairment itself and the reduced interactions resulting from the language impairment can result in ToM deficits that may play a role in the poorer social outcomes of children with SLI, such as their tendency to have poorer social skills, be more socially withdrawn, and be at a higher risk of peer victimization and bullying. Structural language abilities are significant predictors of performance on cognitive ToM tasks (Andrés-Roqueta, Adrian, Clemente, & Katsos, 2013). Numerous studies investigating the performance of children and adolescents with SLI on cognitive ToM tasks have reported a general delay in ToM development (Nilsson & deLópez, 2016). Children with SLI also exhibit deficits on affective ToM tasks that require minimal language. They perform more poorly than typically developing children on tasks that require them to identify emotions in facial expressions or in the prosody of spoken sentences (Fujiki, Spackman, Brinton, & Illig, 2008; Merkenschlager, Amorosa, Kiefl, & Martinius, 2012; Taylor, Maybery, Grayndler, & Whitehouse, 2015). Even when they were able to identify emotional expressions, they had greater problems inferring the appropriate emotion that would be associated with an event context (Ford & Milsoky, 2003). ToM development in SLI appears to follow a trajectory similar to that in typically developing (TD) children but at a different pace and with a lower final level of ToM performance (Nilsson & deLópez, 2016).

These ToM delays or deficits contribute significantly to the social communication difficulties exhibited by children with SLI. Children's scores on ToM tasks predicted nominations as "least-liked" by their peers (Andrés-Roqueta, Adrian, Clemente, & Villanueva, 2016). As a group, children with SLI are less competent in regulating their own emotions, and they experience fewer peer friendships and higher rates of bullying than their typical peers. Persons who accurately express and regulate their own emotions and understand the emotions of others are more successful socially than those who have difficulty with these behaviors (Denham, 1998). To participate effectively in social situations, children must be able to infer and interpret their partners' emotional reactions—a feat that requires an understanding of causal connections. Causal inferences may be based on physical events (e.g., inferring that wet clothes are caused by rain) or mental states (e.g., inferring that forgetting an umbrella might cause someone to be angry). Physical events are observable, but mental states are not; as a consequence, it may be more difficult for children to link events to mental states. Research indicates that children with SLI have difficulty making inferences based on both physical events and mental states

(Adams et al., 2009; Botting & Adams, 2005; Ford & Milosky, 2003; Ryder & Leinonen, 2014). Inability to make these inferences may contribute to the social difficulties children with SLI experience.

Attention-Deficit/Hyperactive Disorder (ADHD)

The DSM-5 criteria for ADHD reveal a set of communication problems characteristic of pragmatic dysfunction (e.g., difficulty awaiting turns, talking excessively, interrupting others, not listening to what is being said, and blurting out answers to questions before they are completed) (Camarata & Gibson, 1999; Westby & Cutler, 1994). Nearly half of children diagnosed with ADHD also have a language disorder, so it is likely that children with ADHD + SLI will have some difficulty with social communication (Mueller & Tomblin, 2012). However, even children with ADHD only (that is, those who do not have a diagnosed language disorder) have pragmatic difficulties (Staikova, Gomes, Tartter, McCabe, Halperin, 2013).

Children with ADHD are likely to talk more than typical children during spontaneous conversations (Barkley, Cunningham, & Karlsson, 1983). When they must organize and generate language in response to specific task demands, however, they are likely to talk less, be dysfluent (using pauses, fillers such as "uh," "er," and "um"), and be less organized (Hamlett, Pelligrini, & Conners, 1987; Purvis & Tannock, 1997; Zentall, 1985). Compared with typically developing children, children with ADHD tend to produce excessive verbal output during spontaneous conversations, task transitions, and in play settings, yet they tend to produce less speech in response to confrontational questioning than children without ADHD do (Baker & Cantwell, 1992; Tannock & Schachar, 1996). They are also less competitive in verbal problem-solving tasks and less capable of communicating task-essential information to peers in cooperative tasks (Whalen, Henker, Collins, McAuliffe, & Vaux, 1979). Children with ADHD exhibit difficulties in introducing, maintaining, and changing topics appropriately, in negotiating smooth interchanges or turn taking during conversation, and in adjusting language to the listener in specific contexts (Hamlett, Pelligrini, & Collins, 1987).

The inattention and hyperactivity symptoms could easily lead to difficulties in conversational situations. Also, because of children's attention difficulties, parents may become more directive, be less elaborative, and prefer to talk using short utterances, which could affect children's pragmatic development. However, not all of the social communication difficulties exhibited by children with ADHD can be explained by the behavioral symptoms. Studies indicate that children and adolescents with ADHD exhibit some delays and differences in cognitive and affective ToM. They have been shown to have less knowledge about social skills and appropriate behavior with others. Although school-age children and adolescents with ADHD pass early cognitive ToM tasks, they are likely to be delayed in developing later cognitive ToM skills. With regard to affective ToM, there is a tendency for children and adolescents with ADHD to exhibit difficulty in accurately identifying emotions in photos or videos and matching emotions to situations (Celestin-Westreich & Celestin, 2013; Shin, Lee, Kim, Park, & Lim, 2008; Yuill, & Lyon, 2007). As a result of these interpersonal ToM deficits, they do not read essential verbal, nonverbal, and situational cues or make decisions based on that evidence in accordance with social expectations. They also have intrapersonal ToM deficits that contribute to their inappropriate behavior. They fail to reflect on their thoughts and behaviors; they seem to lack self-talk critical to the control and organization of social behavior. Lack of private, self-directed speech also affects their ability to modulate their emotional reactions. Because negative emotions prove more socially unacceptable, students' difficulties in managing these emotions is problematic in relationships with teachers, peers, and parents.

▶ Assessing Social-Emotional Bases for Communication

Caregiver–Child Interaction

Children's development of the social-emotional/intentional basis of communication is dependent on their interactions with those around them and on their own personality and abilities. Because communication in infancy is so related to caregiver-child interaction, when a young child is referred for communication evaluation, it is desirable to observe the nature of this interaction. Children require different types of interaction with caregivers at various stages of development. Squires et al. (2014) provide the Social Emotional Assessment/Evaluation Measure (SEAM) that employs child observation and parent interview. The SEAM includes not only scales to evaluate infants, toddlers, and preschool children's social emotional skills and behaviors, but also scales that evaluate the strategies parents use when interacting with their children—how they respond to their child's nonverbal, verbal, emotional, and inappropriate behaviors and the types of activities and routines they engage in with their child. By completing the scales through an interview process with a professional, parents reflect not only on their children's strengths and needs, but also on the ways they interact with their children.

Vigil and Westby (2004) have also proposed a parent-child interaction profile (**TABLE 6-3**). Their scheme differentiates behaviors according to whether caregivers intend to socialize children toward independence or toward interdependence.

Assessment of Children's Communicative Behaviors

The Scope of Practice for the American Speech Language Hearing Association (2016) advocates the use of the World Health Organization's International Classification of Functioning (WHO-ICF; World Health Organization, 2001) for all clinical and research work in speech language pathology. **FIGURE 6-3** shows the

TABLE 6-3 Patterns of Socialization Interaction

Behavior	Definition	Attentional Style	
		Independent (Attention Following)	Interdependent (Attention Directing)
Follow lead	Caregiver attends to the object to which the child shows interest.		■
Direct attention	Caregiver uses vocalization, gesture, or object manipulation to engage the infant with an object or event that they want the child to attend to.	■	
Alternate attention	Caregiver alternates attention between competing events, focusing on one while momentarily stopping progress in another.		■
Simultaneous Attention	Caregiver attends to several activities occurring at the same time. This does not necessarily involve simultaneous action but rather simultaneous attention.	■	
Descriptives	An utterance in which information is given about an ongoing activity or behavior performed by either the caregiver or the child.		■
Attentional directives	Caregiver attempts to elicit the infant's attention to self or object through vocalization (i.e., "Look, look here").	■	
Behavioral directives	Utterance that elicits or constrains the physical behavior of the infant by commanding, requesting, and encouraging the child to do or desist from doing something (i.e., "Put your hand here").		■
Holds object	Caregiver holds object to support playing but does not manipulate the object or the child's hands.	■	
Manipulates object or child	Caregiver manipulates an object to direct the child's play (i.e., shows child how to play with the toy).		■

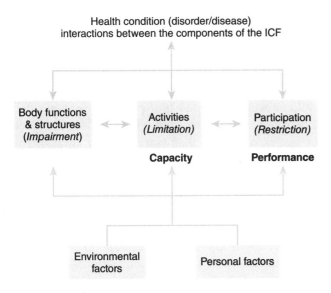

Health condition (disorder/disease)
interactions between the components of the ICF

Body functions
& structures
(*Impairment*)

Activities
(*Limitation*)
Capacity

Participation
(*Restriction*)
Performance

Environmental
factors

Personal factors

FIGURE 6-3 Interactions between the components of the ICF.

ICF framework. When evaluating a child using the ICF framework, clinicians note if the child has an impairment in body structure (e.g., missing ears, cleft palate) or body function (e.g., unintelligible speech, delayed language), ask whether this impairment limits the child from executing activities (e.g., respond to receptive/expressive language test items), and then asks whether the limitation in activities restricts a child's ability to participate in life activities (e.g., play with other children). The ICF distinguishes between the *capacity* to execute a skill or activity in a standard environment under optimal conditions and the actual *performance* of that skill when participating in social situations. The capacity to execute a behavior does not ensure that the behavior will be performed functionally in life contexts. For example, a child might be able to label pictures of a cookie or a glass or milk yet not use those words to request cookies or milk. Most formal, standardized tools assess children's skills at the activity/capacity level. Yet, the ultimate goal of intervention should be the development of children's communicative participation, i.e., pragmatically appropriate communication in life situations where knowledge, information, ideas, or feelings are exchanged (Eadie et al., 2006).

The ICF also includes two types of contextual factors, environmental and personal, that influence capacity and performance. Environmental factors include the existence of supportive relationships and attitudes towards disabilities that can serve as external barriers or facilitators to development. Personal factors can include temperament, gender, attention, or motivation, which can serve as internal barriers or facilitators to development. The ICF framework (Figure 6-3) is compatible with the SOCIAL model in Figure 6-1 and provides a holistic assessment approach to understanding social-emotional development.

Assessment of children's communicative participation should consider the number of different communicative functions or intentions they use, the proportion of each function, the rate of communicative intentions, and the child's developing theory of mind. The rate of communication may be a particularly useful measure of communicative development in language-impaired children who are using few or no words (Wetherby, Cain, Yonclas, & Walker, 1988). In particular, a lack of developing communicative functions may be a warning sign of broad-based communicative impairment. Assessment of children's communicative participation can include standardized and norm-referenced questionnaires and tests, observation of caregiver-child/teacher-child interactions, interviews of family members and teachers regarding the child's communicative behavior, and observation of children's language use in naturalistic settings and in activities structured to trigger a variety of communicative intentions.

Formal/Standardized Assessments

An increasing number of formal tools, which often employ standardized methods for their administration, have been developed. Standardized, normed tests are useful when there is a need to compare an individual or group to a standard—for example, when screening children at risk of communication deficits. Formal, standardized questionnaires and tests may also be more time-efficient than observational approaches. The use of standardized tests for evaluating pragmatics is, however, controversial. Adults have control in test-like situations, and consequently, children may not produce the same types and range of communicative intentions that they may produce in more natural situations. This outcome is particularly likely with children who are unfamiliar with test-like situations and unfamiliar with the examiner/examinee roles in testing (Westby, 2000).

Some formal assessment tools are not norm-referenced but provide guidance for determining a child's participation level and ideas for developing intervention goals. Considering the important role of joint attention in the development of the social/emotional bases for communication, it is critical that joint attention be evaluated. Mundy et al. (2003) have provided a protocol, known as the *Early Social Communication Scales* (available at https://education.ucdavis.edu/sites/main/files/file-attachments/escs_manual_2003_2013.pdf), that can be used to evaluate several types of joint attention in children between 8 and 30 months of age. Although joint attention and its related behaviors of emotional sharing, referencing, and co-referencing develop in the first 12–18 months of life, they may not be well developed in older children, particularly those with ASD. Because joint attention is so essential for meaningful communication, it should be evaluated in individuals of all age levels who exhibit deficits in social communication.

FOCUS (Focus on the Outcomes of Children under Six; Thomas-Stonell, Oddson, Robertson, & Rosenbaum, 2010) was developed to monitor communication gains in children from 12 months to 6 years enrolled in intervention programs (available at http://research.hollandbloorview.ca/outcomemeasures/focus). FOCUS is a parent/clinician questionnaire reflective of the ICF structure with items evaluating capacity and performance/ participation (available for free download at www.focusoutcomemeasurement.ca). Parents or clinicians rate children on seven-point Likert scales. Nearly half of the items assess communicative participation; for example, my child can communicate independently with adults who do not know my child well; my child becomes frustrated when trying to talk with other children; my child can tell adults who do not know my child well about past events; my child talks when playing; my child joins in conversations with peers.

Some formal criterion and normed referenced assessment tools for infants and toddlers include items that evaluate early social-emotional and pragmatic communication development. These tools include the following assessments: *Rossetti Infant-Toddler Language Scale* (Rossetti, 2006); *Ages and Stages Questionnaires: Social-Emotional* (Squires, Bricker, & Twombly, 2015); *Communication and Symbolic Behavior Scales Developmental Profile* (Wetherby & Prizant, 2002).

Some standardized, normed assessments for older children also include assessment of pragmatic behaviors. The *Children's Communication Checklist-2* (CCC-2 Bishop, 2006) is a widely used normed-referenced checklist in clinical practice and research. The CCC-2 is a 70-item checklist of communicative behaviors for children 4–16 years of age. The CCC-2 has 10 scales. Four scales assess structural aspects of language (speech, syntax, semantics, discourse), four assess pragmatics aspects of communication (initiation, scripted language, context, nonverbal communication), and two assess behaviors predictive of ASD (social relations, interests). An adult who has regular contact with the child rates each item on a four-point scale of how often a behavior is observed, from 0 (less than once a week or never) to 3 (more than twice a day or always). The CCC-2 can be used to differentiate children who have structural language impairments from those who have primarily pragmatic impairments or SCD.

The *Clinical Evaluation of Language Fundamentals—Preschool-2* (for ages 3–6 years) (Semel, Wiig, & Secord, 2004) and the *Clinical Evaluation of Language Fundamentals—4* (CELF—5; for ages 5–21 years) (Wiig, Semel, & Secord, 2013) both include a pragmatics profile. Several standardized tests for school age students assess pragmatic aspects of language. For example, *The Test of Pragmatic Language-2* (TOPL, Phelps-Terasaki & Phelps-Gunn, 2007) assesses pragmatic language exclusively and *The Comprehensive Assessment of Spoken Language-2* (CASL; Carrow-Woolfolk, 2017) has several subtests that assess pragmatic understanding. *The Social-Emotional Evaluation* (SEE; Wiig, 2008) was designed to evaluate aspects of emotional and social awareness in children 6–13 years. Formal assessments of pragmatics are problematic, however, because as soon as a task is standardized, natural aspects are removed and the complexity of the situation is reduced.

Standardized, non-normed assessments of pragmatics may use structured or scripted interactions or require judgments of what should be said in particular situations. For example, Creaghead (1984) provided a non-normed, scripted "Peanut Butter Protocol" (reproduced in Paul, 2012). With this tool, the adult attempts to elicit communication with the child while engaged in an activity with cookies, crackers, peanut butter, and jelly. During the evaluation, the adult notes the type and appropriateness of the child's pragmatic acts in response to the adult's comments.

Context	Expected Pragmatic Act
Child enters room.	Greeting
Crackers and cookies are in view but out of reach.	Requests object
Give child tightly closed jar with cookies in it.	Requests action
Ask, "How do you think we can open the jar?"	Hypothesizing
Say, "Do you want (mumble)?"	Requests clarification

Naturalistic Observations

The majority of studies on children's intentional communication have relied on naturalistic social contexts—that is, having children interact with familiar people and allowing children to converse about topics of their choosing (Coggins, Olswang, & Guthrie, 1987). It has been assumed that nonobtrusive observation provides the best opportunity to obtain a representative sample of children's language use. This technique may, however, provide an incomplete picture of a child's capabilities. A combination of both natural, unstructured activities and structured activities designed to elicit particular communicative functions may be the best way of sampling children's capabilities. Children are more likely to use requests in structured conditions and comments during free-play situations (Coggins et al., 1987). In low-structured activities, toys are readily accessible and caregivers follow the child's leads; hence, there is little need for children to request. In such situations, the child is in control and desires to share the experience with the adult. Consequently, the child is more likely to use comments to gain adult attention in unstructured settings and less likely to use requests. Elicitation tasks are adult controlled in nature, with the adult manipulating the materials to direct the child's attention. The child does not need to gain the adult's attention, but to gain access to the materials, the children has to make a request.

Young children will most readily communicate with familiar people in familiar settings. For infants and toddlers, it is best to carry out naturalistic observations of the child during daily routines at home—eating, bathing, or playing. When this is not possible, one can arrange naturalistic activities in a center and have the child's significant others (parents, grandparents, and siblings) carry out activities like they might do at home.

In practice, most clinicians use predetermined categories of communication intents and functions such as those outlined in Tables 6-1 and 6-2. A notation should be made each time a communicative behavior occurs. When using predetermined checklists, however, one should not feel compelled to make the child's responses fit the predetermined categories. The clinician should add new categories as necessary to explain the data. This may be particularly necessary when the child being evaluated is not from the demographic background on which the checklist was developed (DeJarnette, Rivers, Hyter, 2015).

In a completely naturalistic evaluation, children may not show the full range of intentionality of which they are capable. For this reason, one might want to structure the environment and interactions to trigger particular communicative functions. The activity may be loosely structured, in that the adult selects the materials and makes either leading comments or open-ended comments that could lead the child into using a particular communicative function. As adults play with the child, they may attempt to trigger requesting by not providing all the parts of a toy that are necessary; predicting by commenting, *I wonder what the fireman will do?*; projecting feelings by commenting, *I wonder how the baby feels?*; and so on.

The evaluator may want to use an even greater structure and plan to present specific activities and interactions that might trigger specific communicative intentions. For young children or children who exhibit limited initiations, the evaluator can use activities that might tempt the child to communicate (Wetherby & Prizant, 1989). Some suggestions are as follows:

- Eating desired food in front of a child without offering any to the child
- Activating a toy, letting it wind down, and then handing it to the child
- Opening a jar of bubbles, blowing some, and then closing the jar tightly and giving it to the child

Preschool and school-age children's communicative intentions can also be evaluated through the use of observational checklists. For example, the checklist in **TABLE 6-4** (based on Erickson, 1986) assesses both speech acts/communicative functions and discourse skills. Children in school should be observed in several contexts (i.e., reading class, math class, cafeteria, playground) and with both adults and peers.

The intent or function of a gesture or verbalization cannot be determined from the child's behavior alone. One must also take into account both nonverbal and verbal aspects of the interactions and the linguistic and nonlinguistic contexts of the communication in determining communicative intentions and functions. What occurred prior to or following the behavior? How does the act relate to what came before and after? Does it repeat a prior behavior, respond to it, or provide further information? Did the child give clues that they were attempting to communicate, such as orienting their body to another person, looking toward another person or attempting to clarify a behavior? Following the child's behavior, did they wait as though expecting a response?

Assessment of social-emotional bases for pragmatic communication development must go beyond the assessment of communicative intent to how the child participates in communicative interactions. The Targeted Observation of Pragmatics in Children's Conversation (TOPICC) Observation Scale was developed

TABLE 6-4 Analysis of Communicative Competence	
Discourse Skills	**Speech Acts/Communicative Functions**
▪ Starts a conversation ▪ Shows listening behavior ▪ Passes turns ▪ Receives turns/follows ▪ Responds with appropriate content ▪ Interrupts legitimately ▪ Stays on topic ▪ Changes topic appropriately ▪ Appropriately ends conversation ▪ Recognizes listener's viewpoint ▪ Demonstrates topic relevancy ▪ Uses appropriate response length ▪ Comments and gives examples of inappropriate conversational styles	▪ Labels things/actions ▪ Asks for things/actions ▪ Describes things/actions ▪ Asks for information ▪ Gives information ▪ Asks for permission ▪ Promises ▪ Agrees ▪ Threatens ▪ Warns ▪ Apologizes ▪ Protests/argues/disagrees ▪ Shows humor/teases ▪ Gives greetings and leavings ▪ Pleads ▪ Commands/orders ▪ Comments and gives examples of inappropriate language usage

Data from Erickson, J. G. (1986). Analysis of communicative competence. In L. Cole & V. Deal (Eds.), *Communication disorders in multicultural populations*. Washington, DC: American Speech-Language-Hearing Association.

for children 6–11 years of age to document their pragmatics in conversation as an outcome measure of an intervention program (Adams, Lockton, Gaile, & Freed, 2011; available for free download at http://research.bmh.manchester.ac.uk/scip/topicc.pdf and https://www.escholar.manchester.ac.uk/uk-ac-man-scw:83594). The TOPICC is a semi-structured task between an adult and a child that uses pictured photographs of events to elicit and evaluate the overall quality of a child's conversation skill. The TOPICC coding scheme rates 14 aspects of problematic pragmatic behavior, organized into six categories: reciprocity/turn-taking, taking account of listener knowledge, verbosity, topic management, discourse styles, and response problems. Each item is rated on a 0–3 scale, from never observed (typical of an age-appropriate interaction style) to marked evidence of the behavior across conversation that makes a marked impact on the interaction.

Adequate pragmatic interactions with adults do not ensure that children will interact appropriately with peers. The Pragmatics Observation Measure (POM) was developed to measure the pragmatic language performance of children between the ages of 5 and 11 years during peer-peer interactions within naturalistic contexts (Cordier, Munroc, Wilkes-Gillan, Speyer, Pearce, 2014; available for free download at http://www.sciencedirect.com/science/article/pii/S0891422214001498). The POM maps 27 items into five elements of pragmatic language: (1) Introduction

and responsiveness (introducing communication and being responsive to social interactions with peers); (2) Nonverbal communication (interpreting and using nonverbal communication); (3) Social-emotional attunement (understanding and using emotional reactions and intentions of peers); (4) Executive function (using higher-level thinking to promote interaction with peers); and (5) Negotiation (using appropriate negotiation techniques when interacting with peers). Unlike the TOPICC, which evaluates inappropriate behaviors, the POM rates appropriate behaviors on a 4-point scale (1–4) based on the child's consistency of performance ranging from rarely or never observed to almost always observed.

Interviews

A formal observational evaluation—whether it is nonstructured or structured—can be quite useful, but it does not demonstrate the variety and consistency of a child's behavior in familiar environments. Although it may be possible to conduct an evaluation in the child's home or in the classroom, it is not possible to follow children in every aspect of their daily lives.

Interviewing significant others in children's lives can provide one with information regarding their's social emotional competence and how children actually use their language. *The Social Emotional Assessment/Evaluation Measure (SEAM)* (Squires &

Bricker, 2014) employs professional observation with parent interviews to evaluate the social-emotional competence of infants, toddlers, and preschool children in terms of their participation in interactions, the range of emotions they express (displaying, interpreting, labeling, self-regulating), empathy with others, and self-regulation of behavior in activities.

TABLE 6-5 presents an interview format with cue questions and situations to explore five communicative functions that appear early in children's repertoires:

- Requests for affection/interaction
- Requests for adult actions
- Requests for objects or food
- Protests
- Declaratives/comments (Schuler, Peck, Willard, & Theimer, 1989)

Such intentional behaviors may include crying, pulling another's hand, touching/moving another's face, grabbing, walking away, vocalizing, pointing, facial expression, shaking the head yes or no, echoing something someone else said, a single word or single sign, or a phrase or sign combinations. Specific situations are presented and the adult is asked to describe what the child would do.

Assessing Theory of Mind and Emotion Understanding

The assessments discussed so far have focused on the nature of the parent-child interaction and the language functions (reasons for communicating) used by the child. Because intersubjectivity (the ability to appreciate the emotions, intentions, and beliefs of others) is so critical to the social basis of communication, it is useful to evaluate children's ToM: that is, their awareness and understanding of emotions and mental states in themselves and others.

A number of strategies have been used to assess children's ToM. In the preschool and early elementary years, children exhibit a predictable pattern of development of ToM and emotional understanding (Brinton, Spackman, Fujiki, & Ricks, 2007; Peterson, Wellman, & Slaughter, 2012; Pons et al., 2004; Wellman & Liu, 2004). The Theory of Mind Inventory-2 (ToMi-2; Hutchins, Prelock, & Bouyea, 2016) is a questionnaire completed by parents and persons who know the child well. It is normed on children 2–13 years but appropriate for individuals of any age who are at-risk of poor ToM development. The ToMI-2 consists of 60 items designed to tap a wide range of social cognitive understandings.

TABLE 6-5 Interview Questions for Communicative Functions

Requests for Affections/Interaction
What if the child wants:
- Adult to sit near?
- Peer to sit near?
- Nonhandicapped peer to sit near?
- Adult to look at him?
- Adult to tickle him?
- To cuddle/embrace?
- To sit on adult's lap?
- Other

Requests for Adult Action
What if the child wants:
- Help with dressing?
- To read a book?
- To play ball/a game?
- To go outside?
- Other

Requests for Object, Food, or Things
What if the child wants:
- An object out of reach?
- A door/container opened?
- A favorite food?
- Music/radio/TV?
- Keys/toys/book?
- Other

Protest
What if:
- Common routine is dropped?
- Favorite toy/food is taken away?
- Taken for ride with/without desire?
- Adult terminates interaction?
- The child is required to do something they don't want to?

Declaration/Comment
What if the child wants:
- To show you something?
- You to look at something?
- Other

Source: Data from Schuler, A. L., Peck, C. A., Willard, C., & Theimer, K. (1989). Assessment of communicative means and functions through interview: Assessing the communicative capabilities of individuals with limited language. *Seminars in Speech and Language*, 10, 51–62.

Each item takes the form of a statement (e.g., "My child understands whether someone hurts another on purpose or by accident"). The respondent is asked to read a statement and draw a hash mark at the appropriate point along a 20-centimeter continuum anchored by 'definitely not,' 'probably not,' 'undecided,' 'probably,' and 'definitely.' The ToMi-2 includes an interview component. The clinician reviews the protocol and then asks about the items that are expected for a child of that age but that the caregiver believes the child has not acquired, is undecided whether the child has acquired the item, or believes the child has probably but not definitely acquired the item. The scores on the protocol and caregivers' responses in the interview provide guidance for development of the intervention program.

TABLE 6-6 provides a hierarchical list of strategies for assessing some components of affective and

TABLE 6-6 Some Assessment Strategies for Theory of Mind		
Age	**Cognitive Theory of Mind**	**Affective Theory of Mind**
Emergent ToM 3–5 years		*Recognition of emotion:* Name an emotion (happy, sad, mad, surprised, afraid/scared) and ask the child to point to a photo of the person displaying the emotion.
	Knowledge access: The child sees what is in a box and judges (yes/no) the knowledge of another person who does not see what is in the box. The child is shown a small box and asked what is in it. The evaluator opens the box and shows the child a small plastic toy dog. They then produce a toy figure of a girl and tells the child, "Polly has never seen what's inside this box. Here comes Polly. Does Polly know what's inside the box? Did Polly see inside the box?"	*Identification of an external cause of emotion:* The child is shown a picture (without faces on the characters) and given a scenario (e.g., "This boy's dog ran away. He can't find his dog. How is the boy feeling?"). The child selects from photos showing happy, sad, scared, mad, and surprised and labels the emotion.
	Diverse beliefs: Tell the child Linda wants to find her cat. Her cat might be hiding in the bushes or it might be hiding in the garage. Where do you think the cat is? In the bushes or in the garage? If the child chooses bushes say: "Well, that a good idea, but Linda thinks her cat is in the garage. So where will Linda look for her cat?" (Wellman & Liu, 2004).	*Diverse desires:* The child judges that two persons have different desires about the same object. Show the child a scenario with two boys, Mark and Jeff, on either side of a closed box with a moveable flap. Tell the child, "Mark hates carrots. Jeff likes carrots very much." Check to make certain the child remembers this story and then ask the child to open the flap to see the contents of the box. There are carrots in the box. Ask, "How is Mark feeling? How is Jeff feeling?
First Order ToM 4–6 years (predicting what someone thinks or feels)	*False belief cognitive:* The child judges how a person will search, given the person's mistaken belief. The child is shown two dolls, Sally and Ann, and told, "While playing, Sally puts a marble into a basket and then goes outside. [The Sally doll disappears.] When Sally is gone, naughty Ann takes the marble out of the basket and puts it in a box. [Have the Ann doll move the marble from the basket to the box.] Sometime later, Sally comes back and wants to play with her marble. Where will Sally look for her marble?" "Why?" (Baron-Cohen, Leslie, & Frith, 1985).	*False Belief emotion:* The child judges how a person will feel, given a mistaken belief. The child is shown a picture of a rabbit eating a carrot and told that the rabbit likes carrots very much. The child is then asked to lift a flap on the page, which reveals a hidden fox. Tell the child that the fox wants to eat the rabbit. Close the flap and ask the child whether the rabbit knows the fox is there. If the child answers the false belief question correctly, say, "That's right—the rabbit doesn't know the fox is hiding behind the bushes." If the child answers incorrectly, say, "Well, actually the rabbit doesn't know the fox

6–8 years
Second
Order ToM
(predicting
what
someone
thinks
someone
else thinks or
feels; what
someone
wants
someone else
to believe or
feel)

Cognitive False Belief: John and Mary are together in the park. Mary would like to buy ice cream, but she has left her money at home. The ice cream man says, "You can go get your money and buy some ice cream later. I'll be here in the park all afternoon." So Mary goes home. Now John is on his own in the park. He sees the ice cream man leaving the park in his van. "Where are you going?" asks John. The ice cream man says, "I'm going to drive my van to the school. There is no one in the park to buy ice cream; so perhaps I can sell some outside the school." On his way, the ice cream man passes Mary's house. Mary spots the van and runs out to ask the ice cream man where he is going. "I'm going to the school," answers the man. Now John doesn't know that Mary talked to the ice cream man. John goes home. After lunch, John goes over to Mary's house to ask for help with his homework. Mary's mother answers the door. "Is Mary in?" asks John. "Oh," says Mary's mother, "She's just left. She said she was going to get an ice cream." So John runs to look for Mary. Where does he think she has gone? Justification question: Why does he think she has gone to the____? (Perner & Wimmer, 1985).

is hiding behind the bushes." Then ask, "How is the rabbit feeling? Is he happy, just all right, angry, or scared?" (Pons et al., 2004).

Affective False Belief: Joe and Anna are setting the table for dinner. Anna pours Joe a glass of water, but some water spills on his new shirt. Joe says: "It's nothing, I will change the shirt later." Anna puts the glass on the table and goes to look for a paper towel to dry Joe's shirt. When she leaves the dining room, Joe gets furious about the wet shirt and kicks the table. Anna peeks into the dining room, sees what Joe is doing and feels guilty. Anna comes back to the dining room. What does Joe think that Anna feels about the wet shirt when she returns? What does Anna think Joe feels about the wet shirt? (Shamay-Tsoory, Tibi-Elhanany, & Aharon-Peretz, 2007).

Regulation of emotion: The child is shown a picture of Tom with tears in his eyes while looking at a photo of his rabbit. The child is told that Tom is very sad because his rabbit was eaten by the fox. Ask, "What is the best way for Tom to stop himself from being sad? Can Tom cover his eyes to stop himself from being sad? Can Tom go outside and do something else to stop himself being sad? Or is there nothing Tom can do to stop himself being sad?" (Pons et al., 2004).

Hiding emotions: The child recognizes that there are situations where one should hide one's true emotions. The child is shown a picture of Chris and his aunt and told, "This is Chris, and this is Chris's aunt. Chris's aunt brings him a present for his birthday. Chris really wants a new scooter. Chris opens the present. It's a shirt. Chris does not want a shirt. How does Chris feel? What does Chris say to his aunt? What would Chris's parents want him to say?" (Brinton et al., 2007).

(continues)

TABLE 6-6 Some Assessment Strategies for Theory of Mind		(continued)
Age	**Cognitive Theory of Mind**	**Affective Theory of Mind**
8 years + Higher order	*Cognitive Lie:* John hates going to the dentist because every time he goes to the dentist, he needs a filling, and that hurts a lot. But John knows that when he has toothache, his mother always takes him to the dentist. Now John has bad toothache at the moment, but when his mother notices he is looking ill and asks him, "Do you have toothache, John?" John says, "No, Mom". Is what John says to his mother true? Why does John say this? (O'Hare, Bremner, Nash, Happe, & Pettigrew, 2009).	*Affective Lie:* One day, Aunt Jane came to visit Peter. Now Peter loves his aunt very much, but today she is wearing a new hat that Peter thinks is very ugly indeed. Peter thinks his aunt looks silly in it and much nicer in her old hat. But when Aunt Jane asks Peter, "How do you like my new hat?" Peter says, "Oh, it's very nice". Was what Peter said true? Why did he say it? (O'Hare et al., 2009).

cognitive ToM between ages 3–10. One should expect the majority of 4-year-olds to be able to identify the expressions of happy, mad, sad, surprised, and afraid; by age four or five, children they should be able to match expressions to situations that would cause the expressions (Baron-Cohen et al., 2010; Michalson & Lewis, 1985; Pons et al., 2004). Neurotypical 4- to 5-year-olds should also be able to predict what someone thinks or feel; they should be able to pass First Order ToM tasks that involve evaluating understanding of diverse beliefs, knowledge access, and false beliefs (Wellman & Liu, 2004). By early to mid-elementary school, neurotypical developing children pass Second Order ToM tasks that require them to predict what one person thinks another person is thinking or feeling; they also recognize how beliefs affect emotions, how to dissemble or hide emotions, and how to regulate emotions (Brinton et al., 2007; Fujiki, Brinton, & Clarke, 2002). By 9–10 years of age, neurotypical children recognize that persons can have multiple emotions in response to situations (Harter, 1987). They also understand that words can have multiple meanings and that the meaning of words can be different from their literal interpretation, as exhibited by figurative language, lies, and sarcasm.

One can also evaluate children's understanding of emotions by asking them to identify emotions of characters in wordless picture books such as *One Frog Too Many* (Mayer & Mayer, 1975) or *A Boy, a Dog, and a Frog* (Mayer, 1967) or movies (such as the Pixar shorts available on YouTube). One can also ask the child why the characters feel as they do and what they might do next. By age 8 years, the majority of children should be able to explain the reasons for the feelings and predict what the characters will do in response to emotions.

A word of caution about assessment of ToM and emotion understanding: belief understanding does not guarantee emotion understanding; emotion understanding does not guarantee empathy; and empathy does not guarantee that the children will be kind to people they perceive as sad (Davis & Stone, 2003).

▶ Philosophy of Intervention for Social-Communicative Deficits

The social competence that underlies communication develops from the early emotional sharing relationships between caregivers and children. Because joint attention underlies the social interactive competence essential for true communication, interventions should address any deficits in the behaviors and interactions that underlie JA and that result from development of JA. Although IBR can be developed through use of clinician-directed behavioral approaches that use drill and practice, true RJA and IJA cannot. The social competence reflected in RJA and IJA cannot be trained outside of meaningful contexts. Instead, children must be motivated to engage with others in sharing experiences that will foster RJA and IJA. If children with social-emotional deficits are to share experiences with enthusiasm and enjoyment, parents and clinicians must provide them with real pleasures inherent in experience-sharing encounters.

Intervention approaches for social communicative deficits typically use a functional or naturalistic/ecological-based, child-centered framework rather than more directive, clinician-centered approaches. Three aspects of the social use of language are essential components of these language intervention programs: the social context in which intervention occurs, the embedding of communicative goals and objectives in daily activities, and the inclusion of caregivers (or children's significant others [SOs], such as parents, siblings, grandparents, and teachers) in the intervention. Some programs, such as *It Takes Two to Talk* (Pepper & Weitzman, 2004), *More Than Words* (Sussman, 2012), *Floortime* (Davis, Isaacson, & Harwell, 2014; Greenspan, 2006), and *Relationship Development Intervention* (Gutstein, 2009), focus on intervention with family members. Other approaches, such as the milieu approach and activity-based approach, are naturalistic intervention strategies that have been widely used in infant-toddler preschool programs. Milieu teaching uses everyday instances of social-communicative exchanges as opportunities to teach elaborated language and capitalizes on natural consequences as reinforcers (Hancock, Ledbetter-Cho, Howell, & Lang, 2016). Activity-based intervention is similar to milieu teaching but is often directed to a group rather than an individual child and addresses all aspects of development, rather than just communication (Johnson, Rahn, & Bricker, 2015).

All ecologically based programs share some common assumptions:

- The SOs are facilitators, not trainers.
- The interactions should be contextualized and familiar.

As facilitators, SOs do not teach or control interactions with demands or questions. Instead, they follow the child's lead. For children who do not yet intentionally communicate, SOs imitate the infants' behavior. The facilitator looks for behaviors in the child and responds appropriately to the content and intent of the child's behavior. The child controls and initiates the conversational topics. The SO's job is to reinforce and maintain the communication naturally by responding in semantically and pragmatically contingent ways. Responses to children's behavior should be natural consequences. Thus, a request for a cookie should be followed by giving the cookie and by words such as *Okay*, or *Just one*, or *What kind?*, but not by good talking.

The learning context should be meaningful to the child. Facilitatory activities should occur in natural encounters throughout the day in the child's usual environments with familiar people and materials, not in contrived therapeutic settings. Highly routinized sequences of behavior have been shown to promote the development of intentional communication (Goetz, Gee, & Sailor, 1985). A strategy termed *interrupted behavior chain* can be used to trigger communicative behaviors. With this approach, the SO participates with the child in a familiar activity, such as eating cereal, washing hands, or putting a doll to bed. The SO interrupts the behavior chain by delaying the presentation of an item necessary for completion of the routine, placing a needed item just out of the child's reach, or preventing the child from obtaining the desired object or person (e.g., by holding an object down, stepping back out of the child's reach, or preventing the child from going outside by putting a hand on the child). For example, the child may begin the handwashing activity by turning on the water, picking up the soap, and getting, say, their hands wet and soapy. The adult may then turn off the water before the child rinses their hands. Because the routine is highly familiar, the child is likely to comment that they have not rinsed their hands, complain that her hands are sticky, or request that the water be turned back on. Adults must be conscious of a wide range of communicative functions and model them contingently in response to the child's behavior.

For young children with social-communicative deficits, ecologically based programs have the following goals:

- *Establish interactional functions.* Turn-taking is essential for communication. SOs begin to establish turn-taking routines by attending to a child's behavior, responding to it, pausing and waiting for the behavior to recur, and then responding again. Turn-taking can occur in games in which the SO nuzzles the infant; stops; watches for the infant to smile, vocalize, or laugh; and then nuzzles the infant again. With older children, this may occur in play exchanges in which the SO and child roll a car back and forth, take turns stacking blocks, or take turns placing rings on a stand or dropping blocks in a bottle.

- *Establish a clear intentional signaling system.* SOs treat an observed infant behavior as intentional (even when it isn't) and respond accordingly. If the infant looks toward a toy, the SO may say, *You want your teddy. Here it is*, as the SO brings the toy to the infant. If the infant moves its arms, the SO may say, *You want up*; raise the infant's arms; and then pick the infant up. By responding consistently, children discover that they have an effect on their environment. In time, their gestures and sounds acquire meaning because they elicit a predictable response.

- *Develop socially appropriate and conventionalized signals.* After the child is indicating intentions through gaze, vocalizations, or reaching, the adult begins to shape the behaviors by modeling appropriate gestures and words.

- *Increase the variety and frequency of communicative intentions.* As the child becomes successful in indicating intentionality, SOs provide communicative temptations that will encourage active participation of the child.

These goals cannot be achieved unless children and SOs are engaging in activities in ways that promote *emotional sharing, social referencing*, and *coordination/ coregulation* (i.e., ongoing mutual social referencing of the participants involved in social interactions). When playing with children, adults can provide surprising turns of events that promote heightened anticipation and excitement; adults can also amplify the shared emotion through facial expressions, gestures, and vocal tone. Development of social referencing can be promoted by creating simple decision points, such as moving forward or stopping where the only way for the child to determine subsequent actions is to reference the partner's emotional reactions (i.e., is the partner smiling and nodding or frowning and shaking their head?).

Adults can encourage coordination/coregulation by setting up activities that require the child to continually check whether the partner is ready to participate or continue interacting. For example, if playing ball, the child must check whether the partner is ready to catch the ball. Adults can also alter their own actions in relation to anticipated actions of their children. They can also gradually introduce activities where coordination begins to break down, and the child must notice this fact and repair the breakdown. For example, when playing catch, the adult may move so far away so that it is difficult for the child to catch the ball. The child must realize this fact and move closer. Or when walking, the adult can vary the pace so that the child must modify their pace to stay with the adult.

Emotional sharing, social referencing, and coordination/coregulation lay the foundation for the development of autobiographical episodic memory. This type of memory enables mental time travel to the past and the future. Mental time travel to the past involves recollecting happenings and events from the past. Mental time travel to the future involves using information from past memories to project anticipated events into one's future (Tulving, 2005). Autobiographical episodic memory enables individuals to make predictions—and hence make inferences in social interactions and text comprehension. Autobiographical episodic memory and ToM are interdependent. Interventions to increase parental reflection on shared experiences has been shown to improve the child's growing autobiographical episodic memory and sense of self (Reese & Newcombe, 2007). As children develop awareness of the relationship between their own feelings and experiences, they also begin to conceptualize the notion that others might have feelings about experiences. Beyond the early years,

autobiographical episodic memory and ToM form the cognitive underpinnings for social competence and pragmatic language skills.

Because ToM provides a foundation for much social-emotional/social cognitive development, it is an important component to intervention. **TABLE 6-7** shows a hierarchy of ToM skills in each of the four ToM dimensions. The goal of intervention is not to teach children to pass the ToM tasks but to use their performance on the tasks to understand how they understand social interactions and teach the language and social skills that are foundational for that ToM level. In infancy, birth to about 18 months, there is no clear differentiation among the ToM dimensions; hence, all interactions likely contribute to the development of precursors for each ToM dimension. During infancy, development is most obvious in the affective ToM dimension. The distinction between cognitive/affective and interpersonal/intrapersonal ToM becomes more evident after 18 months. Children develop the ability to pretend, which requires that what they are thinking or doing is not the same as reality. Furthermore, they develop a *sense of self*. One indication of this sense of self-awareness is that children recognize themselves in a mirror or photograph. A *sense of self* can be assessed by surreptitiously putting a small mark on a child's forehead, such as by kissing them while wearing lipstick. Children cannot feel the mark, but they can see it if they look in a mirror. If children have a sense of self, they will reach up to touch the mark when shown a mirror, indicating that they equate the mirror image with their own body.

During the preschool years, children rapidly expand their vocabularies. Emotional vocabulary and mental state vocabulary (e.g., think, know, remember, forget, wonder, and so on) provide children with information that promotes the development of interpersonal cognitive and affective ToM. Between 4 and 5 years of age, most typically developing children have acquired First Order ToM. They can predict what a person is thinking or feeling; they understand that a person may have false belief and that the person will act on that false belief. By 7 years, children have typically acquired Second Order ToM; they are able to predict what a person might think about what another person is thinking or feeling. The thinking and working memory skills associated with higher order ToM are critical for the increasingly complex social interactions expected of school-age children. During the school years, performance on higher order ToM tasks is highly correlated with peer social skills (Peterson, Slaughter, Moore, & Wellman, 2015).

TABLE 6-7 Interventions for Developing Theory of Mind

Characteristics of ToM Levels	Objectives: Develop			
	Intrapersonal Cognitive	Intrapersonal Affective	Interpersonal Cognitive	Interpersonal Affective
Stage 1: ■ Primary and secondary intersubjectivity	■ Motor imitation and imitation with objects	■ Emotional sharing, referencing, coregulation ■ Affective imitation	■ Motor imitation and imitation with objects	■ Emotional sharing, referencing, coregulation ■ Affective imitation
Stage 2: Pre-ToM, ■ Sense of self ■ Pretend skills ■ Language skills	■ Pretend behaviors ■ Awareness of physical and psychological self	■ Foundations for autobiographical memory by reminiscing ■ Identification of nonsocial emotions in self	■ Pretend skills ■ Descriptive language skills ■ Basic mental state and emotional vocabulary	■ Identification of nonsocial emotions in others ■ Identification of emotions associated with situations
Stage 3: First-order ToM ■ Passes false belief tasks ■ Mental time travel; autobiographical memory and future thinking	■ Awareness of what one knows, doesn't know, remembers, forgets ■ Cognitive flexibility; more than one way to do a task; cognitively reappraise situation	■ Autobiographical memory by sharing personal stories ■ Identification of nonsocial emotions in self ■ Strategies to regulate one's behavior/ emotions	■ Expansion of mental state and emotion words ■ Ability to determine how others cognitively appraise a situation	■ Identification of nonsocial emotions in others ■ Inferring persons'/ characters' emotions from situations ■ Predicting persons' emotions in a situation
Stage 4: Second-order ToM and higher ■ Metacognitive strategies ■ Nonliteral language ■ Conversational skills	■ Reflection on one's knowledge ■ Strategies for learning (e.g., thinking aloud; questioning the author) ■ Goal-directed planning, problem solving	■ Vocabulary for social emotions ■ Reflection on one's nonsocial and social emotions ■ Strategies for regulating behavior/ emotions	■ Multiple meanings for words ■ Recognition of multiple contextual factors that contribute to person's appraisal of situation ■ Rules for conversational interactions	■ Attention to multiple contextual cues to interpret emotions ■ Recognition of complex and subtle emotions; nuances of emotions ■ Recognition of cues for turn taking/ responding in conversations

▶ Summary

Parents, clinicians, and researchers are increasingly becoming aware of the social/pragmatic deficits exhibited by many children with a variety of language, learning, and behavioral difficulties. Age-level syntax, vocabulary, and semantic/procedural memory do not guarantee effective communication and academic success. Emergence of true communication and language depends on social-emotional competence and the motivation or goal to share emotional experiences. Then, developing language further promotes the development of social-emotional competence, which is essential for achieving friendships, working effectively with others, and comprehending narrative discourse.

The significance of the emergence of intentional communication in infants and toddlers has been recognized for some time. In recent years, research has provided insight into what underlies early social-emotional competence and what caregivers can do to promote this competence. Less attention has been given to the significance of social-emotional competence for older children. In fact, some school districts do not permit treatment of social-emotional/pragmatic deficits unless the clinician can show how these deficits affect academic performance. Nevertheless, such deficits in communicative competence have long-term consequences that affect all aspects of an individual's life.

The World Health Organization's International Classification of Functioning-Children and Youth (ICF-CY; WHO, 2007) serves as the framework for the scope of research and clinical practice for speech-language pathologists and audiologists (ASHA, 2007). The ICF views disability as the product of person-environment interaction and provides a multidimensional framework for assessing persons' impairments in body functions and structures, limitations in activities, restrictions in participation, and environmental factors. A focus of the ICF is the child's ability to participate in everyday life situations. The degree to which children participate in events or communicate with others in the home, school, and community is dependent not only on the child's specific cognitive and linguistic skills, but also on their social-emotional and pragmatic skills and the support for participating they receive from others in their environment.

Study Questions

- Describe the components of the Beaucamp and Anderson conceptualization of social competence.
- Define and give examples of each of the theory of mind dimensions.
- Describe the horizontal and vertical development of children's social communication from birth through the preschool years.
- Explain how children's temperaments, attachment factors, and cultural differences in child-rearing practices may influence the development of children's language and social communicative competence.
- Explain the significance of theory of mind in the development of children's language and social communication skills. In what ways can aspects of theory of mind be evaluated in infants, toddlers, and preschool children?
- In what ways do different types of developmental disabilities affect children's social communicative competence?
- How should a clinician approach intervention for a child's social communicative deficits?

References

Abu-Akel, A., & Shamay-Tsoory, S. (2011). Neuroanatomical and neurochemical bases of theory of mind. *Neuropsychologia, 49,* 2971–2984.

Adams, C., Clarke, E., & Haynes, R. (2009). Inference and sentence comprehension in children with specific or pragmatic language impairments. *International Journal of Language and Communication Disorders, 44,* 301–318.

Adams, C., Lockton, E., Freed, J., Gaile, J., Earl, G., McBean, K., ... Law, J. (2012). The Social Communication Intervention Project: A randomized controlled trial of the effectiveness of speech and language therapy for school-age children who have pragmatic and social communication problems with or without autism spectrum disorder. *International Journal of Language & Communication Disorders, 47*(3), 233–244.

Adams, C., Lockton, E., Gaile, J., & Freed, J. (2011). TOPIC-CAL applications: Assessment of children's conversation skills. *Speech and Language Therapy in Practice*, Spring, 7–9.

Ainsworth, M. D. S., Blehar, M. C., Waters, E., & Wall, S. (1978). *Patterns of attachment: A psychological study of the strange situation.* Hillsdale, NJ: Erlbaum.

Alessandri, S. M., & Lewis, M. (1996). Development of the self-conscious emotions in maltreated children. In M. Lewis & M. W. Sullivan (Eds.), *Emotional development in atypical children* (pp. 185–202). Mahwah, NJ: Erlbaum.

American Psychiatric Association. (2000). *Diagnostic and statistical manual of mental disorders* (4th ed.). Washington, DC: American Psychiatric Association.

American Psychiatric Association. (2013). *Diagnostic and statistical manual of mental disorders* (5th ed.). Arlington, VA: American Psychiatric Publishing.

American Speech-Language-Hearing Association. (2016). *Scope of Practice in Speech-Language Pathology.* Retrieved from www.asha.org/policy

Andrés-Roqueta, C., Adrian, J. E., Clemente, R. A., & Katsos, N. (2013).Which are the best predictors of theory of mind delay in children with specific language impairment? *International Journal of Language and Communication Disorders, 48,* 726–737.

Andrés-Roqueta, C., Adrian, J. E., Clemente, R. A., & Villanueva, L. (2016). Social cognition makes an independent contribution to peer relations in children with Specific Language Impairment. *Research in Developmental Disabilities, 49,* 277–290.

American Speech-Language-Hearing Association. (2007). *Scope of Practice in Speech-Language Pathology.* Retrieved from www.asha.org/policy.

Austen, S. (2010). Challenging behaviour in deaf children. *Educational & Child Psychology, 27,* 33–39.

Baker, L., & Cantwell, D. P. (1987). A prospective psychiatric follow-up of children with speech/language disorders. *Journal of the American Academy of Child and Adolescent Psychiatry, 26,* 546–553.

Baker, L., & Cantwell, D. P. (1992). Attention deficit disorder and speech language disorders. *Comprehensive Mental Health Care, 2*(1), 3–16.

Bakermans-Kranenburg, M. J., & van IJzendoorn, M. H. (2006). Gene-environment interaction of the dopamine D4 receptor (DRD4) and observed maternal insensitivity predicting externalizing behavior in preschoolers. *Developmental Psychobiology, 48,* 406–409.

Barkley, R. A., Cunningham, C., & Karlsson, J. (1983). The speech of hyperactive children and their mothers: Comparisons with normal children and stimulant drug effects. *Journal of Learning Disabilities, 16,* 105–110.

Baron-Cohen, S., Golan, O., Wheelright, S., Granader, Y., & Hill, J. (2010). Emotion word comprehension from 4 to 16 years old: A developmental study. *Frontiers in evolutionary neuroscience, 2,* 1–8.

Baron-Cohen, S., Leslie, A. M., & Frith, U. (1985). Does the autistic child have a 'theory of mind'? *Cognition, 21,* 37–46.

Bates, E. (1976). *Language in context.* New York, NY: Academic Press.

Bates, E., Bretherton, I., Beeghly-Smith, M., & McNew, S. (1982). Social bases of language development: A reassessment. In H. W. Reese & L. P. Lipsett (Eds.), *Advances in child development and behavior* (Vol. 16, pp. 7–75). New York, NY: Academic Press.

Beauchamp, M., & Anderson, V. (2010). SOCIAL: An integrative framework for the development of social skills. *Psychological Bulletin, 136,* 39–64.

Begeer, S., Dik, M., voor de Wind, M. J., Asbrock, D., Brambring, M., & Kef, S. (2014). A new look at theory of mind in children with ocular and ocular-plus congenital blindness. *Journal of Visual Impairment and Blindness, 108,* 17–27.

Bertenthal, B., & Longo, M. (2007). Is there evidence of a mirror system from birth? *Developmental Science, 10,* 526–529.

Bishop, D. V. M. (2006). *Children's Communication Checklist* (2nd ed., U.S. ed. 2). San Antonio, TX: Harcourt Assessment.

Bishop, D. V. M., Snowling, M. J., Thompson, P. A., Greenhalgh, T., & CATALISE-2 consortium (2017, March 30). Phase 2 of CATALISE: A multinational and multidisciplinary Delphi consensus study of problems with language development: Terminology. *Journal of Child Psychology and Psychiatry.* Published online. doi:10.1111/jcpp.12721.

Bloom, L. (1993). *The transition from infancy to language: Acquiring the power of expression.* New York, NY: Cambridge University Press.

Botting, N., & Adams, C. (2005). Semantic and inferencing abilities in children with communication disorders. *Journal of Language & Communication Disorders, 40,* 49–66.

Bretherton, I. (1991). Intentional communication and the development of an understanding mind. In D. Frye & C. Moore (Eds.), *Children's theories of mind* (pp. 49–75). Hillsdale, NJ: Erlbaum.

Bretherton, I., & Beeghly, M. (1982). Talking about internal states: The acquisition of an explicit theory of mind. *Developmental Psychology, 18,* 906–921.

Brinton, B., & Fujiki, M. (1993). Language, social skills, and socioemotional behavior. *Language, Speech, and Hearing Services in Schools, 24,* 194–198.

Brinton, B., Spackman, M. P., Fujiki, M., & Ricks, J. (2007). What should Chris say? The ability of children with specific language impairment to recognize the need to dissemble emotions in social situations. *Journal of Speech, Language, Hearing Research, 50,* 798–811.

Brown, A. D., Dorfman, M. Marmar, C. R., & Bryant, R. A. (2012). The impact of perceived self-efficacy on mental time travel and social problem solving. *Consciousness and Cognition, 21,* 299–306.

Bruner, J. (1983). *Child's talk.* New York, NY: W. W. Norton.

Bruner, J. (1986). *Actual minds, possible worlds.* Cambridge, MA: Harvard University Press.

Camarata, S. M., & Gibson, T. (1999). Pragmatic language deficits in attention-deficit hyperactivity disorder (ADHD). *Mental Retardation and Developmental Disabilities Research Reviews, 5,* 202–214.

Capps, L., Kehres, J., & Sigman, M. (1998). Conversational abilities among children with autism and children with developmental delays. *Autism, 2,* 325–344.

Carrow-Woolfolk, E. (2017). *Comprehensive assessment of spoken language-2.* San Antonio, TX: Pearson.

Celestin-Westreich, S., & Celestin, C. P. (2013). ADHD children's emotion regulation in FACE-Perspective (Facilitating adjustment of cognition and emotion): Theory, research and practice. In C. Banerjee (Ed.), *Attention deficit hyperactivity disorder in children and adolescents* (pp. 243–283). Rijeka, Croatia: InTech. Retrieved from https://www.intechopen.com/books/how-to-link/attention-deficit-hyperactivity-disorder-in-children-and-adolescents

Chapman, R. (1981). Exploring children's communicative intents. In J. F. Miller (Ed.), *Assessing language production in children* (pp. 111–138). Austin, TX: Pro-Ed.

Chen, X., & Rubin, K. H. (Eds.) (2011). *Socioemotional development in cultural context.* New York, NY: Guilford.

Coggins, T. E. & Carpenter, R. L. (1981). The communicative intention inventory: A system for observing and coding children's early intentional communication. *Applied Psycholinguistics, 2*(3), 235–51.

Coggins, T. E., Oslwang, L. B., & Guthrie, J. (1987). Assessing communicative intents in young children: Low structured observation or elicitation tasks? *Journal of Speech and Hearing Disorders, 52,* 44–49.

Conti-Ramsden, G., Moka, P. L. H., Pickles, A., & Durkin, K. (2013). Adolescents with a history of specific language impairment (SLI): Strengths and difficulties in social, emotional and behavioral functioning. *Research in Developmental Disabilities, 34*, 4161–4169.

Cordier, R., Munroc, N., Wilkes-Gillan, S., Speyer, R., & Pearce, W. M. (2014). Reliability and validity of the Pragmatics Observational Measure (POM): A new observational measure of pragmatic language for children. *Research in Developmental Disabilities, 35*(7), 1588–1598.

Creaghead, N. (1984). Strategies for evaluating and targeting pragmatic behaviors in young children. *Seminars in Speech and Language, 5*, 241–252.

Davis, A., Isaacson, L., & Harwell, M. (2014). *Floortime strategies to promote development in children and teens.* Baltimore, MD: Brookes.

Davis, M., & Stone, T., (2003). Synthesis: Psychological understanding and social skills. In B. Repacholi & V. Slaughter (Eds.), *Individual differences in theory of mind: Implications for typical and atypical development* (pp. 306–352). New York, NY: Psychology Press.

Dejarnette, G., Rivers, K. O., & Hyter, Y. D. (2015). Ways of examining speech acts in young African American children. *Topics in Language Disorders, 35*, 61–75.

Denham, S. A. (1998). *Emotional development in young children.* New York, NY: Guilford.

de Villiers, P. (2005). The role of language in theory-of-mind development: What deaf children tell us. In J. W. Astington & J. A. Baird (Eds.), *Why language matters for theory of mind* (pp. 266–297). New York, NY: Oxford University Press.

de Villiers, P. A., & de Villiers, J. G. (2012). Deception dissociates from false belief reasoning in deaf children: Implications for the implicit versus explicit theory of mind distinction. *British Journal of Developmental Psychology, 30*, 188–209.

Dore, J. (1975). Holophrases, speech acts and language universals. *Journal of Child Language, 2*, 21–40.

Dore, J. (1978). Requestive systems in nursery school conversations: Analysis of talk in its social context. In R. Campbell & P. Smith (Eds.), *Recent advances in the psychology of language: Language development and mother-child interaction* (pp. 271–292). New York, NY: Plenum Press.

Dyck, M. J., Farrugia, C., Shochet, I. M., & Holmes-Brown, M. (2004). Emotion recognition/understanding ability in hearing or vision-impaired children: Do sounds sights, or words make the difference? *Journal of Child Psychology and Psychiatry, 45*, 789–800.

Eadie, T. L., Yorkston, K. M., Klasner, E. R., Dudgeon, B. J., Deitz, J., Baylor, C. R., … Amtmann, D. (2006). Measuring communicative participation: A review of self-report instruments in speech-language pathology. *American Journal of Speech-Language Pathology, 15*, 307–320.

Erickson, J. G. (1986). Analysis of communicative competence. In L. Cole & V. Deal (Eds.), *Communication disorders in multicultural populations.* Washington, DC: American Speech-Language-Hearing Association.

Ervin-Tripp, S. & Gordon, D. (1986). The development of requests. In. R. L. Schiefelbusch (Ed.), *Language competence: Assessment and intervention* (pp. 61–95). San Diego, CA: College-Hill.

Field, T., Sostek, A. M., Vietze, P., & Leiderman, P. H. (1981). Culture and early interactions. Hillsdale, NJ: Erlbaum.

Fivush, R. (2011). The development of autobiographical memory. *Annual Review of Psychology, 62*, 559–582.

Ford, J. A., & Milosky, L. M. (2003). Inferring emotional reactions in social situations: Differences in children with language impairment. *Journal of Speech, Language & Hearing Research, 46*, 21–30.

Fujiki, M., Brinton, B., & Clarke, D. (2002). Emotion regulation in children with specific language impairment. *Language, Speech, and Hearing Services in Schools, 33*, 102–111.

Fujiki, M., Brinton, B., Isaacson, T., & Summers, C. (2001). Social behaviors of children with language impairment on the playground: A pilot study. *Language, Speech, and Hearing Services in Schools, 32*, 101–113.

Fujiki, M., Brinton, B., & Todd, C. M. (1996). Social skills of children with specific language impairment. *Language, Speech, and Hearing Services in Schools, 27*, 195–202.

Fujiki, M., Spackman, M. P., Brinton, B., & Illig, T. (2008). Ability of children with language impairment to understand emotion conveyed by prosody in a narrative passage. *International Journal of Language and Communication Disorders, 43*, 330–345.

Garello, V., Viterbori, P., & Usai, M. C. (2012). Temperamental profiles and language development: A replication and extension. *Infant Behavior & Development, 35*, 71–82.

Giddan, J. J. (1991). School children with emotional problems and communication deficits: Implications for speech-language pathologists. *Language, Speech, and Hearing Services in Schools, 22*, 291–295.

Gillespie-Lynch, K., Sepeta, L., Wang, Y., Marshall, S., Gomez, L., Sigman, M., & Hutman, T. (2012). Early childhood predictors of the social competence of adults with autism. *Journal of Autism & Developmental Disorders, 42*, 161–174.

Goberis, D., Beams, D., Dalpes, M., Abrisch, A., Baca, R., & Yoshinaga-Itano, C. (2012). The missing ling in language development of deaf and hard of hearing children: Pragmatic language development. *Seminars in Speech and Language, 33*, 297–309.

Goetz, L., Gee, K., & Sailor, W. (1985). Using a behavior chain interruption strategy to teach communication skills to students with severe disabilities. *Journal of the Association of Persons with Severe Handicaps, 10*, 21–30.

Gordon, D., & Ervin-Tripp, S. (1984). Structure of children's requests. In R. L. Schiefelbusch & J. Pickar (Eds.), *The acquisition of communicative competence* (pp. 295–322). Baltimore, MD: University Park Press.

Gray, C., Hosie, J., Russell, P., Scott, C., & Hunter, N. (2007). Attribution of emotions to story characters by severely and profoundly deaf children. *Journal of Developmental and Physical Disabilities, 19*, 145–159.

Greenaway, R., & Dale, N. J., (2017). Congenital visual impairment. In L. Cummins (Ed.), *Research in clinical pragmatics* (pp. 441–469). London, UK: Springer.

Greenfield, P. M., & Cocking, R. R. (1994). *Cross-cultural roots of minority child development.* Hillsdale, NJ: Erlbaum.

Greenspan, S. (2006). Engaging children: Using the floortime approach to help children relate, communicate, and think. Cambridge, MA: Da Capo Press.

Gutstein, S. E. (2009). *The RDI book.* Houston, TX: Connections Center Publishing.

Halliday, M. A. K. (1975). *Learning how to mean: Explorations in the development of language.* London, UK: Edward Arnold.

Hamlett, K. W., Pellegrini, D. S., & Connors, C. K. (1987). An investigation of executive processes in the problem solving of attention deficit disorder-hyperactive children. *Journal of Pediatric Psychology, 12*, 227–240.

Hamlett, K. W., Pelligrini, D. S., & Conners, C. K. (1987). An investigation of executive processes in the problem-solving of attention deficit disorder-hyperactivity children. *Journal of Pediatric Psychology, 12,* 227–240.

Hancock, T. B., Ledbetter-Cho, K., Howell, A., & Lang, R. (2016). Enhanced milieu teaching. In R. Lang, T. B. Hancock, & N. Singh (Eds.), *Early intervention for young children with autism spectrum disorders* (pp. 177–218). Cham, Switzerland: Springer.

Harris, P. L. (2008). Children's understanding of emotions. In M. Lewis, J. M. Haviland-Jones, & J. F. Bartlett (Eds.), *Handbook of emotions* (3rd ed., pp. 320–331). New York, NY: Guilford.

Harter, S. (1987). Children's understanding of the simultaneity of two emotions: A five-stage developmental acquisition sequence. *Developmental Psychology, 23,* 388–399.

Heath, S. B. (1983). *Ways with words.* Cambridge, MA: Cambridge University Press.

Hewitt, L. E. (1994). Narrative comprehension: The importance of subjectivity. In J. F. Duchan, L. E. Hewitt, & R. M. Sonnenmeier (Eds.), *Pragmatics: From theory to practice.* (pp. 88–104). Englewood Cliffs, NJ: Prentice-Hall.

Hollo, A., Wehby, J. H., & Oliver, R. M. (2014). Unidentified language deficits in children with emotional and behavioral disorders: A meta-analysis. *Exceptional Children, 80,* 169–186.

Hurtig, R., Ensrud, S., & Tomblin, J. B. (1982). The communicative function of question production in autistic children. *Journal of Autism and Developmental Disorders, 12,* 57–69.

Hutchins, T. L., Prelock, P. A., & Bouyea, L. B. (2016). Theory of mind inventory-2. Retrieved from http://www.theoryofmind-inventory.com/

James, D. M., & Stojanovik, V. (2007). Communication skills in blind children: A preliminary investigation. *Child: Care, Health and Development, 33,* 4–10.

Johnson, J., Rahn, N. L., & Bricker, D. (2015). *An activity-based approach to early intervention* (4th ed.), Baltimore, MD: Brookes.

Johnston, J. R., & Wong, M. Y. A. (2002). Cultural differences in beliefs and practices concerning talk to children. *Journal of Speech, Language, and Hearing Research, 45,* 916–926.

Laible, D. (2004). Mother-child discourse in two contexts: Links with child temperament, attachment security, and socioemotional competence. *Developmental Psychology, 40,* 979–992.

Legerstee, M. (2005). Infants' sense of people: Precursors to a theory of mind. New York, NY: Cambridge University Press.

Lewis, M. (2014). *The rise of consciousness and the development of emotional life.* New York, NY: Guilford.

Loveland, K. A., Landry, S. H., Hughes, S. O., Hall, K. K., & McEvoy, R. E. (1988). Speech acts and the pragmatic deficits of autism. *Journal of Speech and Hearing Research, 31,* 593–604.

Ludlow, A., Heaton, P., Rosset, D., Hills, P., & Deruelle, C. *(2010). Emotion* recognition in children with profound and severe deafness: Do they have a deficit in perceptual processing? Journal of Clinical & Experimental Neuropsychology, 32, 923–928.

Lynch, E. W., & Hanson, M. J. (2004). *Developing cross-cultural competence.* Baltimore, MD: Paul Brookes.

Main, M. (1996). Introduction to the special section on attachment and psychopathology: 2. Overview of the field of attachment. *Journal of Counseling and Clinical Psychology, 64,* 237–243.

Mayer, M. (1967). *A boy, a dog, and a frog.* New York, NY: Dial Press.

Mayer, M., & Mayer, M. (1975). *One frog too many.* New York, NY: Dial Press.

McGurk, H. (1983). Effective motivation and the development of communicative competence in blind children. In A. E. Mills (Ed.), *Language acquisition in the blind child: Normal and deficient.* (pp. 114–132). San Diego, CA: College-Hill.

Meltzoff, A., & Moore, W. (1977). Imitation of facial and manual gestures by human neonates. *Science, 198,* 75–78.

Merkenschlager, A., Amorosa, H., Kiefl, H., & Martinius, J. (2012). Recognition of face identity and emotion in expressive specific language impairment. *Folia Phoniatrica et Logopaedica, 64,* 73–79.

Michalson, L., & Lewis, M. (1985). What do children know about emotions and when do they know it. In M. Lewis & C. Saarni (Eds.), *The socialization of emotions* (pp. 117–139). New York, NY: Plenum.

Mills, A. (1993). Visual handicap. In D. V. M. Bishop & K. Mogford (Eds.), *Language development in exceptional circumstances* (pp. 150–164). Hove, UK: Erlbaum.

Moore, V., & McConachie, H. (1994). Communication between blind and severely visually impaired children and their parents. *British Journal of Developmental Psychology, 12,* 491–502.

Mueller, K. L., & Tomblin, J. B. (2012). Examining the comorbidity of language disorders and ADHD. *Topics in Language Disorders, 32,* 228–246.

Mundy, P. (2016). *Autism and joint attention: Development, neuroscience, and clinical fundamentals.* New York, NY: Guilford.

Mundy, P., Delgado, C., Block, J., Venezia, M., Hogan, A., & Seibert, J. (2003). *Early social communication scales.* Miami, FL: University of Miami. Retrieved from http://www.ucdmc.ucdavis.edu/mindinstitute/ourteam/faculty_staff/escs.pdf

Mundy, P., Sigman, M., & Kasari, C. (1994). Joint attention, developmental level, and symptom presentation in a young child with autism. *Developmental and Psychopathology, 6,* 389–401.

Mundy, P., & Thorp, D. (2006). The neural basis of early joint-attention behavior. In T. Charman & W. Stone (Eds.), *Social and communicative development in autism spectrum disorders* (pp. 296–336). New York, NY: Guilford.

Netten, A. P., Rieffe, C., Theunissen, S., Doede, W., Dirks, E., Briaire, J. J., & Frijns, J. H. M. (2015). Low empathy in deaf and hard of hearing (pre)adolescents compared to normal hearing controls. *PLOS One.* doi:10.1371/journal.pone.0124102

Nilsson, K. K., & de López, K. J. (2016). Theory of mind in children with specific language impairment: A systematic review and meta-analysis. *Child Development, 87,* 143–153.

Northoff, G., Heinzel, A., de Greck, M., Felix, B., Dobrowolny, H., & Panksepp, J. (2006). Self-referential processing in our brain: A meta-analysis of imaging studies on the self. *Neuro-Image, 31,* 440–457.

O'Hare, A. E., Bremner, L., Nash, M., Happe, F., & Pettigrew, L. (2009). A clinical assessment tool for advanced theory of mind performance in 5 to 12 year olds. *Journal of Autism & Developmental Disorders, 39,* 916–928.

O'Reilly, K., Peterson, C. C., & Wellman, H. M. (2014). Sarcasm and advanced theory of mind understanding in children and adults with prelingual deafness. *Developmental Psychology, 50*(7), 1862–1877.

Ozonoff S. J. (2012). Editorial Perspective: Autism Spectrum Disorders in DSM-5—An historical perspective and the need for change. *Journal of Child Psychology and Psychiatry, 53,* 1092–1094.

Paul, R. (2012). Language disorders from infancy through adolescence. St. Louis, MO: Elsevier Mosby.

Paul, R., Orlovski, S., Marcinko, H., & Volkmar, F. (2009). Conversational behaviors in youth with high-functioning ASD and Asperger syndrome. *Journal of Autism & Developmental Disorders, 39,* 115.

Pepper, J., & Weitzman, E. (2004). *It takes two to talk: A practical guide for parents of children with language delays.* (3rd ed.). Toronto, ON: The Hanen Centre.

Perner, J., & Wimmer, H. (1985) "John thinks that Mary thinks that . . ." Attribution of second order beliefs by 5- to 10-year-old children. *Journal of Experimental Child Psychology, 39,* 437–471.

Perry, P. D. (1997). Incubated in terror: Neurodevelopmental factors in the "cycle of violence." In J. D. Osofsky (Ed.), *Children in a violent society* (pp. 127–149). New York, NY: Guilford.

Peterson, C. C. (2009). Development of social-cognitive and communication skills in children born deaf. *Scandinavian Journal of Psychology, 50,* 475–483.

Peterson, C. C. (2016). Empathy and theory of mind in deaf and hearing children. *Journal of Deaf Studies and Deaf Education, 21,* 141–147.

Peterson, C. C., Peterson, J. L., & Webb, J. (2000). Factors influencing the development of a theory of mind in blind children. *British Journal of Developmental Psychology, 18,* 431–447.

Peterson, C., Slaughter, V., Moore, C., & Wellman, H. M. (2015). Peer social skills and theory of mind in children with autism, deafness, or typical development. *Developmental Psychology, 52,* 46–57.

Peterson, C. C., Wellman, H. M., & Slaughter, V. (2012). The mind behind the message: Advancing theory-of-mind scales for typically developing children, and those with deafness, autism, or Asperger Syndrome. *Child Development, 83,* 469–485.

Phelps-Terasaki, D., & Phelps-Gunn, T. (2007). *Test of pragmatic language* (2nd ed.). Austin, TX: Pro-Ed.

Pons, R., Harris, P., & de Rosnay, M. (2004). Emotion comprehension between 3–11 years: Developmental periods and hierarchical organization. *European Journal of Developmental Psychology, 1,* 127–152.

Purvis, K. L., & Tannock, R. (1997). Language abilities in children with attention deficit hyperactivity disorder, reading disabilities, and normal controls. *Journal of Abnormal Child Psychology, 25,* 133–144.

Reese, E., & Newcombe, R. (2007). Training mothers in elaborative reminiscing enhances children's autobiographical memory and narrative. *Child Development, 78,* 1153–1170.

Reese, E., & Sutcliffe, E. (2006). Mother-child reminiscing and children's understanding of mind. *Merrill-Palmer Quarterly, 52,* 17–43.

Rice, M. L. (1993). "Don't talk to him; He's weird." A social consequences account of language and social interactions. In A. P. Kaiser & D. B. Gray (Eds.), *Enhancing children's communication: Research foundations for intervention* (pp. 139–158). Baltimore, MD: Paul H. Brookes.

Rieffe, C., Terwogt, M. M., & Smit, C. (2003). Deaf children on the causes of emotions. *Educational Psychology, 23,* 159–168.

Roch-Levecq, A. C. (2006). Production of basic emotions by children with congenital blindness: Evidence for the embodiment of theory of mind. *British Journal of Developmental Psychology, 24,* 507–528.

Rossetti, L. (2006). *The Rossetti infant-toddler language scale.* East Moline, IL: Linguisystems.

Rutter, M., & Garmezy, N. (1983). Developmental psychopathology. In E. J. Hetherington (Ed.), *Handbook of child psychology, Vol. IV: Socialization, personality, and social development.* (pp. 601–616). New York, NY: Wiley.

Ryder, N., & Leinonen, E. (2014). Pragmatic language development in language impaired and typically developing children: Incorrect answers in context. *Journal of Psycholinguistic Research, 43,* 45–58.

Sak-Wernicka, J. (2016). Exploring theory of mind use in blind adults during natural communication. *Journal of Psycholinguistic Research, 45,* 857–69.

Salmon, K., & Reese, E. (2016). The benefits of reminiscing with young children. *Current Directions in Psychological Science, 25,* 233–238.

Schaffer, H. R. (1984). *The child's entry into a social world.* New York, NY: Academic Press.

Schuler, A. L., Peck, C. A., Willard, C., & Theimer, K. (1989). Assessment of communicative means and functions through interview: Assessing the communicative capabilities of individuals with limited language. *Seminars in Speech and Language, 10,* 51–62.

Schulte-Ruther, M., Markowitsch, H. J., Fink, G. R., & Piefke, M. (2007). Mirror neuron and theory of mind mechanisms involved in face-to-face interactions: A functional magnetic resonance imaging approach to empathy. *Journal of Cognitive Neuroscience, 19,* 1354–1372.

Sebastian, C. L., Fontaine, N., Bird, G., Blakemore, S. J., De Brito, S. A., McCrory, E. J. P., & Viding, E. (2012). Neural processing associated with cognitive and affective Theory of Mind in adolescents and adults. *SCAN, 7,* 53–63.

Semel, E., Wiig, E., & Secord, W. (2004). *Clinical Evaluation of Language Fundamentals—Preschool 2. (CELF—P2).* San Antonio, TX: Harcourt Assessment.

Shamay-Tsoory, S., Tibi-Elhanany, Y., & Aharon-Peretz, J. (2007). The ventromedial prefrontal cortex is involved in understanding affective but not cognitive theory of mind stories. *Social Neuroscience, 1,* 149–166.

Sheinkopf, S., Mundy, P., Claussen, A., & Willoughby, J. (2004). Infant joint attention skill and preschool behavioral outcomes in at-risk children. *Developmental Psychopathology, 16,* 273–291.

Siegel, D. (2012). *The developing mind: How relationships and the brain interact to shape who we are.* New York, NY: Guilford.

Shin, D.W., Lee, S.J., Kim, B.J., Park, Y., & Lim, S. W. (2008). Visual attention deficits contribute to impaired facial emotion recognition in boys with attention-deficit/hyperactivity disorder. *Neuropediatrics, 39*(6), 323–3277.

Slaughter, V., & De Rosnay, M. (2017). *Theory of mind development in context.* New York, NY: Routledge.

Snow, C. E., & Ferguson, C. A. (1977). *Talking to children: Language input and acquisition.* Cambridge, UK: Cambridge University Press.

Sonksen, P. M., & Dale, N. (2002). Visual impairment in infancy: Impact on neurodevelopmental and neurobiological processes. *Developmental Medicine and Child Neurology, 44,* 782–791.

Squires, J., Bricker, D., & Twombly, L. (2015). *Ages and stages questionnaires: Social-emotional (2nd ed.)* Baltimore, MD: Brookes.

Squires, J., Bricker, D., Waddell, M., Funk, K., Clifford, J., & Hoselton, R. (2014). *Social-emotional assessment/evaluation measure (SEAM™), Research Edition.* Baltimore, MD: Brookes.

Staikova, E., Gomes, H., Tartter, V., McCabe, A., & Halperin, J. M. (2013). Pragmatic deficits and social impairment in children with ADHD. *Journal of Child Psychology and Psychiatry, 54,* 1275–1283.

St. Clair, M. C., Pickles, A., Durkin, K., & Conti-Ramsden, G. (2011). A longitudinal study of behavioral and social difficulties in individuals with a history of specific language impairment (SLI). *Journal of Communication Disorders, 44,* 186–199.

Stern, D. (1977). *The first relationship: Infant and mother.* Cambridge, MA: Harvard University Press.

Sussman, F. (2012). *More than words: The Hanen program for parents of children with autism spectrum disorders*. Toronto, ON: The Hanen Centre.

Tadic, V., Pring, L., & Dale, N. (2010). Are language and social communication intact in children with congenital visual impairment at school age? *Journal of Child Psychology & Psychiatry, 51*, 696–705.

Tager-Flusberg, H., Paul, R., & Lord, C. (2005). Language and communication in autism. In F. Volkmar, R. Paul, A. Klin, & D. Cohen (Eds.), *Handbook of autism and pervasive developmental disorders: Vol. 1: Diagnosis, development, and neurobiology* (pp. 335–363). New York, NY: Wiley.

Tannock, R., & Schachar, R. (1996). Executive dysfunction as an underlying mechanism of behaviour and language problems in attention deficit hyperactivity disorders. In J. H. Beitchman, N. J. Cohen, M. M. Konstantareas, & R. R. Tannock (Eds.), *Language learning and behavior disorders: Developmental, biological, and clinical perspective* (pp. 128–155). New York, NY: Cambridge University Press.

Taumoepeau, M., & Reese, E. (2013). Maternal reminiscing, elaborative talk, and children's theory of mind: An intervention study. *First Language, 33*, 388–410.

Taylor, L. J., Maybery, M. T., Grayndler, L., & Whitehouse, W. J. O. (2015). Evidence for shared deficits in identifying emotions from faces and from voices in autism spectrum disorders and specific language impairment. *International Journal of Language and Communication Disorders, 40*, 42–466.

Thomas, A., & Chess, S. (1977). *Temperament and development*. New York, NY: Brunner/Mazel.

Thompson, R. A. (2014). Socialization of emotion and emotion regulation in the family. In J. J. Gross (Ed.), *Handbook of emotion regulation* (2nd ed., pp. 173–186). New York, NY: Guilford.

Thomas-Stonell, N., Oddson, B., Robertson, B., & Rosenbaum, P. (2010) Development of the FOCUS (FOCUS on the Outcomes of Communication Under Six), a communication outcome measure for preschool children. *Developmental Medicine and Child Neurology, 52*, 47–53.

Todd, J. T., & Dixon, W. E. (2010). Temperament moderates responsiveness to joint attention in 11-month-old infants. *Infant Behavior & Development, 33*, 297–308.

Toe, D., Rinaldi, P., Caselli, M. C., Paatsch, L., & Church, A. (2016). The development of pragmatic skills in children and young people who are deaf and hard of hearing. In M. Marschark, V. Lampropoulou, & E. K. Skordilis (Eds.), *Diversity in deaf education* (pp. 247–269). New York, NY: Oxford University Press

Tomasello, M. (1995). Joint attention as social cognition. In C. Moore & P. Denham (Eds.), *Joint attention: Its origins and role in development* (pp. 103–130). Hillsdale, NJ: Erlbaum.

Tronick, E. (2007). *The neurobehavioral and social-emotions development of infants*. New York, NY: W.W. Norton.

Tulving, E. (2005). Episodic memory and autonoesis: Uniquely human. In H. S. Terrace & J. Metcalfe (Eds.), *The missing link in cognition: Origins of self-reflective consciousness* (pp. 3–56). New York, NY: Oxford University Press.

Urwin, C. (1984). Communication in infancy and the emergence of language in blind children. In R. L. Schiefelbusch & J. Pickar (Eds.), *The acquisition of communicative competence* (pp. 479–520). Baltimore, MD: University Park Press.

van Agt, H., Verhoeven, L., van den Brink, G., & De Koning, H. (2010). The impact on socio-emotional development and quality of life of language impairment in 8-year-old children. *Developmental Medicine & Child Neurology, 53*, 81–88.

van Balkom, H., Verhoeven, L., & van Weerdenburg, M. (2010). Conversational behaviour of children with developmental language delay and their caretakers. *International Journal of Communication Disorders, 45*, 295–319.

Vigil, D. C. (2002). Cultural variations in attention regulation: A comparative analysis of British and Chinese-immigrant populations. *International Journal of Language & Communication Disorders, 37*, 433–458.

Vigil, D., & Westby, C. E. (2004). Caregiver interaction style. *Perspectives on Language Learning and Education, 11*(2), 10–14.

Volkmar, F., & Klin, A. (2005). Issues in classification of autism and related disorders. In F. Volkmar, R. Paul, A. Klin, & D. Cohen (Eds.), *Handbook of autism and pervasive developmental disorders: Vol. 1: Diagnosis, development, and neurobiology* (pp. 5–41). New York, NY: Wiley.

Vostanis, P., Hayes, M., Du Feu, M., & Warren, J. (1997). Detection of behavioural and emotional problems in deaf children and adolescents: Comparison of two rating scales. *Child Care, Health, & Development, 23*, 233–246.

Wang, Q. (2013). *The autobiographical self in time and culture*. New York, NY: Oxford.

Waxman, S., Fu, X., Ferguson, B., Geraghty, K., & Leddon, E. (2016). How early is infants' attention to objects and actions shaped by culture? New evidence from 24-month-olds raised in the US and China. *Frontiers in Psychology, 7*, 97. doi:10.3389/fpsyg.2016.00097

Wellman, H. M., & Liu, D. (2004). Scaling of theory-of-mind tasks. *Child Development, 75*, 523–541.

Westby, C. E. (2000). Multicultural issues in speech and language assessment. In J. B. Tomblin, H. L. Morris, & D. Spriesterbach (Eds.), Diagnosis methods in speech-language pathology (pp. 35–62). San Diego, CA: Singular.

Westby, C. E. & Cutler, S. (1994). Language and ADHD: Understanding the bases and treatment of self-regulatory behaviors. *Topics in Language Disorders, 14*, 58–76.

Wetherby, A. M., Cain, D. H., Yonclas, D. G., & Walker, V. G. (1988). Analysis of intentional communication in normal children from the prelinguistic to multiword stage. *Journal of Speech and Hearing Research, 31*, 242–252.

Wetherby, A. M., & Prizant, B. M. (1989). The expression of communicative intent: Assessment guidelines. *Seminars in Speech and Language, 10*, 77–91.

Wetherby, A. M., & Prizant, B. M. (2002). *Communication and symbolic behavior scales developmental profile*. Baltimore, MD: Brookes.

Whalen, C., Henker, B., Collins, B., McAuliffe, S., & Vaux, A. (1979). Peer interactions in a structured communication task. Comparison of normal and hyperactive boys and methylphenidate (Ritalin) and placebo effect. *Child Development, 50*, 338–401.

Whiting, B. B., & Edwards, C. P. (1988). *Children of different worlds*. Cambridge, MA: Harvard University Press.

Widen, S. C., & Russell, J. A. (2010). Children's scripts for social emotions: Causes and consequences are more central than are facial expressions. *British Journal of Developmental Psychology, 28*, 565–581.

Wiefferink, C. H., Rieffe, C., Ketelaar, L., De Raeve, L., & Frijns, J. H. M. (2013). Emotion understanding in deaf children with a cochlear implant. *Journal of Deaf Studies and Deaf Education, 18*, 175–186.

Wiig, E. (2008). *The social-emotional evaluation (SEE)*. Greenville, SC: Super Duper.

Wiig, E., Semel, E., & Secord, W. (2013). *Clinical evaluation of language fundamentals—5*. San Antonio, TX: Pearson.

Wilton, A. P. (2011). Implications of parent-child Interaction for early language development of young children with visual impairments. *Insight: Research & Practice in Visual Impairment & Blindness, 4,* 139–147.

World Health Organization. (2001). *International classification of functioning, disability and health (ICF).* Geneva, Switzerland: Author.

World Health Organization (WHO). (2007). *International classification of functioning, disability, and health—Children and youth.* Geneva, Switzerland: Author.

Yuill, N., & Lyon, J. (2007). Selective difficulty in recognising facial expressions of emotion in boys with ADHD. General performance impairments or specific problems in social cognition? *European Child & Adolescent Psychiatry, 16*(6), 398–404.

Zentall, S. S. (1985). A context for hyperactivity. In K. D. Gamow & I. Bailer (Eds.), *Advances in learning and behavioral disabilities* (Vol. 4, pp. 273–343). Greenwich, CT: JAI Press.

Zlatev, J., Racine, T. P., Sinha, C., & Itkonen, E. (Eds.) (2008). *The shared mind: Perspectives on intersubjectivity.* Philadelphia, PA: John Benjamins.

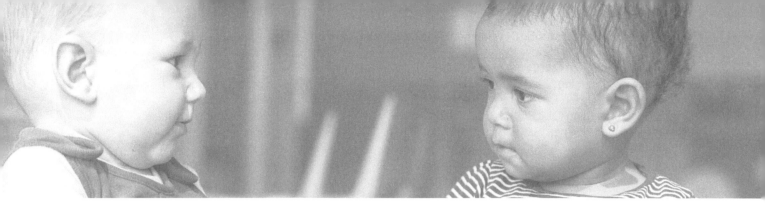

CHAPTER 7

Early Semantic Development: The Developing Lexicon

Nina Capone Singleton, PhD, CCC-SLP
William O. Haynes, PhD, CCC-SLP

OBJECTIVES

- To learn the milestones of early semantic development
- To understand factors that influence word learning in children
- To understand theories of word learning and retrieval in children
- To identify a common measure of word use from a spontaneous language sample

KEY TERMS

Action words
Basic-level terms
Breadth
Central executor
Configuration
Decontextualization
Depth
Distributed neural network
Emergentist coalition model
Engagement
Episodic buffer
Expressive language learnersFast mapping
Function words
Functional core hypothesis

General nominals
Hierarchical organization of the lexicon
Indeterminate errors/responses
Innate biases
Late bloomers
Late talkers
Lexeme
Lexical representation
Lexical-semantic network
Modifiers
Natural partitions hypothesis
Neighborhood density
Nominal insight

Novel name-nameless category principle (N3C)
Ordering of word classes
Ordinate terms
Overextension
Perseverative errors
Personal-social words
Phonetically consistent form (PCF)
Phonological errors
Phonological loop
Phonotactic probability
Principle of conventionality
Principle of extendibility
Principle of mutual exclusivity
Principle of reference

▶ Introduction

The child spends a year preparing for his first word with a variety of developments across motor, pragmatic, cognitive, and phonological domains. For example, stability in the trunk muscles supports sitting at approximately 6 months of age. The child's ability to develop fine motor movements of the hand and mouth depends on this gross motor development in the body. A stable base allows for mobility in the hands to explore objects and for the muscles of the mouth to babble and for later word productions. Mature babbling shares phonemes (i.e., sounds) with first words.

On average, by 12 months of age, the child's first word emerge. Subsequent utterances remain one word in length for several months. By 16 months, words are combined with gesture in the form of pointing in combination with a single word (e.g., point to dog + "doggie"). From the time first words emerge until the first 50 words are accrued, word learning is gradual (Nelson, 1973). The 50-word lexicon accrues some time between 18 and 24 months of age (Fenson et al., 1993). The lexicon refers to our store of words. Once approximately 50 words have been amassed, the child has a *word spurt* (Bates et al., 1994; Goldfield & Reznick, 1990). The word spurt is characterized by the fast learning of many new words.

It seems as though children have become expert word learners at this point! Children are saying many new words and a third milestone emerges—word combinations. With all these new words, the child links ideas into short utterances that reveal their relationships with each other through systematic combinations. A verb spurt then occurs around the second birthday, and many word classes are being mapped in memory after this as the child heads toward 30 months of age. This chapter presents developments and theories within the domain of semantics from infancy through childhood.

▶ Preparing the First Year: Perlocution Stage

Bates (1976) defined the development of communicative functions as consisting of three stages: *perlocution,*

illocution, and *locution.* These three stages are a pragmatic concept. From birth to approximately 8 to 10 months of age, babies are in the perlocution stage of communication development. In this stage, the infant produces vegetative sounds (e.g., burping), sound play (e.g., coo-goo), and other prelinguistic behaviors (e.g., eye gaze) to which the adult infers a communicative intent. For instance, a child looks at a toy and the adult infers that the child wants it. Communication has taken place even though the child has not necessarily conveyed a specific message to the adult. Vegetative sounds such as cries and burps are also interpreted by the adult as having communication intent. The adult responds to these with language ("*Oh, you're hungry*"). The child then associates the intention (pragmatics), the meaning (semantics), and the form (phonology, morphology, and syntax) of language over the course of time as many of these events recur. Three important pragmatic behaviors that are necessary for successful communication throughout the life span are already observed during the perlocution stage, namely eye *contact, joint attention,* and *turn-taking.*

Prelinguistic speech behaviors are also observed during this stage of development, including vocal play and babbling. These speech behaviors do not have meaning or intention to communicate. Nevertheless, a number of studies have shown that certain types of babbling have connection to later lexical development (e.g., de Boysson-Bardes & Vihman, 1991; Stoel-Gammon & Cooper, 1984; Vihman, 1996; Vihman, Macken, Miller, Simmons, & Miller, 1985).

▶ Intent to Communicate: Illocution Stage

The second stage of communication is illocution. In this period, the child displays the intention to communicate with gestures and nonlinguistic vocalizations. Words have not yet emerged in the infant's spoken repertoire, although they are understood. Receptively, the infant understands at least 50 words by 10 months of age (Paul & Norbury, 2012). A major difference between the perlocution stage and the illocution stage is that the child has a clear intention to communicate in the illocution stage. The adult is not inferring intention. The infant communicates the intention. Gestures and vocalizations are necessary in the transition to using spoken language to communicate. It is important to remember this when working with clinical populations. Communicating with gestures and vocalizations is a natural and necessary stage of development. They build the continuing foundation for spoken language. Gestures and vocalizations from the child do not hinder spoken language; they are part and parcel of developing spoken language (Capone & McGregor, 2004; Capone Singleton & Saks, 2015).

Around the time first words are going to emerge, a vocalization that is word-like in form but is not an actual word may be used. These word-like vocalizations are *protowords* (Halliday, 1975), also referred to as *phonetically consistent forms* (PCF; Dore, Franklin, Miller, & Ramer, 1976). Protowords are not attempts at word approximations, but they are child-specific. One child might say "tata!" every time they protest, but another child may produce a different vocalization for protest, such as "zuzu!" The vocalization will be similar for each protest situation and the same for an individual child but not shared between children.

▶ The First Word: Locution Stage

The locution stage of communication begins on average at 12 months of age, when the hearing child utters their first word. 12 months is only the average age. Children typically vary in this milestone from 10 to 14 months of age. The child might say "*ba*" to indicate a bottle or say "*da*" to direct the adult's attention to an oncoming canine. Before that, though, an infant may babble "mamamama" and parents might say "she says 'mamma!'" when actually it was not purposeful. For words to be valid word forms, there needs to be:

- Semantic context
- Phonetic consistency
- Pragmatic intent
- Overlap with the adult word form
- Replication over time
- Replication across contexts

Meeting these factors indicates that there is stability and validity of word form.

Nelson (1973) reported that the mean age of a 10-word vocabulary is 15 months with a range of 13 to 19 months of age. During the time that children are acquiring these first 10 words, their vocabulary is somewhat unstable. That is, words tend to appear and then disappear. This phenomenon should not be confused

with vocabulary regression, which can be reported by parents in the history of children with language disorders. In typical development, it is not uncommon for children to use a word for a few weeks and then stop using it. In typical development, the disappearance of a word is exchanged with new words being used. In the case of vocabulary regression, new words do not appear; rather, children with language impairments may experience a loss of using words more generally.

Nelson (1973) reported that the mean age for acquisition of the 50-word lexicon (i.e., vocabulary) was 19.75 months—though children vary around that milestone as well with a range of 15 to 24 months of age. Word learning is fairly slow in the first half of the second year compared to the second half of that same year and beyond. The 50-word lexicon milestone is important, however, because two key milestones follow it. Around the time the child accumulates 50 words, they enter the rapid period of word acquisition discussed at the start of the chapter (i.e., the word spurt) and begins to combine words into short utterances. Read **BOX 7-1** for an opposing opinion of one scientist regarding the word spurt.

The timely acquisition of these early vocabulary milestones—first word, 50-word milestone, word spurt, and word combinations, is important for continued language development. Marchman and Bates (1994) suggest that the size of the lexicon must reach

---

BOX 7-1 Is the *Word Spurt* a Myth?

Bloom (2004) argues that word spurt is a "myth" (p. 205) because other factors could account for the findings of an increase in the rate of word learning. Two possible reasons Bloom suggests for the observed word spurt are the child's general talkativeness and the way in which the researcher of a study defines a word spurt (e.g., a child may be defined as having a word spurt when they acquire 12 new words in a 2-week period). On the first point, it is possible that the number of words children produce is simply a function of how much they talk, not how many new words they know. Put another way, the more one talks, the more words a researcher is likely to find (p. 213). On the second point, Bloom argues that researchers may define a child as having had a word spurt when 12 new words were acquired within a 2-week period but do not reference how many words were acquired the previous 2 weeks. The child may have learned 10 new words and then 12 new words in each respective time period, indicating a gradual increase in vocabulary rather than a sudden shift in word learning. These ideas are controversial, so it is wise to remember that children start out learning words slowly and then get better at it.

a necessary threshold if other language domains are to fully develop particularly morphology and syntax. For example, word spurt and two-word combination milestones tend to emerge after children have a threshold of at least 50 words in their lexicon. Nelson (1973) also found that vocabulary size at 2 years of age was related to mean length of utterance (MLU—a measure of syntactic development) at 30 months of age.

Vocabulary development is an important predictor of school readiness (Scheffner Hammer et al., 2017) and literacy (National Early Literacy Panel, 2008). Children who do not meet early vocabulary milestones in a timely manner are referred to as late talkers or children with late language emergence (e.g., Rice, 2012). While many late-talking toddlers appear to outgrow their early delay, recent data suggests this characterization is not so cut-and-dry (Capone Singleton, 2018). For example, even though some late talkers perform within an average range on language tests, other areas of development that rely on strong oral language skills are problematic for them by kindergarten (Aro, Laakso, Määttä, Tolvanen, & Poikkeus 2014). These problematic areas include socialization with peers, attention skills, and behavior regulation needed for learning and success in school. Scheffner Hammer et al. (2017) tied the odds of being ready for school by 5 years of age to a small expressive vocabulary at 2 years of age (i.e., to being a late talker) and to a small receptive vocabulary at 4 years of age. Having a small expressive vocabulary at 2 years of age and a small receptive vocabulary at 4 years of age increased the odds of facing low reading performance by school entry. Scheffner Hammer et al. (2017) explored the relationships further among variables of socioeconomic status, vocabulary, and school-readiness. They found that low socioeconomic status (versus middle or higher) increased the odds of children accruing a small vocabulary at the 2-year mark. What aspects of lower socioeconomic status accounted for toddlers having difficulty learning to use words? It was their birthweight being lower than children from higher socioeconomic levels, the quality of parenting, the amount of time in daycare, and that children from a low socioeconomic level had a different attention style for learning.

Studies such as the Scheffner Hammer et al. (2017) study are important to understand because some of these variables are amenable to intervention. Intervention that bolsters vocabulary at 24 months of age has the potential to influence a child's learning and performance across childhood (Capone Singleton, 2018). Rescorla (2009) followed a group of late talkers from the age of identification in toddlerhood through 17 years of age. Their vocabulary size at 2 years accounted for 17% of the variance between children

on several tasks, including vocabulary, grammar, and memory tasks. In addition to preventative prenatal care, parent coaching models that aim to nurture early vocabulary have the potential to bolster a child's performance over time across a variety of domains.

▶ Case Studies

To see how this development is assessed, consider the early semantic milestones of the three case studies. Johnathon was reported to speak his first word at 12 months, Josephine did not speak her first word until 15 months, and Robert's first word emerged at 18 months. Therefore, at the time of each evaluation, Josephine and Robert already had a history of delayed semantic development in expressive vocabulary. Josephine was 22-months old at evaluation and had only 7 words in her vocabulary. Robert was 27-months old at evaluation and had only 14 words in his vocabulary, some of which were sound effects. Only Johnathon was using new words and combining words. Josephine and Robert were both delayed for learning new words regularly and for combining words. Josephine and Robert have a history of delay that is persisting into toddlerhood. Their semantic delay could now be characterized as having (1) a small expressive vocabulary size for their age, (2) too few new words being added to their expressive vocabulary, and (3) a delay in combining words. Finally, while Johnathon relies on words to communicate, Josephine and Robert still rely on gestures and nonlinguistic vocalizations. Johnathon is evaluated as typical for his age, whereas Josephine and Robert show delays in vocabulary development that place them in a category of language delay. During this time in development, we refer to them as late talkers or as children with late language emergence (Rice, 2012).

▶ A Preponderance of Nouns

Nelson (1973) analyzed the word classes present in the first 50-word lexicon using the classification system of *specific nominals* (i.e., nouns), *general nominals*, *action words*, *modifiers*, *personal-social words*, and *function words*. (Refer to **TABLE 7-1** for definitions of these terms.) The proportion of total vocabulary that each word class (e.g., noun, action) represents in the early lexicon is remarkably similar across children. General nominals are common nouns. They make up the largest proportion of the lexicon, accounting for 51% of the vocabulary words. Action words and specific nominals each account for 14% of the lexicon. Modifiers and personal-social words each represent 9% of

TABLE 7-1 Word Classifications

Word Class	Definition
Specific nominals	These words refer to a specific exemplar of a category, whether or not it is a proper name (e.g., mommy, daddy, pet's name).
General nominals	These words refer to all members of a category and include classes such as objects, substances, animals, people, letters, numbers, pronouns, and abstractions.
Action words	These words are used to describe or demand an action.
Modifiers	These words refer to properties or qualities of things or events, such as attributes, states, locations, or possessives.
Personal-social words	These words express affective states and social relationships, such as assertions (e.g., no, yes, want) and social expressive words (e.g., please, ouch).
Function words	These words refer to items that serve a grammatical function in relation to other words (e.g., what, is, for, to).

Source: Data from Nelson, K. (1973). Structure and strategy in learning to talk. *Monographs of the Society for Research in Child Development, 143*(38).

the lexicon. Only 4% of the vocabulary is made up of function words. This same classification system is used today in clinical analyses of early language (e.g., Retherford, 2000).

Despite significant differences in language and culture, children learning a variety of languages (e.g., Mandarin Chinese, Japanese, Kaluli, German, Italian, Hebrew, and Turkish) have more nouns than other word classes in their early vocabularies (Caselli et al., 1995; Gentner, 1982; Goldfield, 1993; Kim, McGregor & Thompson, 2000). A noun preference in early vocabularies appears to be somewhat universal. A good question is "why?" For example, is there a frequency effect? That is, are nouns spoken more often than verbs? This is unlikely because even though adults use more nouns than other word classes, there is also a larger variety of nouns. This means that individual nouns are used *less* frequently than the smaller lexicon of verbs in a language (Goldfield, 1993). With fewer verbs to use, adults will use each verb more often. Put another way, the pattern should be reversed (more verbs than nouns in the early lexicon) because children actually hear each of the smaller number of verbs more often than each of the larger number of nouns.

Another explanation might lie in the way parents teach language to their children. When speaking to their child, do adults organize their language around naming objects? American parents largely put a focus heavily on naming objects with their children (Nelson,

Hampson, & Shaw, 1993). However, in Kaluli, parents are not particularly interested in teaching object names to their children, and Korean-speaking parents tend to focus their interactions around actions and activity (Kim et al., 2000). With little difference in the early lexicons of children from these disparate cultures, it would appear that this is not a salient factor in noun acquisition.

Two factors that have received attention for their part in this phenomenon are (1) the ordering of word classes in a sentence of a language and (2) conceptual differences between nouns and other word classes. The ordering of word classes in a sentence generally refers to the order of nouns in subject (S) and object (O) position and verbs (V). In English, we might say *The girl is reading a book,* where *The girl* is the noun phrase that occupies the subject position, *a book* is the noun phrase that occupies the object position, and *is reading* is the verb phrase that occupies the verb position. In English, nouns occupy the most salient positions in sentences. For example, the speech signal tends to change at the end of sentences and clauses (e.g., greater stress, elongated vowel, or fricative duration), making the words and morphemes that occur in this position more salient for the listener. It is possible that children acquire more nouns early on because they occur in salient sentence positions, particularly in final sentence position. However, languages such as Korean, German, Kaluli, and Turkish have verbs, not nouns, in the final position of sentences (S–O–V; O–S–V), yet children learning these languages have vocabularies that are predominantly made up of nouns as well.

Gentner (1982, 2006) proposes that concrete nouns promote more rapid learning than other word classes—particularly verbs—because they allow for greater transparency of the mapping between word label and semantic information (natural partitions hypothesis; Gentner, 1982, p. 327). Nouns represent more perceptually stable entities than other word classes. Other word classes (verbs, prepositions, modifiers) are acquired more slowly because relationships among them are less spatially cohesive and far less concrete than they are for objects. Verbs, for example, have a more ambiguous relationship with the perceptual world. Verb meanings are harder to glean in a single exposure. Finally, because object concepts are concrete, they allow children to bootstrap into the language system. *Bootstrapping* is a term that refers to the child's use of known information to infer unknown information. In essence, knowing object concepts gives children a foothold in the speech stream, and it creates a scaffold from which one can learn other word classes. Simply put, learning nouns helps you learn verbs and other word classes.

It is likely that both language input and conceptual factors, such as perceptual salience, contribute to the universal pattern of noun learning. Kim et al. (2000) set out to compare early vocabularies of English- and Korean-speaking children to confirm or refute the claim that nouns dominate early vocabularies universally and to explore why that might be. Specifically, their study followed eight English-speaking and eight Korean-speaking mother-child dyads to examine the influence of maternal language on the child's early vocabulary. Children were followed from 16 months of age to 21 months of age, just before or around the time they reached their 50-word milestone. Kim et al. (2000) found that both Korean- and English-learning children acquired significantly more nouns than verbs over time. This dominance of nouns over verbs was found for Korean-speaking children even though their caregivers tended to emphasize verbs in their interactions with them. As expected, English-speaking caregivers tended to emphasize nouns in their talk to the children. These results suggest that children tend to come to the task of early word learning with a strong predisposition toward linking nouns to objects.

In addition to noun preference, there was also an influence of the frequency and saliency of verbs in the Korean-speaking input. Even though Korean-speaking children had more nouns than verbs in their vocabulary, they had a greater proportion of verbs in their vocabulary compared to the number of verbs in

the English-speaking children's vocabulary. Therefore, while children appear to have some universal predisposition for noun learning, their environment also shapes the rest of their developing lexicon to some extent. In this case, the environmental variables include social activity and the surface structure of the grammar that the child hears.

This pattern of noun learning over other word-class learning continues to be observed in the development of preschool and early school-age children, with and without language impairments. For example, Rice et al. (Oetting, Rice, & Swank, 1995; Rice, Buhr, & Nemeth, 1990) examined word learning after just a brief exposure to vocabulary items from a cartoon video. Both studies found that typically developing children and children with language disorders showed a preference for learning object terms over other word-class items, including action, attribute, and affective terms. Because non-object labels are difficult to map in a single exposure, more experience and varied contexts may be needed to map the meanings and linguistic specifications of these word classes (Oetting et al., 1995; Waxman, 1994). We discuss the idea of the richness of experience as an influence on acquisition of words later in the chapter. First, we return to the early lexicon and the importance of noun learning.

▶ Expressive Versus Referential Language Learners

When Nelson (1973) analyzed the infant's first 50-word lexicon, she found that although the majority of children had a preponderance of general nominals, there was a small group of children for which this was not the case. Nelson classified children as *referential language learners* if general nominals accounted for more than 50% of their total vocabulary. Those children with general nominals accounting for less than 50% of their lexicon were referred to as *expressive language learners*. The expressive language learners used many personal-social words, whereas the referential language learners used many nouns (see also Bates, Bretherton, & Snyder, 1988; Bloom, 1973; Goldfield, 1986, 1987; Snyder, Bates, & Bretherton, 1981). Snyder et al. (1981) found the expressive-referential distinction in children as young as 13 months of age, when the children had only 10–12 words in their lexicons. Note that expressive language learners and referential language learners should not be viewed as dichotomous categories. Indeed, most authorities indicate that children who are categorized as expressive versus referential probably represent extreme points on a continuum rather than separate classifications or typologies of language-developing children (Bates et al., 1988; Nelson, 1981).

In addition to lexical composition, other characteristics in the language of referential and expressive language learners have been observed. For instance, referential language learners were reported to develop language earlier and more rapidly than expressive language learners did (Bates et al., 1988; Horgan, 1979; Nelson, 1973; Ramer, 1976). Bates et al. (1988) noted that referential language learners had larger vocabularies and reached grammar milestones sooner than expressive language learners. Referential language learners had a word spurt, whereas expressive language learners tended to learn words at a slow and steady pace without a word spurt. Referential language learners showed greater growth of verb vocabulary at 20 months and more productive control over function words (e.g., determiners, prepositions) by 28 months. Initially, expressive language learners had more function words in their lexicon because they used phrases as holistic chunks. They did not appear to analyze the words of a phrase as individual words but rather as one larger lexical item. A U-shaped curve in function word development was observed. Once expressive language learners began analyzing individual words in their phrasal productions, the function words dropped out and reappeared later as productive forms. Also, referential language learners tended to use words in context-flexible ways (e.g., saying *cup* to refer to many cups, not just their cup). They would *decontextualize* their word use by talking about absent objects. Decontextualization refers to the gradual distancing of a symbol from the original referent or learning context (Werner & Kaplan, 1963). The ability to decontextualize language is important for spoken and written language development as the child ages, particularly for social, emotional, academic, and vocational success.

The relationship between the size of the object vocabulary and overall vocabulary growth was also observed in the late talkers studied by Rescorla, Mirak, and Singh (2000). Even among late talking children, if they had larger vocabularies (although smaller than is typical), the children tended to have greater growth in total vocabulary size over time than the children who had the smallest vocabularies did.

▶ Innate Biases Make Word Learning Efficient

If children relied on explicit teaching (i.e., "this is a *cup*," "this is another *cup*") to learn each word-to-object pairing of their language, language learning would be a laborious, effortful, and inefficient task. Luckily, children come to the task of word learning with some innate *biases* (also referred to as *constraints* or *principles* of word learning) that help them narrow down the many possible referents that could be paired with a word that they hear. For example, if mother says, "Oh, I see the *dax*," where *dax* is a word they have never heard before, the child must figure out which of the many objects, parts of objects, actions, and events going on in the room *dax* refers to.

Several biases can help the child achieve this feat. First, the child must differentiate between spoken language and other sounds as labels. The *principle of reference* states that words—but not other sounds—label objects, actions, and events (Hollich et al., 2000). When Balaban and Waxman (1997) presented 9-month-olds with objects paired with either a tone or a word, the infants showed a preference to link a word—but not a tone—with an object. This occurred even though both tones and words captured their attention in the learning phase.

Three related biases that help the child map a new word to the right referent are the *novel name-nameless category principle* (N3C; Golinkoff, Mervis, & Hirsh-Pasek, 1994), the *principle of mutual exclusivity*, and the *whole-object bias* (Markman, 1989). The principle of mutual exclusivity states that if the child already has a name for an object (*cup*, *comb*), it cannot receive another name. The flip side of this bias is the N3C principle, which states that a novel word will be taken as the name for a previously unnamed object. For example, in experiments that examine how children map novel words to unfamiliar objects, an array of three objects may be presented to the child: a cup, a comb, and a novel object previously unseen or unnamed. When the experimenter states, "Give me the *dax*," the child will hand over the novel object because they already have names for the other objects. Children choose objects in this way even though they have never been explicitly taught, "This is a *dax*." Finally, the whole-object bias guides the child to infer that the word label refers to the entire object and not just a part, an attribute, or its motion. For example, the child knows that the word *car* refers to the whole entity and not just the wheels, windows, or steering wheel of the vehicle.

Children also come to language learning armed with a *principle of conventionality* (Clark, 1993). That is, children know that there are culturally agreed-upon names for things and that these names do not change. Our use and understanding of language would be quite chaotic if the names given to things were ever-changing. Children make this assumption early on.

Two additional biases that make word learning efficient for the child are the *principle of extendibility*

(Hollich et al., 2000) and the *shape bias* (e.g., Clark, 1973; Landau, Smith, & Jones, 1988). These issues are addressed again later in the chapter, so they are mentioned only briefly here. Put simply, the principle of extendibility states that a word does not refer to only one object but rather to a category of objects, events, or actions if they share similar properties. A word will label all instances of an object if all of those instances have the same shape and/or function ("ball" refers to all balls, not just the child's first ball). The shape bias constrains word extension based on shared perceptual features of the original referent and the novel exemplar.

We can readily see the shape bias at work in some of the children's naming errors. For example, a child may look at the moon and say *ball* because both moon and ball are round. The shape bias has been extensively studied in terms of its relationship with word learning (Booth & Waxman, 2002; Gershkoff-Stowe & Smith, 2004; Jones, 2003). Gershkoff-Stowe and Smith (2004) found a positive parallel relationship in toddlers' increasing use of the shape bias and an increase in their expressive noun vocabulary—the more nouns they accrued in their vocabulary the greater accuracy they had in the lab on a task of shape bias testing.

Furthermore, three groups of children with individual differences in vocabulary development do not show a shape bias (Collison, Grela, Spaulding, Rueckl, & Magnuson, 2014; Jones, 2003; Tek, Jaffery, Swensen, Fein, & Naigles, 2012):

- Children with specific language impairment now referred to as having a language disorder
- Toddlers who are late talkers
- Children with autism spectrum disorder

Even though one basis for word extension is whether or not two objects share a similar shape, a shared function between objects also indicates that two objects will share the same name (Booth & Waxman, 2002; Clark, 1973; Kemler Nelson, 1999). For example, Kemler Nelson (1999) assessed the role of shared function in word extensions made by 28-month-olds. These toddlers heard the names of objects and had opportunities to enact their functions. They were then tested on word extension for four types of objects:

- Similar shape-similar function
- Similar shape-dissimilar function
- Dissimilar shape-similar function
- Dissimilar shape-dissimilar function

In this study, toddlers were able to transcend shape similarities and extend words based on shared function. That is, they used the same name for two objects if the function was the same, even for objects that did not look alike.

Size, Animacy, and Color

Other object features, such as the size of an object, have not been shown to influence extension decisions (Jones, Smith, & Landau, 1991). For example, children label a real car and a toy car both as *car* despite the obvious difference in size (and texture). Even though the size difference between their parent's car and their Fisher-Price miniature car is quite large, children call both *car* because the items share shape properties that include four wheels, doors, seats, windshield, steering wheel, and other salient features.

Toddlers are also quite smart about adjusting their shape bias within the context of certain features they have had experiences in. When Jones et al. (1991) placed eyes on their objects, children accepted shape changes and extended a word label to another object that shared texture (e.g., fur). In this case, the presence of eyes signaled that the object was an animate entity, and animate entities tend to share material (e.g., bears have fur, humans have skin, birds have feathers) and change shape (i.e., we change shape as we move). Therefore, children appear to adapt to and integrate multiple perceptual cues to make inferences about what something is or is not.

For some object categories, color, in addition to shape, can be defining (Perry & Saffran, 2017). For example, red can be important to *strawberry* but not *car*, or green may be defining of *grass* but not *plate*. Perry and Saffran (2017) showed that toddlers as young as 19 to 22 months of age were accurate in identifying a pictured object (e.g., cow) if the color matched their expectation of the object's color, but identification was disrupted if there was a mismatch between object and color (e.g., a pink cow).

▶ The Emergent Coalition Model of Word Learning

As stated earlier, little of language learning is accomplished by direct and explicit teaching. Instead, much of what the child learns is a result of what they infer about the language that the child hears and what is going on around them. The previous section discussed the innate principles or biases that the child brings to the word-learning task. Other cues in the environment also scaffold word learning for the child—for example, a parent's point or eye gaze, the grammatical structure of the language model, the perceptual salience of the object. The emergentist coalition model (ECM; Hollich et al., 2000) describes how children coalesce environmental cues and innate biases to learn new words. In addition to the interaction between cues and strategies, the ECM posits that children calculate their success and failure rate of mapping words to referents. This error signal feeds back into the learning system to improve the reliability of coalescing these cues and strategies as the child develops.

A full range of cues is always available to the child, though they weigh each cue differently over time. With development and experience, the child learns which cues are more reliable indicators of word-referent pairings. In turn, the child's accuracy in linking words to referents becomes more efficient. When a parent produces a word label, the child recruits attentional cues (e.g., perceptual salience of objects), social cues (e.g., eye gaze, pointing), and linguistic cues (e.g., regularities in syntax) in the environment to further constrain the possibilities of which referent that word is labeling. Infants 12 to 18 months of age initially consider perceptual salience (e.g., a moving object) to be a more important cue about what is being labeled than a social cue (e.g., eye gaze or pointing to it). Therefore, the child infers that the interesting moving object is what is being labeled even though the parent may be looking at the boring object. By ages 18 to 24 months, children have learned that the social cue is a more reliable indicator of the word to referent mapping. Now when they hear a word, they pay attention to the adult's gesture and eye gaze to ensure that a reliable word-to-referent mapping occurs. Put simply, by toddlerhood, children can accurately map the names of the boring objects as well as the interesting ones (Golinkoff & Hirsh-Pasek, 2006).

▶ Learning a Word

Learning a word is not an all-or-nothing phenomenon. As Carey (1978) described it, word learning is a gradual and long-term process. Learning a word grossly encompasses learning the lexeme (word form or label), the semantic representation (word meaning), and grammatical specifications (e.g., word-class information), plus making connections between these various representations. As children encounter words in a variety of contexts over time, their knowledge of individual words is enriched. Our experiences with words differ. Therefore, the *breadth* of words we know and our *depth* of word knowledge will vary. Breadth is how many words you know. Depth is how well or how

much we know about each word. We might refer to depth as richness of word knowledge. In the clinical evaluation of children's vocabulary, we tend to focus on the breadth of words known to a child. A formal test of vocabulary size will be included in the evaluation repertoire, such as the Expressive Vocabulary Test (EVT; Williams, 1997). The EVT is a predetermined set of words to be tested at various age intervals. **BOX 7-2** and **TABLE 7-2** detail another analysis of vocabulary breadth, known as the Type:Token Ratio (TTR; Templin, 1957). The TTR examines the diversity of words being used spontaneously by the child in a functional context (e.g., play conversation).

Fast Mapping and Slow Mapping

Carey (1978) delineated two phases of word learning: *fast mapping* and *slow mapping*. A word is considered fast mapped if there is an initial association made between word and referent. A related phenomenon has been termed *quick incidental learning* (QUIL; Oetting et al., 1995; Rice, Buhr, & Oetting, 1992). QUIL reflects more naturally occurring word-learning situations that offer minimal environmental support with multiple cues in ongoing scenes. In experimental studies of QUIL, many new words may be presented as part of a cartoon program prior to the test of word learning. In contrast, the fast mapping phenomenon is often measured after a more explicit or structured task. The former scenario may better reflect the child's natural word-learning experiences. What is important for the reader to keep in mind is whether a study is discussing fast mapping or QUIL, the trace of a word left in memory is newly formed. A child will not know much about a newly formed word trace. Lexical and semantic information are weakly represented in memory after such a brief exposure. Therefore, the child needs a few to several exposures of a word, depending on the word, to truly discern the subtleties of its meaning. Discerning the subtleties of meaning happens during the slow mapping phase of word learning.

Slow mapping is the process of enriching lexical-semantic representations that have been retained in memory. The child's word representations are enriched through increased frequency of exposures (i.e., quantity) and through richer quality of exposure. This process has significant implications for the clinical practice of speech-language pathologists. Specifically, intervention provides the child with increased frequency of exposure to language and a richer quality of language learning. Quality of learning is enriched through the therapeutic scaffolds used by the clinician.

BOX 7-2 Type-Token Ratio Analysis by Mildred C. Templin

The Type-Token Ratio (TTR; Templin, 1957) is an index of how diverse a child's word use is in spontaneous language (i.e., lexical diversity). In other words, this is an analysis of how many different words the child uses given the overall number of words they have said in a sample of conversation. The analysis is specifically for children between the ages of 3 and 8 years and must be calculated from 50 consecutive utterances only. Be sure to note that we are using 50 utterances, not 50 words. This is an important point to underscore because in other language analyses (e.g., morpho-syntax), 100 utterances or 25 utterances can be used. Using 100 or 25 utterances works out fine because averages are calculated in the grammar analyses. However, the TTR analysis is taken from raw frequencies of words, and so 50 utterances is an exact number of utterances (not words) that must be used. I tell students that the TTR measure complements a formal vocabulary test well because performance on the test tells the examiner about the size of a child's vocabulary. The TTR and in particular the numerator—Number of Different Words (NDW)—illustrates how the child is using the words they have.

Calculation

The TTR is calculated from two numbers—the number of different words (NDW) in the 50 utterances and the Number of Total Words (NTW) in the 50 utterances. The calculation is:

$$NDW/NTW = TTR$$

For example, in the following example, some utterances are taken from a 50-utterance sample:

Types and Tokens[1] Sample	
Child: momma, make a train.	momma, make[1,1], a[1,1], train[1]
Child: okay.	okay[1]
Child: make a train!	
Child: with this one!	with, this, one
Child: I'll make it.	I[1], 'll, it
Child: okay.	
Child: there's the track.	there, 's, the, track
Child: I need a boxcar.	need, boxcar

Words that are used for the first time are Types, and words used thereafter are marked by a superscript 1 to indicate a Token of an already noted word Type said. You can observe that the word Type make has three Tokens (including the first Type). Thus far in this child's eight utterances, we can start with 17 in the numerator as Types, and 24 to the denominator as Tokens to set up the TTR calculation: 17 NDW/24 NTW = TTR, where NDW = number of different words and NTW = number of total words.

The following are the rules for counting the number of different words (NDW; Templin, 1957):

1. Subject-verb contractions are counted as two different word Types as in the example above. Also, when a word is uncontracted, it is also a different word Type from the contracted form. So, *I'll* and *I will* have three word Types (I, 'll, will) and four word Tokens (I, 'll, will).
2. Bound morphemes and inflections (noun, verb) are not separated the way they are in the MLU calculation. They are kept bound to their root word. Therefore, *walks* is one word Type, *walking* is another word type. Articles (*a*, *the*) are one word Type each.
3. Contracted negatives such as *can't* or *don't* are one word Type.
4. Verb tenses containing several helping verbs are each an individual word Type. Therefore, *had been walking* contains three word Types.
5. Hyphenated and compound nouns are one word Type (e.g., *sunshine* is one word Type).
6. Phrases or expressions that are learned or function as a unit are one word Type (e.g., *all right*, *night-night*).
7. Interjections are one word Type (*oh*, *uh*, *um*).

Such therapeutic scaffolds could include the explicit use of verbal models of the word *label* being repeated with greater frequency for the child or visual cues such as gesturing the shape of the object to highlight this salient feature, gesturing the function of the object while labeling it, or organizing objects by category to help the child build connections between related vocabulary items.

TABLE 7-2 Normative Data to be used When Calculating Vocabulary Diversity using Type-Token Ratio (*N* = 480)					
	Different Words		Total Words		Type-Token Ratio
Age	Mean	SD	Mean	SD	Different Words/Total Words
3.0	92.5	26.1	204.9	61.3	0.45
3.5	104.8	20.4	232.9	50.8	0.45
4.0	120.4	27.6	268.8	72.6	0.45
4.5	127	23.9	270.7	65.3	0.47
5.0	132.4	27.2	286.2	75.5	0.46
6.0	147.	27.6	328.	65.9	0.45
7.0	157.7	27.2	363.1	51.3	0.43
8.0	166.5	29.5	378.8	80.9	0.44

At any given time, words may vary in the richness of their lexical-semantic representations simply because some words are encountered more often than others. For example, as you and the student are learning the vocabulary of speech-language pathology, education, or psychology, you are mapping many new terms into memory. Your knowledge of these terms is still weak compared to that of the master-level student who is about to enter the profession. The master-level student has had many more exposures through additional coursework and advanced reading as well as richer quality of each experience through clinical practice. The richness of these professional terms in your own vocabulary will evolve over time as you move through undergraduate and graduate study. Conversely, if this is the only class you take in the field, your lexical-semantic knowledge of these terms will remain sparse and perhaps weaken as other words in your lexicon are continually updated and strengthened with repeated exposure.

Some interesting new studies have looked at other variables that might affect how richly young children map new words. One relevant context of word learning is the young child's interest in having books read to them. Horst, Parsons, and Bryan (2011) examined whether preschool children map and then retain novel words better if they hear new words in the *same* story read to them repeatedly or if they hear new words read to them in a variety of *different* stories. In these experiments, preschoolers hear new words the same number of times. The context differs in that they hear those words repeatedly in the same story or repeatedly across different story contexts. Results over the experiments revealed:

1. Preschoolers fast mapped more words if they heard them in the same story repeatedly.
2. Preschoolers retained words over time if they heard them in the same story repeatedly.

So, be sure to oblige a child who asks to have a story read to them over and over again! We may wonder, "why would a child want to hear that story again?" Much like the older infant who gains new vocabulary by bootstrapping into routines, songs, and rhymes, children appear to utilize the familiarity of a story to make connections to new words. Put another way, familiarity with the story surrounding new words may act as a template to scaffold learning.

▶ Triggering, Configuring, and Engaging a Lexical-Semantic Representation

In the fast mapping phase, a child needs to recognize a word as unknown in order to map a referent to it.

We read about the N3C bias in the biases section, but the N3C bias is used to determine the *referent* as novel when hearing a novel label. How do children become aware that a *word* they just heard is new? Under the Associationistic account, a new word representation is triggered when there is a mismatch between what was heard in the environment (i.e., the novel word) with a search in the internal lexicon (Li, Farkas, & MacWhinney, 2004). A novel word should *trigger* a new lexical-semantic representation in memory.

In the slow mapping phase, the lexical-semantic representation will be configured. *Configuration* is happening in long-term memory with phonological detail, multimodal meaning, and syntactic specifications (Leach & Samuel, 2007). The third action of a word representation is engagement. *Engagement* can only happen when a lexical-semantic representation is fully developed. The term refers to engaging other words in a process of competing activation within the lexicon. Leach and Samuel (2007) showed that a word needs to be well configured with its referent and that semantic representations need to be developed if other word representations are to be engaged with it. Engagement is considered a sign of a fully functioning (or developed) lexical-semantic representation.

▶ ## Phonotactic Probability and Neighborhood Density

There are two additional variables that influence word learning—*phonotactic probability* and *neighborhood density*. Phonotactic probability is the frequency with which a sound or sound sequence occurs in the language (Vitevitch & Luce, 1999). It takes word position into account. For example, "si" as in *sit* is a frequent sound sequence in English, whereas the sound sequence /θæ/ is rare, and "ngi" never occurs in the English language. Phonotactic probability influences word learning (e.g., Storkel, 2001). For example, when taught words were made up of low-phonotactic-probability sequences and others consisting of high-phonotactic-probability sequences, Storkel (2001) found preschoolers learned the high-phonotactic words faster. Depending on the probability level, phonotactic probability indicates to the learner:

- Which novel words heard are "acceptable" given the child's language
- When a word they hear is novel

As phonotactic probability increases—indicating high frequency sounds/sound sequences, words become easily detected as acceptable in the language. However, triggering a novel word representation may be easier at lower probabilities, where novelty is apparent and acceptability is at a threshold of recognition (Storkel, Bontempo, Aschenbrenner, Maekawa, & Lee, 2013).

Neighborhood density is a measure of how many words or neighbors a target word has in memory when only one phoneme varies (Vitevitch & Luce, 1999). Some neighbors of *cat* (i.e., /kæt/) might be *cab, cot, hat, mat, at, kit,* and *rat*. If there are many words that result from this variance, the target word is said to reside in a dense neighborhood. Conversely, a sparse neighborhood contains few neighbors around target words. Children find words from dense neighborhoods easier to learn than from sparse neighborhoods (Storkel & Morrisette, 2002; Storkel et al., 2013). Neighborhood density influences configuration of representations in long-term memory. The lexical neighbors support the new word as it is established in memory by sharing connections with it (see below).

Interestingly, neither phonotactic probability nor neighborhood density influences lexical engagement with other words! Why is this? Phonotactic probability and neighborhood density are a phonological variable and a lexical variable, respectively. Engagement between word representations invokes the semantic representation (Leach & Samuel, 2007; Storkel et al, 2013).

▶ ## A Connectionist Account of Lexical-Semantic Representations

According to connectionist accounts, lexical and semantic information are stored and linked within a distributed neural network in the brain (Barsalou, 1999a, 1999b; Plunkett, Karmiloff-Smith, Bates, Elman, & Johnson, 1997). For example, the concept of *bone* comprises visual information (shape, color), thematic associates (dogs chew bones), actions (chewing), the proprioceptive-tactile experience of feeling its weight and rough texture, and its lexeme (/bon/). Lexemes are further divisible into phonemes (/b/, /o/, and /n/). Each of these is a node of information (semantic, phonological, lexical) in the network; connections within and between representations, in

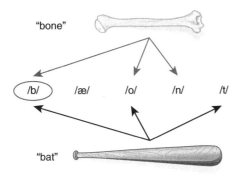

FIGURE 7-1 Competing objects and word representations.

turn, allow for spreading of neural activation among semantic and lexical nodes. For example, when you see a bone, your shape of the bone has perceptual nodes that are activated. Through connections between representations of that word in the network, there is activation of the other nodes as well. This includes the lexeme /bon/. What happens when you see /bæt/? These objects may share overall shape and some phonological and phonetic features (**FIGURE 7-1**). Before the child has rich representations that differentiate these two objects, they may misname one for the other by saying "bat" for "bone." This will be particularly true if the child has more experience with one object (e.g., bat) over the other.

Information recall from memory is determined by the activation weights of nodes and connections between them. Frequency of exposure, for example, can influence the baseline—resting activation of a lexical representation (Storkel & Morrisette, 2002). Therefore, a frequently said word makes it easier to retrieve from memory than an infrequently encountered one. When a semantic representation is richer, it has many connected nodes of information, which leads to a greater number of connections to the word form. This richer quality and quantity of connections provides an activation strength that will subsequently stimulate the word label's threshold when needed for retrieval.

Each node and connection pair carries an activation weight (excitatory or inhibitory). Fast-mapped words or infrequently encountered words tend to have few nodes with weak activation weights. These lexical-semantic representations are not distinct from other weakly represented words that share some, but not all, features. It is through the slow mapping phase that lexical-semantic representations are enriched. Richer lexical-semantic representations are distinct because a greater number of nodes and connections are present within and between lexical-semantic representations and because their activation weights

are stronger. When semantic activation weights and connections to the word form are richer, then the likelihood of recalling the word (i.e., activating it in memory) is quite good.

Let's consider another example. Upon seeing an image of a pig, the child may activate several lexical-semantic representations that are weak if they have little experience with farm animals. These representations perhaps all have two ears, four legs, and a tail—pig, horse, and cow may all be retrieved. However, as the child enriches their knowledge of pigs, horses, and cows, only the relevant word will be activated when the child sees one of these because the distinct semantic features are being activated for one of them. As part of this process, the unique feature nodes activate the correct lexeme for retrieval. When pig gets activated, inhibitory signals are also sent to horse and cow nodes to forestall their activation.

Before the child develops a richer representation, they are likely to fail to retrieve the name of an intended word (Capone Singleton, 2012; Capone & McGregor, 2005; McGregor & Appel, 2002; McGregor, Freidman, Reilly, & Newman, 2002a; McGregor, Newman, Reilly, & Capone, 2002b). For example, the child may say *doggie* instead of *cow*, where *cow* is the intended target word. The next sections deal with the issue of naming errors in children.

CLINICAL APPLICATION EXERCISE

In this clinical exercise, we will form a plan for Anthony, a 5-year-old child who on evaluation produced many indeterminant words, such as *thing*, *that*, and *it* in his spontaneous language sample while playing with his mom and the examiner. On formal vocabulary testing, Anthony got a score that indicated a small vocabulary for his age. Errors on testing were again largely indeterminate errors (*I don't know*) but also superordinate terms (*animal* instead of *bear*, *toy* instead of *race car*) or circumlocutions (*stuff I wear* instead of *pants* or *shirt*). Plan a treatment goal that targets vocabulary. This will require you to choose a category or two that is underdeveloped to target separately. List 5–10 vocabulary words to teach in each category. Finally, consider the sections of the chapter on connectionist networking and quantity and quality of word learning with regards to setting up a rich lexicon. Plan a hands-on intervention activity to teach your vocabulary targets.

▶ Overextension and Underextension

Parents and researchers have noted for decades that children often misuse the words in their vocabularies. The early lexicon is in an almost continual state of flux and begins to stabilize only after the child's word spurt (Gershkoff-Stowe, 2001; Nelson, 1973). When a child calls a cow *doggie,* they are exhibiting the limitations of his vocabulary. Limitations can take the form of either weak knowledge (as discussed above) or an immature retrieval process (Gershkoff-Stowe, 2002).

When a child uses a word too broadly to refer to referents that may be similar in perceptual feature or function, the error is referred to as an *overextension.* Some examples might be calling the moon a *ball* or calling a strange man *daddy.* Conversely, the child may also produce *underextensions.* Underextended words have too narrow a meaning. An example is the use of the word *dog* only when referring to the child's pet, and not when referring to other dogs. Clark (1973) has estimated that overextensions and underextensions occur frequently and can represent as much as one-third of a child's early vocabulary between the ages of 1 and 2 years. Two traditional theories attempt to explain extension errors.

First, the *semantic feature hypothesis* (Clark, 1973) states that children classify and organize referents in terms of perceptual features such as size, shape, animacy, and texture. This phenomenon could explain some overextensions in which a child generalizes a word based on perceptual similarity (e.g., *ball-moon*).

Second, the *functional core hypothesis* (Nelson, 1974) states that words are overextended because of the actions or functions performed on objects rather than the perceptual features of the referents. Thus, a child may say the word *rake* when a person is sweeping because the actions are similar.

Aspects of each of these traditional theories are present in the current theories of word retrieval in children. While it is true that children organize categories around perceptual (e.g., shape) or functional features, several other factors also influence word learning and retrieval. These factors include the phonological make-up of the word (e.g., high versus low phonotactic probability; Storkel, 2001), the frequency with which the word is encountered and/or practiced (Dell, 1990; Gershkoff-Stowe, 2002), and the richness of the word's semantic representation (Capone Singleton, 2012; Capone & McGregor, 2005; McGregor et al., 2002a). The next section delves into the nature of word retrieval and naming errors.

▶ Naming Errors

The retrieval errors that children (and adults) make are often logically related to the word that was targeted for expression. That is, we do not mistakenly say "fork" for "car" because there is no relationship between the two. Instead, we say "fork" for "spoon" because both are utensils and often appear together. Therefore, errors in word retrieval reflect how a speaker's knowledge is organized in memory (Dell, 1990; Dell, Reed, Adams, & Meyer, 2000; McGregor, 1997).

For example, as the child's vocabulary grows in size, the semantic system begins to take on a hierarchical organization. Children acquire *basic-level* (or *ordinate terms)* lexical items first (e.g., *dog*) and later develop a hierarchy of *superordinate* (e.g., *animal*) and *subordinate* (e.g., *collie*) terms. If a target word is *dog,* the child's error is more likely to be *animal* than *spoon* because *dog* and *animal are* more closely related (or connected) in the lexicon than *dog* and *spoon.* These items are rarely, if ever, associated together in our experiences.

Word retrieval errors can relate to their targets in several ways:

- Phonologically—for example, saying *chicken* instead of *kitchen* or *miracleride* for *merry-go-round*
- Semantically—for example, saying *key* for *door* or *skating* for *skiing*
- Phonologically and semantically—for example, saying *elevator* for *escalator*
- An indeterminate response—for example, saying *thing* or *I don't know*
- A perseverative response—that is, using the same word to label different objects within a brief time interval
- A visual misperception—for example, saying *lollipop* for *balloon*

McGregor (1997) found that the most prevalent type of word retrieval errors were semantic errors and indeterminate errors. These errors indicate that retrieval failure is likely related to a weak or missing semantic representation of the target word or weak links between semantic knowledge and word labels (see also Capone Singleton, 2012; Capone & McGregor, 2005; Gershkoff-Stowe, 2001; Lahey & Edwards, 1999; McGregor, 1997; McGregor et al., 2002b; Plunkett et al., 1997). McGregor showed that preschoolers with and without language impairments make the same types of word retrieval errors (predominately semantic errors), but more importantly, children with language impairments make more of those errors than typically developing children.

During the word spurt, the toddler begins mapping many new words into memory. This age is a good developmental time for examining word retrieval errors because many errors are being made (Gershkoff-Stowe, 2002; Gershkoff-Stowe & Smith, 1997). Gershkoff-Stowe and Smith (1997) found that during this shift toward rapidly learning new words, toddlers were also producing many more naming errors. As their word acquisition increased rapidly, they also had a sudden but temporary increase in naming errors when naming words they had already named previously. Consistent with the findings of other studies, these naming errors were most often semantically related to the target word, although perseverative errors were also prevalent. Phonological errors were significantly less common.

Perseverative errors subsequently decline in the post-spurt period (Gershkoff-Stowe, 2002). Gershkoff-Stowe and Smith (1997) suggest that such errors reflect a general fragility in the retrieval process and/or a weakness of word representations, reflecting the fact that children of this age are new word learners. In contrast, semantic errors persist in the post-spurt period. This relationship is to be expected because the retrieval process itself has stabilized, yet new words are continually fast mapped. As a consequence, the child will always have a continuum of weak to richer representations. As the child practices saying words (i.e., retrieving them) and continues to enrich word meanings, the child may make fewer errors on those words that are repeatedly encountered and enriched (Gershkoff-Stowe, 2002).

Word Representations Vary by Experience

Go back to the connectionist and associationistic theories of the lexical-semantic system. We can think of lexical-semantic representations as existing along a continuum of representations from weak to richer forms, depending on the quantity and quality of experience with a particular word (Capone & McGregor, 2005).

Gershkoff-Stowe (2002) manipulated toddlers' frequency of experience in saying words via two conditions of naming practice. In one condition, toddlers had practice naming pictures from a picture book; in the second condition, toddlers had extra practice naming the same pictures (i.e., book, picture cards). Toddlers in the extra-practice condition produced fewer naming errors than the low-practice condition.

Storkel (2001) found low phonotactic probability words are prone to error more than high phonotactic probability words. She hypothesized that high phonotactic probability words are learned faster, which most likely allows the child to map and integrate semantic information better for these words than for low phonotactic probability words. That is, high phonotactic probability words are less prone to error because they are more richly represented in memory than low phonotactic probability words.

The quality of semantic information represented in memory also influences word retrieval (Capone Singleton, 2012; Capone & McGregor, 2005; McGregor et al., 2002a, b). McGregor and colleagues have studied the richness of semantic representation associated with both accurate naming and naming errors by typically developing children and those with language disorder (previously referred to as specific language impairment; SLI). Children with language disorder are known for having difficulty with word retrieval (McGregor, 1997). In the studies conducted by McGregor et al. (2002a, b), children were asked to name a set of pictures to assess naming accuracy and then were subsequently asked to draw pictures of the target words and define the target words. A group of adults rated pictures and definitions for quality and quantity of information, respectively. The results showed that for both groups of children, when they produced naming errors on target words, the corresponding drawings and definitions of those words were weak. Specifically, drawings were rated as poor in quality and definitions contained fewer pieces of semantic information than drawings and definitions of accurately named targets. Drawings and definitions of accurately named targets contained more information in both drawings and definitions, indicating richer representations of these words. In summary, richer semantic knowledge was associated with accurate word retrieval for naming, while weaker semantic knowledge was associated with naming errors.

Semantic Enrichment

Experience with words is a key factor in creating a richer lexical-semantic network. Having more experience with certain words can lead to retrieval of them despite other factors that are often associated with expressive word use, such as older age and higher IQ (Bjorklund, 1987). Experience can be enriched via quantity (or frequency) of experience or via quality of each experience (e.g., through scaffolding). For example, in the Gershkoff-Stowe (2002) study discussed earlier, frequency of experience was manipulated by increasing practice in saying words; this extra practice had a positive effect on retrieving words for naming.

Capone and McGregor (2005) examined the influence of enriched quality of semantic learning for its effect on word retrieval. In their study, the frequency of word exposure was controlled but the semantic knowledge was enriched via representational gesture cues. Frequency of word exposure was controlled by ensuring that the training objects and words were novel and the objects were labeled the same number of times in each condition. Semantic teaching varied by three conditions: *shape, function,* and *control.* In the shape condition, toddlers heard the word label and also saw a gesture that highlighted the shape of the object. In the function condition, toddlers heard the word label and also saw a gesture that highlighted the function of the object. In the control condition, no gesture cues accompanied the word label. By the study's end, toddlers had learned the same number of words under all three learning conditions, but the quality of learning differed by condition. Toddlers retrieved more words for naming (i.e., to say them) when semantic teaching (shape, function) was provided than when words were learned without it (control). Indeed, when semantic learning was assessed, toddlers knew more about the objects in the shape and function conditions than in the control condition.

In a follow-up study, Capone Singleton (2012), replicated this finding by showing that semantic enrichment not only supported naming of taught words, but also supported naming other untaught exemplars of teaching objects. Specifically, when children were taught words with a gesture that highlighted the shape of the object, children went on to name two additional objects from that category that were never named or gestured toward. Semantic teaching helped the children extend learned words correctly in a naming task. A second interesting finding was that when children did make errors, they rarely made overextension errors with semantic teaching. Instead, many of the errors in the semantic teaching conditions conveyed the function of the object. When a child (or adult) expresses some aspect of a word's meaning instead of the word label, this is a special type of semantic error called a *circumlocution error.* Circumlocution errors indicate that children had retrieved the correct word representation but that the link to the word form had failed. Therefore, semantic teaching appears to reduce the number of overextension errors children make when they make errors.

▶ Working Memory

Our discussion thus far has largely referred to learning and retrieving words within the long-term memory system. Long-term memory is where information is stored after learning. Another memory system, known as working memory (Baddeley, 2000; Baddeley & Hitch, 1974), also plays a key role in word learning. The working memory system is involved in active, online processing of information; it allows temporary storage of information while it is being manipulated or processed. Working memory has a limited capacity of resources

to process information, so there is always a trade-off in terms of where those resources are being directed. For example, when the child sees an unknown referent and hears a novel word, they engage in a process of linking the word to the referent, but the child also fast-maps phonological and semantic information and integrates the entire picture with what they already know (i.e., information from long-term memory). This kind of processing is termed *online processing.* Working memory is the system that allows us to process information online. It is the system that's used to make sense of new information and integrate new information with known information stored in long-term memory.

Several distinct components constitute the working memory system. First, two workspaces process visual and verbal information. The workspace for verbal information, which is called the *phonological loop,* encodes, maintains, and manipulates speech-based input. The second workspace, called the *visuo-spatial sketchpad,* manipulates visual information for visual recognition and orientation of stimuli. These two subsystems compete for the limited processing resources available in the working memory system. The third component of the system, known as the *central executor,* acts as the overseer. It maximizes the processing of visuo-spatial and phonological information by allocating processing resources to one or the other of the two workspaces or by splitting the resources between the two. The central executor modulates attention to each type of information. A fourth component of the working memory system, the *episodic buffer,* provides a place for integration of information to occur after the initial processing. It allows temporary representations to be integrated (new and old information) prior to that final integrated representation being sent for storage in long-term memory (Baddeley, 2000).

The integrity of the phonological loop is critical for vocabulary development (Gathercole & Baddeley, 1989, 1990; Gathercole, Willis, Emslie, & Baddeley, 1992; Jarrod & Baddeley, 1997). For example, Gathercole and Baddeley (1989) showed that the size of a child's receptive vocabulary was positively related to their ability to remember phonological information. Four- and five-year-olds were better at repeating nonwords when they had larger, rather than smaller, vocabularies. A child's performance accuracy in nonword repetition is a common measure of integrity of the phonological loop. Of course, all new words to the child are nonwords initially, until they make a connection with their referents; therefore, nonword repetition is a good measure of the phonological loop's capacity for processing new words. Gathercole et al. (1992) identified the same relationship between the integrity of the phonological loop and vocabulary development in children 4–8 years of age.

Conversely, children with language learning impairments (e.g., SLI, Down syndrome) have been found to have poor nonword repetition and smaller vocabularies than typically developing children (Gathercole & Baddeley, 1990; Jarrod & Baddeley, 1997). Therefore, the relationship is the same: good nonword repeaters have larger vocabularies and poor nonword repeaters have smaller vocabularies.

▶ Later Lexical Development

Word learning continues across the life span (Nippold, 2007). During the first half of the second year, the infant's vocabulary consists largely of nouns. As they pass into toddlerhood, the child's verb vocabulary expands. The size of other word classes grows as the child moves through the preschool years and beyond (e.g., spatial terms, temporal terms, pronouns, conjunctions). As the child enrolls in school, word-learning opportunities expand from oral to include written. The school-age child begins to learn many new vocabulary items via academic and social readings. Children are directly taught words or make an inference about words from the surrounding context and/or through morphological analysis bound to the word (Nippold,

2007). The child relies largely on inferences from the context that surrounds new words to glean their meanings. There is also some more direct teaching through instructors and text reading. For example, definitions (i.e., direct explanations) are stated explicitly for some words. In **BOX 7-3**, the reader is given a glimpse of the scaffolding a father gives his son around several specific nominals but also general nominal—buccaneer, stadium. The words in bold illustrate a potential connectionist network forming around the theme of *football*. Box 7-3 is accompanied by a video of the interaction, which can be found in the online materials.

One of the most significant accomplishments for the child from preschool to school age and into adolescence and adulthood is the ability to learn and use more abstract language. The child develops a flexibility in understanding that words can have multiple meanings and that sometimes these meanings are concrete (e.g., *cold* refers to temperature), and sometimes they are more abstract (e.g., *cold* refers to a person's temperament). More concrete meanings are learned first, in the preschool years; later, the psychological and abstract meanings are acquired. Also, the child expands the type of lexical items learned by including figurative language (e.g., metaphors, idioms, slang terms). Metaphors, idioms, and slang terms are extensions of lexical

---

BOX 7-3 Contextual Scaffolding to Learn New Words in Conversation about Football Teams between a Father and His Son

Father's Spoken Transcript	Contextual Scaffold Used
It's a **football team** that **plays** in **Philadelphia**.	Definition of the Philadelphia Eagles.
I like the **Greenbay Packers**.	Semantic connection to a thematic neighbor. The Eagles and the Packers are both football teams.
That's a **football team**.	Provides direct explanation.
And they have a **yellow helmet with a big G** on it (dad *gestures* a G while saying "G")	Semantic connection by providing features of the team and visual cue with gesture.
And they **play** in **a state** called **Wisconsin**.	Semantic connection by providing a salient feature and direct explanation that Wisconsin is a state.
But I also like – I'm from **Tampa**, right. Tampa has a team called the Tampa Bay Buccaneers. The **Buccaneers** is another name for **Pirates**. And their **stadium** has a **pirate ship** <u>IN</u> it (dad *gestures* while saying pirate ship in it) (son repeats what dad says) There's a **pirate ship** in their **stadium**, where they're **playing** You'll have to see it some time.	Semantic connection Semantic connections Direct explanation Prosodic cues with pause between *pirate, ship*, and emphasis on "IN" and semantic connections Vocal manual monitoring by dad who repeats what son said Semantic connection

*Bolded words are a semantic network woven around the topic of FOOTBALL with a new word *Buccaneer* and perhaps *stadium* introduced.

development. For example, idioms (e.g., *It's raining cats and dogs*) are believed to function as a single word. These constructs convey a single meaning that differs from the meaning that the words convey in isolation. Children's understanding of figurative language follows its own developmental course, with literal meanings being learned earlier (preschool and early school age) and figurative meanings being acquired later as the child moves through middle school, adolescence, and adulthood. Mastery of figurative language is essential for social and academic success. For example, humorous play on words is often a device used in advertising. Even in adulthood, however, performance on figurative language tasks does not reach a ceiling of 100% accuracy. Therefore, lexical acquisition and figurative language use are lifelong in their development.

▶ Summary

Word learning is a lifelong, complex, and dynamic process. The child comes equipped with certain tools (i.e., biases) to help them jump into the word-learning system; many scaffolds are also available for the child in the environment (e.g., mother's talk, mother's eye gaze, gestures). The child readily takes advantage of these aids. The child spends a full year preparing for their first word. Although word learning is slow to start, by toddlerhood, the child is a word-learning machine.

The early lexicon largely consists of nouns. As the child moves through toddlerhood and into the preschool years, however, vocabulary expands to include many other word classes, including verbs, prepositions, pronouns, conjunctions, and adjectives. The lexicon also expands to include words with multiple and figurative meanings as well as larger language units that function as a single lexical item.

The process of learning a single word is an extended process that moves from an initial fast mapping to a longer period of slow mapping that enriches the lexical and semantic representation of the word. The richness of lexical-semantic representation is related to the likelihood of whether the child will retrieve that word from memory. Speech-language intervention provides the child with increased frequency and richer quality of word-learning experiences, thereby narrowing the gap between a child with language impairments and the child's typically developing peers.

Study Questions

- Describe lexical development from first words to two-word combinations, including the word class that predominates in this early lexicon.

- What are the benefits in language learning for the referential language learner when compared to the expressive language learner?

- Define the principles of word learning and explain how they aid the young child in learning words.

- Contrast the breadth and depth of word learning. What factors in the slow mapping period contribute to the depth of learning a word?

- What is the effect of how richly a word is represented on retrieval of the lexeme?

- Describe working memory and explain how it relates to word learning.

References

Aro, T., Laakso, M., Määttä, S., Tolvanen, A., Poikkeus, A. M. (2014). Associations between toddler-age communication and kindergarten-age self-regulatory skills. *Journal of Speech, Language & Hearing Research, 57*(4), 1405–1417.

Baddeley, A. (2000). The episodic buffer: A new component of working memory? *Trends in Cognitive Sciences, 4*(11), 417–423.

Baddeley, A. D., & Hitch, G. J. (1974). Working memory. In G. Bower (Ed.), *The psychology of learning and motivation* (Vol. 8, pp. 47–90). New York, NY: Academic Press.

Balaban, M. T., & Waxman, S. R. (1997). Do words facilitate object categorization in 9-month-old infants? *Journal of Experimental Child Psychology, 64*(1), 3–26.

Barsalou, L. W. (1999a). Perceptual symbol systems. *Behavioral and Brain Sciences, 22*(4), 577–660.

Barsalou, L. W. (1999b). Language comprehension: Archival memory or preparation for situated action? *Discourse Processes, 28*(1), 61–80.

Bates, E. (1976). *Language in context: The acquisition of pragmatics.* New York, NY: Academic Press.

Bates, E., Bretherton, I., & Snyder, L. (1988). *From first words to grammar: Individual differences and dissociable mechanisms.* New York, NY: Cambridge University Press.

Bates, E., Marchman, V., Thal, D., Fenson, L., Dale, P., Reznick, J. S., ... Hartung, J. (1994). Developmental and stylistic variation in the composition of early vocabulary. *Journal of Child Language, 21*(1), 85–123.

Bjorklund, D. F. (1987). How age changes in knowledge base contribute to the development of children's memory: An interpretive review. *Developmental Review, 7*, 93–130.

Bloom, L. (1973). *One word at a time.* The Hague: Mouton.

Bloom, P. (2004). Myths of word learning. In G. Hall & S. Waxman (Eds.), *Weaving a lexicon* (pp. 205–224). Cambridge, MA: MIT Press.

Booth, A. E., & Waxman, S. R. (2002). Object names and object functions serve as cues to categories for infants. *Developmental Psychology, 38*(6), 948–957.

Capone, N. C., & McGregor, K. K. (2004). Gesture development: A review for clinical and research practices. *Journal of Speech, Language, Hearing Research, 47*(1), 173–186.

Capone, N. C., & McGregor, K. K. (2005). The effect of semantic representation on toddlers' word retrieval. *Journal of Speech, Language, and Hearing Research, 48*(6), 1468–1480.

Capone Singleton, N. (2012). Can semantic enrichment lead to naming in a word extension task? *American Journal of Speech-Language Pathology, 21,* 279–292.

Capone Singleton, N. (2018). Late talkers: Why the wait-and-see approach is outdated. *Pediatric Clinics of North America* on Pediatric Speech and Language: Perspectives on Inter-Professional Practice, *65*(1), 13–29. doi:10.1016/j.pcl.2017.08.018.

Capone Singleton, N., & Saks, J. (2015). Co-speech gesture input as a support for language learning in children with and without early language delay. Invited article in *Perspectives on Language Learning and Education, 22,* 61–71.

Carey, S. (1978). The child as word learner. In M. Halle, J. Bresnan & G. A. Miller (Eds.), *Linguistic theory and psychological reality* (pp. 264–293). Cambridge, MA: MIT Press.

Caselli, M. C., Bates, E., Casadio, P., Fenson, J., Fenson, L., Sanderl, L., & Weir, J. (1995). A cross-linguistic study of early lexical development. *Cognitive Development, 10*(2), 159–199.

Clark, E. (1973). What's in a word? On the child's acquisition of semantics in his first language. In T. Moore (Ed.), *Cognitive development and the acquisition of language* (pp. 65–110). New York, NY: Academic Press.

Clark, E. (1993). *The lexicon in acquisition.* Cambridge, England: Cambridge University Press.

Collison, B. A., Grela, B., Spaulding, T., Rueckl, J. G., & Magnuson, J. S. (2014). Individual differences in shape bias in preschool children with specific language impairment and typical language development: Theoretical and clinical implications. *Developmental Science,* 1–16. doi:101111/desc.12219.

de Boysson-Bardes, B., & Vihman, M. (1991). Adaptation to language: Evidence from babbling and first words in four languages. *Language, 67*(2), 297–319.

Dell, G. S. (1990). Effects of frequency and vocabulary type on phonological speech errors. *Language and Cognitive Processes, 5,* 313–349.

Dell, G. S., Reed, K. D., Adams, D. R., & Meyer, A. S. (2000). Speech errors, phonotactic constraints, and implicit learning: A study of the role of experience in language production. *Journal of Experimental Psychology, 26*(6), 1355–1367.

Dore, J., Franklin, M., Miller, R., & Ramer, A. (1976). Transitional phenomena in early language acquisition. *Journal of Child Language, 3,* 13–28.

Fenson, L., Dale, P., Reznick, J. S., Thal, D., Bates, E., Hartung, J. P., … Reilly, J. S. (1993). *MacArthur communicative development inventories.* San Diego, CA: Singular.

Gathercole, S. E., & Baddeley, A. D. (1989). Evaluation of the role of phonological STM in the development of vocabulary in children: A longitudinal study. *Journal of Memory and Language, 28*(2), 200–213.

Gathercole, S. E., & Baddeley, A. D. (1990). Phonological memory deficits in language disordered children: Is there a causal connection?. *Journal of Memory and Language, 29,* 336–360.

Gathercole, S. E., Willis, C. S., Emslie, H., & Baddeley, A. D. (1992). Phonological memory and vocabulary development during the early school years: A longitudinal study. *Developmental Psychology, 28*(5), 887–898.

Gentner, D. (1982). Why nouns are learned before verbs: Linguistic relativity versus natural partitioning. In S. Kuczaf (Ed.), *Language development: Volume 2: Language, thought and culture* (pp. 301–334). Hillsdale, NJ: Lawrence Erlbaum.

Gentner, D. (2006). Why verbs are hard to learn. In K. Hirsh-Pasek & R. M. Golinkoff (Eds.), *Action meets word: How children learn verbs* (pp. 544–564). New York, NY: Oxford University Press.

Gershkoff-Stowe, L. (2001). The course of children's naming errors in early word learning. *Journal of Cognition and Development, 2*(2), 131–155.

Gershkoff-Stowe, L. (2002). Object naming, vocabulary growth, and the development of word retrieval abilities. *Journal of Memory and Language, 46*(4), 665–687.

Gershkoff-Stowe, L., & Smith, L. B. (1997). A curvilinear trend in naming errors as a function of early vocabulary growth. *Cognitive Psychology, 34*(1), 37–71.

Gershkoff-Stowe, L., & Smith, L. B. (2004). Shape and the first hundred nouns. *Child Development, 75*(4), 1098–1174.

Goldfield, B. (1986). Referential and expressive language: A study of two mother–child dyads. *First Language, 6,* 119–131.

Goldfield, B. (1987). The contributions of child and care-giver to referential and expressive language. *Applied Psycholinguistics, 8*(3), 267–280.

Goldfield, B. (1993). Noun bias in maternal speech to one-year-olds. *Journal of Child Language, 20*(1), 85–99.

Goldfield, B. A., & Reznick, J. S. (1990). Early lexical acquisition: Rate, content and the vocabulary spurt. *Journal of Child Language, 17*(1), 171–283.

Golinkoff, R. M., & Hirsh-Pasek, K. (2006). Baby word-smith: From associationist to social sophisticate. *Current Directions in Psychological Science, 15*(1), 30–33.

Golinkoff, R. M., Mervis, C. V., & Hirsh-Pasek, K. (1994). Early object labels: The case for a developmental lexical principles framework. *Journal of Child Language, 21,* 125–155.

Halliday, M. (1975). *Learning how to mean.* New York, NY: Elsevier.

Hollich, G. J., Hirsh-Pasek, K., Golinkoff, R. M., Brand, R. J., Brown, E., Chung, H. L., … Rocroi, C. (2000). Breaking the language barrier: An emergentist coalition model for the origins of word learning. *Monographs of the Society for Research in Child Development, 65*(3), i–vi, 1–123.

Horgan, D. (1979). *Nouns: Love 'em or leave 'em.* New York, NY: Address to the New York Academy of Sciences.

Horst, J. S., Parsons, K. L., & Bryan, N. M. (2013). Get the story straight: Contextual repetition promotes word learning from storybooks. *Frontiers in Psychology, 2*(17), 1–11. doi:10.3389/fpsyg.2011.00017

Jarrod, C., & Baddeley, A. D. (1997). Short-term memory for verbal and visuospatial information in Down's syndrome. *Cognitive Neuropsychiatry, 2*(2), 101–122.

Jones, S. S. (2003). Late talkers show no shape bias in a novel name extension task. *Developmental Science, 6*(5), 477–483.

Jones, S. S., Smith, L. B., & Landau, B. (1991). Object properties and knowledge in early lexical learning. *Child Development, 62,* 499–516.

Kemler Nelson, D. G. (1999). Attention to functional properties in toddlers' naming and problem solving. *Cognitive Development, 14,* 77–100.

Kim, M., McGregor, K. K., & Thompson, C. K. (2000). Early lexical development in English- and Korean-speaking children: Language-general and language-specific patterns. *Journal of Child Language, 27*(2), 225–254.

Lahey, M., & Edwards, J. (1999). Naming errors of children with specific language impairment. *Journal of Speech, Language, and Hearing Research, 42*(1), 195–205.

Landau, B., Smith, L. B., & Jones, S. S. (1988). The importance of shape in early lexical learning. *Cognitive Development, 3,* 299–321.

Leach, L., & Samuel, S. G. (2007). Lexical configuration and lexical engagement: When adults learn new words. *Cognitive Psychology, 55,* 306–353.

Li, P., Farkas, I., & MacWhinney, B. (2004). Early lexical development in a self-organizing neural network. *Neural networks, 17,* 1345–1362.

Marchman, V. A., & Bates, E. (1994). Continuity in lexical and morphological development: A test of the critical mass hypothesis. *Journal of Child Language, 21*(2), 339–366.

Markman, E. M. (1989). *Categorization and naming in children: Problems in induction.* Cambridge, MA: MIT Press.

McGregor, K. K. (1997). The nature of word-finding errors of preschoolers with and without word-finding deficits. *Journal of Speech and Hearing Research, 40*(6), 1232–1244.

McGregor, K. K., & Appel, A. (2002). On the relation between mental representation and naming in a child with specific language impairment. *Clinical Linguistics and Phonetics, 16*(1), 1–20.

McGregor, K. K., Friedman, R. M., Reilly, R. M., & Newman, R. M. (2002a). Semantic representation and naming in young children. *Journal of Speech, Language, and Hearing Research, 45*(2), 332–346.

McGregor, K. K., Newman, R. M., Reilly, R. M., & Capone, N. C. (2002b). Semantic representation and naming in children with specific language impairment. *Journal of Speech, Language, and Hearing Research, 45*(5), 998–1014.

National Early Literacy Panel. (2008). *Developing early literacy: Report of the National Early Literacy Panel.* Washington, DC: National Institute for Literacy.

Nelson, K. (1973). Structure and strategy in learning to talk. *Monographs of the Society for Research in Child Development, 143*(38).

Nelson, K. (1974). Concept, word, and sentence: Interrelations in acquisition and development. *Psychological Review, 81,* 267–285.

Nelson, K. (1981). Individual differences in language development: Implications for development and language. *Developmental Psychology, 17,* 170–187.

Nelson, K., Hampson, J., & Shaw, L. K. (1993). Nouns in early lexicons: Evidence, explanations and implications: Erratum. *Journal of Child Language, 20*(2), 228.

Nippold, M. A. (2007). *Later language development: School-age children, adolescents, and young adults* (3rd ed.). Austin, TX: Pro-Ed.

Oetting, J., Rice, M., & Swank, L. (1995). Quick incidental learning (QUIL) of words by school-age children with and without SLI. *Journal of Speech and Hearing Research, 38,* 434–445.

Paul, R., & Norbury, C. F. (2012). *Language disorders from infancy through adolescence. Listening, speaking, reading, writing, and communicating* (4th ed.). St. Louis, MO: Elsevier.

Perry, L. K., & Saffran, J. R. (2017). Is a Pink cow a cow? Individual differences in toddlers' vocabulary knowledge and lexical representations. *Cognitive Science, 41,* 1090–1105.

Plunkett, K., Karmiloff-Smith, A., Bates, E., Elman, J. L., & Johnson, M. H. (1997). Connectionism and developmental psychology. *Journal of Child Psychological Psychiatry, 38*(1), 53–80.

Ramer, A. (1976). Syntactic styles in emerging language. *Journal of Child Language, 3,* 49–62.

Rescorla, L. (2009). Age 17 language and reading outcomes in late-talking toddlers: Support for a dimensional perspective on language delay. *Journal of Speech, Language & Hearing Research, 52*(1), 16–30.

Rescorla, L., Mirak, J., & Singh, L. (2000). Vocabulary growth in late talkers: Lexical development from 2;0 to 3;0. *Journal of Child Language, 27*(2), 293–311.

Retherford, K. (2000). *Guide to analysis of language transcripts* (3rd ed.). Eau Claire, WI: Thinking Publications.

Rice, M., (2012). Toward epigenetic and gene regulation models of specific language impairment: Looking for links among growth, genes, and impairments. *Journal of Neurodevelopmental Disorders, 4*(1), 27.

Rice, M. L., Buhr, J. C., & Nemeth, M. (1990). Fast mapping word learning abilities of language-delayed preschoolers. *Journal of Speech and Hearing Disorders, 55,* 33–42.

Rice, M. L., Buhr, J. C., & Oetting, J. B. (1992). Specific-language-impaired children's quick incidental learning of words: The effect of a pause. *Journal of Speech and Hearing Research, 35,* 1040–1048.

Scheffner Hammer, C., Morgan, P., Farkas, G., Hillemeier, M., Bitetti, D., & Maczuga, S. (2016). Late talkers: A population-based study of risk factors and school-readiness consequences, *1–20.*

Snyder, L., Bates, E., & Bretherton, I. (1981). Content and context in early lexical development. *Journal of Child Language, 8,* 565–582.

Stoel-Gammon, C., & Cooper, J. (1984). Patterns of early lexical and phonological development. *Journal of Child Language, 11*(2), 247–271.

Storkel, H. (2001) Learning new words: Phonotactic probability in language development. *Journal of Speech, Language, and Hearing Research, 44*(6), 1321–1337.

Storkel, H., Bontempo, D. E., Aschenbrenner, A. J., Maekawa, J., & Lee, S. (2013). The effect of incremental changes in phonotactic probability and neighborhood density on word learning by preschool children. *Journal of Speech-Language-Hearing Research, 56,* 1689–1700.

Storkel, H. L., & Morrisette, M. L. (2002). The lexicon and phonology. *Language, Speech and Hearing Services in the Schools, 33,* 24–37.

Tek, S., Jaffery, G., Swensen, L., Fein, D., & Neigles, L. R. (2012) The shape bias is affected by differing similarity among objects. *Cognitive Development, 27,* 28–38.

Templin, M. C. (1957). *Certain language skills in children: Their development and interrelationships* (Institute of Child Welfare Monograph Series No. 26). Minneapolis, MN: University of Minnesota Press.

Vihman, M. (1996). *Phonological development: The origins of language in the child.* Oxford, UK: Basil Blackwell.

Vihman, M., Macken, M., Miller, R., Simmons, H., & Miller, J. (1985). From babbling to speech: A reassessment of the continuity issue. *Language, 61,* 397–445.

Vitevitch, M. S., & Luce, P. A. (1999). Proabilistic phonotactics and neighborhood activation in spoken word recognition. *Journal of Memory and Language, 40,* 374–408.

Waxman, S. R. (1994). The development of an appreciation of specific linkages between linguistic and conceptual organization. *Lingua, 92,* 229–257.

Werner, H., & Kaplan, B. (1963). *Symbol formation.* New York, NY: John Wiley & Sons.

Williams, K. T., (1997). *Expressive vocabulary test.* Circle Pines, MN: American Guidance Services.

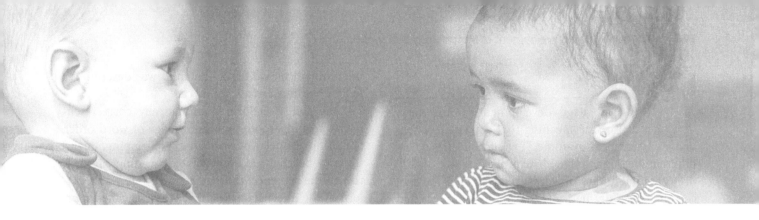

CHAPTER 8

The Development of Morphology and Syntax

Sandra L. Gillam, PhD, CCC-SLP
Jamie Mecham, MS, CCC-SLP
Ronald B. Gillam, PhD, CCC-SLP

OBJECTIVES

- Provide an overview of morphological and syntactic development
- Identify difficulties in morphological/grammatical learning in late talkers and children with specific language impairment (SLI)
- Familiarize students with theoretical accounts of syntactic difficulties associated with language impairments
- Describe clinical applications of morphological and syntactic development

KEY TERMS

Bound morpheme
C-unit
Derivational morphemes
Emergent account of language
  acquisition
Extended optional infinitive
  account

Free morpheme
Late-talker
Linguistic account
MLU
Morphology
Obligatory context
Phonological short-term memory

Procedural memory
Processing account
Prosody
SLI
Statistical or probabilistic
  learning
Syntax

▶ Introduction

During language development, words carry much of the meaning (or "content") of sentences. For example, "I want milk" has a very different meaning than, "I hate milk." The size of children's mental library of words (referred to as the lexicon) increases dramatically over their lifetime as new experiences lead to the discovery of knowledge about new objects, concepts, ideas, and words. As children develop more complex concepts and ascertain the words they use to express them, they formulate more complex things to say, which, in turn, requires them to string words together into longer and more complex sentences. This requires the integration of multiple linguistic systems, including morphology and syntax, which is what this chapter will address.

The relationships between words in sentences express much more multifaceted and precise meanings than words alone. Children progress from naming objects (*ball*), to talking about actions and objects (*throw ball*), to talking about agents, actions, and objects (*The boy is throwing the ball*), to talking about attributes of objects (*The boy is throwing the red ball*). By the time children go to school, they are able to produce very complex sentences such as, "The boy threw the red ball to the girl who was waiting to catch it."

All languages have conventions or rules for the way to combine words into sentences. In linguistics, this is referred to as syntax. Knowledge of syntax, or word order, matters because the same words denote different meanings when their order is changed. For example, if I said, "Mary helped Billy," we would agree that Mary was the helper and Billy was the person who was helped. That isn't the same thing as, "Billy helped Mary." Knowledge of the word-order conventions of language, in this case "Subject–Verb–Object," makes it possible for us to indicate who did what to whom. For meaningful communication to occur, speakers and listeners need to agree not only on the meanings of particular words, but also on meanings that are conveyed by word order.

Grammar (language form) is somewhat independent of meaning (language content). Even when speakers use word order incorrectly, their sentences may still be interpretable. For example, a sentence such as, "Her holded baby kitty," is ungrammatical because an object pronoun (*Her*) is used in place of the subject, the regular past tense marker is applied to the word *hold* that should be produced in the irregular form (*held*), and the child omitted an article (*the* or *a*) before the object noun phrase (*baby kitty*). Even though the sentence is ungrammatical, we know the child was describing a female holding a small, young cat.

The ability to form grammatically correct sentences requires more than knowledge of word order. Sometimes, aspects of words (i.e., zip, zipping, unzip) need to be changed somewhat depending on their role in the sentence. In linguistics, the allowable pattern of the internal structure of words is called morphology. A morpheme is the smallest grammatical unit that has meaning. For example, the word *dog* is a morpheme because it cannot be divided into individual parts that carry meaning (neither "d" nor "og" has any meaning). *Dog* is a free morpheme because it can stand alone as a word. In contrast, the plural marker *-s* is a bound morpheme. Plural *-s* is considered to be bound because it cannot stand alone. The plural *-s* is a grammatical tag or marker in English. When the grammatical morpheme *-s* is added to the word *dog*, it indicates that there is more than one dog. The plural marker *-s* is considered to be grammatical because the sentence, "The dogs were barking" would be ungrammatical without the *-s* on the word *dog* (e.g., *The dog were barking*). Other examples of grammatical morphemes include inflections such as the past tense marker *-ed* and the progressive tense marker *-ing*. In English, most bound morphemes are suffixes that are placed on the ends of words.

There are derivational morphemes, such as *-un* (e.g., *uninteresting*). Derivational morphemes are usually prefixes that are placed at the beginning of a word. Some derivational morphemes are suffixes, such as the *-ly* in *honestly*. This derivational morpheme changes a noun (*I am honest*) to an adverb (*He answered honestly*). The use of derivations requires sophisticated knowledge of the lexical, phonological, and syntactic aspects of language. Derivational morphology is acquired well into the school-age years and plays a role in academic success (Jarmulowicz & Hay, 2009; Jarmulowicz, Taran, & Hay, 2007). Morphological awareness, or the explicit knowledge and use of morphological markers, significantly contributes to literacy, vocabulary, sight-word reading, decoding, reading comprehension, and spelling abilities (Wolter & Pike, 2015). Various types of bound morphemes are illustrated in **TABLE 8-1**.

▶ Learning About the Development of Morphology and Syntax

Much of what we know about language development is based on the careful analysis of language

TABLE 8-1 Types of Bound Morphemes		
Derivational		**Inflectional**
Prefixes	**Suffixes**	
*un*usual	eas*ily*	Lisa*'s* movie
*in*sufficient	larg*est*	runn*ing*
*pre*term	bold*er*	crash*ed*
*trans*continental	warm*ness*	sit*s*

samples in which the words said by the adult and child are transcribed (written down) and then analyzed to determine the complexity of the vocabulary, morphology, and syntactic constructions that were used. To obtain a language sample, an investigator or clinician video- or audio-records a child talking to an adult or another child. In the past, researchers and clinicians have collected language samples that were approximately 15 minutes in length and/or 100 utterances long (Evans & Craig, 1992). Recent research has shown that samples do not necessarily have to be 100 utterances or 15 minutes in length to capture and assess language in naturalistic contexts. Heilmann, Nockerts, and Miller (2010) have shown that a 5-minute conversational sample yielding 40–50 utterances was sufficient to obtain meaningful information about these aspects of the language system in adolescents.

In a more recent study, Pavelko and Owens (2017) obtained 50 utterance conversational language samples from 270 typically developing children ages 3;0–7;11 (years;months). Their protocol is referred to as Sampling Utterances and Grammatical Analysis Revised (SUGAR). They transcribed and then analyzed the samples for mean length of utterance, total number of words, total number of clauses per sentence, and number of words per sentence. Results indicated that there were statistically significant age-related increases in the metrics, and that the process for elicitation, transcription, and analysis required only 20 minutes of time. More research is needed to generalize these findings to younger children.

Language sample analysis was the primary method used in a seminal study of morphological and syntactic development conducted about 40 years ago by a Harvard psychologist named Roger Brown (1973). Brown and a group of his students collected language samples from three children (Adam, Eve, and Sarah) at regular intervals over a 4-year period. Through careful analysis of the language transcripts, Brown and his research team tied changes in linguistic development to increases in utterance length, which they measured using a metric called *mean length of utterance* (MLU). Key milestones in morphological and syntactic development, which are still valid today, are shown in **TABLE 8-2**.

MLU is the average number of morphemes per utterance. It is calculated by counting the number of free and bound morphemes contained in each utterance and dividing the total morphemes by the total number of utterances in the sample. MLU is a general metric of language productivity because longer utterances tend to be more complex. So, computing MLU is a relatively quick way to estimate where a child is in the language development process. In addition, there are types of morphological and sentence forms that tend to occur at different levels of MLU. Therefore, once MLU is obtained, clinicians and researchers can assess whether the child is using the kinds of utterances that would be expected for a particular MLU level.

MLU is considered to be a *moderate* predictor of the complexity of a child's language, although in the past, this measure was considered only fairly reliable until MLU reached 4.0 or 5.0. Beyond the ages of 4;0 or 5;0, internal complexity and variability may increase without necessarily adding length to an utterance. That is, children may demonstrate linguistic complexity based on the types of words used rather than by stringing more words together (Owens, 2008). Beginning at age 18 months, when MLU is somewhere between 1.0 and 2.0, it increases by approximately 1.2 morphemes per year until age 5 years. This progression roughly correlates with 1-year-old children having a predicted MLU of approximately 1.0, 2-year-olds having an MLU of approximately 2.0, and so on (Scarborough, Wyckoff, & Davidson, 1986).

Computing MLU

The general rules for counting morphemes in utterances are shown in **TABLE 8-3**. After transcribing children's speech into utterances, clinicians and researchers count the number of free and bound morphemes in each utterance. Utterances that are incomplete or unintelligible are excluded from the analysis. False starts, repetitions, and fillers (*uh*) are not counted because they do not add to the meaning of the utterance and including them in the morpheme count would tend to inflate the child's MLU.

TABLE 8-2 Key Milestones in Morphologic and Syntactic Development

Age (yrs;mos)	Brown's Stage	Range for Predicted MLU	Morphology	Syntax
0–8 months				
8–12 months				
1;0–1;6				
1;7–1;10	Early I	1.01–1.49	Occasional use	Two-word utterances, Consistent word order, *What* + this/that
1;11–2;2	Late I	1.50–1.99	Occasional use	Agent + Action Action + Object Entity + Recurrence Negation + Entity Action + Locative *What/where* + NP or VP No/not + Noun or Verb
2;3–2;7	II	2.0–2.49	*-ing*, plural *-s*, irregular past tense, preposition *in*; occasional use of copula *is*, possessive *-s*,	NP + V + NP NP + Modal + Verb What + (NP) + Verb Where + (NP) + Verb
2;8–2;11	III	2.5–2.99	regular past *-ed*, preposition *on*; third person present *-s*, auxiliary & copula *is*, *am*, *are*	NP + Aux + V-*ing* + NP + Prep Ph, *Why/Who* + Sentence Aux + neg in sentences
3;0–3;6	IV	3.0–3.49	Auxiliary and copula *was/were*; Auxiliary Do (*do, does, did*) Modal verbs (*can, might, could*)	Conjoining with *and*; Simple infinitives Aux inversion in questions Clausal complements
3;7–3;11	V	3.5–4.49	Definite and indefinite articles, Contractible auxiliaries	Adverbial clauses Relative clauses (object modifying), Sentences containing conjoined and embedded clauses
4;0–4;11	V+	4.5–5.63	Auxiliary *have* (*have, has, had*) Present perfect with auxiliary marked	Sentences with multiple conjoined and embedded clauses Relative clause (subject modifying) Use of the conjunctions *because, when, so* Gerunds

5;0–6;11	5.64–8.10		Understanding of passive sentences and exceptions to grammatical rules Use of tag questions Negative interrogatives
7;0–8;11	8.10–9.28	*-er* suffix	Accurate judgments of grammaticality
9;0–11;11	9.28–11.14		Uses *tell, promise, ask, definitely, probably, possibly, if, though*
12;0–13;11	11.14–11.73		Use of perfect aspect (*have, had*) More prevalent Written syntactic complexity Outdistances oral syntactic Complexity
14;0–18;0	11.73–13.00		Use of modal auxiliaries become more prevalent

Sources: Data from Brown, R. (1974). *A first language*, Cambridge, MA: Harvard University Press; Johnston, J., Ammon, M. S. & Kamhi, A. (1988). Appendix in early syntactic development: Simple clause types and grammatical morphology. *Topics in Language Disorders*, 8(2), 42–43; Larson, V., & McKinley, N. (2003). Communication solutions for older students: Assessment and intervention strategies. Eau Claire, WI: Thinking Publications; Paul, R. (2007). Language disorders from infancy through adolescence: Assessment and intervention (3rd ed.). St. Louis, MO: Mosby; and Retherford, K., (2000). Guide to analysis of language transcripts (3rd ed.). Eau Claire, WI: Thinking Publications.

TABLE 8-3 Rules for Counting Morphemes in Utterances

General Rule	Example
1. The utterance must be completely intelligible and complete; fillers and singing are not counted	And Bingo *ah se* name-o. = 0 morphemes
2. Morphemes are assigned to repetitions only when they are used for emphasis or clarification, not when used in false starts or dysfluencies	He is not my friend, *NOT* my friend. = 8 morphemes He was not, is not my friend. = 5 morphemes
3. Compound words, proper nouns, diminutive forms, and formulated reduplications are counted as single words	John Smith wore a goofy cowboy hat. = 6 morphemes
4. Auxiliary verbs, catenative forms, common derivational affixes, inflectional morphemes, and inflections marked on gerunds and predicate adjectives are counted as 1 morpheme. Incorrect use of a form (*walkded*) is counted as 1 morpheme rather than 2	I *will* go. = 3 morphemes. I'm *gonna* go. = 4 morphemes They are going. = 4 morphemes The ball was *taken*. = 5 morphemes. They *tooked* the ball. = 4 morphemes
5. Count negative contractions as two morphemes only if both parts are used separately in the sample	He *isn't* my friend. = 5 morphemes She *is not* my friend. = 5 morphemes
6. Nonnegative contractions should be counted as two morphemes	*You're* my friend. = 4 morphemes

Source: Adapted from Brown, R. (1973). *A first language: The early stages*. Cambridge, MA: Harvard University Press.

Using the guidelines from Table 8-3, we would analyze the following utterances as:

Leave it in the water	5 morphemes
That's dirty	3 morphemes
Happy birthday Mommy	3 morphemes
I hafta clean my shoe s	6 morphemes
Play ing with my toy s	6 morphemes
Go night-night	2 morphemes
He fell down	3 morphemes

Although the preceding sample of seven utterances is far smaller than the number of utterances that would provide a truly representative sample of a child's language, we can compute the MLU for it as an exercise. By adding the total number of morphemes in the sample, we obtain a sum of 28 morphemes. That is divided by the number of utterances, which is 7, and it results in an MLU for this brief sample of 4.0.

Clinicians often use MLU as a quick way to assess the progress that children make during language intervention. Researchers sometimes use MLU to form groups of children with and without language impairments (Rice, Redmond, & Hoffman, 2006) that are matched according to their language productivity. For example, a 6-year-old child with a language impairment may have an MLU of 4.2. A researcher might find a "match" for that child by locating a 4-year-old who also has an MLU of 4.2. This is a good method for comparing the language complexity and the types of errors in children with and without language impairments.

The remainder of this chapter focuses on the development of two components of language form: morphology and syntax. We discuss the abilities that support the acquisition of syntax and describe some of the important milestones in morphological and syntactic development from the early preschool years through adolescence. For the purposes of this chapter, we will divide syntactic development into two periods: early syntactic constructions built by combining words into short sentences (ages 2–4), and later syntactic constructions built by combining phrases and clauses (later preschool years through adolescence).

▶ Precursors to Syntax

There are a number of cognitive and linguistic prerequisites for the development of syntax. Children often

exhibit combinations of actions within symbolic play, before they start combining words in utterances. An example would be pretending to pour liquid into a cup and then pretending to put the cup to a stuffed animal's mouth. Remember, in the case studies, there was mention that Johnathon and Josephine used objects symbolically with Johnathon talking on a "key" phone and Josephine "blowing on pretend hot food," whereas Robert was observed to engage mostly in banging and shaking of objects.

Between 18 months and 2 years of age, children begin to produce two-word utterances such as "Cara stay" or "Stay here." These word combinations are traditionally described by semantic relations such as Agent + Action and Action + Location. As noted by Tomasello (2003), children at the pre-syntactic stage of language development are learning concrete patterns of words that co-occur frequently. An example of this would be the child who says utterances like, "Mommy go, Daddy go, doggy go, car go," etc. It is clear that the child who produces these utterances knows that different things have the ability to "go," and this can be expressed by matching the word for the goer (the Agent) plus the word *go* (the Action).

It is likely that children learn these two-word patterns by remembering combinations of words that are heard repeatedly. In this way, the child's linguistic environment provides the basic elements (sequences of words) needed for them to form ideas about how to combine words. For example, a child whose parents talk about sitting at the table at dinner (e.g., *Mommy's sitting, Daddy's sitting, Grandma's sitting*) is likely to say something like, "Me sitting."

These two-word utterances are not considered to be syntactic. Syntax requires an understanding of abstract categories such as subject. The key to syntactic development is an important discovery that a child makes about the position of words and phrases in sentences. On different days and in different contexts, a child may hear the following utterances spoken about the child's cat: "Fluffy is scratching the couch. The cat is scratching the couch again. Stop scratching the couch, Fluffy. Is the cat scratching the couch?" As the child begins to analyze the similarities and differences in these utterances, the child comes to realize that different sequences of words can express similar relationships between actors and actions (*The cat scratched the couch*, and *Stop scratching the couch, Fluffy*). The ability to recognize that similar meaning relationships can be expressed by different word orders is called *distributional analysis* (Tomasello, 2003). When children begin to remember different forms of the same relationships between actors (*Fluffy*), actions (*scratching*), and objects (*the couch*), they come to realize that the actor in the previous sentences (Fluffy) can be expressed as a name (*Fluffy*) or as a phrase (*the cat*) and can appear at the beginning of the sentence (as in, *Fluffy is scratching the couch* and *The cat is scratching the couch again*), in the middle of the sentence (as in, *Is the cat scratching the couch?*), or at the end of the sentence (as in, *Stop scratching the couch, Fluffy*). Distributional analysis makes it possible for children to create an understanding of subjects of sentences, which is an abstract category.

Early Syntactic Development: Combining Words into Sentences

Between 2 and 3 years of age, children advance from using one- or two-word utterances to using sentences that can contain up to five or six words. Declarative sentences are expressed first using simple Subject + Verb + Object constructions such as "Mommy eat cookie" (refer to **FIGURE 8-1**). As the number and type of meanings that children want to express increase, it becomes necessary for them to use specific kinds of grammatical morphology and syntactic structures. For example, in order to say what happened, who did it, and where it happened, a speaker would have to combine a subject noun phrase (*The boy*), a verb phrase (*was riding*), an object noun phrase (*his bike*), and a prepositional phrase (*down the street*). This requires knowledge of abstract syntactic categories (Subject Noun Phrase + Verb Phrase + Object Noun Phrase + Prepositional Phrase) and grammatical morphology (adding a determiner).

Roger Brown and his students identified 14 grammatical morphemes that appeared relatively frequently in young children's language. The 14 grammatical morphemes are listed in Table 8-1 and are illustrated in Figure 8-1. Some of the earliest grammatical

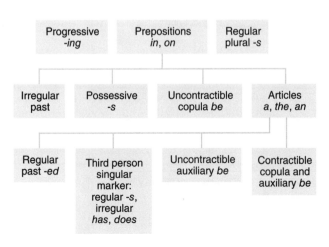

FIGURE 8-1 Brown's 14 morphemes.

morphemes to emerge are inflectional in nature and include plural -*s* (*The ducks swim*), possessive -*s* (*The cat's yarn*), and progressive -*ing* (*The boys are running*). Children begin to mark verb tense using third person singular -*s* (e.g., *The baby cries*) or past tense -*ed* (e.g., *The rabbit jumped*) at around the age of 3. This corresponds to Brown's Stage III, a time associated with a great deal of morphological and syntactic development in the lives of young language learners. Copula and auxiliary forms of "be" as in "Mommy *is* a nurse" (a copula form) or "She *is* laugh*ing*" (an auxiliary form) are used later as children produce increasingly more complex utterances to express new concepts and experiences.

There are certain conditions under which a particular morphological form must be used. It is called an obligatory context because use of the morpheme is "obligated" in the utterance. For example, when a number is used before a noun (*two duck*), the noun must be pluralized (*two ducks*). In this example, plural -*s* is obligatory for the utterance to be grammatical. Figure 8-1 illustrates the approximate developmental order of acquisition for the 14 morphemes identified by Brown (1973) that appear in Stage II and continue to be mastered until well after Stage V.

In addition to learning that inflectional morphemes occur in obligatory contexts, children must learn that there are phonological variations that occur on inflectional markers that are also obligatory but do not change the nature of the inflection. For example, in some plurals, the phoneme /z/ is required (as in the word *dogs*), and in others, the phoneme /s/ is required (as in the word *cats*). Different phonemes that express the same morphological meaning (past tense) are called allomorphs. Similar rules apply for past tense -*ed*. The /t/ allomorph is the past tense inflection for the verbs *walk* and *jump*, while the /d/ allomorph is the past tense inflection for the verbs *learn* and *happen*. If you are like the first author of this chapter, you may need to say the words in the previous two sentences out loud to fully understand the concept of allomorphs.

The Developmental Sequence

As noted in Table 8-2, early syntactic structures typically appear between 2 years, 3 months of age (2;3) and 2 years 7 months of age (2;7) when children's MLUs vary between 2.0 and 2.49 (Brown's Stage II). At this point, children start producing Subject–Verb–Object utterances like, "I got a ball," "That boy like me," and "Fluffy scratched me." These sentences represent the construction Noun Phrase + Verb Phrase + Noun Phrase (NP + VP + NP). At this stage, children also produce utterances like "He is big," "Daddy is sad," and "I'm happy" (NP + copula + Complement) and ask early questions like "What he doing?" and "Where Daddy going?" At the same time, the present progressive -ing (playing), plural -s (dogs), the prepositions in and on, the copula is (Mommy is happy), and possessive -s (John's ball) emerge. Simple yes/no (That mommy?) and wh- questions predominate early in language development (e.g., Where doggy? What that?). Negative forms at this state include utterances such as "Mommy no eat," "No eat cake," "No mommy eat cake" and even more complex utterances such as "Mommy is not happy" or "Mommy is not going." The developmental sequence for these sentence types is shown in **FIGURE 8-2**.

Children enter Brown's Stage III between the ages of 2 years, 8 months and 2 years, 11 months (2;8–2;11), when their MLUs vary between 2.5 and 2.99. In Stage III, we begin to see increased verb elaboration and the emergence of auxiliary verbs (is, am, are + verb -ing). This is also the time when most of the grammatical morphemes and why questions emerge. Children at this stage produce utterances like, "I am playing a game" (NP + Aux +V-ing + NP), "Mommy is cooking in the kitchen" (NP + VP + NP + Prepositional Phrase),

and "Why Daddy going in the car?" (Why + Sentence). At this time, regular past tense -ed (tripped), third person present indicative -s (jumps), and auxiliary verbs (is going, am going, are going) emerge. At this point in development, children are producing a variety of complete sentences.

The Developmental Process

There are two kinds of theories of early syntactic development: generativist theories and usage-based constructivist theories. Generativist theories of language acquisition hold that an innate universal grammar (UG) provides children with an understanding of abstract syntactic categories such as verb tense (present, past, future) and agreement (person and number) and the abstract operations needed to create a variety of grammatical constructions (Pinker & Ullman, 2002).

According to usage-based constructivist theories of early syntactic development, children's early linguistic productions reflect their knowledge of word sequences that occur frequently in the language that children hear (Tomasello, 2003). The theory predicts that children generate their own knowledge of abstract

Declarative	Interrogative	Negative
subj + v + obj	Wh-, yes/no using single words with rising intonation	Rejection, nonexistence, prohibition, denial of statement or question (neg + X)
subj + aux + v + obj	Wh-, yes/no using single words with subject & predicate	subj + neg + v
subj + aux + v + cop + comp	Sub/verb inversion	neg + v + obj
subj + v + indirect obj + obj	Auxiliary inversion	neg + subj + v + obj
subj + v + obj + to + indirect obj	Tag questions	subj + cop + neg + adv
	Negative interrogatives	subj + aux + neg + v

FIGURE 8-2 Development of sentence types.

Data from Gerken, L. (2007). Acquiring Linguistic Structures. In Hoff, E., & Shatz, M. (Eds). Blackwell Handbook of Language Development. Malden, MA: Blackwell; and Owens, R. (2008). Language development: An introduction (7th ed.). Boston, MA: Pearson.

syntactic categories like "subject" over time. Children start with a store of lexically based constructions such as "Doggy go." Over the course of development, children begin to recognize the overlap in the semantic roles expressed in various constructions (e.g., *Doggy go* and *Horse is running*) and build abstract links between them. Thus, correct use of a variety of constructions should emerge slowly after a significant amount of lexical learning. To date, we do not have compelling evidence that either the generativist or constructivist theories of syntactic development are correct (Rowland & Theakston, 2009; Theakston & Rowland, 2009).

An interesting phenomenon called regression occurs during early morphological development. Children sometimes increase their use of a new structure and later appear to lose the new skill. To illustrate, it is not uncommon for children to use irregular past tense verbs such as *cut* early on (*I cut my finger*), only to over-regularize them, saying "cutted" as they begin to learn past tense *-ed* in earnest during Brown's Stage III. This apparent regression appears to represent a step backward in morphological development. However, research suggests that this phenomenon may be explained as an instance in which *rote learning* precedes *rule learning*. That is, children may learn the irregular past verb forms as unanalyzed units through rote learning and memorization, while past tense *-ed* must be learned through the process of applying an abstract rule. As children learn how to express past tense in many different verb phrases, they may overgeneralize their new understanding of *-ed* to all verbs (*cutted*, *runned*). As children learn more and more verbs, they cease to overgeneralize past tense *-ed* and start using both regular and irregular past tense forms fairly accurately.

It is interesting that typically developing preschoolers are grammatically accurate only about 72% of the time, according to a recent study by Eisenberg, Guo, and Germezia (2012). These authors found that the typically developing 3-year-olds who participated in their study produced error rates as high as 25% for regular plurals, 40% for tense marking, and 50% for subject case pronouns (e.g., *he* for *she*). This study highlights the fact that the acquisition of grammar is highly variable. Although we would like to be able to place morphological and syntactic behaviors neatly into phases or stages, there is a wide range of individuality that is still considered typical.

Some of the variability in the findings reported by Eisenberg et al. (2012) may be related to the role of linguistic input on the development of specific grammatical forms. For example, Finneran and Leonard (2010) investigated the role of linguist input in the

acquisition of third person singular *s* for 16 33- to 36-month-old, typically developing (TD) children. In the study, children were asked to learn 16 single-syllable, novel verbs that, when inflected with third person singular *-s*, required the addition of either the /z/ or /s/ allomorph. Children heard third-person singular *-s* in contexts that required the finite form be used (*The tiger heens*) and in contexts obligating the nonfinite form (*Will the tiger heen?*) a total of three times for each context. Children were asked to produce the novel verbs in contexts that obligated the use of the finite form or the nonfinite form. Interestingly, the researchers also gathered data on children's' ability to produce third person singular *-s* in familiar verbs as well. Children were more likely to produce the finite verb form after being exposed to it in contexts obligating the finite and nonfinite forms, but only for novel verbs, not for the familiar verbs. That is, children used the finite forms accurately and overgeneralized their use to nonfinite contexts for novel verbs but showed no measurable change in their use of the finite form in familiar verbs. The results suggest the powerful role of linguistic input on the use of specific verb forms.

In a more recent study with slightly younger children, Hadley, Rispoli, Fitzgerald, and Bahnsen (2011) investigated the role of linguistic input on morphosyntactic growth for 15 21-month-old children. Parent speech input during spontaneous conversations was analyzed for language productivity and MLU as well as for instances in which parents marked tense in their speech to children. For example, when parents produced utterances that contained overt past tense markers such as "You missed," the verb was coded as +T (+tense). However, when utterances produced by parents did not contain information related overtly to tense (*You* need *more blocks*), the verb form was coded as −T (-tense). The percentage of overt +T forms was divided by the total number of verb forms coded as either +T or −T to yield a measure of "input informativeness." Morphosyntactic growth was calculated using a number of different words (NDW) and MLU in words and also by calculating a tense productivity score when children were 21, 24, 27, and 30 months of age.

Tense productivity was calculated by determining whether children's use of tense morphemes such as third person singular *-s*, past *-ed*, auxiliary *do*, copula and auxiliary *be* were judged sufficiently differently over time. That is, verb inflections such as third person singular *-s* that were used on different lexical verbs, and copula and auxiliary *be* and *do* used in different subject-tense morpheme combinations were judged as "different" from one time to another. A statistical technique called growth curve modeling was used to estimate each child's morphosyntactic growth from 21 to 30 months of age. There was a great deal of variability across parents for all of the measures of interest, including input informativeness for tense that ranged from 33% to 70%. Results suggested that input informativeness was positively associated with growth early on (1 year, 9 months) and predicted children's later performance. There was a moderately large positive correlation between parent use of overt tense marking (+T) and growth in children's tense productivity at 2 years, 6 months of age. Similarly, when parents' input contained fewer instances of overt tense marking (−T) children at 2 years, 6 months of age demonstrated slower growth in tense productivity.

A follow-up study by Fitzgerald, Hadley, and Rispoli (2013) addressed variations in parent interaction styles and language input. The purpose was to discern the relationship between parent interaction style and children's language development. In examining the relationships between children's language development and parent's use of question forms and various kinds of verbs, the researchers found that children's grammatical growth can be accelerated as parents use more descriptions of their children's actions.

Oja and Fey (2014) studied children's responses to telegraphic (short, grammatically incomplete phrases like "That doggy.") vs. grammatically complete prompts ("That's a doggy.") provided to elicit speech imitations. They studied children between 30 and 51 months of age in the early stages of combining words to determine whether they were more likely to respond to prompts that were telegraphic or prompts that were grammatically complete. In this study, children were just as likely to respond to telegraphic and grammatically complete prompts. Therefore, it is important to teach parents to use short, grammatically correct utterances when talking to their children. Clearly, parent input plays an important role in early syntactic and morphological development.

A correlational meta-analysis conducted by Sandbank and Yoder (2016) examined the relation between parental utterance length and child language outcomes for various populations of children with disabilities. Their findings suggested that for students with SLI, Down syndrome, intellectual disability, or combined disabilities, there was a small, positive trend for an association between length of parental input and MLU produced by the student. However, for children with autism spectrum disorder (ASD), the length of the parental utterance was strongly and positively associated with MLU. These results suggest that children with ASD may benefit greatly from hearing longer parental utterances. Clearly, parental input plays an important

role in early syntactic and morphological development; however, this may vary depending on the population.

Later Syntactic Development: Combining Phrases and Clauses

As children string more and more words together, they start using phrases, clauses, and complex sentences. Noun and verb phrase development involves distinct rules of word order and syntactic marking that become more complex over time. For example, noun phrases include elements such as initiators (*only, a few, less than, almost*), determiners (quantifiers, articles, possessives, demonstratives), adjectives (possessive nouns, ordinals, attributes), nouns (subject, object and reflexive pronouns, nouns), and modifiers (prepositional phrases, adjectivals, adverbs, embedded clauses). The order of developmental acquisition for noun phrase elaboration is illustrated in **TABLE 8-4**.

Similarly, as illustrated in **TABLE 8-5**, verb phrase development results in increasingly more complex sentences as children learn to use transitive verbs (a verb that takes a direct object), intransitive verbs (verbs that do not take the passive form or direct objects), and stative verbs (verbs that are followed by a complement). Verb phrases may include modal auxiliaries (*may, shall, would*), perfective auxiliaries (*have, has, had*), *be* verbs (*am, is, are*), negatives (*not*), passives (*been*), main verbs (*jog, drink, listen*), prepositional phrases (*in the box*), noun phrases (*the girl*), noun complements (*a carpenter*), and adverbial phrases (*walk quickly*).

Children progress from elaborating noun and verb phrases to producing complex sentences through the processes of phrasal and clausal conjoining and embedding. Phrases differ from clauses in that phrases are utterances that do *not* contain both a subject and a verb. Thus, a phrase must be embedded within a sentence to be grammatical. For example, the phrase *with my mother* cannot stand alone. To be grammatical, this phrase must be combined with a subject and a verb as in, *I went to the store with my mother*. Clauses contain subjects (nouns) and predicates (verbs) and are grammatical in and of themselves. Clauses can be as short as two words as in *She went*.

Sentences may contain multiple clauses. Sometimes, two main clauses are joined with a coordinating conjunction (*for, and, nor, but, or, yet, so*) to form a compound sentence (*Sara was working, and she dropped her hammer*). Later, children produce subordinated clauses by embedding one clause within a main clause as in *The girl who had red hair pushed the boy on the swing*. In this case, the main clause is, *The girl pushed the boy on the* swing. The clause *The*

TABLE 8-4 Development of Noun Phrases from Preschool to School-Age	
Noun Phrase Development	Indefinite article *a* & demonstrative *that*
	Subject pronouns (*I, he, she, we, they*)
	Object pronouns (*me, him, her, us, them*)
	Reflexive pronouns (*myself, himself, herself, ourselves*)
	Possessives, quantifiers, physical attributes
	Elaboration in subject and object positions using adjectives
	Relative clauses that modify nouns
	Multiple noun phrases used in succession
	Postnoun modifiers in embedded phrases and clauses

Source: Data from Gerken, L. (2007). Acquiring linguistic structures. In Hoff, E., & Shatz, M. (Eds). Blackwell Handbook of Language Development. Malden, MA: Blackwell; Owens, R. (2008). Language development: An introduction (7th ed.). Boston, MA: Pearson.

TABLE 8-5 Development of Verb Phrases from Preschool to School-Age	
Verb phrase development	Transitive and intransitive verbs in single word utterances
	Morphological modifications including the use of progressive -ing, infinitives, and auxiliary verbs with overgeneralizations;
	Modal auxiliaries; subject + auxiliary + verb + object
	Regular past, irregular past, third person singular, contractible copula
	Auxiliary inversion, use of do; subject + auxiliary + copula + complement
	Forms of *be*, past tense modals, auxiliaries; subject + verb + indirect object + object (or indirect object)
	Passives; noun + be/get + verb (-ed) + object

Source: Data from Gerken, L. (2007). Acquiring linguistic structures. In Hoff, E., & Shatz, M. (Eds). Blackwell Handbook of Language Development. Malden, MA: Blackwell; Owens, R. (2008). Language development: An introduction (7th ed.). Boston, MA: Pearson.

girl had red hair is embedded into the main clause to clarify just who the subject was. Generally speaking, children conjoin two main clauses before they begin to produce more complex constructions that involve embedding. **TABLE 8-6** provides examples of a number of different kinds of complex sentences.

At the same time that children are producing sentences containing multiple phrases and clauses, they are also creating more complex questions. Yes-no questions require the use of auxiliary inversion in which the auxiliary verb is moved in front of the subject as in, "Are you going to school?" Although not extensively used in the English language, tag questions begin to appear about the same time children create multiple clause utterances. Tag questions include the use of simple (*Let's play in the snow, okay?*) and more complex syntactic utterances (*She is really pretty, isn't she?*).

During the school-age years (ages 5;0 to adolescence), children are required to use more complex language to talk about things they are learning about. An important part of language development during the school-age years is learning literate language structures. Literate language is the style of language that is used in academics. Oral language is used in daily communication. An example of oral language is, "She is pretty." The same basic message using literate language might be conveyed as, "Her beauty is outshined only by her grace." It has been theorized that children who use literate language styles reach teacher expectations more often than children who use other oral language styles only.

There are four language structures that comprise literate language: conjunctions, elaborated noun phrases, mental and linguistic verbs, and adverbs (Greenhalgh & Strong, 2001). Conjunctions are words that are used to clarify the relationship between events and objects. There are three categories of conjunctions that are often targeted for literate language use, including temporal conjunctions, causal conjunctions, and coordinating conjunctions. Temporal conjunctions (e.g., *when, while,* and *after*) provide a background for the events in a narrative. For example, "*When* Tom woke up, he leaned over his bed to say good morning to the frog." Causal conjunctions present a physical or psychological motivation for the events in the narrative. This includes conjunctions such as *because* or *so that* as in, "The bees were angry *because* the hive fell to the ground." Coordinating conjunctions such as *so,*

TABLE 8-6 Examples of Complex Syntactic Structures
Coordinated Clauses

You can go <u>and</u> John can go with you.
I want to buy it <u>but</u> my mom won't let me.
You can buy it <u>or</u> you can go without it.
You should come over <u>so</u> we can play.

Subordinated Clauses

Noun Clauses
He said, don't ever do that again.
I don't believe <u>what you said</u>.
<u>What you want</u> is not what I want.
Adverbial Clauses
I bought the dog <u>because he was cute</u>.
I ran over there after I got home from school.
<u>If you want to catch me</u>, you'll have to run fast.
<u>When you called me</u>, I was eating dinner.
Relative Clauses
That's the boy <u>who took my bicycle</u>.
The boy <u>who stole my bicycle</u> was caught by the
   police.
My mom liked the flowers <u>that my dad bought for her</u>.
Comparative Clauses
My dad is fatter <u>than your dad is</u>.
I picked up as many coins <u>as I could get my hands on</u>.

but, and *however* are used to demonstrate opposition. For example, "She ran fast, *but* she didn't win the race."

Elaborated noun phrases (ENPs) are words or series of words used to add further description to the elements of the narrative. Elaboration may be accomplished by using noun modifiers (e.g., *the old, dead log*), qualifiers (e.g., the rabbit ran into a *hole in the ground*), relative clauses (e.g., the boy took the baby *that liked him* home), and appositives (e.g., this boy, *Tom*, had a dog) (Eisenberg et al., 2008). Eisenberg et al. (2008) examined noun phrase elaboration in children ages 5–11 by asking them to tell stories using single scene and picture sequences. Their stories were evaluated for different levels of noun phrase use, such as simple designating noun phrases (one pre-noun element—*the* boy), simple descriptive noun phrases (a descriptive element and a determiner—*a small* girl), complex descriptive noun phrases (two or more descriptive elements and a determiner—*the crazy yellow* bus), and complex noun phrases (i.e., noun postmodification—a face like aliens, a girl named Amanda). Eisenberg et al. found that children used more noun phrase elaboration when they told stories using a single scene prompt as compared to stories that were told about sequences of pictures. The researchers also found that

the most complex types of noun phrase elaboration may not be present until age 11.

Mental and linguistic verbs (ML) demonstrate that characters are thinking while linguistic verbs demonstrate different ways that characters use speech/language in a narrative (e.g., Tom *called* out the window). Adverbs indicate time, manner, or degree (e.g., the deer stopped *quickly* at the edge of the cliff).

Literate language features are directly linked to reading and writing development and are used by children to make their language more complex. When children are deficient in their use of literate language, their ability to convey a specific meaning may be limited and their literacy acquisition may be affected. Children who use less literate language also tend to score lower on measures of language productivity such as MLU (Greenhalgh & Strong, 2001).

The Developmental Sequence

As noted in Table 8-2, syntactic structures begin to appear around 3 years of age when children's MLUs vary between 3.0 and 3.49 (Brown's Stage IV). At this point, children have become adept at using auxiliary *be* verbs (e.g., *They* <u>were</u> *going to the park; Tommy* <u>is</u> *washing dishes*). Now, children start using auxiliary *do* (*I don't drink tea*) and modal verbs such as *can, should*, and *could* (e.g., *I could walk over there*). They start combining sentences with *and* (e.g., *She ran home, and her dog followed her*), and they use simple infinitive forms (e.g., *I like* <u>to eat</u> *fried chicken*). Finally, children discover how to ask questions that require auxiliary inversion (*Are you coming over to my house? Why is he looking at me?*).

Late in their third year of life, when their MLUs are between 3.75 and 4.5 (Brown's State V), children begin to use a variety of complex sentences. They conjoin clauses with *but* and *so*, and they start to produce a variety of adverbial clauses (refer to Table 8-6 for examples). At the same time, children are using the definite and indefinite articles (*the, a*) consistently and are using contracted forms of auxiliary verbs (*They're going home now*).

During the fourth year of life (MLU = 4.5–5.63), children produce subjective relative clauses (*The man* <u>who laughed at me</u> *broke his ankle)*, the conjunctions *because, when*, and *so*, and gerunds (<u>Skiing</u> *is my favorite sport*). Children also begin to produce utterances with multiple phrases and clauses (*I told my friend Sherry to play by the swings*).

After children enter kindergarten, they begin to understand and use passive forms (*The cat* <u>was chased</u> *by the dog*), tag questions (*The teacher told you to put that away,* <u>didn't she?</u>), and perfect tense (*has, had, will have*). Children's use of literate language structures (conjunctions, adverbs, cognitive and linguistic verbs, adjectives in elaborated noun phrases) increases markedly during the elementary school-age years.

As children learn to write, the syntactic and morphological complexity of the oral language is greater than the syntactic and morphological complexity of their written language. However, between the ages of 12 and 14 years, there is a remarkable shift, as their written language becomes more complex than their oral language. By adolescence, children should have adult-like syntax and morphology in their speaking and their writing.

The Developmental Process

There are three important influences on later syntactic development: exposure to written language, an increase in working memory capacity, and new ways of relating language to thought. Written language tends to contain more elaborated noun and verb phrases and a greater variety of complex sentences than oral conversational language (Greenhalgh & Strong, 2001). As children hear stories read to them and learn to read stories themselves, they encounter a wide variety of complex sentences. Therefore, it is no accident that the development of complex language co-occurs with increased exposure to narrative (stories) and expository (instructional) texts.

The ability to conjoin and embed phrases and clauses into complex sentences requires the ability to hold multiple pieces of information in mind as new information is added. Essentially, this is a working memory problem. Working memory (WM) refers to the mental processes that are responsible for keeping information actively accessible for use in cognitive tasks (Baddeley & Hitch, 2000). Gillam, Montgomery, Gillam, and Evans (2017) explained how learning language relies on a variety of WM processes related to focusing attention on the speaker, associating the words that are heard with their meanings, and relating the meanings to knowledge in long-term memory. If the sentence that was spoken contains a complex syntactic structure that is unfamiliar to the child, the child needs to remember the sequence of words, any grammatical morphemes that were attached to the words, the context that the sentence was spoken in, and ideas about the role the words may have played in the utterance (subject, verb, object, modifier, etc.). Most children manage to process and store all this complex information in ways that allow them to remember a great deal of information about the new construction and make a good guess about its meaning.

As children's memory capacity increases, they are able to remember longer sequences of words and

the grammatical morphemes that are attached to the words. They can hold that information in mind as they try to decipher the meaning of the sentence. The next time children hear a similar sequence of words, they begin to recognize patterns across the two utterances. This enables children to discover how words, grammatical morphemes, phrases, and clauses can be combined (Maratsos, 1990; Mintz, Newport, & Bever, 2002; Redington, Chater, & Finch, 1998). For example, Montgomery, Magimairaj, and Finney (2010) reported that PSTM functions as an important language learning device and enables children to establish stable, long-term phonological representations of new words, enabling them to store these words in long-term memory. They also report that children with greater WM capacity have greater comprehension and processing speed. This allows children to gradually start using less frequently encountered combinations of phrases and clauses (Tomasello, 2003).

Between 4 and 5 years of age, as children become more skilled at understanding and telling stories, they begin to use language differently. Nelson (1986) observed that 2- and 3-year-old children primarily use language in the context of ongoing activities. What is said is closely tied to actions that the child or others in the immediate environment are engaged in. Late in the preschool years and early in the school-age years, children start to tell stories that depict events that have already occurred or that have never occurred (as in the case of fictional stories). New, more complex language structures are needed to describe events that are not present. There seems to be a relationship between the need to create contexts with language and the development of complex utterances. According to Westby and Culatta (2016), producing complex narratives supports social and psychological well-being as well as students' ability to meet academic demands.

▶ Morphological/Grammatical Learning in Late Talkers and Children with Developmental Language Disorders (DLD)

Unfortunately, not all children learn language easily or well. Children with language impairments have difficulty understanding what other people say and/or have difficulty expressing themselves in ways that would be expected for their age. These children may have smaller vocabularies, they may use less complex sentence forms, and/or they make more grammatical errors. The next sections of the chapter provide some

Preschool

Sometimes, it becomes apparent that a preschool child is not acquiring aspects of language form, content, or use as quickly or efficiently as their peers. This was the case with Robert and Josephine, who were described in the case studies. When this happens, we may label them a "late talker" rather than as someone having language impairment. The term *late talker* or slow expressive language development (SELD) generally refers to the 10%–15% of toddlers and preschoolers who demonstrate slower than usual expressive language development, as evidenced in delayed production of early words and word combinations, or who continue to demonstrate grammatical errors when their peers no longer do so (Rescorola & Turner, 2015).) Late talkers may be reliably identified when children have vocabularies of fewer than 50 words and are not producing 2-word utterances by 2 years of age. The prevalence of late talkers ranges from 7% to 18%, depending on the study.

Remember from the case study presented earlier in the book that Josephine's mother reported her to have produced her first words later than most children (around 15 months), and she had a small vocabulary for her age. Late talkers generally do not demonstrate problems related to cognitive, sensory, emotional, or environmental deficits and often eventually "catch up" with their peers. This was the case with Josephine, as her evaluation revealed typical cognitive skills. There is some evidence to suggest that children who were labeled as late talkers in preschool may not manifest difficulties in higher-level linguistic skills such as phonological awareness or reading when they reach school age (Paul, Murray, Clancy, & Andrews, 1997).) Many late talkers catch up to age expectations for expressive language by the time they reach kindergarten (Rescorla, 2002, 2013). Other studies suggest that as many as 50% of children with SELD will not acquire proficiency in language production without intervention (Shevell, Majnemer, & Webster, 2005; Snowling, Bishop, & Stothard, 2006).

Given the conflicting findings in the research, it is difficult to know for sure that early difficulties in language acquisition will not continue into the school years and impact social, emotional, psychological, and academic performance. This represents a compelling problem for SLPs who work with preschool children when they must make decisions about whether or not to recommend intervention for children identified as late talkers or SELD. The clinician in our case study

example judged Josephine's prognosis to be good on the basis of the presence of typical prelinguistic abilities, play, receptive language, and gestural imitation skills. However, in the case of Robert, the findings were much more straightforward. The presence of a receptive delay is always concerning, and in Robert's case, there is a history of other problems that accompany his language delay. Given this information, it is much more likely that Robert will be diagnosed as having language impairment later on.

The terms *specific language impairment (SLI)* and *developmental language disorder (DLD)* have been used to refer to preschoolers who have unusual difficulties understanding and/or using vocabulary or grammar in age-appropriate ways. These children's language difficulties cannot be attributed to other conditions such as intellectual disability, hearing impairment, neurological disorders, motor disfunctions, or other medical conditions. While some researchers have used the term SLI to refer to children who primarily have grammatical problems, most researchers and clinicians recognize that these children face language-based deficits as well as cognitive deficits in areas such as attention, perception, and memory. Recently, to avoid confusion with the more narrow definition of SLI, there has been a shift in the literature for the label DLD (American Psychiatric Association [APA], 2013; Reilly, Bishop, & Tomblin, 2014). Approximately 7% of preschoolers face DLD.

As we noted earlier, linguistic proficiency is commonly measured in young preschool children by eliciting a conversational sample and calculating MLU and other metrics. Procedures for calculating MLU have been discussed earlier in this chapter. The validity and stability of using MLU as a measure of linguistic proficiency has been debated over the years, particularly for use in children over the age of 4 or 5. Rice et al. (2006) investigated the concurrent validity and temporal stability of MLU equivalency for children with specific language impairment (SLI) and children developing typically (TD). In their first study, 124 archival conversational samples elicited from 39 children with SLI (5;0 years;months), 40 MLU equivalent children developing typically (3;0), and 45 age equivalent (AE) controls were studied. The researchers examined whether MLUs corresponded with other well-accepted measures of linguistic ability such as developmental sentence scoring (DSS) and the index of productive syntax (IPSyn). They reported high correlations among MLU, DSS, and IPSyn measures.

In a second study, 205 archival conversational samples representing 5 years of longitudinal data collected from 20 children with SLI (5;0) and 18 MLU matches (3;0) were analyzed using growth curve modeling. Growth curve modeling is a useful statistical method for estimating growth trajectories over time. As in study 1, MLU was associated with high levels of temporal stability over the 5-year period studied, suggesting that it is a reliable and valid index of general language development for use by clinicians and an appropriate grouping variable for use by researchers, specifically when children are between the ages of 3 and 10.

In a more recent study, Rice, Smolik, Perpich, Thompson, Rytting and Blossom, (2010) report age referenced MLU data obtained at 6-month intervals for 306 children ages 2;6–9;0 with and without SLI. They examined MLU for 170 students with SLI and 136 who were developing typically. In their article, MLU was reported in words and in morphemes. MLU data from this project across four different age ranges is shown in TABLE 8-7. It is clear that at each age range, the lower range of MLU values for the typically developing children are above the upper range of values for the children with SLI. Therefore, calculations of MLU in either words or morphemes can be very helpful for tracking language development in children with SLI as well as children developing typically.

Speech language pathologists use MLU in words and morphemes (refer to Table 8-2) along with other measures of linguistic ability to make decisions about whether to recommend intervention for late talkers or children with DLD. That is, MLU, along with an analysis of vocabulary use, verb use, social skills, and the consideration of other risk factors such as prolonged otitis media, socioeconomic status, and familial history of language and learning problems is considered in a comprehensive language assessment protocol (Olswang, Rodriguez, & Timler, 1998). Examination of other language abilities, such as vocabulary knowledge, in combination with MLU, may give practitioners more confidence in making predictions about who may or may not "grow out" of early language delay. In a longitudinal investigation, Moyle, Ellis-Weismer, Evans, and Lindstrom (2007) examined the relationship between vocabulary and grammar proficiency for 60 children ranging in age from 2;0 to 5;6, half of whom were identified as late talkers. They found that measures of vocabulary were highly correlated with measures of grammar over time. Furthermore vocabulary skill was shown to be a strong, consistent predictor of later grammatical skills; grammatical impairments are a known risk factor for language impairment.

While historically, MLU has been used to characterize the language development of late talkers and children with DLD, MLU may underestimate a child's language skills if children produce a large number of one-word utterances in their conversational sample

TABLE 8-7 MLU Ranges

Age Range (years; months)	Mean MLU (Words)	Mean MLU (Morphemes)
Children with SLI		
2;6–3;11	2.37–3.10	2.59–3.36
4–5;11	3.31–3.64	3.64–4.34
6–7;11	4.18–4.33	4.38–4.77
8–8;11	4.36–4.49	4.80–4.97
Children Developing Typically		
2;6–3;11	2.91–3.71	3.23–4.09
4–5;11	4.10–4.47	4.57–4.96
6–7;11	4.57–4.92	5.07–5.45
8–8;11	5.08–4.99	5.67–5.51

Rice, M., Smolik, F., Perpich, D., Thompson, T., Rytting, N., & Blossom, M. (2010). Mean length of utterance levels in 6-month intervals for children 3 to 9 with and without language impairments. *Journal of Speech Language and Hearing Disorders, 53,* 333–349.

(e.g., "yes", "nope", "hello", "bye") even when they are capable of producing longer utterances. This has been shown to occur across the preschool years. Therefore, another measure that shows promise in predicting whether children are late talkers is length of the longest utterance (LLU). Smith and Jackson (2014) conducted a study to evaluate the efficacy of using LLU to approximate MLU and to predict later MLU for late talkers and children developing typically. Correlations between LLU and MLU at 30 months were significant and LLU predicted MLU at 42 months for 43 late talkers and 33 age-matched children who were TD. This is an efficient measure, calculated by averaging the three longest utterances in a conversational sample.

Another tool that may be useful for identifying language impairments in young children was proposed by Eisenberg and Guo (2013). They compared the diagnostic accuracy of three grammaticality measures in accurately differentiating between young preschool children with and without language impairments. They compared the percentage of grammatical utterances (PGU) to a measure that excluded utterances that did not contain a subject and/or a main verb (PSP: percentage sentence point) and a measure that included only verb tense errors (PVT: percentage verb tense usage).

PGU is calculated by subtracting the number of ungrammatical C-units from the total number of C-units and then dividing it by the total number of C-units. PSP is calculated the same way, except utterances that do not have subjects or main verbs are not included. To calculate PVT, all of the verb contexts that obligate tense must be marked, including copula, auxiliary be, auxiliary do, regular past, regular third person singular, irregular past, and third-person verb forms. PVT is calculated by subtracting the total number of tense marker errors from the total number of obligatory contexts for tense marking in all C-units and then dividing it by the total number of obligatory contexts for tense marking.

Their study included 34 3-year-olds, half of whom demonstrated language impairment. Language samples were elicited from the children by asking them to talk about pictures that either contained an obvious problem (e.g., children fighting in the sandbox) or pictures that contained three or more characters involved in familiar activities (e.g., a family cooking breakfast). The best cut-off score for differentiating between children with and without language impairments was 58.32% for PGU, 67.46% for PSP, and 85.48% for PVT. All of the measures demonstrated very high levels of diagnostic accuracy. Their findings support the use of PGU as a screening measure for identifying young children with language impairment.

Recent research suggests that short, highly structured language intervention programs, even those that involve parents as the primary interventionists, may result in positive outcomes for very young late talkers and young children with DLD (Buschmann et al., 2009). This was the recommendation made for Josephine, who was diagnosed as a late talker. The clinician suggested that her parents be trained in the use of language facilitation techniques so that they might assist Josephine in acquiring the language skills she needs during her daily interactions with others.

School-Age

Many preschoolers who have been diagnosed with DLD continue to have difficulty with oral language during the school-age years. DLD occurs in approximately 7.4% of the kindergarten population and refers

---

CLINICAL APPLICATION EXERCISE

Watch the video entitled "Story Retell," available with the online materials, and then answer the following questions about this short narrative language sample.

C: So, the frog escapeded from the jar
C: And this is how he did it
C: Put one foot out and then the other foot out
C: And then he go to his frog and fish family
C: And the kid didn't know where he at
C: But when he looks there he keeps on yelling right when he after looks
C: And then he found the frog with his frog family and his fish family
C: And that's the end

1.   There are eight utterances in this sample. How many are grammatically correct?
     a.   1–3
     b.   4–6
     c.   6–8
     d.   None
     e.   All

2.   How many of the utterances contain complex syntax?
     a.   1–3
     b.   4–6
     c.   6–8
     d.   None
     e.   All

3.   If you had to make a decision, would you say this child has a developmental language delay or not? She is 5.
     a.   Yes
     b.   No

to a state in which children demonstrate significant language learning difficulties in the absence of cognitive, hearing, oral-motor, emotional, or environmental deficits (Leonard, 1998; Tomblin et al., 1997). The young Robert will likely be among this population of school-age children when he grows older. Often, children with DLD demonstrate significant weaknesses in the development of morphology, semantics, vocabulary, phonology/articulation, and complex syntax. In addition, these children have sentence comprehension difficulties as well as poor attention skills, slower speed of processing, and reduced WM capacity. Language disorder affects receptive language, expressive language, or both. Receptive language relates to an individual's ability to comprehend linguistic information, whereas expressive language relates to an individual's ability to formulate and produce linguistic information.

Children with DLD also demonstrate a great deal of difficulty organizing stories and using appropriate vocabulary and linguistic forms to understand and formulate them. Analysis of oral narratives or stories may be used to document linguistic proficiency for school-age children because increasing grammatical and syntactic abilities are related to improvements in the overall organization of narratives (Gillam & Johnston, 1992; Heilmann, Miller, Nockerts, & Dunaway, 2010).

Typically, examination of language form and content for school-age children is accomplished by asking them to retell or generate a story of their own. The narrative sample is generally segmented into C-units, much like conversational samples, and individual utterances are analyzed for linguistic form and content. Total number of words (TNW), NDW, MLU in words and morphemes, and percentage of complex sentences (those that contain a main clause and a subordinate clause) may be calculated and compared to databases such as the one illustrated in **TABLE 8-8**.

A diagnosis of a language disorder is usually made by showing that a child's language development is significantly below age expectations to the extent that it interferes with communicative, social, and academic functioning. A DLD cannot be caused by an intellectual or sensory impairment or some other medical problem. Looking across a number of studies of children with language disorders, many investigators identify language disorder by performance that is -1 or more standard deviations below the mean on multiple tests or subtests of receptive or expressive language (Gillam, Gillam, Holbrook, & Orellano, in press).

What Causes DLD?

There are two broad categories of causal explanations for DLD: linguistic accounts and processing accounts. Linguistic accounts of DLD traditionally highlight problems children have in learning grammatical morphology. Perhaps the most popular of the linguistic theories is the extended optional infinitive (EOI) account (Rice, Hoffman, & Wexler, 2009). The

TABLE 8-8 Means (SDs) for Narrative Measures by Age					
Age (years)	TNW	NDW	MLU-W	MLU-M	Percent Complex
5	68 (47)	39 (20)	6.8 (1.7)	7.6 (1.8)	0.33 (0.2)
6	77 (54)	43 (22)	7.5 (1.6)	8.3 (1.6)	0.37 (0.2)
7	96 (74)	52 (28)	8.5 (3.8)	9.5 (4.3)	0.38 (0.2)
8	137 (77)	69 (27)	8.1 (1.4)	9 (1.5)	0.45 (0.2)
9	162 (96)	79 (30)	8.4 (1.4)	9.4 (1.6)	0.51 (0.2)
10	237 (196)	101 (49)	8.9 (2.1)	10 (2.4)	0.55 (0.2)
11	167 (70)	84 (27)	8.7 (1.4)	9.6 (1.6)	0.5 (0.2)
12	148 (95)	67 (36)	8.8 (1.9)	9.7 (2.1)	0.5 (0.2)

Sources: Adapted from Justice, L. M., Bowlels, R., Kadaravek, J. N., Ukrainetz, T. A., Eisenberg, S. L., & Gillam, R. B. (2006). The index of narrative micro-structure (INMIS): A clinical tool for analyzing school-age children's narrative performance. *American Journal of Speech-Language Pathology, 15,* 177–191.

EOI posits that children advance through a stage of language acquisition during which they inconsistently mark tense in main clauses because they do not quite realize that to do so is obligatory. While developmentally, this seems to apply for all children, even those developing typically, children with SLI continue to mark tense inconsistently long after children developing typically cease to do so. The most compelling evidence for the EOI account comes from studies that show that tense markers (e.g., past tense *-ed*) rather than those unrelated to tense (plural markers, progressive *-ing*) were most problematic for children with SLI and continued to be produced in error well after children entered school (Conti-Ramsden, 2003).

There is increasingly more evidence to suggest that DLD be associated with deficits in PSTM or WM, both of which may be inherited or genetic in nature (Falcaro et al., 2008). Falcaro et al., (2008) investigated the involvement of chromosomes 16q and 19q on performance on PSTM and tense marking tasks for 93 probands and their first-degree relatives. PSTM is proposed to be responsible for temporarily storing and processing verbal information (Gathercole & Baddeley, 1990). PSTM was measured by asking participants to repeat a series of 28 nonwords that varied in length and complexity (*brufid, shimitet, dexiptecastic*). Grammatical morphology was measured by asking participants to fill in missing words requiring the use of regular and irregular verbs. There was a significant relationship between scores obtained on the PSTM task for first-degree relatives and probands but not for scores on the grammatical morphology task.

Processing capacity limitation explanations of SLI, such as the ability to store and manipulate verbal information by PSTM or WM, have gained more support over the years. Processing accounts propose that general and/or specific limitations in information processing may explain the problems that children with SLI experience in learning the morphology of the language (Gathercole & Baddeley, 1990; Kail, 1994; Montgomery, 1995). If children have difficulty processing incoming information quickly and efficiently, it will affect their ability to detect and process inflectional morphemes or to make judgments about grammaticality (Wulfeck & Bates, 1995). Typically, tasks that measure speed of processing are used to support processing accounts of SLI, the assumption being that processing speed will determine how much information may be processed during a given amount of time. There is considerable evidence to suggest that children with DLD demonstrate slowed response times on a variety of tasks (Leonard et al., 2007; Miller, Kail, Leonard, & Tomblin, 2001).

Some have argued that processing efficiency rather than processing speed is the cause of problems experienced by children with DLD (Gillam, Cowan, & Day, 1995). This position is supported in studies that show that children with SLI take longer to accomplish more difficult tasks than easier ones or that they perform more poorly when tasks require manipulation of verbal information as opposed to nonverbal information (Mainela-Arnold & Evans, 2005; Montgomery, 2000, 2004; Montgomery & Windsor, 2007). In a typical PSTM task, as measured using nonword repetition, children must remember an unfamiliar sound sequence so that they may recall and produce it. This requires processing and temporary storage of each sound in a specific order for accurate recall. There are many studies that have shown that children with SLI perform significantly more poorly on nonword repetition tasks than their age-matched peers and younger children matched for language ability in English, and in other languages even after they no longer demonstrate overt language difficulties (Conti-Ramsden & Durkin, 2007; Montgomery, 1995; Reuterskiold-Wagner, Sahlen, & Nyman, 2005).

Ullman and Pierpont (2005) have proposed the Procedural Deficit Hypothesis (PDH), which suggests that impairments in procedural memory account for the problems experienced by children with DLD. Procedural memory refers to the ability to learn new skills over many trials without conscious effort or awareness. Under the PDH, children with DLD have deficiencies in their ability to recognize and store "patterns," and/or events that "occur together," making it difficult for them to learn to pair inflectional morphemes with their uninflected verb forms. The PDH proposes that DLD is the result of abnormal functioning of the frontal-basal ganglia neurological circuits that support procedural learning. In support of this hypothesis, a recent meta-analysis conducted by Lum, Conti-Ramsden, Morgan, and Ullman (2014) showed that, across a number of studies, DLD has been associated with impairments in procedural learning.

It is likely that the language learning problems experienced by children with SLI are the result of some combination of both linguistic deficits and processing limitations. Explanations that highlight limitations in WM as causal correlates for language impairment are congruent with linguistic accounts because remembering and sorting out the rules for tense and agreement places more demands on the listener than conceptually easier aspects of language, such as nonfinite markers. The nature of the relationship between linguistic and processing explanations is complex and will continue to be a source of rich debate for years to come.

One theoretical account of language impairment for children with DLD that is of particular relevance for practicing SLPs is known as emergentism. This theory suggests that language acquisition is an emerging process by which children simultaneously integrate sources of acoustic, linguistic, social, and communicative information that they encounter within daily, naturally occurring interactions. Emergentists posit that language is a dynamic, evolving system that may be represented as a distribution of probabilistic information. That is, children purportedly focus on the inherent regularities or statistical properties of a language in order to learn it. For children with DLD, reduced processing capacity or speed may place them at a linguistic disadvantage when learning those features of the language that occur with low frequency or are more difficult to discern because of a lack of overt salience. An emergentist account of language impairment is important for the field of speech language pathology for a number of reasons but perhaps most importantly because it takes under consideration the role of the environment in informing language acquisition. Under this account, consistent, intensive, and stable exposure to problematic linguistic forms during intervention should result in their eventual acquisition (Evans, 2001).

Clinical Implications

Studies investigating approaches to improving morphology and syntax for children with language problems are generally met with positive outcomes, particularly in preschool. For example, Leonard, Camarata, Pawlowska, Brown, and Camarata (2006) investigated the use of focused stimulation in facilitating the use of third-person singular -s and auxiliary *is, are, was* for 25 children with DLD. Focused stimulation is a technique that employs the use of repetitive overt models to highlight specific forms that are the target of instruction. For example, an SLP might say, "This *is* a baby, *Is* this a baby, This *is*" to highlight copula *is* during a teaching session. The preschool children ranged in age from 3:0 to 4:4 ($M = 3;5$) and were assigned to a treatment condition focusing either on third person singular ($n = 15$) or auxiliary *is, are, was* ($n = 10$). During each session, children listened to stories while the SLP acted out the events using toys and props and provided restated or recasted utterances during play to emphasize correct use of target forms. The instruction was conducted twice daily, two times per week, over a 12-week period. Children in both treatment conditions made significant gains in their use of the targeted form.

Very few studies have been conducted that have examined language outcomes as a result of intervention

for school-age children with language impairment (Cirrin & Gillam, 2008). In one study, Ebbels, van der Lely, and Dockrell (2007) studied two approaches to improving verb argument structure for 27 school-age (11–16 years of age) children with DLD. Children were randomly assigned to one of three groups. Children in Group 1 received syntactic-semantic therapy that involved the use of shapes, colors, and coding schemes to highlight parts of speech and/or morphology. Children in Group 2 received semantic therapy that targeted semantic aspects of verbs (i.e., *This is pouring*). Children assigned to Group 3, a control group, did not receive intervention targeting verb argument structure but rather received it on their ability to formulate inferences. All of the children participated in assessment sessions prior to beginning intervention, immediately after intervention, and a follow-up session 3 months after intervention. Children who received instruction in verb argument structure, whether in syntactic-semantic or semantic therapy, demonstrated measurable gains in morphology and syntax over the control groups that were maintained over time.

In a meta-analysis, Goodwin and Ahn (2010) investigated the impact of morphological instruction on outcomes for school-age children with reading, learning, and language disabilities, children learning English as a second language, and struggling readers. Morphological treatment strategies included affix and root word instruction, building words from morphemes, compound word instruction, distinguishing between morphemes and pseudomorphemes, using context, teaching morphological patterns and rules, word family instruction, identification of words by analogy, instruction in word origins, word sorts, and word mapping. Findings revealed that morphological instruction made the largest impact on phonological awareness (the awareness of the sounds in the language), morphological awareness (awareness of the morphological components of a language such as past tense -ed), and vocabulary outcomes; small effects on reading comprehension and spelling; and no measureable impact on decoding or the ability to "sound out" words in print.

Cleave, Becker, Curran, Owen Van Horne, and Fey (2015) conducted a systemic review and meta-analysis investigating the research evidence on the effectiveness of conversational recasts in grammatical development for children with language impairments. A conversational recast is a response to a child's utterance in which the clinician repeats parts or all of the utterance spoken by the child while highlighting a certain aspect of the utterance. For example, the child might say "Her want baby", to which the clinician might say "Yes, she wants the baby." emphasizing the correct pronoun

"She" as compared to "Her." Their findings support the use of recasts as a key component of interventions designed to facilitate the use of specific grammatical targets for children with SLI.

▶ Summary

The study of language acquisition has evolved over the years. Early in the history of our field, research focused primarily on whether language was innate or learned and how language was acquired by "typical children." Recently, science has shifted its focus onto studying how differences in biological make-up, brain development, and/or cultural and environmental experiences shape the way children learn and use language. Knowledge about how children acquire language in the context of these factors may better inform our attempts to assess and intervene when children demonstrate difficulty.

Study Questions

- According to linguistic accounts, why do children with SLI have difficulty learning grammatical morphology?
- Why is it so difficult to be certain that children are developing typically when it comes to grammatical and syntactic development? What factors influence acquisition?
- How is MLU calculated? Why is it useful? Can it be misleading? If so, when? Why?

- What is LLU? What advantages does it have over calculating MLU?
- What does it mean when children demonstrate a growth pattern that appears to indicate regression in the acquisition of past tense?
- Children form longer and more complex sentences using a number of strategies. Discuss some of these strategies.

References

American Psychiatric Association [APA]. (2013). *Diagnostic and Statistical manual of mental disorders* (5th ed.). Arlington, VA: American Psychiatric Association.

Baddeley, A. D., & Hitch, G. J. (2000). Development of working memory: Should the Pascual-Leone and the Baddeley and Hitch models be merged? *Journal of Experimental Child Psychology, 77*(2), 128–137.

Brown, R. (1973). *A first language: The early stages.* Cambridge, MA: Harvard University Press.

Buschmann, A., Jooss, B., Rupp, A., Feldhusen, F., Pietz, J., & Philippi, H. (2009). Parent based language intervention for 2-year-old children with specific expressive language delay: A randomized controlled trial. *Archives of Disease in Childhood, 94*, 110–116.

Cirrin, F., & Gillam, R. B. (2008). Language intervention practices with school-age children with spoken language impairments: A systematic review. *Language, Speech, and Hearing Services in Schools, 39*(1), S110–S137.

Cleave, P., Becker, S., Curran, M., Owen Van Horne, A., & Fey, M. (2015). The efficacy of recasts in langage intervention: A systematic review and meta-analysis. *The American Journal of Speech Language Pathology, 24*, 237–255.

Conti-Ramsden, G. (2003). Processing and linguistic markers in young children with specific language impairment (SLI). *Journal of Speech and Hearing Research, 46*, 1029–1037.

Conti-Ramsden, G., & Durkin, K. (2007). Phonological short-term memory, language and literacy: Developmental relationships in early adolescence in young people with SLI. *Journal of Child Psychology & Psychiatry, 48*(2), 147–156.

Ebbels, S., van der Lely, H., & Dockrell, J. (2007). Intervention for verb argument structure in children with persistent SLI: A randomized control trial. *Journal of Speech, Language, and Hearing Research, 50*(5), 1330–1349.

Eisenberg, S., & Guo, L. (2013). Differentiating children with and without language impairment based on grammaticality. *Language, Speech and Hearing Services in Schools, 44*, 20–31.

Eisenberg, S. L., Guo, L, & Germazia, M. (2012). How grammatical are 3-year-olds? *Language, Speech and Hearing Services in Schools, 43*, 36–52.

Eisenberg, S. L., Ukrainetz, T. A., Hsu, J. R., Kaderavek, J. N., Justice, L. A., & Gillam, R. B. (2008). Noun phrase elaboration in children's spoken stories. *Language Speech and Hearing Services in Schools, 39*(2), 145–157. doi: 10.1044/0161-1461(2008/014)

Evans, J. (2001). An emergent account of language impairments in children with SLI: Implications for assessment and intervention. *Journal of Communication Disorders, 34*(1–2), 39–54.

Evans, J. L., & Craig, H. K. (1992). Language sample collection and analysis: Interview compared to freeplay assessment contexts. *Journal of Speech & Hearing Research, 35*(2), 343–353.

Falcaro, M., Pickles, A., Newbury, D., Addis, L., Banfield, E., Fisher, S., Monaco A., Simkin, Z., Conti-Ramsden, G., & the SLI Consortium. (2008). Genetic and phenotypic effects of phonological short-term memory and grammatical morphology in specific language impairment. *Genes, Brain and Behavior, 7*(4), 393–402.

Finneran, D., & Leonard, L. (2010). Role of linguistic input in third person singular -s use in the speech of young children. *Journal of Speech, Language, and Hearing Research, 53*(4), 1065–1074.

Fitzgerald, C., Hadley, P., & Rispoli, M. (2013). Are some parents' interaction styles associated with richer grammaitcal input? *American Journal of Speech-Language Pathology, 22*, 476–488

Heilmann, J., Miller, J., & Nockerts, A. (2010). Using language sample databases. *Language, Speech, Hearing Services in the Schools, 41*, 84–95.

Gathercole, S., & Baddeley, A. (1990). Phonological memory deficits in language disordered children: Is there a causal connection? *Journal of Memory and Language, 29*, 336–360.

Gillam, R., Cowan, N., & Day, L. (1995). Sequential memory in children with and without language impairment. *Journal of Speech and Hearing Research, 38*(2), 393–402.

Gillam, R., Gillam, S., Holbrook, S., & Orellano, C. (in press). Language disorder. In S. Goldstein & M. DeVries (Eds). *Handbook of DSM 5 childhood disorders*. Manhattan, NY: Springer Publishers.

Gillam, R., & Johnston, J. (1992). Spoken and written language relationships in language/learning-impaired and normally achieving school-age children. *Journal of Speech and Hearing Research, 35*, 1303–1315.

Gillam, R., Montgomery, J., Gillam, S., & Evans, J. (2017). Memory and attention in children with language impairments. In R. G. Schwartz (Ed), *Handbook of child language disorders* (2nd ed., pp. 213–237). New York, NY: Psychology Press.

Goodwin, A., & Ahn, S. (2010). A meta-analysis of morphological interventions: Effects on literacy achievement of children with literacy difficulties. *Annals of Dyslexia, 60*(2), 183–208.

Greenhalgh, K., & Strong, C. (2001). Literate language features in spoken narratives of children with typical language and children with language impairments. *Language, Speech, and Hearing Services in Schools, 32*(2), 114–125.

Hadley, P., Rispoli, M., Fitzgerald, C., & Bahnsen, A. (2011). Predictors of morphosyntactic growth in typically developing toddlers: Contribution of parent input and child sex. *Journal of Speech, Language, and Hearing Research, 54*(2), 549–566.

Heilmann, J., Miller, J., Nockerts, A., & Dunaway, C. (2010). Properties of the narrative scoring scheme using narrative retells in young school-age children. *American Journal of Speech-Language Pathology, 19*(2), 154–166.

Jarmulowicz, L., & Hay, S. (2009). Derivational morphophonology: Exploring errors in third graders' productions. *Language, Speech, and Hearing Services in Schools, 40*(3), 299–311.

Jarmulowicz, L., Taran, V., & Hay, S. (2007). Third graders' metalinguistic skills, reading skills, and stress production in derived English words. *Journal of Speech, Language, and Hearing Research, 50*, 1593–1605.

Kail, R. (1994). A method of studying the generalized slowing hypothesis in children with specific language impairment. *Journal of Speech and Hearing Research, 37*(2), 18–421.

Leonard, L. (1998). *Children with specific language impairment*. Cambridge, MA: MIT Press.

Leonard, L., Camarata, S., Pawlowska, M., Brown, B., & Camarata, M. (2006). Tense and agreement morphemes in the speech of children with specific language impairment during intervention: Phase 2. *Journal of Speech, Language, Hearing Research, 49*(4), 749–770.

Leonard, L., Ellis Weismer, S., Miller, C., Francis, D., Tomblin, J., & Kail, R. (2007). Speed of processing, working memory, and language impairment in children. *Journal of Speech, Language, and Hearing Research, 50*(2), 408–428.

Lum, J., Conti-Ramsden G., Morgan A., & Ullman M. (2014). Procedural learning deficits in specific language impairment (SLI): A meta-analysis of serial reaction time task performance. *Cortex; A Journal Devoted to the Study of the Nervous System and Behavior, 51*(100):1–10. doi:10.1016/j.cortex.2013.10.011.

Mainela-Arnold, E., & Evans, J. (2005). Beyond capacity limitations: Determinants of word recall performance on verbal working memory span tasks in children with SLI. *Journal of Speech, Language, and Hearing Research, 48*, 897–909.

Maratsos, M. (1990). Are actions to verbs as objects are to nouns? On the differential semantic bases of form, class, category. *Linguistics, 28*, 1351–1379.

Miller, C., Kail, R., Leonard, L., & Tomblin, B. (2001). Speed of processing in children with specific language impairment. *Journal of Speech, Language, and Hearing Research, 44*(2), 416–433.

Mintz, T. H., Newport, E. L., & Bever, T. G. (2002). The distributional structure of grammatical categories in speech to young children. *Cognitive Science, 26*, 393–424.

Montgomery, J. (1995). Examination of phonological working memory in specifically language-impaired children. *Applied Psycholinguistics, 16*, 355–378.

Montgomery, J. (2000). Verbal working memory and sentence comprehension in children with specific language impairment. *Journal of Speech, Language, and Hearing Research, 43*(2), 293–308.

Montgomery, J. (2004). Sentence comprehension in children with specific language impairment: Effects of input rate and phonological working memory. *International Journal of Language and Communication Disorders, 39*(1), 115–133.

Montgomery, J., Magimairaj, B., & Finney, M. (2010). Working memory and specific language impairment: An update on the relation and perspectives on assessment and treatment. *American Journal of Speech Language Pathology, 19*, 78–94.

Montgomery, J., & Windsor, J. (2007). Examining the language performances of children with and without specific language impairment: Contributions of phonological short-term memory and speed of processing. *Journal of Speech, Language, and Hearing Research, 50*(3), 778–797.

Moyle, M., Ellis-Weismer, S., Evans, J., & Lindstrom, M. (2007). Longitudinal relationships between lexical and grammatical development in typical and late-talking children. *Journal of Speech, Language, and Hearing Research, 50*(2), 508–528.

Nelson, K. (1986). *Event knowledge: Structure function in development*. Hillsdale, NJ: Lawrence Erlbaum Associates.

Oja, B., & Fey, M. (2104) Children's response to telegraphic and grammatically complete prompts to imitate. *American Journal of Speech-Language Pathology, 23*(1), 15–26.

Olswang, L., Rodriguez, B., & Timler, G. (1998). Recommending intervention for toddlers with specific language learning difficulties: We may not have all the answers, but we know a lot. *American Journal of Speech-Language Pathology, 7*(1), 23–32.

Owens, R. (2008). *Language development: An introduction* (7th ed.). Boston, MA: Pearson.

Paul, R., Murray, C., Clancy, K., & Andrews, D. (1997). Reading and metaphonological outcomes in late talkers. *Journal of Speech Language and Hearing Research, 40*(5), 1037–1047.

Pavelko, S., & Owens, R. (2017). Sampling utterances and grammatical analysis revised (SUGAR): New normative values for language sample analysis measures. *Language, Speech, and Hearing Services in Schools, 48*, 197–215.

Pinker, S., & Ullman, M. T. (2002). The past and future of the past tense. *Trends in Cognitive Sciences, 6*(11), 456–463.

Redington, M., Chater, N., & Finch, S. (1998). Distributional information: A powerful cue for acquiring syntactic categories. *Cognitive Science, 22*(4), 425–469.

Reilly, S., Bishop, D., & Tomblin, B. (2014). Terminological debate over language impairment in children: Forward movement and sticking points. *International Journal of Language and Communication Disorders, 49*, 452–462.

Rescorla, L. (2002). Language and reading outcomes to age 9 in late-talking toddlers. *Journal of Speech Language and Hearing Research, 45,* 360–371.

Rescorla, L. (2013). Late talkers: Do good predictors of outcomes exist? *Developmental Disabilities Research Reviews, 17,* 141–150.

Rescorola, L., & Turner, H. (2015). Morphology and syntax in late talkers at age 5. *Journal of Speech, Language and Hearing Research, 58,* 434–444

Reuterskiold-Wagner, C., Sahlen, B., & Nyman, A. (2005). Non-word repetition and non-word discrimination in Swedish preschool children. *Clinical Linguistics & Phoniatrics, 19*(8), 681–699.

Rice, M., Hoffman, L., & Wexler, K. (2009). Judgments of omitted BE and DO in questions as extended finiteness clinical markers of specific language impairment (SLI) to 15 years: A study of growth and asymptote. *Journal of Speech, Language, and Hearing Research, 52,* 1417–1433.

Rice, M., Redmond, S., & Hoffman, L. (2006). Mean length of utterance in children with specific language impairment and in younger control children shows concurrent validity and stable and parallel growth trajectories. *Journal of Speech, Language, and Hearing Research, 49,* 793–808.

Rice, M., Smolik, F., Perpich, D., Thompson, T., Rytting, N., & Blossom, M. (2010). Mean length of utterance levels in 6-month intervals for children 3-9 years with and without language impairments. *Journal of Speech Language Hearing Research, 53,* 333–349.

Rowland, C. F., & Theakston, A. L. (2009). The acquisition of auxiliary syntax: A longitudinal elicitation study. Part 2: The modals and auxiliary DO. *Journal of Speech, Language, and Hearing Research, 52*(6), 1471–1492.

Sandbank, M., & Yoder, P. (2016). The association between parental mean length of utterance and language outcomes in children with disabilities: A correlational meta-analysis. *American Journal of Speech Language Pathology, 25,* 240–251.

Scarborough, H., Wyckoff, J., & Davidson, R. (1986). A reconsideration of the relationship between age and mean utterance length. *Journal of Speech and Hearing Research, 29*(3), 394–399.

Shevell, M., Majnemer, A., & Webster, R., (2005). Outcomes at school age of preschool children with developmental language impairment. *Pediatric Neurology, 32*(4), 264–269.

Smith, A., & JackinsJackson, M. (2014). Relationship between longest utterance and later MLU in late talkers (2014). *Clinical Linguistics & Phonetics, 28,* 143–152.

Snowling, M., Bishop, D., & Stothard, S. (2006). Psychosocial outcomes at 15 years of children with a preschool history of speech-language impairment. *Journal of Child Psychology and Psychiatry, 47*(8), 759–765.

Theakston, A. L., & Rowland, C. F. (2009). The acquisition of auxiliary syntax: A longitudinal elicitation study. Part 1: Auxiliary BE. *Journal of Speech, Language, and Hearing Research, 52*(6), 1449–1470.

Tomasello, M. (2003). *Constructing a language: A usage-based theory of language acquisition.* Cambridge, MA: Harvard University Press.

Tomblin, B., Records, N., Buckwalter, P., Zhang, X., Smith, E., & O'Brien, M. (1997). Prevalence of specific language impairment in kindergarten children. *Journal of Speech Language and Hearing Research, 40,* 1245–1260.

Ullman, M., & Pierpont, E. (2005). Specific language impairment is not specific to language: The procedural deficit hypothesis. *Cortex, 41,* 399–433.

Westby, C., & Culatta, B. (2016). Telling Tales: personal event narratives and life stories. *Language, Speech and Hearing Services in Schools, 44,* 260–282

Wolter, J., & Pike, K. (2015) Dynamic assessment of morphological awareness and third-grade literacy success. *Language, Speech, and Hearing Services in Schools, 46,* 112–126

Wulfeck, B., & Bates, E. (1995). *Grammatical sensitivity in children with language impairment.* Technical Report CND-9512. Center for Research in Language, University of California at San Diego.

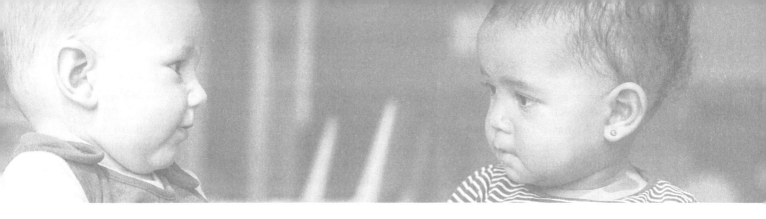

CHAPTER 9

Speech Sound Disorders: An Overview of Acquisition, Assessment, and Treatment

Lynn K. Flahive, MS, CCC-SLP, BCS-CL
Barbara W. Hodson, PhD, CCC-SLP

OBJECTIVES

- To demonstrate basic knowledge and skills in the area of speech sound disorders
- To differentiate the parts of the speech mechanism and describe their purposes
- To identify and categorize phonemes, noting differences based on place, manner, and voicing as well as typical ages of acquisition
- To identify phonological deviations in children's speech productions
- To specify goals of an evaluation to assess a child for a possible speech sound disorder
- To write goals and procedures for a lesson plan for a child with highly unintelligible speech

KEY TERMS

Articulation
Consonants
Cycles phonological remediation
  approach
Phoneme

Phonological awareness
Phonological deviations
Phonological intervention
Phonological patterns
Phonology

Sound system development
Speech mechanism
Speech sound disorders
Vowels

Introduction

The American Speech-Language-Hearing Association (ASHA) has recommended using the term *speech sound disorders* to refer to problems in producing the sounds of a language. As noted by Prezas and Hodson (2007), the term *articulation,* which refers to the process of producing speech sounds, is often used in conjunction with a child who has difficulty with only a few sounds (e.g., articulation disorder or delay). Children with a *phonological impairment* experience challenges with the speech sound system of language. Children with a phonological impairment have difficulties that involve more than one sound that are error patterns in the phonological system. A child who omits an /s/ in consonant clusters (e.g., *smoke* → [mok]) is said to have a phonological impairment because the production of /s/ may occur in non-cluster contexts. *Childhood apraxia of speech* (CAS) refers to problems with motor planning.

Although these terms are often used interchangeably, an articulation problem generally is considered to be mild to moderate in severity, and the child typically is understood most of the time. By comparison, children with disordered phonological systems and/or apraxia tend to have highly unintelligible speech and are considered to have a severe-to-profound disorder. ASHA (2008) reported that 80% of children diagnosed with a speech sound disorder have a condition severe enough to warrant intervention.

Several different approaches to addressing speech sound disorders are possible. One can examine the speech mechanism for structural problems and/or for muscle weakness, muscle incoordination, and/or other motor problems. One can also evaluate for signs of CAS. Alternatively, some speech-language pathologists (SLPs) address speech sound errors through the use of oral motor exercises, even though evidence regarding the effectiveness of that method is lacking.

Although all of these approaches are currently used, this chapter focuses on a linguistic approach, one of phonology—that is, the sound system of language. It includes the study of (1) syllable/word shapes/structures, (2) phonemes and allophones, and (3) prosody/suprasegmentals (Hodson, 2010). Phonological substitutions tend to be consistently produced in a child's language once they pass the earliest stage of lexical acquisition (Bernthal, Bankson, & Flipsen, 2013). The remediation process focuses on reorganizing the child's phonological system by helping the child learn to produce and acquire phonological patterns (e.g., word endings/final consonants).

This chapter provides an overview of speech, including how it is produced, an exploration of the sounds of English, and a review of the general stages of development. It also describes phonological patterns and explores their importance in assessing and treating young children. Although treatment for speech sound disorders may utilize a motor-based approach, a linguistic approach, or a combination of the two, this chapter focuses mostly on linguistic or phonologically based approaches. Regardless of which approach an SLP uses when working with young children with speech sound disorders, they always need a solid foundation of this particular body of information.

The Speech Mechanism

Six major organs/subsystems are used in the production of speech. The respiratory system, which pertains to where the airflow is generated, includes the lungs, airways, ribcage, and diaphragm. The diaphragm is the chief muscle of inhalation. Speech begins here when the diaphragm moves air through the respiratory system. Air is pushed through the thoracic cavity, past the trachea, to the larynx.

The larynx, often referred to as the "voice box," is composed of various cartilages and muscles. It is the chief structure for the production of sound. The vocal folds are found in the larynx. When the vocal folds vibrate as air flows through them, the sound is voiced. If the vocal folds remain open and do not vibrate, the consonant produced is voiceless.

The air stream then enters the velopharyngeal area, which contains the velum, also known as the *soft palate.* This area separates the oral and nasal cavities. Thus, air may go through the nasal cavity, through the oral cavity, or both. Nasal sounds are produced in the nasal cavity. The oral cavity contains the articulators. The tongue, which is the major articulator, is composed of muscles and can be divided into five parts: tip (apex), blade, back (dorsum), root, and body. After the air flows over the tongue, it crosses the teeth and lips. The lips are the most visible articulators. The jaws are bony structures that support the tissues of the tongue, teeth, and lips.

Phonemes

A *phoneme* is the smallest arbitrary unit of sound in a given language that can be recognized as being distinct from other sounds in that language (Nicolosi, Harryman, & Kresheck, 1996). Phonemes are the sounds of a language that combine to form words. American English has 44 symbols that are denoted in the International Phonetic Alphabet (IPA). English phonemes are divided into *consonants, vowels,* and *diphthongs.* **TABLE 9-1** lists the consonants with examples of each.

TABLE 9-1 Phonemes

Phoneme	Key Word	Place	Manner	Voicing
/p/	pie	bilabial	stop	Voiceless
/b/	book	bilabial	stop	Voiced
/t/	type	alveolar	stop	Voiceless
/d/	dog	alveolar	stop	Voiced
/k/	cape	velar	stop	Voiceless
/g/	go	velar	stop	Voiced
/f/	face	labiodental	fricative	Voiceless
/v/	vote	labiodental	fricative	Voiced
/θ/	thumb	interdental	fricative	Voiceless
/ð/	them	interdental	fricative	Voiced
/s/	sun	alveolar	fricative	Voiceless
/z/	zoo	alveolar	fricative	Voiced
/ʃ/	shoe	palatal	fricative	Voiceless
/ʒ/	treasure	palatal	fricative	Voiced
/tʃ/	chip	palatal	affricative	Voiceless
/dʒ/	jump	palatal	affricative	Voiced
/l/	lip	alveolar	liquid	Voiced
/r/	run	palatal	liquid	Voiced
/m/	map	bilabial	nasal	Voiced
/n/	nose	alveolar	nasal	Voiced
/ŋ/	wing	velar	nasal	Voiced
/w/	win	bilabial	glide	Voiced
/j/	yes	palatal	glide	Voiced
/h/	hat	glottal	fricative	voiceless

The position of the consonant in the word is described by the terms *initial, medial,* and *final.* When a consonant is described by its position in a word relative to the vowel, the terms *prevocalic, intervocalic,* and *postvocalic* are used. If the consonant is at the beginning of the word (e.g., <u>n</u>ose), it is in the initial position. This also can be considered prevocalic because it precedes the vowel. Consonants that occur in the middle of a word are in the medial position. If the consonant is between two vowels (e.g., *bunny*), it also is referred to as intervocalic. Consonants that are the last sound in a word are said to be in the final position. If the consonant also follows a vowel in the word-final position, it is postvocalic (e.g., *can*).

The 24 consonants of American English are typically described by their place, manner, and voicing. *Manner* refers to what happens to the airflow through the resonance and articulatory systems (Scherz & Edwards, 2010). Consonants that involve some type of constriction of the airflow are *obstruents,* which include stops, fricatives, and affricates. *Sonorant consonants,* which include nasals, glides, and liquids, are made with a relatively open vocal tract. When a complete closure of the vocal tract occurs at some point so that there is no airflow, thereby allowing pressure to build and then be released, the sound is considered to be a *stop.* Stops /p, b, t, d, k, g/ are sometimes called plosives or stop-plosives. *Fricatives,* which include /f, v, s, z, ʃ, ʒ, θ, ð, h/, are noisy sounds caused by a turbulent airflow as the air stream goes through a narrow constriction. *Affricates* /ʧ, ʤ / include two components: a stop and a fricative release. The sound begins with a stop and then ends with the air stream going through a narrow constriction.

The *nasals* /m, n, ŋ / are sounds in which the airflow goes through the nasal cavity. The *glides* /w, j/ are sometimes referred to as semivowels because of the relatively open vocal tract during production. *Liquids* /l, r/ are similar to glides but have a bit more vocal tract obstruction than the glides or vowels. The only lateral sound in American English is /l/; the airflow goes over the sides of the tongue with an opening near the middle. The /r/ can be produced in many different ways (Secord, Boyce, Donohue, Fox, & Shine, 2007). A retroflex or rhotacized /r/ has the tongue tip curled back and up near the palate. The other major position involves bunching of the tongue near the back of the palate.

When discussing manner, the terms *sibilants* and *stridents* also are useful categories. Sibilants, which include /s, z, ʃ, ʒ, ʧ, ʤ /, are consonants where the air stream going through the constriction produces a "hissing" sound. Strident sounds, which are created when the air stream hits the back of the teeth, include /f/ and /v/ as well as sibilants.

Consonants may also be described by noting which articulators are used to produce the sound. Typically, the place of articulation is the location along the vocal tract where the air stream constriction occurs. *Bilabials* /p, b, m, w/ are produced by the two lips coming together with some lip rounding. *Labiodentals* /f, v/ are created by the lower edge of the upper incisors coming into contact with the upper edge of the lower lip, thereby creating a slight constriction in the airflow. *Interdentals* / θ, ð/ are formed when the tongue tip protrudes slightly and touches the edges of the upper incisors, creating a slight constriction over the tongue tip.

Alveolars /t, d, s, z, l, n/ involve constriction created by the tongue tip coming into contact with the alveolar ridge. Interestingly, alveolars are the sounds most frequently produced (50%) in American English, with /t/ being the most commonly occurring of all sounds. *Palatals* /ʃ, ʒ, ʧ, ʤ, r, j/ are formed when some part of the tongue comes into contact with the hard palate. The *velars* /k, g/ are made by elevating the back of the tongue to the soft palate. The *glottal* /h/ is created by the air stream going through a partial opening of the vocal folds.

Besides describing the place and manner by which the sound is formed, consonants may also be designated as voiced or voiceless. This characteristic is based on the movement of vocal folds. If the vocal folds are vibrating during a sound production, the resulting sound is *voiced.* Voiced sounds include /b, d, g, ð, z, v, ʒ, ʤ, m, n, r, l, r, w, j/. When the vocal folds are not vibrating during production, the sound is said to be *voiceless* (i.e., /p, t, k, θ, s, f, θ, ʃ, ʧ, h/). Sounds in the English language that vary only in terms of voicing are referred to as *cognates* (e.g., /p, b/).

Vowels and diphthongs are the other groups of sounds in the English language. There are 12 vowels and three phonemic diphthongs in mainstream American English. During their production, the tongue typically does not come in contact with any of the other articulators. Vowels are always voiced and typically are not nasalized. Additionally, they are created with a relatively open vocal tract and have no point of constriction. Thus, vowels are sonorants—without constriction. Vowels can be described by identifying where the tongue is in relation to the palate using the terms *high, mid,* or *low.* They are also described by whether the tongue is near the front, middle (central), or back of the mouth. Finally, vowels may be distinguished as either lax or tense. *Lax* vowels are shorter in duration, indicating they are produced with less muscle effort. *Tense* (long) vowels have a longer duration and require more effort to produce.

Diphthongs are formed when two vowels are blended together, creating a change in the vocal tract (e.g., /ɔɪ/). Although a diphthong incorporates two vowels, it is only one phoneme.

All syllables must have a vowel, diphthong, or a vocalic/syllabic consonant to form the nucleus.

Vowels are sometimes referred to as *syllabics* because they are necessary for syllable formation. Typically, a consonant combines with a vowel to make a syllable. When a syllable ends with a vowel (e.g., CV), it is an *open syllable*. If the syllable ends with a consonant (e.g., VC, CVC), it is a *closed syllable*.

▶ Speech Sound System Development

To determine the age of acquisition of the sounds of language, researchers use two different methodologies. In a *cross-sectional* study, which is the type of investigation often carried out by SLPs, children of different ages are tested on their abilities to produce speech sounds at a given point in time. *Longitudinal* studies involve testing children's productions over a period of time. Comparing the results of the various studies can be difficult because various levels of mastery and means of eliciting responses have been used by different researchers. In some studies, a child needed to produce a sound correctly 100% of the time in order to consider that the child had mastered it; in others, the criterion was 75%. Studies varied in children's responses from spontaneous production to direct imitation of the examiner. To further complicate the situation, some investigators required the

mastery level to be met in all three positions, whereas others were concerned only with the initial and final positions.

Despite the variability in criteria, SLPs have reached some general agreement about the progression in which individual sounds are acquired (see **FIGURE 9-1**). Nasals /m, n, ŋ)/, stops /p, b, t, d, k, g/, and glides /w, j/ are acquired earliest, followed by the fricatives /f, v, θ, ð, s, z, ʃ, ʒ, h/, affricates /ʧ, ʤ/, and then the liquids /l, r/ (Sander, 1972). Sander's (1972) analysis of previous studies also noted that /θ, ð, ʒ / were generally the latest phonemes children acquired.

▶ Acquisition

Prelinguistic Stages

The *prelinguistic* stage includes the time before the child's first true word. The early skills demonstrated in this stage—speech perception, infant speech production, and the transition from babbling to meaningful speech—lay the foundation for phonological development (Kelman, 2010).

Speech perception involves the identification of phonemes—that is, the vowels and consonants of language—largely from acoustic cues and the recognition of phonemes in combination as a word (Nicolosi et al., 1996). Being able to perceive the differences in

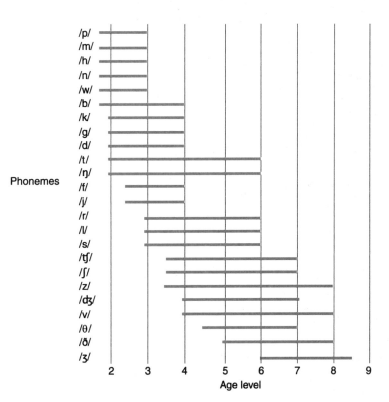

FIGURE 9-1 Ages at which phonemes typically are acquired.

Sander, E. (1972). When are speech sounds learned? *Journal of Speech and Hearing Disorders, 37*(1), 55–63.

speech sounds is critical to comprehending and developing language and is also an essential precursor to speech production. Speech scientists have hypothesized that babies come "prewired" to perceive minimal differences in speech sounds (Kelman, 2010). This ability occurs across languages. To acquire a given language, children's brains must differentiate their particular language from that of others. The sounds a child hears frequently become strengthened and are established as the basis for the individual's language (Cheour et al., 1998).

At birth, infants cry and soon make a variety of vocalizations that eventually become strings of consonant-vowel syllables. These vocalizations, which eventually resemble adultlike timing and intonation patterns, fall into two general categories: reflexive and nonreflexive vocalizations. *Reflexive vocalizations* include cries, coughs, and hiccups. *Nonreflexive vocalizations* are the sounds that will eventually be shaped into the adult form of words (Oller, 1980).

Oller's work serves as the basis for understanding prelinguistic stages of vocalizations. He found that regardless of the linguistic community in which they reside, all infants go through the same stages of vocal development. Although a certain time frame is identified for each stage in the following sections, it should be noted that these stages are not definitive; rather, they tend to overlap and be fluid.

Stage 1: Phonation Stage (Birth to 1 Month)

During the phonation stage, the infant exhibits reflexive vocalizations such as crying, fussing, coughing, burping, and sneezing. These sounds are similar to syllabic nasals and vowels.

Stage 2: Coo and Goo Stage (2–3 Months)

In the coo and goo stage, the productions are acoustically similar to back vowels or to syllables consisting of back vowels and consonants. They are considered primitive because of the immature timing of the vocalizations, and they are the precursors to consonants.

Stage 3: Exploration and Expansion Stage (4–6 Months)

The exploration and expansion stage is one of vocal plays in which the child's productions range from repetitions of vowel-like elements to squeals, growls, yells, "raspberries," and friction noises. The infant begins to produce some sequences of CV syllables in which the vowels have better oral resonance, are more adultlike, and are considered marginal babbling.

Stage 4: Canonical Babbling Stage (7–9 Months)

In *canonical babbling*, which includes *reduplicated babbling* (e.g., /bababa/ or /dududu/) and variegated babbling (e.g., /dubamə/), the child's vocalizations become longer and consist of CV syllables whose timing closely approximates adult speech. It is not uncommon during this stage to hear the infant say [mama], although there is no sound-to-meaning relationship. At this time, the infant commonly uses stops, nasals, and glides, as well as lax vowels (e.g., /ə, æ/).

Stage 5: Jargon Stage (10–12 Months)

In the jargon stage, a greater variety of consonants and vowels is used. At this point, the child's utterances take on sentence-like intonation patterns, especially as the child approaches the first birthday. The consonant and vowel inventories increase dramatically during this stage.

Later Stages

As children approach their first birthday, they begin the transition from babbling to meaningful speech, referred to as the *first word stage*. The first word appears around the age of 12 months. By age 15 months, the child typically has a 15-word vocabulary. During this time, the child produces whole units rather than sequences of sounds. The first word stage continues until approximately 18 months. During this phase of development, the child has a rapidly increasing vocabulary and is developing a systematic relationship between the adult model and the child's pronunciation (Stoel-Gammon & Dunn, 1985).

It is also at this time that a child will use *protowords*, which are well-defined, meaningful sound patterns produced by young children that apparently are not modeled on any adult words (Nicolosi et al., 1996). Protowords are not considered to be the first "true" words but rather tend to be simple CV shapes that are not necessarily related phonetically to the adult form. An example is a child who says [mi] for their favorite blanket. Yet [mi] does not have any phonemic characteristics of the adult word, *blanket*. Protowords are the link between babbling and adultlike speech.

During the next stage of phonemic development, from 18 months to 4 years, the child's vocabulary of true words increases rapidly from approximately 50 words around 18 months to approximately 1,000 words by 36 months (Fenson et al., 1991). It is at this time that syllabic structures become more complex, with consonant clusters and multisyllabic productions beginning to appear.

Porter and Hodson (2001) noted various steps of phonological acquisition that serve as a guide during this time. During the first period, at approximately 12 months of age, the child does canonical babbling and uses vocables. By 18 months, the typically developing child has recognizable words, produces CV structures, and produces stops, nasals, and glides. By age 2 years, the child uses final consonants, communicates with words, and has "syllableness." The 3-year-old's speech involves an expansion of the child's phonemic repertoire, including /s/ clusters (although distortions are common) and anterior-posterior contrasts. By age 4, omissions are rare, most simplifications (e.g., stopping, fronting) are suppressed, and the child's speech sounds are "adultlike." The child's phonemic inventory typically stabilizes between 5 and 6 years of age. Liquids become consistent, with /l/ typically appearing by age 5 years and /r/ by 6 years. By 7 years of age, most children produce sibilants without lisps and are able to produce the "th" sounds unless there is a dialect factor. The child is considered to have "adult standard" speech before 8 years of age (Creaghead, Newman, & Secord, 1989).

Of importance during the stabilization process is the fact that at approximately 5 years of age, the child is introduced to two important skills: reading and writing. Development of these skills helps provide an extension of the understanding of the phonemic nature of the sound system and can add another modality for enhancing the child's phonemic repertoire.

▶ Phonological Deviations

Speech sounds can also be discussed in terms of phonological patterns, which are accepted groupings of sounds within an oral language (Hodson, 2010, 2011). Speech pattern errors have been referred to as *phonological processes* (Ingram, 1976) or *deviations* (Hodson, 2004, 2010). According to Grunwell (1982), the concept of phonological "processes" in the clinical assessment of a child's speech is applied primarily as a descriptive device that identifies or analyzes systematic patterns in a child's pronunciations by comparing it with the targeted adult model. Phonological deviations can be viewed in terms of omissions, major substitutions, major assimilations, and syllable-structure/context-related changes (Hodson, 2004, 2010).

Omissions

Omissions at the syllable level include simplification of the word to one syllable (e.g., *rabbit* → [ræ]). With weak syllable deletion, an unstressed syllable is omitted (e.g., *banana* → [nænə]). "Multisyllabicity" problems involve difficulty producing all the syllables and sounds in a multisyllabic word (e.g., *ambulance* → [æmsən]).

Singleton consonant omissions can occur at the end of a word or postvocalic (e.g., *bat* → [bæ]), in the middle of a word or intervocalic (e.g., *happy* → [hæ i]), or at the beginning of a word or prevocalic (e.g., *pot* → [ɑt]). Prevocalic singleton omissions are not common in children who speak English. By contrast, final consonant omissions are common in children with disordered phonological systems.

Omissions are frequently observed in consonant clusters/sequences. A *consonant sequence* consists of all contiguous consonants in a word (e.g., [θbr] as in *toothbrush*), whereas a *consonant cluster* comprises adjacent consonants in the same syllable (e.g., [br] as in *toothbrush*). Consonant cluster reduction indicates that one (or more) consonant(s) is omitted in a syllable (e.g., *spoon* → [pun]). Consonant cluster deletion would denote the omission of all consonants in the cluster, (e.g., *tree* → [i]). Consonant cluster reductions, which are common in the speech of highly unintelligible children, often influence children's morphologies.

Substitutions

In *fronting,* a sound made at the back of the mouth is substituted by a sound produced in the front. For example, the word *cup* would become [tʌp]. Anterior consonants include /p, b, m, w, t, d, s, z, n, l, f, v, θ, ð/, and posterior consonants are /k, g, r, h/.

Backing is the reverse of fronting. In backing, an anterior sound (i.e., made at the front of the mouth) is replaced by a back or posterior sound (i.e., made at the back of the mouth). Thus, the word *tie* becomes [kaɪ]. It should be noted that this not a common deviation.

Stopping refers to the use of a stop /p, b, t, d, k, g/ for a "nonstop" consonant, such as a glide, fricative, liquid, or nasal. An example is *sun* being said as [tʌn].

Gliding is another substitution pattern where the /w/ or /j/ is used for another consonant, typically a liquid. For example, *light* becomes [jaɪt].

Vowelization is the substitution of a pure vowel for a vocalic liquid. An example would be *paper* → [pepo].

In *palatalization* and *depalatiziation,* the palatal feature is added or omitted, respectively. This pattern typically occurs with sibilants. If the child says [sip] for the word *sheep*, the sibilant was depalatalized. If the child says [ʃi] for *see,* the sibilant is palatalized.

Affrication and *deaffrication* refer to addition or loss of the combination of a stop and fricative, respectively. If *chair* → [tɛə] or [ʃɛə], deaffrication has occurred. If *she* → [ʧ], affrication occurred.

Major Assimilations

Assimilation involves a sound in a word taking on a characteristic of another sound in the same word. This change can occur even if the sound that caused the change is omitted. Although labial assimilation is common in young children, children with expressive phonological impairments tend to use it excessively (Hodson, 2010). An example of labial assimilation would be *soap* → [pop] or [po]. Velar assimilation is also common; it occurs when a sound in a word containing a velar is replaced with a velar, such as *doggie* → [gɔgi]. Alveolar assimilation happens when an alveolar is used for a nonalveolar because of another alveolar in the word; for example, the word *fight* would be [taɪt].

Glottal Stop Replacement

Glottal stops are used by some children to "mark" the final consonant in a word until the sounds are developed. Children with repaired cleft palates and other structural anomalies often use glottal stops.

Syllable-Structure/Context-Related Changes

Metathesis occurs when two sounds or syllables in a word change places (e.g., *ask* → [æks]). In *migration*, only one sound moves within the word (e.g., *snake* → [neks]). *Coalescence* occurs when two sounds in a word are replaced by a single sound, which has the features of the two replaced sounds but is neither of the original sounds. An example is *spoon* → [fun]: the /f/ has the stridency of /s/ and the labial component of /p/. *Reduplication* is the repetition of phonemes or syllables that young children demonstrate as a typical part of developing language (e.g., *bottle* → [baba]). *Epenthesis* is the insertion of a sound. The most common form of epenthesis is the addition of /ə/ between two consonants in a cluster, such as *black* → /[balæk]. The *diminutive* in English involves the addition of /i/ at the end of words (e.g., *pig* → [pɪgi]).

▶ Suppression of Phonological Processes

Stoel-Gammon and Dunn's report (1985) now serves as a classic reference for suppression of phonological processes. As noted in **TABLE 9-2**, these processes are divided into those that typically disappear by the age of 3 years and those that commonly persist past 3 years of age.

TABLE 9-2 Age of Suppression of Phonological Processes

Processes that Disappear by 3 Years of Age	Processes that Persist After 3 Years of Age
Unstressed syllable deletion	Cluster reduction
Final consonant deletion	Epenthesis
Doubling	Gliding
Diminutization	Vocalization/ Vowelization
Velar fronting	Stopping
Consonant assimilation	Depalatalization
Prevocalic voicing	Final devoicing
Reduplication	

Source: Stoel-Gammon, C., & Dunn, C. (1985). Normal and disordered phonology in children. Austin, TX: Pro-Ed.

TABLE 9-3 Age of Acquisition of Phonological Patterns/Phonemes

Phonological Pattern	Age in Years
All consonant categories except liquids; "syllableness" and singleton consonants (syllable/word structures)	3
Consonant clusters/sequences (two or more contiguous consonants without omissions)	4
Liquid /l/	5
Liquid /r/	6

Source: Data from Porter, J. H., & Hodson, B. W. (2001). Collaborating to obtain phonological acquisition data for local schools. Language, Speech, and Hearing Services in Schools, 32(3), 165–171.

Porter and Hodson (2001) evaluated phonological patterns and phonemes used by children ages 3–6 years. The study results in **TABLE 9-3** indicate the age of acquisition for phonological pattern/phonemes.

▸ Phonological Awareness

Phonological awareness—a term that began to appear in the literature in the 1970s—refers to the child's knowledge that words are made up of smaller, discernable units (Gillon, 2004). The development of this skill indicates that a person has an awareness of the sound structure, or phonological structure, of spoken words independent of their meaning. Research has indicated that there is a strong link between literacy and phonological awareness (Gillon, 2004). The understanding of a word's sound structure enables a child to sound out, or decode, a word in print. Phonological awareness may also be referred to as *metaphonological awareness* because it is one aspect of the broader category of metalinguistics (Hodson, 2010). *Metalinguistic knowledge* refers to the child's ability to reflect on and discuss aspects of language separate from its meaning.

Phonological awareness can be separated into syllable awareness, onset-rime awareness, and phoneme awareness. *Syllable awareness* requires knowledge that a word can be divided into large parts (i.e., syllables). Five tasks are included in this area:

1. *Syllable segmentation* is the ability to tell how many syllables are in a word (e.g., *elephant* has three syllables/parts).
2. *Syllable completion* is the ability to complete a word when one or more parts are provided (e.g., Show the child a picture of a *computer* and ask the child to finish the word when you say, "Finish this word, *compu____*.")
3. *Syllable matching* is the ability to discern which syllables are the same in two similar words. An example is asking the child to tell which part of *telephone* and *telegraph* is the same.
4. *Syllable/word manipulation* includes: (1) substitution—for example, substitute *foot* for *base* in *baseball* to yield *football*; (2) deletion—for example, *baseball* without *base* would be *ball*; and (3) transposition—for example, reversing the syllables in *ballbase* yields *baseball*.
5. *Syllable/word blending* pertains to putting two or more syllables together to make a word. Words that yield compound words are generally easier than meaningless syllables (e.g., *base* plus *ball* yields *baseball*).

Another level of phonological awareness pertains to *onset-rime*. This level of phonological awareness is typically tested through rhyming tasks. This skill indicates the child knows that words share a common/same ending (rime) and understands that the beginning sound or sounds of the word are what differentiate them. The rime is the part of the word from the vowel to the end. The onset includes the consonant(s) before the vowel (e.g., *st* in *stun*). Alliteration involves only the beginning consonant (e.g., *s* in *stun*). Three tasks of onset-rime awareness follow:

1. *Judgment*: The ability to tell whether two words rhyme (e.g., "Do *ball* and *call* rhyme?").
2. *Oddity*: The ability to tell which word does not rhyme, given a set of words (e.g., "Which word does not rhyme—*car, ball*, or *far*?").
3. *Rhyme generation/supply*: The ability to provide a word or a number of words that rhyme when a word is presented.

A third level is that of *phonemic awareness*. At this level, the child is able to break a word down into its smallest parts, the individual phonemes or sounds. Tasks at this level include these:

- *Alliteration*, also referred to as phoneme detection, is tested by asking the child to tell which words have a different sound at the beginning (initial alliteration).
- *Phoneme matching* asks the child to indicate which words have the same sound at the beginning when given a set of words. An example is, "Which words begin with the same sound as *bat—ball, horn*, or *bone*?"
- *Phoneme isolation* is being able to tell which sound is heard in a specific position within a word (e.g., "What sound do you hear at the beginning of *cat*?").
- *Phoneme completion* is the ability to provide a missing sound (e.g., "Finish the word '*gla___*.'").
- *Phoneme blending* is a skill in which the child puts sounds given separately together to form a word (e.g., the child blends /k æ n/ to *can*).
- *Phoneme segmentation* is the ability to tell how many sounds are in a word (e.g., *neck* has three sounds: /n, ɛ, k/).
- *Phoneme deletion* is the ability to remove a specified sound from a word (e.g., "Say *boat*. Now say it without /t/.").
- *Phoneme reversal* refers to changing positions of sounds in words (e.g., /ti/ becomes /it/).
- *Phoneme substitution* implies changing a sound within a word (e.g., "Say *hop*. Now change the /*a*/ to /ɪ/." [*hip*]).
- *Spoonerisms* involve changing the first sound in two words (e.g., "*top man*" becomes "*mop tan*").

Phonological awareness skills are influenced by many factors, including vocabulary development, early language experiences, and the child's native language (Gillon, 2004). Research has shown that the size of a child's vocabulary is positively correlated with phonological awareness tasks, including onset-rime and phoneme-level skills. In addition, early language experiences appear to influence phonological awareness skills in children. Studies examining differences in these skills in children from different socioeconomic groups have found that children from middle-income families perform better on phonological awareness tasks than children from low-socioeconomic homes (Lonigan, Burgess, Anthony, & Barker, 1998).

Researchers also have noted the importance of exposure to alphabetic knowledge and print referencing activities (Justice & Ezell, 2004). Both of these activities have been shown to help children understand the sound structure of words. Native languages that are alphabetic, such as English, Spanish, and French, support the progression of the skills outlined by Gillon (2004). Research involving children whose first language is Cantonese or Japanese indicates phonological awareness skills are poorer in these children because they have not had exposure to alphabetic scripts (Cheung, Chen, Lai, Wong, & Hills, 2001; Holm & Dodd, 1996). School-age children with moderate-to-severe expressive phonological impairment typically perform poorly on phonological awareness tasks (Bird, Bishop, & Freeman, 1995; Hodson, 2004; Webster & Plante, 1992). Justice and Schuele (2004) provided three tentative conclusions based on current studies, while noting that further study is needed in this area:

1. Children with expressive phonological impairment are more likely to have difficulty with phonological awareness tasks and literacy skills.
2. Children with expressive phonological impairment who also have receptive and/or expressive language difficulties are at greater risk than children with only phonological impairment.
3. Some children with phonological impairment may have problems acquiring phonemic awareness, but they may not show obvious signs of difficulty in the early stages. As the academic demands placed on these children increase, however, their phonological awareness problems become apparent.

ASHA issued a document outlining the roles and responsibilities of SLPs with respect to reading and writing. It noted that "as many as half of all poor readers have an early history of spoken-language disorders" (ASHA, 2001). Many of these children are part of the caseloads of SLPs who work in schools. Thus, the SLP needs to make a focused effort to promote literacy skills for these children to help them succeed in school. Moreover, working on both expressive phonology and phonological awareness should improve both areas (Carson, Gillon, & Boustead, 2013).

▶ Evaluation of Children with Speech Sound Disorders

Major Etiological Factors

The acquisition of speech is affected by factors that relate to the structure and function of the speech mechanism as well as other variables. Effects on speech sound productions may vary considerably. In addition, many variables often overlap.

Hearing

Adequate hearing is needed so that children are aware of the speech and language being used in their homes and surroundings. A hearing loss can affect the child's ability to hear, which in turn may affect the acquisition of speech. Additionally, hearing is needed so that the children can monitor their speech as it is developing. Of children with disabilities (ages 6–21) served in the schools, approximately 1.2% receive services for a hearing loss (ASHA, 2008).

The age of onset of a loss affects both speech and language acquisition. Children with severe/profound hearing losses since birth have a difficult time acquiring speech and language. If the hearing loss occurs later, the child may maintain some skills learned up to that point, but these skills typically deteriorate over time. Better language development is associated with early identification of hearing loss and early intervention (Yoshinaga-Itano, Sedey, Coulter, & Mehl, 1998).

Hearing loss and its effects on speech can be evaluated by noting the degree of loss. Individuals who are "hard of hearing" have some residual hearing, which may assist them with speech and language acquisition. The less severe the loss, the less impact it typically has on speech and language.

Additionally, the type of loss will be accompanied by differing problems. A sensorineural loss involves a pathology of the inner ear or neural pathways. This type of loss may be helped by the use of a hearing aid; alternatively, the individual may be a candidate for a cochlear implant. A conductive loss, which occurs in the outer or middle ear, usually can be treated medically.

The prevalence of mild, moderate, or severe unilateral hearing loss (UHL) in the "worse" ear and "normal" hearing in the better ear was estimated at 4.9% and 5.7% in children 6–19 years of age in 1976 and 1994, respectively (National Institute on Deafness and Other Communication Disorders [NIDCD], 2006). Speech is audible for children with UHL, but it may not always be understandable, depending on the listening environment (Oyler & McKay, 2008).

A common cause of conductive loss is otitis media—that is, infection/inflammation with an accumulation of fluid in the middle ear. Studies indicate that among children who have had an episode of acute otitis media, as many as 45% have persistent fluid after 1 month (Thrasher & Gregory, 2005). Approximately 5% of children between the ages of 2 and 4 years have hearing loss due to middle ear effusion that lasts 3 months or longer. The prevalence of otitis media with effusion is highest in those age 2 years or younger, but sharply declines markedly in children older than 6 years (Thrasher, 2007).

Oral Mechanism

Individuals can also have anomalies of the structures used for speech production, such as the lips, teeth, tongue, and palate. These abnormalities can vary from slight to considerable; likewise, their impact on speech sound acquisition can range from negligible to severe. For this reason, it is important that SLPs examine the structure and function of the oral mechanism and evaluate the effects of any variation on speech production.

Personal Factors

Do gender, age, intelligence, socioeconomic levels, and birth order have some effect on speech sound acquisition? Statistics indicate that males are at higher risk of speech and language difficulties than females (Peña-Brookes & Hegde, 2015). Several studies have explored the age of acquisition of various phonemes. The ages identified vary across the studies, but all agree that by the age of 8 years, a child should have speech that is similar to an adult's. Therefore, children typically have fewer speech sound errors as they age.

Intelligence does not have a direct correlation to speech sound acquisition. That is, scores on articulation tests do not correlate with an individual's intelligence. When intelligence falls into the cognitively delayed range (e.g., intelligence quotient [IQ] <70), however, there does tend to be a correlation: the lower the IQ, the higher the prevalence and frequency of speech sound errors (Peña-Brooks & Hegde, 2015).

Currently, no data indicates that birth order has an effect on speech sound acquisition. The same is true in regard to socioeconomic status.

Ethnocultural Considerations

The 2010 U.S. Census indicated that 381 languages were spoken in the United States at that time (Ryan, 2011). Some of these languages are indigenous to the United States, whereas others are languages that immigrants used when they came to this country. Given this diversity, SLPs will most likely work with individuals whose English has been influenced by another language.

ASHA has published several technical reports and other documents that address cultural and linguistic diversity. Its social dialects position paper (ASHA, 1983) stated that "no dialectal variety of English is a disorder or a pathological form of speech or language."

The SLP needs to know about the child's background and consider cultural and linguistic issues during evaluations. As noted by Peña-Brooke and Hegde (2015), children may speak: (a) a language other than English, (b) English as a second language, (c) a dialectal variation of English (e.g., African American English), or (d) a different form of English (e.g., British English).

It is imperative that SLPs recognize that the use of standardized tests may not be appropriate for a given child, depending on the individuals on which the test was performed. Likewise, it is important that individuals who speak English as a second language or a variation of English are not misdiagnosed simply because of that fact. The SLP needs to know: (a) which language is used and what the phonological characteristics of the other/primary language are, (b) how the first language affects the learning of the second language, and (c) how to determine whether there is a speech sound disorder in the primary language, the second language, or both (Peña-Brooks & Hegde, 2015).

Assessment

To fully assess the child's language in its cultural context, Bernthal et al. (2013) suggested that the SLP should take the following steps:

1. Sample the speech of adults in the child's linguistic community.
2. Obtain information from interpreters/support personnel.
3. Become familiar with dialectal and language features of the child's linguistic community.

The monolingual SLP may need the assistance of a bilingual SLP in some cases. Given the diversity of the languages that can be encountered, however, it may be necessary to train an aide or interpreter. When that is not possible, the SLP will need to conduct the assessment using alternative strategies such as establishing an interdisciplinary team involving another professional (e.g., an educational diagnostician who is bilingual [ASHA, 1985]).

Evaluation is the process followed by the SLP to determine the presence or absence of a disorder. If a disorder is present, its characteristics are described and possible causes are explored. A screening can be done with a large number of children in a short period of time to determine whether a more in-depth evaluation is necessary.

If a formal evaluation is needed, it will typically include a case history, an oral peripheral exam, administration of a standardized test, evaluation of stimulability in differing contexts, and a hearing evaluation. The case history can be obtained by written and oral methods. The goal is to obtain information about the child as well as pertinent developmental, medical, familial, and social information that may affect the child's speech. Physical factors that should be considered include syndromes, sensory deficits, structural anomalies, and neurophysiological involvement (Hodson, 2010).

Tests

A standardized test of speech sounds should be administered as part of the evaluation. Most tests will assess the child's production of the various sounds in single-word productions. The test an SLP chooses should be based on several factors, including the amount of time it takes to administer the test, the stimulus materials, the difficulty of scoring, and the type of analysis. Testing results should aid the SLP in determining whether a disorder exists and, if so, in formulating treatment goals (Bernthal et al., 2013). Norm-referenced tests allow for comparison of

a child's score in terms of speech sound productions with scores of children who are the same age.

Many phoneme-oriented tests are used for this purpose (see **TABLE 9-4** for examples). These instruments are designed to evaluate how the child says a targeted sound in each position of a specified word. Typically, omissions, additions, substitutions, and distortions are noted on the form but not differentiated in the final score (Prezas & Hodson, 2007).

Other assessment instruments focus more on phonological processes/deviations (see **TABLE 9-5**). These tests examine the child's sound system in terms of possible phonological deficiencies in an attempt to determine patterns that need to be targeted. Individual sounds also are assessed with these instruments.

In addition to assessment via a standardized test, the child's speech should be examined by collecting a continuous conversational speech sample. The speech of a child who is highly unintelligible, however, may be difficult or impossible to analyze. If analysis of the sample is possible, it allows the SLP to study the child's speech in a natural way. Note, however, that a continuous conversational sample may have a restricted range of phonemes (Stoel-Gammon & Dunn, 1985).

Stimulability also should be addressed when conducting a comprehensive speech evaluation. This measure indicates the degree to which a misarticulated sound can be produced correctly by imitation (Nicolosi, Harryman, & Kresheck, 2006). To assess stimulability, the SLP typically provides a model first to see whether the child can imitate correctly, and then, if necessary, gives the child simple instructions for where to place the articulators. Additional assists (e.g., amplification) are added as needed. This procedure provides valuable information when making a prognostic statement about the treatment process.

Another part of the assessment should examine how intelligible the child is to the listener. When a child uses phonological deviations, speech intelligibility is

TABLE 9-4 Phoneme-Oriented Tests			
Test	**Author(s)**	**Publisher**	**Age Range (Years)**
Arizona Articulation Proficiency Scale, Third Edition	Fudala (2000)	Western Psychological Services	1:5–18:0
Goldman-Fristoe Test of Articulation, Third Edition	Goldman and Fristoe (2015)	American Guidance Service, Inc.	2–21
Photo Articulation Test, Third Edition	Lippke, Dickey, Selmar, and Soder (1997)	ProEd	3–8

TABLE 9-5 Tests that Assess Phonological Processes/Deviations

Test	Author(s)	Publisher	Age Range (Years)
Bankson-Bernthal Test of Phonology	Bankson and Bernthal (1990)	Harcourt Assessment, Inc.	3–9
Diagnostic Evaluation of Articulation and Phonology	Dodd, Hua, Crosbie, Holm, and Ozanne (2006)	Pearson Assessment	3–8:11
Hodson Assessment of Phonological Patterns, Third Edition	Hodson (2004)	Pro-Ed	3:0–8:0
Khan-Lewis Phonological Analysis, Third Edition	Khan and Lewis (2015)	Pearson Assessment	2–21

usually reduced. Various studies have been done over the years to assess what level of intelligibility a child should have at various ages. Peña-Brooks and Hegde (2015) note that intelligibility will vary from child to child, but suggest that a 19- to 24-month-old child should be 25–50% intelligible, a child 2–3 years of age should be 50–75% intelligible, a 3- to 4-year-old should be 75–90% intelligible, and a child 5 years or older should be 90–100% intelligible. Of course, children older than age 5 years may still evidence some speech sound errors, but these typically do not affect the listener's ability to understand the child.

Hearing

Another area that is assessed is the hearing of the child. An SLP can, for example, screen the hearing of a child to determine whether the child needs to be referred to an audiologist for a complete hearing evaluation (ASHA, 2007).

Oral Mechanism

The various structures of the oral mechanism and their functions should be assessed. Typically, the SLP views the size and symmetry of the oral mechanism as well as the movements of the lips, tongue, and velum. "[O]nly gross abnormalities interfere with speech production" due to the flexibility and adaptability of the speech mechanism (Bleile, 2002).

Reporting

After all assessment is completed, the SLP writes an evaluation report. Often, the information contained in this report is explained orally to the client's parent(s) as well. This report becomes the official documentation of the evaluation results and recommendations. It should summarize pertinent case history information, hearing screening results, oral mechanism examination findings, test results, and recommendations.

▸ Intervention

Phoneme-Oriented Approaches

Treatment of children with speech sound disorders can be approached in many different ways. Some approaches emphasize articulatory placement and motor or movement components, such as phonetic placement, motokinesthetic, or sensory-motor. Perhaps the most commonly used approach in this area is Van Riper's "stimulus" approach, which is often referred to as the "traditional" approach. Charles Van Riper (1939) brought together principles from various techniques and published his approach in 1939, with revisions following in later editions of his textbook, *Speech Correction: Principles and Methods* (Bernthal et al., 2013). Van Riper advocated for an approach that used placement techniques combined with sensory-perceptual training. The stimulus approach proceeds through five stages: (1) auditory training, (2) elicitation of the sound, (3) stabilization of the sound, (4) carry-over, and (5) maintenance. As Bernthal et al. (2013) noted, this approach has "withstood the test of time."

Contextual testing should be included as a part of the treatment process. Such an evaluation assesses the context, and its results may help the child produce the misarticulated sound. For example, certain vowels that follow the targeted sound make it easier for the child to produce the consonant; the vowels /i, ɪ, e/ after an /r/, for instance, may make it easier for the child to produce the consonant correctly. The information yielded from this kind of contextual analysis allows the SLP to make decisions about the consistency of errors and to decide which sounds should be targeted first. This information can be used as a starting point for treatment or in combination with other techniques (Secord et al., 2007).

Linguistic-Based Approaches

Linguistic-based approaches recognize phonology as a component of the child's language system (Edwards, 2010; Hodson, 2010; Hodson & Paden, 1983, 1991; Stoel-Gammon & Dunn, 1985). Although these methods improve the child's speech sounds, intelligibility is increased by helping reorganize the child's phonological system. At the same time, the processing of phonological information is enhanced (Grunwell, 1985; Strattman, 2010). Through these approaches, an awareness of patterns is developed.

The *cycles phonological remediation approach* was developed for use with children who have highly unintelligible speech. A *cycle* refers to the period of time required for the child to successfully focus on deficient patterns (Hodson & Paden, 1991). The length of the cycle depends on the number of patterns that need to be targeted and the number of phonemes that are stimulable within the pattern. Each phoneme or consonant cluster is targeted for approximately 60 minutes. Most patterns need to be recycled one or more times.

Hodson and Paden (1991) based this approach on seven principles, some of which reflect the natural acquisition of a child's sound system. The first principle notes that phonological acquisition is a gradual process (Ingram, 1976). With the cycles approach, the child is given quick but limited exposure to a target, and the SLP typically recycles the pattern during the second cycle and sometimes the third. This approach allows the child to internalize, sort, experiment with, and do self-rehearsal as a typically developing child does. Thus the concept of a cycle is used.

The second principle notes that children with normal hearing typically acquire the adult sound system primarily by listening (Van Riper, 1939). Most children with adequate hearing develop their speech sounds/patterns without any special assistance.

The third principle notes that as children gain new speech patterns, they associate kinesthetic with auditory sensations that help with later self-monitoring (Fairbanks, 1954). These two modalities—kinesthetic and auditory—need to be "synchronized" if the child is to develop self-monitoring.

The fourth cycles approach principle states that phonetic environment can facilitate or inhibit correct sound production (Buteau & Hodson, 1989; Kent, 1982). In other words, it is easier to produce some sounds in certain words than in others. As a part of the clinical process, words are initially chosen with facilitative phonetic environments.

Children need to be actively involved in their phonological acquisition, as indicated in the fifth principle. Children with disordered phonological systems need to be active (rather than passive) participants in their treatment.

The sixth principle states that children tend to generalize new speech production skills to other targets (McReynolds & Bennett, 1972). This principle implies that not all sounds in a pattern need to be targeted; rather, a few sounds can be taught, with time then allowed for their generalization.

The seventh principle explains the need for an optimal match to facilitate the child's learning (Hunt, 1961). With this approach, the SLP finds the child's current functioning level and then begins work one step above that level. Complexity is increased gradually so that the child is challenged yet experiences success and gains satisfaction (Hunt, 1961).

An eighth principle regarding enhancing metaphonological awareness has been added in recent years to help children who are at risk of literacy difficulties. Children with highly unintelligible speech often have major delays in the area of literacy.

Using these principles, the SLP can work on the speech of highly unintelligible children using the Cycles Phonological Remediation Approach. Through this process, the child's sound system is reorganized. The child learns new rules to use in producing the sounds of the words of their language.

The primary strength of the cycles approach is its efficiency (Hodson, 1982, 1997, 2004, 2010; Hodson & Paden, 1991). Indeed, many preschoolers require less than a year of this type of phonological intervention to become intelligible. Typically, three to four cycles (30–40 hours of SLP contact time) are required for the child to become intelligible via the cycles approach (Hodson, 2010).

To decide which patterns should be targeted, the *Hodson Assessment of Phonological Patterns, Third Edition* (HAPP-3; Hodson, 2004) is administered. Patterns identified as deficient through this tool's results then become possible targets. Early-developing patterns are often first targets and include "syllableness" and singleton consonants (for omissions), followed by /s/ clusters, posterior-anterior contrasts, and liquids (Hodson, Scherz, & Strattman, 2002).

Syllableness is a first target when deficient because most young children are readily able to sequence at least two syllables. When this area is targeted, the emphasis is on the appropriate number of syllables rather than the specific consonants. This pattern is particularly important for language because it has a direct relationship with increasing length of utterances. When children use syllableness, they can put words together.

Improved production of /s/ clusters can have a beneficial impact on morphology. Examples include plurals (e.g., *hats*), third-person present verb tense (e.g., *eats*), and possessives (e.g., the *cat's*).

An intervention session using the cycles approach uses an easy-to-follow structure. Each session begins with a period of auditory stimulation, using slight amplification, in which the SLP reads a list of words that contains the day's target. Next, approximately five picture cards are provided with the child's target. With this treatment, words (rather than nonsense syllables) are always used. During the first cycles, monosyllabic words with facilitative phonetic environments are selected (Hodson, 2010). Semantic considerations during this stage may also include the use of verbs, such as *spin* for /s/ clusters. Actual objects are also used with preschoolers. In later cycles, minimal pairs are often incorporated to ensure the child understands the semantic differences between the error and the target productions (Hodson, 2010).

Experiential-play and production-practice activities follow the listening activities, with these exercises incorporating the child's picture cards into the session's activity. This part of the session allows the child to practice the targeted pattern during a play-based task. The next step is to check stimulability for the next session's target patterns/phonemes. This testing is followed by a brief metaphonological activity (e.g., rhyme). The session ends with a repeat of the listening activity.

Daily home practice is also a component of the cycles approach. Both the reading list and the picture cards used that day are sent home for practice (approximately 2 minutes per day).

A metaphonological activity is incorporated because research has indicated that children with disordered expressive phonological systems have greater difficulty completing phonological awareness tasks than their typically developing peers. Metaphonological deficiencies tend to hinder development of adequate decoding and spelling skills.

Focused Auditory Input/Stimulation

For children who are functioning below the age of 3 years, *focused stimulation* serves to lay the foundation for acquiring language aspects. According to Weismer and Robertson (2006), through this intervention, "the child is provided with concentrated exposures of specific linguistic forms/functions/uses within naturalistic communicative contexts" (p. 175). Focused stimulation differs from general stimulation in that specific patterns are targeted during each session.

For example, a common goal is helping a child become aware of and eventually produce word endings. During the first session for this goal, the final /p/ is often targeted, with the room being filled with objects and activities for final /p/ (e.g., *up, hop, top, jump, mop, cup*). The SLP demonstrates /p/ and models the words (with a slight emphasis on the /p/) during parallel play but does not at this time ask the child to imitate. After a few months of focused auditory stimulation, the child is normally ready for production-practice activities for target patterns (Hodson, 2010).

▶ Case Studies

When assessing the speech sound system of young children, required information includes the phonemic inventory, including both consonants and vowels, syllable shapes, and intelligibility. It also is important to identify each child's common phonological deviations and their phonemic inventory.

One of the best ways to assess these parameters is to have the parent and the child play together. This natural interaction typically elicits speech from the child. During the playtime, the parent can gloss the child's utterances; that is, the parent can restate what the child said to aid in identification of words.

🔍 CASE STUDY: JOHNATHON (TD)

The case study of Johnathon, 25 months of age, indicates that he is at least 60% intelligible; has a solid phonemic inventory, including stops, nasals, and glides; and shows varied syllable shapes. Although some phonological deviations are being used, they are developmentally appropriate. The recommendation for the mother to return to the clinic if she has further concerns is appropriate.

🔍 *CASE STUDY: JOSEPHINE (LB)*

The second case study, involving 22-month-old Josephine, indicates that she has a restricted consonant and vowel inventory. Josephine does use a good variety of syllable shapes with limited reduplicated babbling. Her intelligibility was judged to be 50%. If possible, the SLP also will record notations about any phonological deviations that occurred. The 12-item-screening portion of the HAPP-3 could be administered to do this. If Josephine does not respond to the items spontaneously, modeling could be used, preferably incorporating delayed imitation. The screening portion of the HAPP-3 assesses early-developing patterns. The recommendation for the mother to enroll her child in an early intervention program is appropriate. Josephine's speech skills should be reevaluated in approximately 6 months to assess her progress.

🔍 *CASE STUDY: ROBERT (LT)*

Robert presents some interesting challenges. At 27 months of age, he appears to have global developmental delays. Notably, he appears to have a unilateral hearing loss. When evaluating a child for speech sound disorders, this type of deficiency may be a contributing factor. Robert's intelligibility level, which is less than 25%, is cause for concern. Moreover, he has a restricted consonant inventory. His syllable shapes are also limited.

It would be helpful to screen Robert for potential phonological deviations using the HAPP-3 preschool screening instrument. Modeling could be used, if needed, during the assessment. This screening information could provide a temporary baseline for deficient phonological patterns and assist in the selection of initial treatment goals. Enrolling Robert in speech and language intervention is recommended. Treatment should focus on developing both his speech and language, as this approach would allow for work to be done in both language and phonology. The use of a play-based focused stimulation approach incorporating words with patterns that are deficient and need to be targeted (e.g., syllableness, final consonants, /s/ clusters, velars, and liquids) would be appropriate. Robert's parents should be included in the treatment process and be given home assignments.

▶ Summary

Phonology, which is one of the five components of language, is important for morphology, syntax, and semantics. The process of acquiring speech sounds begins at birth, when the child expresses wants and needs through reflexive vocalizations, such as crying, burping, and coughing. From birth, the speech sounds are formed and improved. The sounds are acquired at different ages, with all sounds being a part of a typically developing child's phonemic inventory by 8 years of age. The sounds of our language can be differentiated by noting their place, manner, and voicing. Phonological patterns/deviations can also be used for classification.

A variety of factors may affect speech sound acquisition. In particular, hearing difficulties influence speech acquisition. Ethnocultural considerations must also be taken into account.

The assessment of children with possible speech sound disorders should include a standardized test that examines sounds and phonological patterns. A connected-speech sample should also be obtained and analyzed, if possible, to determine the percentage of intelligibility and to note the consistency with which errors occur. The oral mechanism and hearing should be evaluated. This information is then analyzed, and the results are summarized in a written report.

Treatment for children with speech sound disorders can take either a motor-based approach or a linguistic-based approach, or it may involve a combination of these strategies. Children whose speech is highly unintelligible are best treated with a phonological approach. The Cycles Phonological Remediation Approach is an effective means of working with children with disordered phonological systems.

Study Questions

- What are the six principal organs/subsystems of speech production? Discuss each part as well as the progression and flow of speech through it.

- Discuss the prelinguistic stages of speech development. Name the stage, define the age range at which each is expected to occur, and describe the expected characteristics of speech at each stage.

- Identify different phonological awareness tasks, giving an example of each skill addressed by the task.
- Phonemes are described by their place, manner, and voicing. List the 24 consonants and note the place, manner, and voicing for each.
- Phonological deviations can be designated by syllable/word structure omissions and consonant category deficiencies as well as substitutions and assimilations. Note patterns/deviations that would be classified by each of these descriptors.

- Discuss how hearing loss relates to speech sound acquisition.
- What is the purpose of an evaluation? Which steps are taken during an evaluation?
- Which factors would an SLP consider in selecting a test for evaluating speech sound productions?
- Briefly outline the structure of a session using the Cycles Phonological Remediation Approach for phonological remediation.

References

American Speech-Language-Hearing Association (ASHA). (1983). Social dialects and implications of the position on social dialects. *ASHA, 25*(9), 23–27.

American Speech-Language-Hearing Association (ASHA). (1985). *Clinical management of communicatively handicapped minority language populations* [position statement]. Retrieved from www.asha.org/policy.

American Speech-Language-Hearing Association (ASHA). (2001). *Roles and responsibilities of speech-language pathologists with respect to reading and writing in children and adolescents* (position statement, executive summary of guidelines, technical report). ASHA *Supplement, 21*, 17–27. Rockville, MD.

American Speech-Language-Hearing Association (ASHA). (2007). *Scope of practice in speech-language pathology* [position statement]. Retrieved from www.asha.org/policy.

American Speech-Language-Hearing Association (ASHA). (2008). Incidence and prevalence of communication disorders and hearing loss in children. Retrieved from www.asha.org/members/research/reports/children.

Bankson, N. W., & Bernthal, J. E. (1990). *Bankson-Bernthal test of phonology.* San Antonio, TX: Harcourt Assessment, Inc.

Bernthal, J., Bankson, N., & Flipsen, P. (2013). *Articulation and phonological disorders: Speech sound disorders in children* (7th ed.). Boston, MA: Pearson Education, Inc.

Bird, J., Bishop, D., & Freeman, N. (1995). Phonological awareness and literacy development in children with expressive phonological impairments. *Journal of Speech and Hearing Research, 38*, 446–462.

Bleile, K. (2002). Evaluating articulation and phonological disorders when the clock is running. *American Journal of Speech-Language Pathology, 11*(3), 243–249.

Buteau, C., & Hodson, B. (1989). *Phonological remediation targets: Words and primary pictures for highly unintelligible children.* Austin, TX: Pro-Ed.

Carson, K. L., Gillon, G. T., & Boustead, T. M. (2013). Classroom phonological awareness instruction and literacy outcomes in the first year of school. *Language, Speech, and Hearing Services in Schools, 44*(2), 147–160.

Cheour, M., Ceponiene, R., Lehtokoski, A., Luuk, A., Allik, J., Alho, K., & Näätänen R. (1998). Development of language-specific phoneme representations in the human brain. *Nature Neuroscience, 1*(5), 351–353.

Cheung, H., Chen, H. C., Lai, C. Y., Wong, O. C., & Hills, M. (2001). The development of phonological awareness: Effects of spoken language experience and orthography. *Cognition, 81*(3), 227–241.

Creaghead, N., Newman, P., & Secord, W. (1989). *Assessment and remediation of articulatory and phonological disorders* (2nd ed.). New York, NY: Macmillan.

Dodd, B., Hua, Z., Crosbie, S., Holm, A., & Ozanne, A. (2006). *Diagnostic evaluation of articulation and phonology.* Bloomington, MN: Pearson Assessment.

Edwards, M. L. (2010). Phonological theories. In B. W. Hodson (Ed.), *Evaluating and enhancing children's phonological systems* (pp. 145–170). Wichita, KS: PhonoComp Publishing.

Fairbanks, G. (1954). Systematic research in experimental phonetics: A theory of the speech mechanisms as a servosytem. *Journal of Speech and Hearing Disorders, 19*, 133–139.

Fenson, L., Dale, P., Reznick, J. S., Thal, D., Bates, E., Hartung, J. P., … Reilly, J. S. (1991). *Technical manual for MacArthur communicative development inventories.* San Diego, CA: San Diego State University Department of Psychology.

Fudala, J. B. (2000). *Arizona articulation proficiency scale* (3rd ed.). Los Angeles, CA: Western Psychological Services.

Gillon, G. (2004). *Phonological awareness: From research to practice.* New York, NY: Guilford Press.

Goldman, R., & Fristoe, M. (2015). *Goldman-Fristoe test of articulation* (3rd ed.). Circle Pines, MN: American Guidance Service, Inc.

Grunwell, P. (1982). *Clinical phonology.* Rockville, MD: Aspen.

Grunwell, P. (1985). *Phonological assessment of child speech.* Windsor, UK: NFER-Nelson.

Hodson, B. (1982). Remediation of speech patterns associated with low levels of phonological performance. In M. Crary (Ed.), *Phonological intervention: Concepts and procedures* (pp. 91–115). San Diego, CA: College-Hill.

Hodson, B. (1997). Disordered phonologies: What have we learned about assessment and treatment? In B. Hodson & M. Edwards (Eds.), *Perspectives in applied phonology* (pp. 197–224). Gaithersburg, MD: Aspen.

Hodson, B. (2004). *Hodson assessment of phonological patterns* (3rd ed.). Austin, TX: Pro-Ed.

Hodson, B. (2010). *Evaluating and enhancing children's phonological systems: Research and theory to practice.* Wichita, KS: PhonoComp Publishing.

Hodson, B. (2011). Enhancing phonological patterns of young children with highly unintelligible speech. *The ASHA Leader, 16*(4), 16–19.

Hodson, B., & Paden, E. (1983). *Targeting intelligible speech: A phonological approach to remediation.* Austin, TX: Pro-Ed.

Hodson, B., & Paden, E. (1991). *Targeting intelligible speech: A phonological approach to remediation* (2nd ed.). Austin, TX: Pro-Ed.

Hodson, B., Scherz, J., & Strattman, K. (2002). Evaluating communicative abilities of a highly unintelligible preschooler. *American Journal of Speech-Language Pathology, 11*, 236–242.

Holm, A., & Dodd, B. (1996). The effect of first written language on the acquisition of literacy. *Cognition, 59*(2), 119–147.

Hunt, J. (1961). *Intelligence and experience.* New York, NY: Ronald Press.

Ingram, D. (1976). *Phonological disability in children.* New York, NY: Elsevier.

Justice, L. M., & Ezell, H. K. (2004). Print referencing: An emergent literacy enhancement strategy and its clinical applications. *Language Speech and Hearing Services in Schools, 35*(2), 185–193.

Justice, L. M., & Schuele, C. M. (2004). Phonological awareness: Description, assessment, and intervention. In J. Bernthal & N. Bankson (Eds.), *Articulation and phonological disorders* (5th ed., pp. 376–403). Boston, MA: Allyn & Bacon.

Kelman, M. (2010). Acquisition of speech sounds and phonological patterns. In B. W. Hodson (Ed.), *Evaluating and enhancing children's phonological systems* (pp. 23–41). Wichita, KS; PhonoComp Publishing.

Kent, R. D. (1982). Contextual facilitation of correct sound production. *Language, Speech, and Hearing Services in Schools, 13,* 66–76.

Khan, L. M., & Lewis, N. P. (2015). *Khan-Lewis phonological analysis* (3rd ed.). Bloomington, MN: Pearson Assessment.

Lippke, B. A., Dickey, S. E., Selmar, J. W., & Soder, A. L. (1997). *Photo articulation test* (3rd ed.). Austin, TX: ProEd.

Lonigan, C., Burgess, S., Anthony, J. L., & Barker, T. A. (1998). Development of phonological sensitivity in 2- to 5-year-old children. *Journal of Educational Psychology, 90*(2), 294–311.

McReynolds, L. V., & Bennett, S. (1972). Distinctive feature generalization in articulation training. *Journal of Speech and Hearing Disorders, 37*(3), 462–470.

National Institute on Deafness and Other Communication Disorders (NIDCD). (2006, December). *NIDCD outcomes research in children with hearing loss.* Retrieved from www.nidcd.nih.gov/funding/programs/hb/outcomes/Pages/report.aspx.

Nicolosi, L., Harryman, E., & Kresheck, J. (1996). *Terminology of communication disorders.* Baltimore, MD: Lippincott, Williams and Wilkins.

Nicolosi, L., Harryman, E., & Kresheck, J. (2006). *Terminology of communication disorders* (4th ed.). Baltimore, MD: Williams & Wilkins.

Oller, D. K. (1980). The emergence of the sounds of speech in infancy. In G. Yeni-Komshian, J. Kavanagh, & C. A. Ferguson (Eds.), *Child phonology: Vol.1. production* (pp. 93–112). New York, NY: Academic Press.

Oyler, R., & McKay, S. (2008). Unilateral hearing loss in children: Challenges and opportunities. *ASHA Leader, 13*(1), 12–15.

Peña-Brooks, A., & Hegde, M. N. (2015). *Assessment and treatment of speech sound disorders in children* (3rd ed.). Austin, TX: Pro-Ed.

Porter, J. H., & Hodson, B. W. (2001). Collaborating to obtain phonological acquisition data for local schools. *Language, Speech, and Hearing Services in Schools, 32*(3), 165–171.

Prezas, R., & Hodson, B. (2007). Diagnostic evaluation of children with speech sound disorders. In S. Rvachew (Ed.), *Encyclopedia of language and literacy development* (p. 107). London, Ontario: Canadian Language and Literacy Research Network. Retrieved from www.literacyencyclopedia.ca/

Ryan, C. (2011). Language Use in the United States: 2011. *American Community Survey Reports.* U.S. Department of Commerce.

Sander, E. (1972). When are speech sounds learned? *Journal of Speech and Hearing Disorders, 37,* 55–63.

Scherz, J., & Edwards, H. (2010). Review of phonetics. In B. W. Hodson (Ed.), *Evaluating and enhancing children's phonological systems* (pp. 9–22). Wichita, KS: PhonoComp Publishing.

Secord, W., Boyce, S., Donohue, J., Fox, R., & Shine, R. (2007). *Eliciting sounds: Techniques and strategies for clinicians.* Clinton Park, NY: Thomson Delmar Learning.

Stoel-Gammon, C., & Dunn, C. (1985). *Normal and disordered phonology in children.* Austin, TX: Pro-Ed.

Strattman, K. (2010). Overview of intervention approaches, methods, and targets. In B. W. Hodson (Ed.), *Evaluating and enhancing children's phonological systems* (pp. 23–41). Wichita, KS: PhonoComp Publishing.

Thrasher, R. D. (2007). Middle ear, otitis media with effusion. *EMedicine.* American Academy of Otolaryngology—Head and Neck Surgery. Retrieved February 19, 2008, from www.emedicine.com/ent/topic209.htm.

Thrasher, R. D., & Gregory, C. A. (2005, October). Middle ear, otitis media with effusion. *EMedicine.* American Academy of Otolaryngology—Head and Neck Surgery, University of Colorado School of Medicine, and Ehrling Berquist Hospital. Retrieved October 20, 2007, from www.emedicine.com/ent/topic209.htm.

Van Riper, C. (1939). *Speech correction: Principles and methods.* Englewood Cliffs, NJ: Prentice-Hall.

Webster, P., & Plante, A. (1992). Effects of phonological impairment on word, syllable, and phoneme segmentation and reading. *Language, Speech, and Hearing Services in Schools, 23,* 176–182.

Weismer, S. E., & Robertson, S. (2006). Focused stimulation approach to language intervention. In R. McCauley & M. Fey (Eds.), *Treatment of language disorders in children* (pp. 175–202). Baltimore, MD: Paul H. Brookes.

Yoshinaga-Itano, C., Sedey, A., Coulter, D., & Mehl, A. (1998). Language of early- and later-identified children with hearing loss. *Pediatrics, 102*(5), 1161–1171.

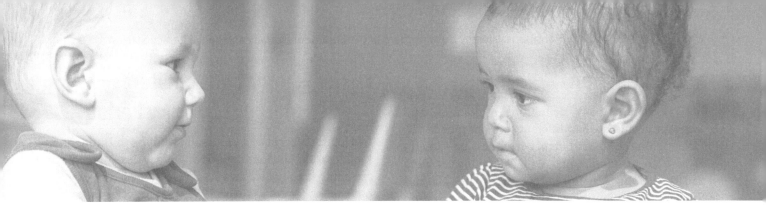

CHAPTER 10

Early Transitions: Literacy Development in the Emergent Literacy and Early Literacy Stages

SallyAnn Giess, PhD, CCC-SLP

▶ Introduction

There are many definitions of literacy, and being literate has different connotations in different cultures. *Literacy* may best be thought of as both a foundational skill of lifelong learning and a lifelong learning process (United Nations Educational, Scientific, and Cultural Organization [UNESCO], 2004). UNESCO (2004) has drafted the following definition:

> Literacy is the ability to identify, understand, interpret, create, communicate, and compute, using printed and written materials associated with varying contexts. Literacy involves a continuum of learning in enabling individuals to achieve their goals, to develop their knowledge and potential, and to participate fully in their community and wider society.
>
> (p. 13)

Within this definition is the fundamental necessity of creating meaning from print. When one thinks of being literate, perhaps the first connotation that comes to mind is being able to read. At a foundational level, reading involves the process of associating a letter sound with a written, orthographic symbol. At a more skilled level, reading involves a complex interaction between the reader and the text as the reader creates meaning from the printed material (Catts & Kamhi, 2005). As the definition put forth by UNESCO illustrates, literacy is a multidimensional, multifaceted construct and one that takes root early in a child's life. How do children come to arrive at this ability? How do they transition from a world where the focus is on language as a spoken event to a world where the focus is on language as a written event? Clearly, children have a great deal to learn as they make this transition.

This chapter considers literacy development along a continuum from the emergent literacy period, typically occurring during the preschool years, through the early literacy period, which consists of the first years of formal schooling. Long before a child enters formal schooling, the foundations of literacy must already be in place; thus, the foundational skills of literacy that develop during the preschool years will be discussed first. The next section will focus on the initial years of a child's formal education, the early literacy years, and the necessary components of effective literacy education. Finally, the three case studies are discussed in line with longitudinal research that has predicted later literacy skills from early speech and language development.

▶ The Foundations of Literacy: The Emergent Literacy Period

During the period of a child's life from birth through kindergarten, the foundations of literacy development are being laid. Justice and Kaderavek (2004a,b) point out that as far back as the 1980s, researchers understood that reading development begins early in life, and recognized early reading and writing experiences as playing a crucial role in the attainment of skilled reading. Teale and Sulzby (1986) introduced the term *emergent literacy* to describe the reading and writing behaviors that precede and develop into conventional literacy. This period occurs before a child learns the formal mechanics of print or to actually decode (i.e., read) a printed word (van Kleeck & Schuele, 1987). Whitehurst and Lonigan (1998) define emergent literacy as "the skills, knowledge, and attitudes that are presumed to be developmental precursors to conventional forms of reading and writing and the environments that support these developments" (p. 849). Although they were first described more than two decades ago, the conclusions Teale and Sulzby (1986) make regarding the underpinnings of emergent literacy are just as relevant today to understanding the foundations of literacy:

- Listening, speaking, reading, and writing abilities develop concurrently and interrelatedly.
- Literacy is a functional activity that develops in real-life settings for real-life activities.
- Children acquire written language skills through active engagement with their world—both in independent activities and through interactions with adults.

Justice and Kaderavek (2004a) point out key areas of emergent literacy attainment, including phonological awareness, print concepts, alphabet knowledge, and literate language; proficiency in each of these areas is critical to successful transition from emergent literacy (prereading) to early literacy (reading). Phonological awareness is the awareness of the sound structure of spoken language at the word, syllable, onset-rime, and phoneme level. Knowledge of print concepts means knowing how print is organized, knowing the terms used to describe print, and understanding how books are organized. Finally, alphabet knowledge refers to knowledge of the features and names of individual letters, and literate language is described as the use of specific syntactic or semantic features such as elaborated noun phrases characteristic of decontextualized written text (Justice & Kaderavek, 2004a).

Looking at emergent literacy in a broader sense, van Kleeck and Schuele (1987) describe two key domains that characterize the emergent literacy period: literacy socialization and language awareness. *Literacy socialization* reflects the social and cultural aspects of reading that a child acquires by being a member of a literate society, whereas *language awareness* focuses on the specific knowledge about the linguistic code that a child needs to master to become literate. The literacy socialization period can be further characterized according to literacy artifacts, literacy events and functions, and literacy knowledge acquired before learning to read (van Kleeck & Schuele, 1987).

Literacy artifacts are those representations of print that enrich a child's environment. Common examples of literacy artifacts include pictures of characters from nursery rhymes and *Sesame Street* that decorate a child's room, clothing, picture books, alphabet blocks, stickers, and even character toothbrushes (van Kleeck & Schuele, 1987). Literacy artifacts also show up in less obvious places. For example, logos on a cereal box, store labels on a grocery bag, and an address on an envelope all expose a child to the importance of print in both their world and the world of their parents.

Although literacy artifacts are certainly important for exposing a child to print, it is the *literacy events and functions* that surround these artifacts that serve as real teaching opportunities during the emergent literacy period. One literacy event that has become part of mainstream American talk about literacy is shared or joint book reading. While joint book reading may not be "the single most important activity for … eventual success in reading" (Commission on Reading, 1985, p. 23), it serves as a rich source of information and opportunity to learn (Whitehurst & Lonigan, 2001). As children engage in joint book reading with a caregiver, they are exposed to a "book-language" way of talking (Mason, 1992) and to routines involving book reading.

In summarizing earlier work, van Kleeck and Schuele (1987) relate the rising expectations parents have for children in shared book reading to the rising expectations teachers have for students' reading curriculum in school. These expectations are reflected in the following developmental progression in questioning and commenting:

- Item labels: What's that? Who is that?
- Item elaborations (labels for subclasses, type, number): What kind of animal is that? How many fish do you see?
- Event: What happened?
- Event elaborations: (talk about already-introduced events by elaborating on location or consequences)
- Motive or cause: Why? How come?

- Evaluation/reaction: What a silly little boy!
- Relation to the real world: That looks just like the fish you caught with Grandpa!

Similar to van Kleeck and Schuele (1987), Whitehurst et al. (1994) also focused on the importance of how adults read to young children in their description of dialogic reading. In dialogic reading, the adult uses strategies that encourage the child to be an active participant in reading and become the storyteller; reading is considered a dialogue between the adult and the child rather than a one-sided monologue. Whitehurst et al. (1994) use the acronym PEER to illustrate the dialogic reading strategy. Using this strategy, the adult:

- Prompts the child to say something about the book.
- Evaluates the child's response.
- Expands the child's response by rephrasing and adding information to it.
- Repeats the prompt to make sure the child has learned from the expansion.

In the video clip, which can be found in the online materials, you will see Mrs. L using a number of strategies as she shares a book with her son, J. Their interaction reflects van Kleeck and Schuele's (1987) developmental expectations and Whitehurst et al.'s (1994) dialogic reading and PEER strategies. For example, Mrs. L consistently comments and questions as she reads with J as she asks him "wh" questions such as "Who is Dad?," "What is he putting on?," and "Who is Seymore?" She reacts with humor and surprise when Dad pours coffee on his cereal and probes J to explain why Dad has a surprised look on his face. Mrs. E's pauses and questions prompt J to say something about the book. She evaluates J's response for the definition of "lad" and adds information to the meaning by associating the story character to J's own father.

These question/answer interactions provide opportunities for children to hear new words in meaningful contexts and build a vocabulary that will be instrumental in the early school years (Mason, 1992). Given the exposure and emphasis placed on shared book reading, one could easily assume that it is the single most important event for literacy success. However, not all researchers support such a belief.

Scarborough and Dobrich (1990) concluded from their review of the literature that while parent–preschoolers shared reading experiences influence language and literacy development, the strength of the influence is variable and may only be modest at best. Factors such as demographics, attitude, and skill level must also be considered important and strong influences on early reading success. Children from lower-socioeconomic backgrounds and low-print homes may experience less benefit from shared book reading but may benefit from other activities that serve a similar function, such as those associated with daily living (e.g., paying bills) and entertainment (e.g., reading a tabloid or television guide). Similarly, a negative attitude about reading may lead to what Scarborough and Dobrich consider a "broccoli effect" (1990, p. 295). Not all young children are interested in books, and forcing an uninterested child to interact in a shared book activity may have the opposite of the desired effect. Catts and Kamhi (2005) stress that a negative attitude and a preference to not read are not the same as an inability to read; thus, negative attitudes may not have long-term effects on literacy achievement.

The third aspect of literacy socialization is the print knowledge children gain from literacy experiences, referred to as *literacy knowledge*. In fact, literacy artifacts and literacy events may be most valuable for providing a context for this learning. By watching, doing, and handling, children learn the spatial orientation of books—that they have covers and backs, that pages turn from left to right, and that there is a right-side-up position. More importantly, children are exposed to fundamental concepts of print—that sentences are read from left to right, that words have boundaries, that there is a spoken counterpart to the orthographic symbol, and that words tell stories. A caregiver sharing an alphabet book with a child is a prime example of how a literacy artifact can be used in a literacy event to teach knowledge of the alphabet principle. As the caregiver says the name of the letter and then the sound that the letter makes while simultaneously pointing to the letter and corresponding picture that represents the sound, the child learns that letters represent sounds in a predictable system and words comprise patterns of letters and corresponding patterns of sounds.

This discussion of print knowledge includes the concept of phonological awareness. While phonological awareness is a skill that develops predominately during the early literacy period (kindergarten and first grade), it also has a place in discussion of emergent literacy skills. *Phonological awareness* is a broad term that refers to an individual's knowledge or sensitivity to the sound structure of words in the absence of print (Pullen & Justice, 2003) and at the emergent literacy level is reflected in activities such as rhyming, word play, and phonological corrections (van Kleeck & Schuele, 1987). For young children who are at risk of developing a reading disability or who come from homes where there is limited opportunity for language play, phonological awareness is a skill whose

development may require explicitly engaging the child in meaningful and enjoyable activities that focus on the internal structure of words.

To this point in the text, the focus has been on the written, or graphic, precursors to literacy development. In fact, oral language skills have also been associated with later reading achievement, especially reading comprehension (Pullen & Justice, 2003). Although children are able to understand and use language long before they begin to read, their early experiences and successes with spoken language serve as the foundation for later reading development (Whitehurst & Lonigan, 1998). Indeed, preschool children's knowledge of vocabulary and grammar accounts for significant variance in later literacy skills. The ability to comprehend and produce increasingly complex syntactic structures influences literacy development. In her investigation of early language deficits of children who later develop dyslexia, Scarborough (1990) identified oral language skills that predicted later reading disability. In a sample of children, she found that syntactic deficits among 2-year-olds and vocabulary deficits among older preschool children corresponded most closely with children's later literacy outcomes. Murphy and Farquharson (2016) recently studied the extent to which preschoolers' knowledge in the domains of orthography, phonology, morphosyntax, and vocabulary (called lexical quality domains) contribute to reading comprehension and identified profiles that predict first grade reading comprehension. Murphy and Farquharson found that below average performance on the four lexical quality domains significantly predicted reading comprehension in the first grade.

Linguistic awareness, which is a metalinguistic skill, also plays a role in emergent literacy and later reading success (Whitehurst & Lonigan, 1998). *Linguistic awareness* is the ability to understand language as a cognitive construct and possess information about the manner in which language is constructed and used. Whitehurst and Lonigan (1998) describe it as awareness that *cat* and *sat* are units of language called words, that words are constructed from units of sound, and that these words differ in one letter but share two other letters. Such sensitivity to phonemes is critical to learning to read, but learning to read also increases one's phonemic sensitivity. Higher levels of linguistic awareness are essential for later reading skills when a child transitions to reading to learn (Whitehurst & Lonigan, 1998).

Van Kleeck and Schuele's (1987) presentation of the literacy socialization period explains some key events that occur during the preschool years and foster later literacy development. However, it does not explain how children become proficient in decoding words, a skill that is at the root of proficient reading. The ability to accurately and effortlessly recognize words is a key—perhaps *the* key—component to proficient reading. Stage theories of reading development are useful in understanding the developmental changes children go through as they become proficient readers.

▶ Stage Theories of Reading Development

Jeanne Chall (1983) introduced her influential *stages of reading development* model based on a theory that reading development resembles cognitive and language development (other influential stage theorists include Linnea Ehri and Uta Frith). Chall based her theory of reading development on several hypotheses that reflect Piaget's cognitive theories of development. Several of Chall's theories are mentioned below:

- Reading stages have a definite structure and differ from one another in qualitative ways, following a hierarchical progression.
- Reading is a problem-solving activity in which readers adapt to their environment.
- Individuals pass through the stages through interactions in their home, school, and community.
- Successive stages are characterized by growth in the ability to read language that is more complex and more abstract.
- As readers advance through the stages, they are required to bring more sophisticated knowledge of the world and the topic to the reading event.
- Readers may get stuck on techniques of an earlier stage, such as the decoding stage, and struggle with the demands of a more difficult stage. (Chall, 1996, pp. 11–12)

According to Lombardino (2012), Chall's framework has particular appeal because it differentiates the developmental milestones of learning to read from reading to learn. The "learning to read" stage occurs from ages 5–6 years (Stage 0 and grades preschool to kindergarten) to ages 7–8 years (Stage 2 and grades 2–3). The stages are hierarchical in nature, do not vary in order of acquisition, and are dependent on the previous stage for development. The *logographic stage* may best be regarded as a prereading stage where children focus on the salient visual features of words. In this stage, children associate unanalyzed spoken words with salient graphic features of printing words and their surrounding context prior to using letter names or associating sounds with letters to decode words (Catts & Kamhi, 2005). As such, the logographic stage

is not considered a prerequisite to reading and may be bypassed in children from low-print homes who go on to become proficient readers. Indeed, Bowman and Treiman (2008) state that the importance of the logographic stage may be overestimated.

In contrast to the logographic stage, the *alphabetic stage* is essential. This stage is characterized by the onset of reading words by processing letter–sound correspondences and may be considered the first step to automatic word recognition. The key event in the alphabetic stage is the development of the *alphabetic principle*—the insight or awareness that letters correspond to sounds and that those same sounds make up our spoken language (Adams, 1994). At this stage, children spend a considerable amount of time phonologically decoding words.

Considering the arbitrariness of the English language, learning letter–sound correspondences is a difficult task for children. Given that phonological decoding is not an exacting strategy for children to use when reading English, orthographic knowledge is necessary for the development of automatic, effortless word recognition. Chall (1966) point outs that orthographic knowledge eventually allows the reader to become "unglued" from the print. When a child reaches the *orthographic stage* of reading, they are able to use letter sequences and spelling patterns to recognize words visually without engaging in the cumbersome task of phonologically decoding each word (Catts & Kamhi, 2005).

A direct visual route to access word meanings, free of phonological mediations, is necessary to develop *automatic word recognition*. To develop this direct route, children must acquire sufficient knowledge of spelling patterns. Such knowledge comes about with repeated encounters with similar letter sequences that are stored in semantic memory.

It is at this point in literacy development that language begins to have a profound effect on the acquisition of written language. To develop automatic word recognition, a child must recognize and understand morphological endings such as *-ing*, *-ed*, and *-able* and function words such as *the*, *a*, and *an*. Understanding the importance and obligatory function of these words in spoken language will facilitate their recognition in written language.

Stage theories of reading development are useful as a framework to explain the knowledge and skills children must have to become accomplished readers, but they fail to explain the actual processes needed to acquire these skills (Catts & Kamhi, 2005). As an alternative to the stage-based theories, Share (1995) and Share and Stanovich (1995) have proposed a self-teaching hypothesis to explain how children learn to read.

▶ The Self-Teaching Hypothesis

In considering direct instruction, contextual guessing, and phonological recoding as possible options for developing a literate lexicon, Share (1995) proposed that only *phonological recoding* (print-to-sound translation, also commonly referred to as *decoding*) offers the most viable means for developing fast, efficient, visual word recognition. The problem with direct instruction as a means to word recognition is that children encounter far too many words in printed text to possibly memorize them. Similarly, the use of semantic, syntactic, and pragmatic cues in written text is far too unreliable to facilitate fast and efficient word recognition (Share, 1995). Thus, Share sees phonological recoding as the only viable means of efficient word recognition in alphabetic languages and the central component to the *self-teaching hypothesis*. According to the self-teaching hypothesis:

Each successful decoding encounter with an unfamiliar word provides an opportunity to acquire the word-specific orthographic information that is the foundation of skilled word recognition. A relatively small number of (successful) exposures appear to be sufficient for acquiring orthographic representations … [in] this way, phonological recoding acts as a self-teaching mechanism or built-in teacher enabling a child to independently develop both (word)-specific and general orthographic knowledge. (p. 155)

The self-teaching hypothesis relies on an item-based role of decoding in development. The process of word recognition depends on the frequency with which a child has been exposed to a word and successful identification of that word. Ehri (2014) describes this as orthographic mapping—a process where letter–sound connections are bonded to the spellings, pronunciations, and meanings of specific words in memory. Because children rapidly acquire orthographic information of a word, they are likely to visually recognize high-frequency words with little effort paid to phonological processing. Words that are encountered less frequently, and thus are less orthographically salient, will be more dependent on phonological processing (Share, 1995). Share describes this as a "phonology by familiarity account" (p. 155).

A second key feature of the self-teaching hypothesis is the lexicalization of phonological recoding (Share, 1995). Young readers initially begin the word recognition process with a basic knowledge of simple letter–sound correspondences that become associated with particular words (i.e., they are "lexicalized"). The early lexicalization of sound–letter correspondences may best be considered a bootstrap or scaffold for developing the "complex, lexically constrained knowledge

of spelling–sound relationships that characterizes the expert reader" (Share, 1995, p. 165). Children modify these simple one-to-one grapheme–morpheme correspondences by using constraints such as context, word position, and morphological endings (a grapheme is a written symbol [letter] that represents a phoneme [sound]). Share recognized that these initial decoding successes are much different than the decoding of the complex words that skilled readers eventually encounter. Nevertheless, according to Share, these early, manageable encounters are enough to kick-start the self-teaching mechanism, which in turn refines itself in light of orthographic knowledge.

Orthography refers to the way a language is represented in print. *Orthographic representation* of a word refers to the way the word is stored visually in one's memory (Torgesen, 2004). Apel (2011) uses the term *orthographic knowledge* to refer to the "information that is stored in memory that tells us how to represent spoken language in written form" (Apel, 2011, p. 592). He supports the belief that children's early development of orthographic knowledge occurs through both implicit and explicit means.

A third key feature of the self-teaching hypothesis relates to the contributions of the phonological and orthographical processes to fluent word recognition. While both processes make independent contributions to fluent word recognition, the phonological component is considered primary, accounting for the majority of individual differences in reading ability (Share, 1995). The ability to store and retrieve word-specific visual/orthographic information depends heavily on the ability to use spelling–sound relationships to identify unfamiliar words.

▶ Early Literacy: The Transition to School

The early literacy years reflect the events surrounding literacy that take place during the first few years of a child's formal education—typically kindergarten through second grade. During this period, children tackle the formidable task of learning how to read. Children arrive at their formal schooling years with different pre-literacy and early literacy experiences. Some may already know how to spell their names and are creatively spelling words; others may be experiencing literacy artifacts (e.g., paper, crayons) for the first time (van Kleeck & Schuele, 1987). Yet, all children face the daunting task of becoming skilled at the same components of early literacy. The ultimate goal in the early literacy period is for a child to develop sufficient orthographic knowledge to allow for automatic, effortless word recognition that eventually leads to the end goal of reading comprehension. A common saying linking learning and reading is "learning to read, reading to learn", with the early school years considered a crucial time for mastering literacy (i.e., learning to read). A number of events, rooted in effective reading instruction, must come together to reach this end goal of comprehension. The National Reading Panel (NRP) identified five areas of reading instruction that are necessary to teach children to read: phonemic awareness, phonics, fluency, vocabulary, and text comprehension (National Institute of Child Health and Human Development [NICHHD], 2000). Skill in each of these areas has a basis in oral language.

Phonemic awareness is the ability to notice, think about, and work with the individual sounds in spoken words (NICHHD, 2000). It is the understanding that sounds of spoken language work together to make words (NICHHD, 2000). Phonemes are the building blocks of spoken words, whereas letters are the building blocks of written words (Ehri & Roberts, 2006). As Ehri and Roberts (2006) state, phonemic awareness is conceptually separate from print; its function is to enable beginning readers to connect speech to print. Without this connection, children will likely struggle with early literacy.

Phonemic awareness is considered necessary, but not sufficient, for the development of word reading accuracy (Phillips & Torgesen, 2006). An example of a phonemic awareness activity is instructing a child to say the word *bat* and then say the word again, replacing the /b/ with the /k/ sound (*cat*). As children develop oral language, they learn about the sounds of English through sound games such as singing the alphabet song and engaging in word play with their caregivers. Eventually, they come to experience these same sounds with their written (i.e., orthographic) counterparts. Repeated exposure to the sounds in words in both their spoken and written forms leads a child to discover the consistency and regularity in words. Knowledge and awareness of this consistency then allows a child to read words that they encounter for the first time in print (Phillips & Torgesen, 2006). Without such awareness, a child would see each printed word as a new experience and would not experience reading as a fluent process. Without the ability to read fluently, reading comprehension will suffer.

Phonics is a second building block of early literacy (NICHHD, 2000). As defined by Adams (1994), "phonics refers to a system of teaching reading that builds on the alphabetic principle, a system of which a central component is the teaching of correspondences between letters or groups of letters and their pronunciations" (p. 50). The connection between spoken and written language is central to phonics. To learn to read, children must understand the linguistic importance of sounds (phonemes) and must know the letters of the alphabet (Adams, 2001). This knowledge, in turn, facilitates reading words both in isolation and in connected text. Perhaps the emphasis on phonemic awareness instructions in early literacy programs can be tied to Juel's (2006) statement that, "without phonemic awareness, phonics instruction is meaningless" (p. 410). Although some children come to school already equipped with this knowledge, explicit instruction in phonics has been shown to be useful for all children (Torgesen, 2004).

Before going on to the other areas identified by the NRP as essential to teaching children to learn to read, it is important to have a good understanding of two similar-sounding terms, phonological awareness and phonemic awareness, and phonics. Scarborough and Brady (2002) provide an excellent tutorial on differentiating the "phon" words. According to Scarborough and Brady (2002), *phonological awareness* is a "broad class of skills that involve attending to, thinking about, and intentionally manipulating the phonological aspects of spoken language, especially the internal phonological structure of words" (p. 312). As such, phonological awareness is considered an umbrella term under which phonemic awareness falls. *Phonemic awareness* refers to the ability to attend to, think about, and purposefully manipulate the individual phonemes within spoken words and syllables. The focus is on the individual phoneme. Finally, *phonics* refers to an approach to reading instruction that focuses on the discovery and understanding of the alphabetic principle (Scarborough & Brady, 2002).

A third component of early literacy is *fluency*. Various definitions of fluency exist (Phillips & Torgesen, 2006) and most include the components of reading text accurately, quickly, and without effort (Meyer & Felton, 1999; NICHHD, 2000). The ability to group words into meaningful phrases, read with prosody, or read with intonation and stress may also be included in a definition of fluency. Phillips and Torgesen (2006) base their understanding of fluency in curriculum-based assessment, defining fluency as rate and accuracy in oral reading. The authors of the NRP report (NICHHD, 2000) differentiate automaticity from fluency. *Automaticity* is the fast, effortless word recognition that is a product of consistent reading practice. Fluent readers, by contrast, read aloud effortlessly and with expression. Automaticity is necessary, but not sufficient, for fluency (NICHHD, 2000).

One skill that facilitates reading fluency is the ability to detect orthographic patterns (Catts & Kamhi, 2005). Young readers learn early on to detect common morphological endings such as -*ed*, -*ing*, and -*s*. Provided a child has a strong foundation in oral language, they will already have encountered words that possess these morphological endings and will know their meanings. Armed with this knowledge, the young reader will read the words quickly and accurately. Common orthographic patterns also come into play with word families or word neighborhoods. For example, *bake*, *cake*, *take*, and *lake* all belong to the same word family because they share the common stem of -*ake*. A child will likely have encountered these words in oral language through word games such as rhyming as well as in emergent literacy activities such as shared book reading. Fluent reading is facilitated through the recognition of these words because the reader does not have to devote cognitive resources to sounding out each word.

In a very broad sense, *vocabulary* can be defined as the words we must know to communicate effectively (NICHHD, 2000). It exists in both the oral and written mode. In the oral mode, vocabulary refers to the words we use when speaking or the words we hear when someone else is speaking. In the written mode, vocabulary refers to the words we recognize or use in print (NICHHD, 2000). According to Biemiller (2006), children require both fluent word recognition skills and at least an average vocabulary to achieve adequate reading comprehension. Children learn vocabulary words directly when an adult tells them the meaning of a word or when they look up the meaning of a word in the dictionary. Most vocabulary learning takes place indirectly. Children learn word meanings indirectly through their exposure to adult conversations, through listening to adults read to them, and by reading on their own (NICHHD, 2000).

Proficiency with phonemic awareness, phonics, vocabulary, and reading fluency—four of the five components of effective literacy instruction—is necessary for the final component of *text comprehension*. Reading comprehension develops from a facility with all aspects of spoken language: vocabulary or word knowledge (semantics); sound-level knowledge (phonology); sentence structure (syntax), including root words, endings, and prefixes; and contextual use of language (pragmatics). Adams (2001) relates the process of text comprehension to a continuum. On one end of the continuum are mental tasks that require a person to invest a maximal amount of mental energy, while on the opposite end of the continuum are mental tasks that require a minimum amount of mental energy and are considered automatic. The task for early readers is to develop the foundational literacy skills that allow them to invest a minimal amount of

energy on phonemic awareness so they can concentrate on text comprehension, a process that requires purposeful and active engagement (NICHHD, 2001).

Reading comprehension—the ultimate goal of reading—is a skill that is highly correlated with listening comprehension in skilled readers (de Jong & van der Leij, 2002). In fact, in Gough and Tunmer's (1986) simple view of reading, listening comprehension combines with word decoding to produce reading comprehension. Beginning readers usually have better listening comprehension skills than reading comprehension skills (Ashby & Rayner, 2006). A strong foundation in phonics and facility with phonemic awareness support automaticity in reading, which in turn helps skilled readers comprehend at a level that is commensurate with their listening comprehension (Ashby & Rayner, 2006). However, successful text comprehension depends on more than accurate and automatic word recognition. Text comprehension suffers if the reader encounters words that are not in their oral vocabulary, if the sentence structure is overly complex, or if the topic is so unfamiliar that the reader cannot make the inferences necessary to understanding the material (Snow, Scarborough, & Burns, 1999).

Snow, Scarborough, and Burns (1999) identified developmental markers of normal written language development for the early preschool period to the early elementary school years. These developmental milestones are useful when considering whether or not a child is at risk of literacy failure.

Three-Year-Olds

- Primary goal: Discover and appreciate the functions and values of written language in the environment
- Interested in signs and labels and their visual image
- Recognize books by cover, orient book, and turn pages
- Understand print is a means of communication (notes, memos, lists)

Four-Year-Olds

- Primary goal: Learn more details about print and words (foundation for understanding alphabetic principle)
- Attend to internal structure of words
- Develop phonological awareness skills
  - Perceive, identify, and separate phonemes (sounds)
  - Differentiate and identify letters accurately

- Engage in inventive writing
  - Practice spelling names
  - Mix letters with scribbling
- Vocabulary is expanding
  - Reflects amount of language to which child is exposed
  - Reflects Access to greater quantities of talk
  - Facilitates more rapid vocabulary development

In the video of Mrs. L and her son J, which can be found in the online materials, you will notice J demonstrating some of these developmental milestones. For instance, Mrs. L engages J in sound blending, a type of phonological awareness skill, when he blends the sounds s-p-l-a-t into the word "splat." J's expanding vocabulary is demonstrated when he provides a definition of "lad," an infrequently used word that J most likely knows because of his enriched language environment and familiarity with the story.

Five-Year-Olds (Kindergarteners)

- Primary goal: Figure out the alphabetic system
  - Example: If shown *hat* and told what it says, may be able to figure out how to exchange letters to spell *bat* and *sat*
- May be able to read regularly spelled words by knowing first and last phonemes
- May be able to recognize very common, familiar sight words
- Able to understand long stories that are read to them
  - Can ask questions about stories read to them

First Graders

- Primary goal: Expected to remember and apply reliable information about sound–letter correspondences to read words
- Should be able to read regular words accurately and automatically
- Should be able to discuss texts they have read or that have been read to them
  - Requires comprehension of new vocabulary terms
  - Requires familiarity and comfort with academic discourse style
- Writing development
  - Both invented and correct spelling
- Example: "vakashun" but also "the," "said"
  - Writing for different reasons

- Stories, journals, personal thoughts, lists about topics
  - Punctuation use is inconsistent
  - Story grammar emerges
- Example: "Once upon a time …"

Second Graders

- Primary goals:
  - Become fluent and automatic readers (fluency and automaticity in reading text)
  - Reading without being aware one is decoding text
- Develop comprehension strategies
- Develop word inference strategies
- Use writing to deepen understanding of literature
  - Book reports, research reports (short reports)
  - Conventional spelling more consistent

Third Graders and Beyond

- Primary goals:
  - Silent independent reading
  - Reading comprehension across subject areas
- Continued refinement of language skills
  - More sophisticated knowledge of syntax, morphology, semantics
  - Facilitates reading comprehension
- Continued development of reading comprehension strategies

It is necessary to have a thorough understanding of emergent and early literacy development before considering factors that put a child at risk of literacy failure. Through longitudinal studies, researchers have identified characteristics of early spoken language development that put a young child at risk of later reading difficulty. Next, these research findings are tied into the case studies presented in this text.

▶ Early Identification of Later Reading Disabilities

Understanding the components of both emergent and early literacy is essential to preventing reading failure in young children. The earlier in a child's education that emergent literacy weakness is identified, the more likely intervention will be successful (Foorman, Breier, & Fletcher, 2003; Snowling & Hayiou-Thomas, 2006). Both Torgesen (1998) and Stanovich (1986) describe the downward spiral that traps young children who get off to a poor start in reading; Stanovich (1986) has used the term *Matthew effect* to describe the lasting effect of early unsuccessful initial experiences with literacy. As Torgesen (1998) warns, children who get off to a poor start in reading rarely catch up to their more able peers. Weak phonological skills make it difficult for such children to identify new, unknown words, and their efforts to decode new words often yield many errors. Fluent reading, which depends on automatic word recognition, then suffers, with difficulties in this area often discouraging a child from engaging in reading. Limited exposure to vocabulary words affects vocabulary growth and negatively affects reading comprehension. Analyzing data from a large, epidemiologic study, Duff, Tomblin, and Catts (2015), applied the *Matthew effect* to vocabulary development and reading. They found a strong relationship between word-reading skill and vocabulary growth with above average readers in 4th grade experiencing a higher rate of vocabulary growth in 10th grade than average readers.

A number of research studies have followed the reading outcomes of preschool children with speech and/or language impairments through school age (Catts, Fey, Tomblin, & Zhang, 2002; Nathan, Stackhouse, Goulandris, & Snowling, 2004; Scarborough, 1990; Scarborough & Dobrich, 1990). Findings from these studies reveal that such children are either at risk of later reading disability or do, in fact, become disabled readers.

Nathan et al. (2004) reported on the early literacy development of preschool children with specific speech difficulties or speech and language difficulties; these children were first examined as preschoolers and followed through kindergarten and first grade. The children were evaluated for receptive language (picture vocabulary, understanding syntactic structure), expressive language (grammar, mean length of utterance [MLU]), output phonology (accuracy of speech production and word repetition), input phonology (auditory discrimination), phonological awareness (rhyme and phoneme manipulation tasks), and literacy skills (letter-name knowledge, word reading, spelling). As compared to a typically developing control group, subjects in both the specific speech only and the speech and language difficulty groups were at a high risk of literacy delay (Nathan et al., 2004). In second grade, subjects with both speech and language delays were more likely to show impairments in literacy skills, including phonological awareness, spelling, and reading. Nathan et al. (2004) also found that

children with the most severe speech difficulties had the poorest literacy outcomes.

Scarborough documented early language deficits in children later identified with specific reading impairments or developmental dyslexia. In her 1990 study, Scarborough examined the oral language proficiency of preschool children at 30 months who were later identified as reading disabled. Formal tests were administered to assess vocabulary recognition, naming vocabulary, and speech discrimination. Scarborough found that the preschool children at age 30 months who later developed reading disabilities were delayed in the length, syntactic complexity, and pronunciation accuracy of their spoken language. At 5 years of age, these children were weak in object-naming, phonemic awareness, and letter–sound knowledge.

Catts et al. (2002) also investigated the reading outcomes in second- and fourth-grade children with language impairments identified while they were in kindergarten. Catts et al. (2002) found that the language-impaired children scored significantly lower than the nonimpaired children (i.e., the control group) on tests of word recognition and reading comprehension in second and fourth grades. The researchers determined that the best kindergarten predictor of reading outcomes was letter identification; however, the grammar composite, nonverbal IQ, rapid naming, and phonological awareness also contributed unique variance in reading achievement at the second and fourth grades.

These research studies provide a context within which to discuss the three children profiled in the case studies. In fact, developing a profile of strengths and weaknesses of young children's early literacy and language skills is key to identifying those who may be at risk of later reading and academic struggles (Lombardino, 2012). Lombardino (2012) developed a multidimensional model to assess and differentiate children at risk of reading and writing disorders that captures both the environmental and neurobiological/neurocognitive factors of reading. As a speech-language pathologist or other practitioner develops a plan to assess a child referred for assessment, they must consider environmental factors such as school instruction and opportunities for literacy exposure and experiences and neurobiological/neurocognitive factors such as genetics and language processing. An assessment to determine a child's strengths and weaknesses in early language and literacy skills will vary according to many things, including the presenting characteristics of the child, the professionals involved, and the professional setting, and may include assessment of spoken language, phonological knowledge, print knowledge, and word level reading depending on the age of the child (Lombardino, 2012).

▶ Case Studies

🔍 CASE STUDY: JOHNATHON (TD)

Johnathon appears to be a typically developing toddler. His speech-language evaluation revealed age-appropriate expressive and receptive language skills. Although Johnathon does not appear to have any risk factors associated with later literacy failure, it is still important for him to be engaged in early literacy experiences and be provided with appropriate instruction when he begins school. Given such experiences, and in combination with his typically developing language skills, there is no reason to expect that he will develop later difficulties with reading.

🔍 CASE STUDY: JOSEPHINE (LB)

Josephine's profile suggests concern for later literacy difficulty. The results of her speech-language evaluation revealed a mild to moderate delay in expressive language and a moderate delay in speech sound development. Josephine is younger than the children in the research studies cited earlier; however, she does possess speech and language delays that could put her at future risk of literacy failure. In the study carried out by Nathan et al. (2004), children with both speech and language delays were at greatest risk of deficits in phoneme awareness at 6 years. If Josephine continues on this path and does not improve and expand her vocabulary knowledge, she may find book reading an unappealing, difficult activity and could enter the downward spiral discussed by Torgesen (1998). If she begins school with a speech-language delay, she may be at risk of future academic struggles. One assessment designed specifically to assess emergent reading and spoken language skills in preschool children is the *Assessment of Literacy and Language* (ALL; Lombardino, Lieberman, & Brown, 2005). The ALL may be used to create profiles of Josephine's strengths and weaknesses in both emergent reading and spoken language domains.

Josephine's background history of early intervention bodes well for her future success. Her continued participation in speech-language therapy that includes early literacy activities such as word games (rhymes, sound–letter matching), shared book-reading, alphabetic activities, and pretend writing will be imperative.

🔍 CASE STUDY: ROBERT (LT)

Of the three children described in the case studies, Robert is at greatest risk of later literacy difficulty. He exhibits delays in expressive language, speech-sound production, and receptive language. In the research studies cited earlier, the children with the most severe delays as preschoolers went on to experience the most severe delays in literacy skills. Given Robert's delays in receptive language as well as play and gesture, his nonverbal language skills may be suspect. The reading outcomes in the Catts et al. (2002) study were poorest for those children who had both nonverbal and language deficits. Scarborough's (1990) report of 30-month-old toddlers who later developed reading disabilities revealed that syntactic deficits most closely corresponded with eventual literacy outcomes; phonological production was also substantially impaired in the children who were later identified as poor readers.

To help Robert, it will be especially important to engage him in early intervention that includes a focus on emergent literacy activities. Robert's caretakers should make sure his home is filled with literacy artifacts and engage him in literacy events using these artifacts. It will be important for Robert to develop a solid understanding of the alphabet and sound–letter correspondences in preparation for his entrance into kindergarten. These activities should be included along with his other prescribed goals for speech and language development.

▶ Summary

Children face a formidable task in learning to read. Even so, most children learn how to read successfully without any conscious effort. Armed with a strong foundation in emergent and early literacy skills, children should be able to successfully navigate the academic curriculum and transition from learning to read to reading to learn.

Study Questions

▪ What important events during the emergent literacy period foster literacy development in young children?

▪ What are the five key components of effective literacy instruction according to the NRP?

▪ Which factors put a child at risk of later literacy failure?

▪ How does language development interact with and facilitate literacy development?

References

Adams, M. (2001). Alphabetic anxiety and explicit, systematic phonics instruction: A cognitive science perspective. In S. B. Neuman & D. K. Dickinson (Eds.), *Handbook of early literacy research* (Vol. 1, pp. 66–80). New York, NY: Guildford Press.

Adams, M. J. (1994). *Beginning to read: Thinking and learning about print.* Cambridge, MA: MIT Press.

Apel, K. (2011). What is orthographic knowledge? *Language, Speech, and Hearing Services in Schools, 42,* 592–603.

Ashby, J., & Rayner, K. (2006). Literacy development: Insights from research on skilled reading. In D. K. Dickinson & S. B. Neuman (Eds.), *Handbook of early literacy research* (Vol. 2, pp. 52–63). New York, NY: Guildford Press.

Biemiller, A. (2006). Vocabulary development and instruction: A prerequisite for school learning. In D. K. Dickinson & S. B. Neuman (Eds.), *Handbook of early literacy research* (Vol. 2, pp. 41–51). New York, NY: Guildford Press.

Bowman, M. & Treiman, R. (2008). Are young children logographic readers and spellers? *Scientific Studies of Reading, 12*(2), 153–170.

Catts, H. W., Fey, M. E., Tomblin, J. B., & Zhang, X. (2002). A longitudinal investigation of reading outcomes in children with language impairments. *Journal of Speech, Language, and Hearing Research, 45*(6), 1142–1157.

Catts, H. W., & Kamhi, A. G. (2005). *Language and reading disabilities* (2nd ed.). Boston, MA: Allyn & Bacon.

Chall, J. S. (1983). *Stages of reading development.* New York, NY: McGraw-Hill.

Chall, J. S. (1996). *Stages of reading development* (2nd ed.). Fort Worth, TX: Harcourt Brace.

Commission on Reading. (1985). *Becoming a nation of readers: The report of the Commissions on Reading.* Washington, DC: National Institute of Education.

de Jong, P. F., & van der Leij, A. (2002). Effects of phonological abilities and linguistic comprehension on the development of reading. *Scientific Studies of Reading, 6*(1), 51–77.

Duff, D., Tomblin, J. B., & Catts, H. (2015). The influence of reading on vocabulary growth: A case for a Matthew effect. *Journal of Speech, Language, and Hearing Research, 58,* 853–864.

Ehri, L. C., (2014). Orthographic mapping in the acquisition of site word reading, spelling memory, and vocabulary learning. *Scientific Studies of Reading, 18*(1), 5–21.

Ehri, L. C., & Roberts, T. (2006). The roots of learning to read and write: Acquisition of letters and phonemic awareness. In D. K. Dickinson, & S. B. Neuman (Eds.), *Handbook of early literacy research* (Vol. 2, pp. 113–131). New York, NY: Guildford Press.

Foorman, B. R., Breier, J. I., & Fletcher, J. M. (2003). Interventions aimed at improving reading success: An evidence-based approach. *Developmental Neuropsychology, 24*(2–3), 613–639.

Gough, P. B., & Tunmer W. E. (1986). Decoding, reading, and reading disability. *Remedial and Special Education, 7*(1), 6–10.

Justice, L., & Kaderavek, J. (2004a). Embedded-explicit emergent literacy intervention I: Background and description of approach. *Language, Speech, and Hearing Services in Schools, 35,* 201–211.

Justice, L., & Kaderavek, J. (2004b). Exploring the continuum of emergent literacy to conventional literacy: Transitioning special learners. *Reading & Writing Quarterly: Overcoming Learning Difficulties, 20,* 231–236.

Juel, C. (2006). The impact of early school experiences on initial reading. In D. K. Dickinson & S. B. Neuman (Eds.), *Handbook of early literacy research* (Vol. 2, pp. 410–426). New York, NY: Guildford Press.

Lombardino, L. (2012). *Assessing and differentiating reading & writing disorders: Multidimensional model.* Clifton Park, NY: Delmar, Cengage Learning.

Lombardino, L., Lieberman, J., & Brown, J. (2005). *Assessment of Literacy and Language (ALL).* San Antonio, TX: The Psychological Corporation.

Mason, J. M. (1992). Reading stories to preliterate children: A proposed connection to reading. In P. B. Gough, L. C. Ehri, & R. Treiman (Eds.), *Reading acquisition* (pp. 215–243). Mahwah, NJ: Lawrence Erlbaum.

Meyer, M. S., & Felton, R. H. (1999). Repeated reading to enhance fluency: Old approaches and new directions. *Annals of Dyslexia, 49*(1), 283–306.

Murphy, K.A., & Farquharson, K. (2016). Investigating profiles in lexical quality preschool and their contribution to first grade reading. *Reading and Writing, 29,* 1745–1770.

Nathan, L., Stackhouse, J., Goulandris, N., & Snowling, M. J. (2004). The development of early literacy skills among children with speech difficulties: A test of the "critical age hypothesis." *Journal of Speech, Language, and Hearing Research, 47*(2), 377–391.

National Institute of Child Health and Human Development (NICHHD). (2000). *Report of the National Reading Panel: Teaching children to read: An evidence-based assessment of the scientific research literature on reading and its implications for reading instruction: Reports of the subgroups (NIH Publication No. 00-4754).* Washington, DC: U.S. Government Printing Office.

Phillips, B. M., & Torgesen, J. K. (2006). Phonemic awareness and reading: Beyond the growth of initial reading accuracy.

In D. K. Dickinson & S. B. Neuman (Eds.), *Handbook of early literacy research* (Vol. 2, pp. 101–112). New York, NY: Guilford Press.

Pullen, P. C., & Justice, L. M. (2003). Enhancing phonological awareness, print awareness, and oral language skills in preschool children. *Intervention in School and Clinic, 39*(2), 87–98.

Scarborough, H. S. (1990). Very early language deficits in dyslexic children. *Child Development, 61*, 1728–1734.

Scarborough, H. S., & Brady, S. A. (2002). Toward a common terminology for talking about speech and reading: A glossary of the "phon" words and some related terms. *Journal of Literacy Research, 34*(3), 299–336.

Scarborough, H. S., & Dobrich, W. (1990). Development of children with early language delays. *Journal of Speech and Hearing Research, 33*(1), 70–83.

Share, D. L. (1995). Phonological recoding and self-teaching: Sine qua non of reading acquisition. *Cognition, 55*(2), 151–218.

Share, D. L., & Stanovich, K. E. (1995). Cognitive processes in early reading development: Accommodating individual differences into a model of acquisition. *Issues in Education: Contributions from Educational Psychology, 1*, 1–57.

Snow, C. E., Scarborough, H. S., & Burns, M. S. (1999). What speech-language pathologists need to know about early reading. *Topics in Language Disorders, 20*(1), 48–58.

Snowling, M. J., & Hayiou-Thomas, M. E. (2006). The dyslexia spectrum: Continuities between reading, speech, and language impairments. *Topics in Language Disorders, 26*(2), 110–126.

Stanovich, K. E. (1986). Matthew effects in reading: Some consequences of individual differences in the acquisition of literacy. *Reading Research Quarterly, 21*(4), 360–406.

Teale, W. H., & Sulzby, E. (1986). Emergent literacy as a perspective for examining how children become writers and readers. In W. H. Teale, & E. Sulzby (Eds.), *Emergent literacy: Writing and reading* (p. 18). Norwood, NJ: Ablex.

Torgesen, J. K. (1998). Catch them before they fall. *American Educator/American Federation of Teachers*, Spring/Summer, 1–8.

Torgesen, J. K. (2004). Leaving no child behind: What every teacher should know. Retrieved from www.fcrr.org/science /pdf/torgesen/Aiken_S_C_keynote.pdf.

United Nations Educational, Scientific, and Cultural Organization (UNESCO). (2004). The plurality of literacy and its implications for policies and programs. Retrieved from http:// unesdoc.unesco.org/images/0013/001362/136246e.pdf

van Kleeck, A., & Schuele, C. (1987). Precursors to literacy: Normal development. *Topics in Language Disorders, 7*(2), 13–31.

Whitehurst, G. J, Epstein, J. N., Angell, A. L., Payne, A. C., Crone, D. A., & Fischel, J. E. (1994). Outcomes of an emergent literacy intervention in Head Start. *Journal of Educational Psychology, 86*(4), 542–555.

Whitehurst, G. J., & Lonigan, C. J. (1998). Child development and emergent literacy. *Child Development, 69*(3), 848–872.

Whitehurst, G. J., & Lonigan, C. J. (2001). Emergent literacy: Development from prereaders to readers. In S. B. Neuman, & D. K. Dickinson (Eds.), *Handbook of early literacy research* (Vol. 1, pp. 11–29). New York, NY: Guildford Press.

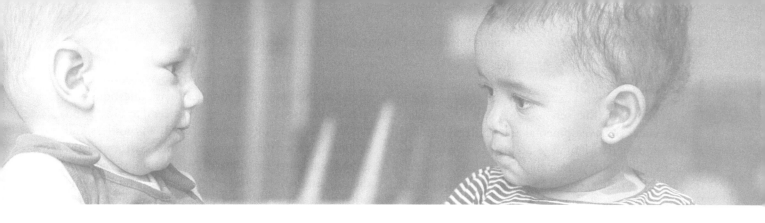

CHAPTER 11

School-Age Language Development: Application of Five Domains of Language Across Four Modalities

Anthony D. Koutsoftas, PhD, CCC-SLP

© santypan/Shutterstock, Inc.

▶ Introduction

Language in the school-age years is complex because of developmental and academic expectations. First, language abilities across all five domains (phonology, morphology, syntax, semantics, and pragmatics) continue to develop through the high school years. For example, although all speech sounds are achieved by 8 years old, children need to use phonological abilities to learn to read and spell. Likewise, although children acquire all sentence types by eight years old, how they comprehend and produce sentences for academic purposes continues to grow. Second, academic demands require language skills across four modalities—listening, speaking, reading, and writing—with an emphasis on the explicit teaching and development of the latter two skills. It is important to consider the relationships between spoken (listening, speaking) and written (reading, writing) forms of language during the school-age years. The purpose of this chapter is to extend foundational knowledge in language development and contextualize it for older children.

▶ Contextualizing Language for Schoolchildren

To understand how language is applied to and through the school-age years, one must consider the context of language use. From birth to 5 years of age, language development is contextualized to the home, parents, primary care providers, daycare centers, and preschools. This means that when children communicate with parents, primary care providers, and preschool teachers, their communication is generally supported by the context of the home or classroom. Children are likely talking about things in their environment, not abstract ideas, as they do during the school-age years. During the school-age years, language is contextualized to school and the academic demands of formal education, but at the same time, language becomes decontextualized from the immediate task at hand. For example, children are asked to read about unusual animals that they themselves have never had experience with or learn about a country located on the other side of the globe. Educational demands play a critical role in how language is used by children between 5 and 21 years old.

Language is at the center of education. Language is used by teachers to provide instruction of academic content but also to regulate classroom behavior and schedules. Language is used by school-age children to negotiate their way around the classroom, the school building, the sports field, and the playground. Children use their language abilities to ask questions and make comments to teachers and peers, to create and develop social interactions, and to understand and produce written language in the classroom. Language is at times the topic of instruction, specifically during English language arts courses, and during other times, it is the tool used by educators to provide instruction in math, science, or social studies. Metalinguistic skill refers to the ability to think about and analyze language in a purposeful manner. Metalinguistic ability plays an important role in language development and use of language during the school-age years. For example, when a child constructs a sentence, they must think about who will read that sentence and how it will be understood. Children with certain kinds of language impairments (e.g., autism, specific language impairment) have difficulty developing metalinguistic skills.

In order to understand the language needs of school-age children in academic settings, one must understand academic expectations. The Common Core State Standards or CCSS (Common Core State Standards Initiative, 2012) represent academic expectations for schoolchildren and are implemented in all but seven states in the United States. These curricular standards for kindergarten through twelfth grade students include expectations for speaking, listening, reading, writing, and language across all content areas (e.g., math, science, social studies, language arts). Content covered in this chapter can support the reader in operationalizing writing, reading, and language standards for schoolchildren.

A brief description of the CCSS (2012) is provided to contextualize the remaining content of the text; however, the reader is directed to the website (www.corestandards.org) for detailed information and grade-level specifics about the standards. The CCSS (2012) were designed to promote College and Career Readiness so that by the end of formal education, U.S. schoolchildren are ready to enter higher education or the workforce. There are two remarkable principles that lay the foundation for the standards, relevant to the content of this chapter. First, the CCSS emphasize interdisciplinary or interprofessional approaches for students' literacy development. These professionals include general and special educators, specialists (e.g. reading, ESL), and related service providers, including speech language pathologists. Second, the CCSS includes an integrated model of literacy addressing reading, writing, listening, speaking, and language. Prior to the CCSS, few curricula addressed the importance of speaking, listening, and language. Language standards expected of schoolchildren are organized into conventions, effective use, and vocabulary across reading, writing, speaking, and listening. That is to say, language instruction is emphasized across modalities rather than one modality (usually writing). A change as such requires interdisciplinary collaboration among educators to ensure schoolchildren meet these standards promoting literacy and supporting College and Career Readiness.

A distinction needs to be made between academic standards, curriculum, and instruction. Academic standards, such as the CCSS (2012) or other state standards, are the skills schoolchildren are expected to gain from their education and are generally prescribed by the grade level. Academic curriculum is the manner in which a state or local education agency achieves academic standards. The curriculum can be designed by states or local education agencies to include content that will be used to meet academic standards. For example, a local education agency (i.e., school district) might opt to use a series of textbooks from a commercially available educational publisher. Likewise, a different local education agency might opt to develop their own curriculum and content to meet the standards. Academic instruction is the manner in which educators deliver curriculum to students. To illustrate this, an educator will use academic standards and state or local curriculum to develop lesson plans and provide instruction to students. Educators include general and special educators, content specialists (e.g., math, science, reading, art, music, etc.), and related service providers, including speech language pathologists. Therefore, when providing language therapy and instruction for school-age children, the speech language pathologist must also consider academic standards and curriculum to which children are exposed.

▶ Language in Four Modalities

Language extends across four modalities: listening, speaking, reading, and writing. Research shows these four modalities are all considered language because of shared processing and production areas of the brain; however, each modality also has unique skills associated with it (Berninger & Abbott, 2010). The commonality between the four modalities is language, and simply stated, language is processed in the brain; what differs is the modality in which this occurs. To be specific, expressive modalities are *speaking* and *writing* and receptive modalities are *listening* and *reading*. Yet, oral modalities are *speaking* and *listening*, whereas written modalities are *reading* and *writing*. **FIGURE 11-1** provides a visual depiction of common and unique skills across the four modalities of language.

The four modalities of language share neural processing areas (i.e., in the brain). These processing

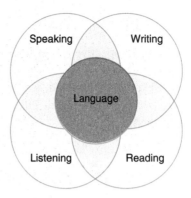

FIGURE 11-1 Visual depiction of language as having shared and unique skills represented across four modalities.

resources of the brain are common to or shared by all four modalities of language. However, the manner in which language is comprehended or expressed embodies unique components as well. For example, one can comprehend language through both auditory and visual input. During a conversation, we primarily listen to language; however, we also comprehend visual cues associated with body language processed through the eye. Another manner of visual input for language is reading, where language is in a written form and is understood by decoding print and using reading comprehension skills to gain meaning. When expressing language orally, we primarily use our mouths to speak the ideas, thoughts, feelings, and so on inside our minds. Similarly, we can formulate ideas in written (print) forms that are expressed through the hand onto paper (for the traditionalists out there) or through hand onto computer (for everyone else!). Notably, different modalities of communication can be used to express language; two examples include the use of an augmentative communication device such as an electronic tablet (e.g., iPad) or the use of manual forms of communication such as American Sign Language.

Unique skills associated with speaking would be the articulation of sounds, words, and sentences for the purposes of communication. Unique skills associated with listening are the processing of acoustic signals by the ear and associated centers of the brain, until the signal is transferred to language centers of the brain. Just as prosodic cues of pitch, tone, and loudness are necessary for conveying information effectively, so are visual cues such as gesture and facial expressions. Unique skills associated with reading include the decoding of words on paper in order to understand the written message. These messages can vary in length, purpose, and academic level and require unique skills associated with visual and cognitive areas of the brain. However, once the message is processed, it must be comprehended, and this happens similarly to the way heard language is comprehended. Unique skills associated with writing include the use of the hand for expression along with spelling abilities and the myriad of other skills associated with writing. Irrespective of the mechanical and cognitive demands of writing, language is at the root of the messages we express at the word, sentence, and text levels (Abbott, Berninger, & Fayol, 2010; Berninger, 2000; Berninger & Abbot, 2010).

▸ Five Domains Across Four Modalities

Remember the five domains of language: phonology, morphology, syntax, semantics, and discourse (pragmatics). Children in the school-age years can be observed to use all five domains of language across four modalities of language. Here, I will expand on the development of the skills required for speaking and listening by focusing on reading and writing using the model depicted in Figure 11-1. At times, it is obvious how each domain of language is utilized across each modality; in other cases, it is not. In some examples, development is confined to one quadrant or one-half of the language modality model, whereas in other examples, it is clear how the five domains of language occur within and across quadrants of the model.

Phonology

Phonemes are the smallest units of language and account for an integral part of school-age language understanding and production. Likewise, the student must listen to speech from teachers and peers during school, which requires phonological processing. The challenge for students in school becomes how phonology relates to reading and writing. Research shows that children with histories of phonological and/or speech sound disorders have more difficulties with acquiring written language skills than nonaffected peers (Catts, 1993; Catts, Fey, Tomblin, & Zhang, 2002). In fact, phonology plays an important role in learning to read and write. To be able to read, the child needs phonological and phonemic awareness skills in order to decode print. The reader is reminded that a translation between phonemes and orthographic symbols is involved in reading and writing. To be able to write, specifically to spell, the child relies on their phonology or understanding of sound to spell words.

Phonological and Phonemic Awareness

Phonemic awareness, the ability to manipulate sounds without print, is a skill that falls under the umbrella term of *phonological awareness* (Cunningham, 2005;

Schuele & Murphy, 2014). During Kindergarten through fifth grades, phonological and phonemic awareness is part of academic standards, namely the CCSS (2012). As part of phonological and phonemic awareness instruction, children are taught to hear the differences between syllables, words, and sounds. Strong phonological and phonemic awareness means that children understand that there is a difference between a sound, a letter, and a word. Without this ability, learning to read is compromised. Think about this: a child tries to read the word *dog* for the first time under the guidance of the teacher. The teacher says, "Sound it out" or perhaps "What's the first sound in the word?" If the child cannot follow that directive without print, how are they supposed to be able to respond accurately with the added stress of print and a teacher standing over their shoulder? Moreover, without intact phonology, the child would not be able to achieve the task of decoding and would require support of the teacher and speech-language pathologist to improve this aspect of language for reading.

Spelling

Phonological ability plays a significant role in the development of spelling. Research shows that when children spell words, they are using phonological, orthographic, and morphological knowledge (Bahr, Silliman, Berninger, & Dow, 2012; Berninger, Abbott, Nagy, & Carlisle, 2006; Silliman, Bahr, & Peters, 2006). Phonological knowledge is the most basic linguistic resource that children use to spell and is defined as "the spelling of a word using the grapheme (letter) that represents the sound." Children learn the letters of the alphabet and gain the knowledge that each letter has a sound. Using their phonological knowledge to spell, they write the letter that best represents the sound they perceive in the word. For example, a child may spell the word *cat* as "kat", where they use a letter that best represents the /k/ sound to spell a word. Similarly, a child may spell the word *lamb* as "lam", where the last sound in the word is /m/, and therefore, it would not make sense to include the letter *b* in that word. Phonology will only get you so far in spelling words in the English language because of the many spelling rules and variations of these rules.

The word *orthography* is Greek for "correct writing" and refers to the written system of a language. Orthographic knowledge, therefore, is the understanding of the written system's rules and variations of rules for spelling purposes. For example, the word *late* has three sounds and could phonologically be spelled as "lat"; however, the silent -*e* at the end of the word is an orthographic spelling pattern that is seen repeatedly in the English language. A child with an intact phonological system would never be able to correctly spell the word *late* without the orthographic knowledge that silent *-e* is required. Another example would be the word *light*, which has three sounds. A child with good phonological abilities might spell the word as "lit" or "lite," both of which are legal spellings in English; neither of which, however, represent the target word. Even with intact phonological abilities, a child would not be able to spell English words without gaining orthographic knowledge of spelling patterns.

Morphology

There are two types of bound morphemes, both of which are relevant to school-age populations: grammatical and derivational. The developmental milestones of the 14 grammatical morphemes identified by Brown (1973) are expected to be well developed before the child enters school at 5 or 6 years of age. Children with language difficulties may not comprehend or produce these morphemes consistently well into the school-age years (Windsor, Scott, & Street, 2000). Because of this, grammatical morpheme comprehension and production needs to be considered in the elementary school years. If you have ever had the pleasure of listening to a child with a language impairment who has difficulties with morphology read out loud to you, you might recall that the child elided the grammatical morphemes *-ed, -ing* and *-s* on more than one occasion despite the visual representation of these morphemes in written text. Windsor et al. (2000) observed this in their sample of fourth and fifth grade students with language-learning difficulties. Specifically, children who produce these grammatical morphemes in spoken narrative and expository samples often omit them when they write. This suggests that grammatical morphology continues to be an area of growth and potential concern for school-age children with language impairments.

Additionally, derivational morphemes play a critical role in the continued development of language, specifically morphological spelling and vocabulary growth. Derivational morphemes are prefixes and suffixes that change the meaning of words and oftentimes their syntactical function as well. We can explore this by looking at the word *happy*. This word by itself is an adjective used to modify a noun and indicate a communally understood level of joy. If one adds the simple prefix *un-* to the word, the meaning is now completely opposite (*unhappy*). Likewise, if one adds the suffix *-ness* to the word (*happiness*), the syntactical category changes from adjective to noun, affecting its place and

purpose in a sentence. Now let's examine the same issue with a more challenging word for a school-age child: *finite*. By definition, this adjective means having bounds or limits. If we add the prefix *in-* to *finite* then the meaning changes to an opposite—limitless or without boundaries (*infinite*). Now if we take the word *infinite* and add the suffix *-y* we have the noun *infinity*. This is a common term used in math and science, meaning a limitless numerical value.

Clearly a strong morphological knowledge is helpful for the school-age child to make meaning of new words with changes in derivational morphemes. There are well over 500,000 words in the English language and hundreds of derivational affixes that can be added to the beginnings or ends of words, resulting in an infinite number of possibilities. Therefore, in the school-age years, knowing the meaning of the word *happy* or *finite* is just as important as knowing the meaning of the derivational morphemes, *un-, in-, -ness*, and *-y*. Having an understanding of the meanings of derivational morphemes is important for both comprehending and producing academic language and should be considered across four language modalities.

Spelling

Returning to spelling, morphological abilities play a critical role in the spelling of words by school-age children. Remember that spelling is dependent upon phonological, orthographic, and morphological knowledge (Bahr et al., 2012; Berninger et al., 2006; Silliman et al., 2006). Morphological spelling is the application of the information presented in the previous section to the spelling of words. For example, a child may have heard the word *unhappy* and knows how to spell *happy* and has seen and used the prefix *un-* in other situations. If the child wants to spell this word for the first time, their knowledge of derivational morphemes would allow for the successful spelling of the word.

Apel and Lawrence (2011) compared children with histories of speech sound disorders to their typical peers on measures of morphological awareness in relation to spelling. Not only did children with typical development score higher on morphological awareness tasks, but these tasks accounted for much of their success in spelling. Bahr et al. (2012) studied the spelling errors of typically developing children from first through ninth grades and found that beyond fifth grade, children continue to make spelling errors that are orthographic and morphological in nature. This suggests that morphological knowledge continues to be an important area of instruction and development for school-age children up to, and likely beyond, ninth grade.

An example of the impact of morphological knowledge on spelling can be observed with the word *light*. If a child were to spell the word as "lit" or "lite," both of which are legal spellings in English, one might consider this an orthographic spelling error because the phonological information is present. However, the intended target word, and thus intended meaning, is not. Because the misspelled words are both legal spellings in English and represent other words with similar phonological information, they are considered morphological spelling errors. This is because the misspelled word represents a different meaning. Another example of this would be the commonly confused *there*, *their*, and *they're*, which all contain the same phonological information with differing orthographic spellings and different meanings. If a child were to replace one with the other, meaning is compromised, but orthography and phonology are intact. Thus, the child has made a morphological spelling error.

Syntax

Syntax is the architecture of words, phrases, and clauses toward the production of the unit known as the sentence (Shapiro, 1997). It is this structure that helps define the relationships between words. During the school-age years, children use syntax across all four modalities of language. For listening, children must understand and derive meaning from sentences heard; in contrast, for speaking, they must produce meaningful sentences for a multitude of reasons. In school, children spend most of their day listening (or so we hope), most often to discourse or connected speech; however, in the context of the classroom, children are often following directions and responding to questions. In this sense, children are processing complex syntax. For example, during a social studies lesson, a teacher likely begins by instructing students to open a particular book to a specific page or to pair up with a classmate to engage in a particular task. These directives are generally complex sentences students must respond to. Likewise, during that same social studies lesson, the teacher will ask wh- and yes/no questions, which the student must process in order to provide an appropriate response. For speaking purposes, children generally respond to questions and ask their own questions throughout the day, another task for which developed and complex syntactic abilities are necessary.

With regard to the reading and writing modalities, children are processing syntax while reading and are producing sentences when writing. To the former, studies of understanding written sentences suggest that sentence-level processing contributes considerably to reading comprehension (e.g., Abbott et al., 2010;

Adams, Clarke, & Haynes, 2009; Berninger et al., 2010; Scott, 2009). To the latter, research in the development of writing suggests that children in the primary grades (first to third) are producing written text at the word and sentence level (Berninger, Whitaker, Feng, Swanson, & Abbott, 1996). During the intermediate years (fourth to sixth) and through junior high and high school, children continue to produce text at the sentence level and moreover connect these sentences to produce meaningful text (Berninger et al., 1996; Whitaker, Berninger, Johnston, & Swanson, 1994). As children write, they must use the knowledge they have of syntax in the oral modalities and apply that to the written modalities, with the additional unique skills associated with writing (e.g., handwriting, spelling, mechanics).

The challenge for all children as they proceed through the school years is that syntax has to grow in both length and complexity to meet the academic demands of school. This is most often observed in spoken and written modalities. To quantify syntactic complexity, researchers have used a variety of different measures to capture the architecture and relationships between words, clauses, and phrases to form sentences. Interestingly, in spoken language, one cannot use the term *sentence* because by definition, a sentence is marked with an initial capital letter and final punctuation. Thus, the term *utterance* is used to describe the syntactical unit of spoken language output.

There are two primary ways to segment spoken utterances into *syntactic units*: communication units (c-units; Loban, 1976) and minimal terminable units (t-units; Hunt, 1970). According to Loban (1976), a c-unit consists of an independent clause with its modifiers and is generally reserved for spoken language analysis. According to Hunt (1970), a t-unit consists of an independent or main clause and all dependent or subordinate clauses and can be used for both spoken and written language. An independent clause can stand on its own, whereas a dependent clause cannot stand on its own. An independent clause generally has both a subject and a verb and there are no subordinating conjunctions within the clause. Dependent clauses generally have verbs but are dependent in two ways. First, the subject of the dependent clause is elided (hidden), but fret not, you can likely find it in the independent clause. Second, the dependent clause has both a subject and verb, but there is a subordinating conjunction within the clause, for example, the word *because* or *when*. The sentence "Because he was hungry" cannot be considered independent. The word *because* requires that two clauses be embedded within the sentence or t-unit. Now that we are clear on the difference between c-units, t-units, and clause types, let's return to the topic at hand: complex syntax.

According to Hunt (1970), to measure syntax, one must be able to quantify both length and complexity. To quantify length, one can count the number of sentences or utterances; however, this often becomes task-dependent. Therefore, syntactic length is better measured by calculating the average words per syntactic unit. Likewise, clause length can be measured by counting the number of words per clause. Combined, both measures provide an index for syntactic length. To quantify complexity, one can count the number of clauses per syntactic unit, referred to as the subordinate clause index. Also, one can calculate the average t-units per sentence in writing, which provides an index of main clause coordination. Syntactic complexity can also be assessed by examining the number of phrases and phrase types within syntactic units (Eisenberg et al., 2008; Scott & Stokes, 1995).

Research shows that syntactic abilities at the clause and phrase levels are necessary for children to produce and comprehend language across the four modalities (Hunt, 1970; Scott & Stokes, 1995). In a seminal paper, Hunt (1970) reported that syntax continues to develop and shows differences in both length and complexity through the high school years. Specifically, Hunt observed that students classified as low-, middle-, and high-performing pupils showed differences in syntactic length and complexity within and across grades in the expected directions. Specifically, the lower performing students produced shorter and less complex sentences, while the high performing students produced longer and more complex sentences. This has been observed to be a function of both development and genre. For example, narratives tend to be associated with less complex syntax, whereas expository genres demonstrate more complex syntax (Koutsoftas & Gray, 2012; Scott & Windsor, 2000). Beers and Nagy (2011) examined the relationships between measures of syntactic complexity and writing genre (narrative, descriptive, compare/contrast, persuasive) in children grades three to seven. Findings from this study suggested that children wrote more complex sentences (i.e., more clauses per t-unit) for persuasive essays and more dense syntax (i.e., words per clause) for descriptive essays. In a different study, Beers and Nagy (2009) examined syntactic complexity and writing quality across two genres (narrative and expository) in the writing samples of adolescents. Findings from this study showed that the words per clause were positively related to quality of expository samples, whereas the clauses per t-unit were positively related to quality for narrative samples. Combined, these findings suggest that syntactic complexity varies greatly due to the genre, age, and manner in which writing samples were collected—all of which should be considered when assessing and treating syntactic deficits in the spoken and written language of school-age children. For example, when assessing a school-age child's writing, a written language sample can be analyzed for the various syntactic measures described above and compared to developmental normative data.

Semantics

Semantic knowledge grows exponentially throughout the school years. Children are constantly bombarded with new vocabulary and must learn the meanings of these new words and how they are related to other words in their vocabulary. Think about the first time you heard the word *photosynthesis*. You were likely in a science class, perhaps biology, and the sound of the word alone was intimidating. Upon the first encounter with this word, an individual is going to make an initial link between the phonetic (word form) and semantic (meaning) information. The process of linking a word to its referent is referred to as fast mapping. Children must hear words multiple times to remember the word well enough to say it. Following initial encounters with the word, slow mapping occurs where the meaning of the word is enriched over time. During your science class, your teacher likely presented the word and explained that it is the procedure whereby plants take sunlight and turn it into food. (Please excuse the over-simplified definition; I am a speech pathologist, not a biologist.) Following the initial definition, you likely spent multiple classes enriching your knowledge of this complex process and thus enriching your knowledge of the word. For example, you may first read about it, then hear the teacher talk about it, and then conduct an experiment to illustrate the process. The initial encounter with the word was an opportunity to fast map the phonological information and the follow-up lessons were opportunities for slow mapping or enriching the meaning of this word.

After learning a word, a child must learn how the word is associated with other words in the lexicon. For example, *photosynthesis* is categorized with science words, specifically ones about plants. The word may also be related to other words with similar phonetic patterns such as *photo* or *synthesis*. Students with rich vocabulary may even be able attempt to understand the meaning of the word by using the knowledge they have about the two root words, *photo* and *synthesis*. Of course this would be impossible without understanding that the word is in the category of plants and sciences.

Semantic development during the school-age years is critical for academic success. In fact, the average high school graduate will have learned approximately 40,000 different words during the school-age years, which is an average of 5–8 new words per day (Nagy & Scott, 2000; Nippold, 2007; White, Power, & White; 1989). Furthermore, vocabulary is a critical factor in reading comprehension and written expression. The National Reading Panel identified vocabulary instruction as one of the top five critical components of reading instruction (National Institute of Child Health and Human Development, 2000). Research has demonstrated that semantic knowledge contributes greatly to reading comprehension (Abbott et al., 2010; Berninger et al., 2010; Wise, Sevcik, Morris, Lovett, & Wolf, 2007). Likewise, studies have demonstrated that semantic ability and vocabulary contribute uniquely to the writing process (Abbott et al., 2010; Berninger et al., 2010; Olinghouse & Leaird, 2009).

Vocabulary has been measured in a variety of different ways from both spoken and written language samples. Similar to syntactic analyses of language, one must be concerned with both length and complexity when it comes to vocabulary and word usage. A child who speaks or writes considerably more than peers when given the same elicitation prompt is likely to have a greater vocabulary; however, the total number of words cannot be the only index used to quantify semantic knowledge. Other considerations include lexical variety, word length, and frequency of the word in the language (Olinghouse & Leaird, 2009). Lexical variety is a common measure used to assess vocabulary complexity and is generally done by measuring the number of different words within a set amount of words. For example, one would measure the number of different root words in the first 50 or 100 words of a language sample. This measure must always be truncated so that it is comparable between students and does not replicate the total number of words produced. Lexical diversity is often affected by genre (Koutsoftas & Gray, 2012) and age (Olinghouse & Leaird, 2009). Longer words tend to represent more complex vocabulary, and so the number of syllables per word has also been used as an indicator of complex or more advanced vocabulary (Olinghouse & Leaird, 2009). The frequency of words used within samples or within a language are also strong indicators of the complexity of vocabulary. For example, in one series of studies, researchers listed all the words used in writing samples by all participants and then rank ordered these words, with the least frequently occurring words receiving higher scores (Berninger et al., 1996; Whitaker et al., 1994). Similarly, a word that is considered high frequency in the English language (e.g., *have, chair, under*) would receive lower scores then less commonly occurring words (e.g., *egress, colloquial, heretofore*) (Olinghouse & Leaird, 2009).

Nippold (2007) identified three primary methods that promote the learning of new words in school-age children: direct instruction, contextual abstraction, and morphological analysis. Direct instruction is simply when a teacher, parent, or peer provides the meaning of a new word for a student. This can be accomplished in many ways, two of which are discussed here. First, the student comes across a word they do not understand and seeks out the definition by asking a teacher, parent, or peer, to which the reply is a definition of the word. Second, the student seeks the definition of a word from a dictionary, either paper form or online. The difficulty with the second option is that one word may have multiple definitions and the student must use the context of the word to select the best definition. A second method that promotes the learning of new words is contextual abstraction, which is the use of context to glean the meaning of a novel word. For example, in the previous sentence, the word *glean* was used and may be novel to the reader of this book. However, using the information within the sentence, that precedes and follows the word, along with information in nearby sentences, the reader is able to figure out the meaning from context. Incidentally, in this context, *glean* means "to learn, discover, or find out." The third method that promotes the learning of new words is morphological analysis. This was previewed earlier in the section on morphology, where I explained that knowing the meaning of affixes such as *un-* and *-ness* would help students glean the meanings of the words *unlikely* or *likeliness*. In addition to knowing the meanings of affixes, students must also understand and identify root words within the morphologically bound words and realize that by adding an affix, the part of speech changes, from noun to adjective, for example. Sometimes, this is obvious or transparent as in the word *unlikely* or *likeliness*. Other times, it is more difficult or opaque, especially when the addition of the affix changes the root word pronunciation or spelling. For example, the suffix *-ate* can be added to the root word *predict*, changing the word to *predicate*, where both the spelling and pronunciation of the root word change form.

It is not likely that a teacher is going to directly present and teach five to eight new words per day across the school-age child's academic career. Therefore, contextual abstraction and morphological analysis play larger roles in how the school-age child's vocabulary grows and develops. To be specific, school-age children are learning most of these five to eight new words per day from reading complex texts across multiple genres and from listening to these words being spoken to them by teachers, parents, and peers.

A challenge for semantic instruction for school-age children is selecting the appropriate words to teach. Beck, McKeown, and Kucan (2002) suggest a three-tiered approach to categorizing words based on their utility. The first tier, tier 1 words, includes basic words that do not require much teaching because they are of high frequency or utility in language. Examples of tier 1 words include *table, walk, picture, computer, sit.* Tier 1 words do not require direct instruction, and children will likely know the meanings of these words without context. The second tier, tier 2 words, includes high frequency words that occur across multiple domains. These are words that are used commonly across all classrooms, subjects, and individuals. Examples of tier 2 words include *essential, conclude, predict, summary.* Tier 2 words may require direct instruction; however, the school-age child is more likely to gain understanding of these words through contextual abstraction and morphological analysis. The third tier, tier 3 words, includes words that are less frequent and more domain-specific. For the school-age child, tier 3 words are subject-specific and represent complex or abstract concepts. Examples of tier 3 words include *photosynthesis, industrialization,* and *exponent.* Tier 3 words generally require direct instruction along with enrichment of the meaning of the word through a variety of teaching strategies in the classroom.

Pragmatics: Discourse

Until now, I have discussed four of the domains of language discretely, separating them from their use in context. Oftentimes, especially with clinical populations, discrete instruction in phonology, morphology, syntax, and semantics is warranted. Students may require instruction for phonological and phonemic awareness, spelling, morphological inflections, syntactic structures, and vocabulary. In reality, language in schools is presented at the discourse level, meaning that language is processed and produced by the school-age child in connected forms that involve stringing sounds together to form words, words to form sentences, and sentences to form discourse.

Discourse is defined as groups of utterances or sustained exchanges combined in cohesive ways to convey meaning (Merritt & Culatta, 1998). Instructional discourse is the particular type of exchange used in schools between teachers and students for the purpose of enhancing knowledge, guiding comprehension, developing skills, and processing connected text (Merritt & Culatta, 1998). In schools, this is observed in a variety of forms. Teachers provide classroom instruction, directions, lectures, and lessons and use discourse levels of language to convey

this information. Students must then comprehend this discourse while listening and attending to instruction. Children must learn that the pragmatics of speaking to a peer differ from the pragmatics of speaking to a teacher.

Discourse can also be observed in written texts or books where information is strung together in a storybook or textbook, in social studies or science, for example. Students produce discourse when speaking to their teachers and classmates and in the written form when writing stories, essays, book reports, and term papers (i.e., expository discourse). Merritt and Culatta (1998) provide a framework for discourse instruction and suggest that organization, content, and genre be considered when understanding how instructional discourse works. These three traits are related and can be observed across all kinds of instructional discourse whether classroom instruction, group discussion, or when read from text.

Organization refers to the complexity of discourse in terms of text elements and topics (Merritt & Culatta, 1998). For example, simple discourse has less complex organization with few levels of subordination and likely follows a sequential order, whereas complex discourse has multiple levels of organization with a great deal of subordination. Considering the other domains of language, specifically syntax and semantics, one would observe less complex syntax and more transparent or tier 1 and tier 2 words in simply organized discourse. Conversely, complex discourse would contain complex and lengthy syntax with multiple subordinating and coordinating clauses and likely contain less frequently observed vocabulary consisting of tier 2 and tier 3 words.

Content refers to the familiarity of concepts and subject matter being taught (Merritt & Culatta, 1998). The content of instructional discourse can vary from concrete and familiar concepts to abstract and unfamiliar concepts. Content is affected by children's background knowledge and motivation. For example, a child who goes to school in a rural farm community brings with them different background knowledge than the child who goes to school in a major city. Even then, background knowledge is variable within the rural or city school community and each child has their own unique experience that informs their background knowledge and how they acquire content. A social studies unit on agriculture and how food is processed would be more concrete for the rural farm student and quite abstract for the city student. Likewise, a social studies unit on public transportation would be familiar to a child schooled in the city and unfamiliar to a child who grows up on a farm.

Genre refers to the type or purpose of text or discourse (Merritt & Culatta, 1998). It can range from informal and personal to formal and impersonal, and this goes across different genre types that include narrative, expository, and persuasive, to name a few. Less formal genres likely contain content familiar to the student with more simply organized text; therefore, the syntax and semantics would be transparent for the student. More formal genres contain unfamiliar or abstract content with more complex organization and thus opaque syntax and semantics. The formality of genre is not dependent upon the type of genre. For example, science and social studies textbooks, which would be considered expository text, can range in how formally the information is presented. Furthermore, narrative texts found in the literature curriculum can range in familiarity from simple sequential stories with few characters to complexly organized epics with multiple generations of characters.

Research shows that both narrative and expository discourse have structures that children must learn (Merritt & Liles, 1987; Nippold, Mansfield, Billow, & Tomblin, 2008; Scott & Windsor, 2000). Narrative retells or stories (whether spoken or written) will include story grammar elements such as initiating events (i.e., problem), attempts to solve the problem, and solutions. Other story grammar elements include settings, internal responses of characters (i.e., feelings), and story endings. Merritt and Liles (1987) found that children construct narratives that include initiating events, attempts, and consequences and that these narratives were judged to be complete. Because children begin telling narratives as early as 2 years old (McCabe & Rollins, 1994), by the time they get to formal schooling, they are quite good at producing oral narratives. A major challenge in school becomes how to produce these in a written form. Expository discourse also has a formal structure; however, these structures vary depending upon the purpose of the discourse (Merritt & Culatta, 1998). Expository structures include topic and detail structures, cause/effect structures, and temporal structures, to name a few. For example, in a history class, one might retell a series of events that would require a temporal structure. An elaboration on these events that provides specific details would be a topic and detail structure. Lastly, if the event caused a noteworthy historical event, then a cause/effect structure might be in order. What differs between narrative and expository discourse is that children are exposed to narrative genres much earlier than expository genres. It is likely that many children only listen to and are asked to produce expository discourse for the first time during the elementary school years. The challenge for all students then becomes learning the different expository structures and then how to comprehend and produce these across all four modalities of language.

As part of the instructional discourse of schools, one must consider the social or pragmatic nature of the classroom too. For example, students are generally expected to raise their hands when they have a comment or question. Yet, we have all observed the student who calls out an answer or asks a question without the expected hand-raise. This student may not be aware of the social pragmatics of the classroom for a variety of reasons. In fact, I have been in elementary school classrooms where hand-raising was not required and the class ran as flawlessly as can be expected. Westby (1997) discusses this in terms of "learning to do school" and suggests that in addition to the academic curriculum of school, students must also learn the social curriculum within the classroom as well as with peers outside of the classroom.

Another important area to consider is nonliteral language. Nonliteral language includes idioms, metaphors, similes, humor, proverbs, and abstraction. Many of us have been exposed to these terms in a language arts classroom and remember simple rules such as "similes use the word *like* or *as* and metaphors do not." What is important to note is that nonliteral language is used by teachers and students throughout the academic day from kindergarten through high school. It is only when we are exposed to the metalinguistic rules presented in a language arts class that we become aware of the structure of this nonliteral language. This is important because children with language impairments, including children with learning disabilities and mild to severe autism, will not comprehend this nonliteral language. So, for example, the kindergarten teacher who uses the idiom "It's raining cats and dogs" may see one or two students walk over to the window to look for a new puppy or kitten.

Discourse levels of language in the school-age years are complex and involve many considerations, from instructional discourse to social pragmatics. Not all of this is obvious or attainable for all students, especially those who struggle with language. By understanding the role discourse plays and that phonological, morphological, syntactic, and semantic abilities are subsumed within discourse and pragmatics, one can identify language deficits that contribute to academic difficulties and target them during intervention.

▶ Written Language

It is important to introduce the reader to a more in-depth look at the written modalities of language (reading and writing). While other sources provide an overview of literacy development, which includes a definition of literacy, development of emergent literacy skills, definitions for what literacy is, and a review of relationships between spoken language deficits and later reading difficulties, this discussion extends that information to further explore the relationships between oral and written language in spoken and written forms and applications of these skills to children in schools.

Written language refers to print—both how we comprehend it (reading) and how we produce it (writing). If "language is a code whereby ideas about the world are expressed through a conventional system of arbitrary signals for communication" (Lahey, 1988, p.2), then the written code may have gone a step further by introducing quite arbitrary shapes to represent sounds (i.e., letters) that are strung together to shape words and sentences, which when combined carry simple to complex meanings. Yet, we are all able to figure out this code and are able to gain meaning from print. In some instances, it just takes a lot more instruction on the code and a whole lot of instruction in comprehending. Let's review current theories about how reading and writing work.

Reading

The *Simple View of Reading* (Hoover & Gough, 1990) is the most prominent theoretical model used to describe reading comprehension. The simple view of reading suggests that reading comprehension is the product of decoding and linguistic comprehension, depicted as follows:

$$\text{Reading Comprehension} = \text{Decoding} \times \text{Linguistic Comprehension}$$

Decoding is the process of translating orthographic symbols into phonemic symbols to decipher the meaning of printed words (Cunningham, 2005). Word attack skills are those a child uses to decode orthographic symbols, and they include decoding individual sounds (phonemes), chunks of words (morphemes), and words within sentences (semantics). For example, the young reader will need to sound out the three phonemes in the word *dog*. More sophisticated readers will use their morphological skills to decode the word *doggy* by delineating the word *dog* and the additional morpheme *-y* in chunks. These word attack skills vary by child and developmental ability.

Linguistic comprehension is what we understand as the comprehension of language at the phonological, morphological, syntactic, semantic, and discourse

(pragmatics) levels. In this way, the simple view of reading suggests that reading comprehension is based on the relationship of both decoding and linguistic comprehension. For example, if a child were to have age-appropriate linguistic comprehension and no decoding ability, there would be no reading comprehension. Likewise, if a child were able to decode print but had poor linguistic comprehension ability, there would be no reading comprehension. Furthermore, if a child is able to decode print at levels at or above their own developmental level, their reading comprehension would still only be as good as what their linguistic comprehension allows.

The National Reading Panel identified five critical areas that should be targeted when providing instruction in reading (National Institute of Child Health and Human Development, 2000). These are phonemic awareness, phonics, fluency, vocabulary, and text comprehension. Relating these areas to the simple view of reading, the skills of phonemic awareness, phonics, and fluency are associated with the decoding portion of the model, while vocabulary and text comprehension are associated with the linguistic comprehension side of the model. Phonological and morphological abilities, as described in previous sections, are also necessary for improving skill in phonemic awareness and phonics, thus contributing to reading fluency. Semantic, syntactic, and pragmatic knowledge is associated with the linguistic comprehension side of the model. Specific skills associated with the five domains of language and reading comprehension are discussed in more detail in the section on the five domains of language.

Writing

When it comes to writing, there are two prominent theoretical models used to explain writing, the writing process model (Hayes & Berninger, 2014) and the simple view of writing (Berninger & Amtmann, 2003). Within the writing process model (Hayes & Berninger, 2014), writing is the end product of planning, translating, and revising. *Planning* includes idea generation, goal setting, and organization. *Translating* includes two subcomponents: transcription and text generation (Berninger, 1999). Transcription includes the skills of handwriting and spelling, whereas text generation includes the production of written language at the word, sentence, and text levels. *Revising* includes the ability to read and edit text that has been written. Research shows that children in the primary grades (first through third) attend to the translating process, but not until the end of the intermediate grades (fourth through sixth) are children able to attend to the planning and revising components (Berninger et al., 1996; Whitaker et al., 1994).

The simple view of writing (Berninger & Amtmann, 2003) suggests that writing involves text generation, transcription, and executive functions. Specifically, *text generation* at the word, sentence, and discourse levels is the result of transcription and executive functions where *transcription* is still defined as handwriting and spelling abilities. Notably, executive functions related to writing are more clearly defined and highlighted in the simple view of writing. *Executive functions* related to writing include conscious attention, planning, reviewing, revising, and self-regulation.

▶ Application to Adam: A Case Study of School-Age Language Demands

This case study provides a common example of how breakdowns in any part of language can disrupt learning.

CASE HISTORY FOR ADAM, A STUDENT WITH A LANGUAGE-LEARNING DISABILITY

Adam is a fifth-grade student who is identified as having a language-based learning disability. His IQ is within normal limits, with his nonverbal performance quotient slightly higher than his verbal performance quotient. According to standardized language testing, his overall language ability falls about 1.5 standard deviations below the mean, with specific difficulties producing complex sentences and explaining the relationships between words that are similar. This testing further suggests that he is able to follow simple two-step directions; however, complex two-step directions that involve temporal or spatial concepts are challenging to him. Adam's language testing results are consistent with his classroom performance.

In the classroom, Adam is always one or two steps behind his classmates when the teacher provides classroom instructions. He is able to spell words he knows with similar accuracy to his classroom peers. New words present two challenges for Adam. First, it takes him more time to learn to spell the word compared to his peers, and second, he is rarely able to recall the words to use in context or provide meanings for these words. Because of this, he rarely passes his weekly spelling and vocabulary tests. When it comes to reading, Adam is able to read classroom material with similar accuracy to his peers; however, his reading fluency is somewhat slower than his classmates. Adam has difficulty understanding what he reads; this is demonstrated by not being able to retell narrative or expository text with similar accuracy to his classmates. Furthermore, he does poorly on multiple choice and short answer questions about the text he reads. Adam enjoys listening to classroom read alouds by his teacher and is able to retell these stories with better accuracy than when he reads stories himself. Unfortunately, as the school year goes on, there is less opportunity for classroom read alouds, especially in the fifth-grade classroom. With regard to writing, Adam is able to produce short narrative stories and expository essays. Although he is able to generate good ideas for his writing, when translating these ideas to paper, his difficulties with spelling, semantics, and syntax become obvious. He generally has difficulty spelling less frequent words and his writing demonstrates less variety in word choice with simple sentences.

Adam does well in mathematics. He is able to perform mathematical operations (addition, multiplication, subtraction, division) of multidigit whole numbers with decimals up to the hundredths place, which is consistent with the fifth-grade math curriculum. In fact, he is really good at this and enjoys math very much because of this. He is able to extend this knowledge to fractions as well and apply his strong math skills to measurement problems. Difficulties are observed when it comes to word problems. He is able to easily extract the numbers from a word problem; however, he often performs the incorrect mathematical operation. This is likely due to two factors: first, his difficulties understanding what he reads, and second, his difficulties with vocabulary.

Adam enjoys art, music, and gym classes tremendously and has quite a few friends in his class and schoolwide. He is what you would call a social butterfly and he gets along well with peers and teachers. His parents are supportive and understand his difficulties with language, and they make ample time to help him with his homework. He receives speech-language therapy twice weekly in a group no larger than five. The school is considering adding a special education support in the form of a resource room to provide Adam additional supports when he struggles academically.

Adam's profile is similar to many of the cases clinicians will face in a school setting where strengths and weaknesses are apparent. Considering the five domains of language and how they are observed across four modalities provides an opportunity to understand the language demands of school for Adam. Adam is considered to have a language-learning disability because his deficits in language negatively impact his academic success and impede learning. As we have learned by now, learning in schools is highly dependent upon language, and breakdowns in language could result in academic failure.

Adam's Language Demands Across Five Domains of Language

Adam's case study provides an opportunity to explore deficits in language across five domains. Adam has general comprehension difficulties with obvious difficulties with semantics and syntax. Regarding phonology, Adam reads somewhat less fluently than peers, suggesting that deficits in language could be affecting his phonemic awareness and thus compromising his decoding. He has phonological deficits in spelling, where Adam has difficulty spelling new words. This, however, could also be related to difficulties with orthographic and morphological knowledge. Morphological deficits could also contribute to Adam's vocabulary deficits. He does not understand many words and has a limited vocabulary. It is possible that his difficulties with language could affect morphological analysis of new words. Further, his difficulty with reading fluently and understanding complex syntax may impede his ability to contextually abstract the meanings of novel words. Although Adam is able to decode text with the same proficiency as peers, his comprehension of this text is an area of weakness. This is likely attributable to general deficits in language. Remember the simple view of reading where comprehension is the product of decoding and linguistic comprehension; given observed difficulties with both aspects of the model, reading comprehension for Adam is compromised.

Adam's syntactic and semantic difficulties likely contribute to his difficulties with writing as well as math. When it comes to writing, Adam has good ideas but has difficulty transforming these ideas to writing. Specifically, his writing lacks lexical variety and consists of simple sentences. These deficits were observed in his spoken language and, consequently, his writing demonstrates these same deficiencies. Because of his limited vocabulary and poor syntax, his writing scores on standardized tests will likely suffer despite his good ideas. When it comes to math, Adam is able to perform mathematical operations that are expected by fifth graders. Where he suffers is when it comes to word problems, which are prevalent in the fifth-grade math curriculum. For example, Adam can easily divide fractions; however, when the same information is presented in text, he cannot identify the type of mathematical operation he needs to perform. This is likely due to his difficulties with reading comprehension, which are rooted in his semantic and syntactic deficits.

Summary

In summary, the five domains of language are evident across all four modalities of language. Moreover, the critical role language plays toward academic success has been unpacked for the early student in language development and disorders. This chapter has described the five modalities of language rather discretely from one another. It is important to understand that these skills are nested together and are dependent upon one another. For example, children cannot spell if they cannot delineate sounds. Likewise, children cannot write a sentence if they cannot formulate one orally. Further, you cannot form a sentence without understanding where in discourse it is to appear and without the use of morphological markers to make meaning certain and precise. The point is that these five domains of language work in concert with the four modalities of language. Lastly, language is the primary tool for academic success and development of school-age children.

Application of this conceptualization of language in the school years provides an insight into the language deficits and how they affect academics in the case example of Adam. The early student in language development and disorders can apply knowledge of the five domains of language across four modalities to the case study of Adam. This allows a better understanding of the critical and important role that language plays during the school-age years and an understanding of the detriments of breakdowns in language function.

Study Questions

- Describe and differentiate the four modalities of language and then describe how the five domains of language are observed across the four modalities.
- Explain the simple view of reading and then indicate which domains of language play a critical role in the process. Do the same for the simple view of writing.
- Identify and describe one unique skill associated with each of the four modalities of language.
- Explain the current academic standards, namely the CCSS (2012), and how these standards are related to the language needs of children during the school years.

References

Abbott, R. D., Berninger, V. W., & Fayol, M. (2010). Longitudinal relationships of levels of language in writing and between writing and reading in grades 1 to 7. *Journal of Educational Psychology, 102,* 281–298.

Adams, C., Clarke, E., & Haynes, R. (2009). Inference and sentence comprehension in children with specific or pragmatic language impairments. *International Journal of Language & Communication Disorders, 44,* 301–318.

Apel, K., & Lawrence, J. (2011). Contributions of morphological awareness skills to word-level reading and spelling in first-grade children with and without speech sound disorder. *Journal of Speech, Language, and Hearing Research, 54*(5), 1312–1327.

Bahr, R. H., Silliman, E. R., Berninger, V. W., & Dow, M. (2012). Linguistic pattern analysis of misspellings of typically developing writers in grades 1 to 9. *Journal of Speech, Language, and Hearing Research, 55,* 1587–1599. doi:10.1044/1092-4388(2012/10-0335)

Beck, I. L., McKeown, M. G., & Kucan, L. (2002). *Bringing words to life: Robust vocabulary instruction.* New York, NY: The Guilford Press.

Beers, S. F., & Nagy, W. E. (2009). Syntactic complexity as a predictor of adolescent writing quality: Which measures? Which genre? *Reading and Writing, 22*(2), 185–200.

Beers, S. F., & Nagy, W. E. (2011). Writing development in four genres from grades three to seven: Syntactic complexity and genre differentiation. *Reading and Writing, 24*(2), 183–202.

Berninger, V. W. (1999). Coordinating transcription and text generation in working memory during composing: Automatic and constructive processes. *Learning Disability Quarterly, 22*(2), 99–112.

Berninger, V. W. (2000). Development of language by hand and its connections with language by ear, mouth, and eye. *Topics in Language Disorders, 20*(4), 65–84.

Berninger, V. W., & Abbott, R. D. (2010). Listening comprehension, oral expression, reading comprehension, and written expression: Related yet unique language systems in grades 1, 3, 5, and 7. *Journal of Educational Psychology, 102*(3), 635–651.

Berninger, V. W., Abbott, R. D., Nagy, W., & Carlisle, J. (2006). Growth in phonological, orthographic, and morphological awareness in grades 1 to 6. *Journal of Psycholinguistic Research, 39*(2), 141–163.

Berninger, V. W., Abbott, R. D., Swanson, H. L., Lovitt, D., Trivedi, P., Lin, S., … Amtmann D. (2010). Relationship of word- and sentence-level working memory to reading and writing in second, fourth, and sixth grade. *Language, Speech, and Hearing Services in Schools, 41,* 179–193.

Berninger, V. W., & Amtmann, D. (2003). Preventing written expression disabilities through early and continuing assessment and intervention for handwriting and/or spelling problems: Research into practice. In H. L. Swanson, K. Harris, & S. Graham (Eds.), *Handbook of learning difficulties* (pp. 345–363). New York, NY: Guilford Press.

Berninger, V., Whitaker, D., Feng, Y., Swanson, H. L., & Abbott, R. D. (1996). Assessment of planning, translating, and revising in junior high writers. *Journal of School Psychology, 54*(1), 23–52.

Brown, R. (1973). *A first language.* Cambridge, MA: Harvard University Press.

Catts, H. W. (1993). The relationship between speech-language impairments and reading disabilities. *Journal of Speech and Hearing Research, 36,* 948–958.

Catts, H. W., Fey, M. E., Tomblin, J. B., & Zhang, X. (2002). A longitudinal investigation of reading outcomes in children with language impairments. *Journal of Speech, Language, and Hearing Research, 45,* 1142–1157.

Common Core State Standards Initiative. (2012). *Common core state standards for English language arts and literacy in history/social studies, science, and technical subjects.* Retrieved from www.corestandards.org

Cunningham, P. M. (2005). *Phonics they use: Words for reading and writing* (4th ed.). New York, NY: Pearson.

Eisenberg, S. L., Ukrainetz, T. A., Hsu, J. R., Kaderavek, J. N., Justice, L. M., & Gillam, R. B. (2008). Noun phrase elaboration in children's spoken stories. *Language, Speech, and Hearing Services in Schools, 39,* 145–157.

Hayes, J. R., & Berninger, V. W. (2014). Cognitive processes in writing: A framework. In B. Arfe, J. Dockrell, & V. W. Berninger (Eds.), *Writing development in children with hearing loss, dyslexia, or oral language problems* (pp. 3–15). New York, NY: Oxford.

Hoover, W. A., & Gough, P. B. (1990). The simple view of reading. *Reading and Writing: An Interdisciplinary Journal, 2,* 127–160.

Hunt, K. W. (1970). Syntactic maturity in schoolchildren and adults. *Monographs of the Society for Research in Child Development, 35*(1), 1–67.

Koutsoftas, A. D., & Gray, S. (2012). Comparison of narrative and expository writing students with and without language-learning disabilities. *Language, Speech, and Hearing Services in Schools, 43*(4), 395–409.

Lahey, M. (1988) *Language disorders and language development.* New York, NY: Macmillan.

Loban, W. (1976). *Language development: Kindergarten through grade twelve* (Report No. 18). Urbana, IL: National Council of Teachers of English.

McCabe, A., & Rollins, P. R. (1994). Assessment of preschool narrative skills. *American Journal of Speech Language Pathology, 3,* 45–56.

Merritt, D. D., & Culatta, B. (1998). *Language intervention in the classroom.* San Diego, CA: Singular.

Merritt, D. D., & Liles, B. Z. (1987). Story grammar ability in children with and without language disorder: Story generation, story retelling, and story comprehension. *Journal of Speech and Hearing Research, 30*(4), 539–552.

Nagy, W. E., & Scott, J. A. (2000). Vocabulary processes. In M. L. Kamil, P. B. Mosenthal, & R. Barr (Eds.), *Handbook of reading research* (Vol. 3, pp. 269–284). Mahwah, NJ: Erlbaum.

National Institute of Child Health and Human Development. (2000). *Report of the National Reading Panel. Teaching children to read: An evidence-based assessment of the scientific research literature on reading and its implications for reading instruction* (NIH Publication No. 00-4769). Washington, DC: U.S. Government Printing Office.

Nippold, M. A. (2007). *Later language development: School-age children, adolescents, and young adults* (3rd ed.). Austin, TX: Pro-Ed.

Nippold, M. A., Mansfield, T. C., Billow, J. L., & Tomblin, J. B. (2008). Expository discourse in adolescents with language impairments: Examining syntactic development. *American Journal of Speech-Language Pathology, 17*, 356–366.

Olinghouse, N. G., & Leaird, J. T. (2009). The relationship between measures of vocabulary and narrative writing quality in second- and fourth-grade students. *Reading and Writing: An Interdisciplinary Journal, 22*, 545–565.

Scott, C. M. (2009). A case for the sentence in reading comprehension. *Language, Speech, and Hearing Services in Schools, 40*(2), 184–191.

Scott, C. M., & Stokes, S. L. (1995). Measures of syntax in school-age children and adolescents. *Language, Speech, and Hearing Services in Schools, 26*, 309–319.

Scott, C. M., & Windsor, J. (2000). General language performance measures in spoken and written narrative and expository discourse of school-age children with language learning disabilities. *Journal of Speech, Language, and Hearing Research, 43*(2), 324.

Schuele, C. M. & Murphy, N. D. (2014). *The intensive phonological awareness program.* Baltimore, MD: Brookes Publishing.

Shapiro, L. P. (1997). Tutorial: An introduction to syntax. *Journal of Speech, Language, and Hearing Research, 40*, 254–272.

Silliman, E. R., Bahr, R., & Peters, M. L. (2006). Spelling patterns in preadolescents with atypical language skills: Phonological, morphological, and orthographic factors. *Developmental Neuropsychology, 29*(1), 93–123.

Westby, C. (1997). There's more to passing than knowing the answers. *Language, Speech, and Hearing Services in Schools, 28*, 274–287.

Whitaker, D., Berninger, V. W., Johnston, J., & Swanson, H. L. (1994). Intraindividual differences in levels of language in intermediate grade writers: Implications for the translating process. *Learning and Individual Differences, 6*(1) 107–130.

White, T. G., Power, M. A., & White, S. (1989). Morphological analysis: Implications for teaching and understanding vocabulary growth. *Reading Research Quarterly, 24*, 283–304.

Windsor, J., Scott, C. M., & Street, C. K. (2000). Verb and noun morphology in the spoken and written language of children with language learning disabilities. *Journal of Speech, Language, and Hearing Research, 43*(6), 1322.

Wise, J. C., Sevcik, R. A., Morris, R. D., Lovett, M. W., & Wolf, M. (2007). The relationship among receptive and expressive vocabulary, listening comprehension, pre-reading skills, word identification skills, and reading comprehension by children with reading disabilities. *Journal of Speech, Language, and Hearing Research, 50*(4), 1093–1109.

Language Development from Unique Perspectives: Neurological, Cultural, and Other Clinical Applications

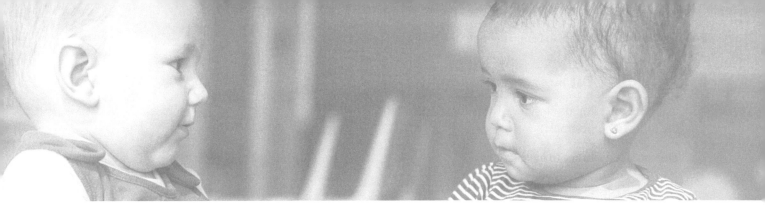

CHAPTER 12

Mapping Language onto the Brain

Nina Capone Singleton, PhD, CCC-SLP

OBJECTIVES

- To learn the history of neurolinguistics
- To understand the anatomy and neural circuitry that subserve language
- To understand the influence of language experience, genetics, and epigenetics on brain development
- To identify the neurolinguistics of language impairments

KEY TERMS

Arcuate fasciculus
Axon terminals
Axons
Broca's area
Brodmann area
Caudal
Cell bodies
Cerebellum
Cerebral cortex
Coronal plane
Corpus callosum
Dendrites
Diencephalon
Dorsal
Epigenetics
Event-related brain potentials (ERP)

Fissure
Frontal lobe
Functional magnetic resonance
 imaging (fMRI)
Gray matter
Gyrus
Inferior parietal lobule
Language transparency
Left anterior front lobe
Longitudinal fissure
Neuron
Occipital lobe
Parietal lobe
Perisylvian language zone
Phenotype
Phrenology

Planum temporale
Primary sensory areas
Prosody
Rostral
Sagittal plane
Sensitive period
Sensory association areas
Soma
Subcortical
Sulcus
Superior longitudinal
 fasciculus
Temporal lobe
Ventral
Wernicke's area
White matter tracts

▶ Introduction

During a professional interview, I was once asked the following question:

"Do you need a brain to have language?"

It was a trick question of sorts only because it was unexpected. The answer is unequivocally "yes". Language—the sounds, words, and structures—is represented in the *cerebral cortex*. Processing language also relies on *subcortical* pathways and *cerebellar* structures. We return to define these terms later.

In this text, we take some of the language behaviors you learned earlier and map them onto the brain. At first, terms may seem overwhelming like learning a foreign language. In fact, many neuroanatomical terms derive from Latin. This text eases unnecessary doubt that the neurology of language can be learned by you, the student of language. I want to be sure that you can identify basic brain structures involved in typical language processing. As in other texts, there are clinical applications.

▶ Making References to the Brain in Direction and Planes

Just as we use terms such as north, south, left, right, up, and down to indicate direction, there are terms to orient the clinical scientist to the brain and its structures. These are *ventral*, *dorsal*, *caudal*, and *rostral* (see **FIGURE 12-1**). The ventral surface refers to the underside of the brain. Dorsal surface refers to the upper surface and continues to the backside of the brain. When identifying structures in relation to one another, *caudal* refers to a structure that is "moving toward the tail" relative to another structure, and *rostral* makes reference to "moving toward the head." For example, when referring to the three structures of the brainstem in Figure 12-1, we can say the pons of the brain stem is caudal to the midbrain, but the pons is rostral to the medulla oblongata.

To find structures that lie deep inside the brain, we visualize the brain in slices or planes. Two of the possible planes used to orient to the brain are—the *sagittal plane* and the *coronal plane*. The sagittal plane slices the brain down the middle into hemispheres so that each eye and each ear falls on either side of the cut, and the nose would slice down the middle (see Figure 12-1). A coronal cut is perpendicular to the sagittal plane. A coronal plane slices the brain like a loaf of bread—behind both eyes, behind both ears,

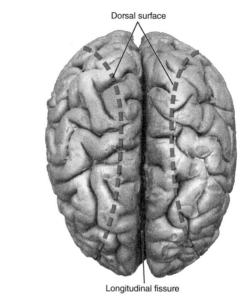

(a)

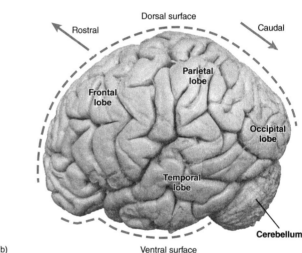

(b)

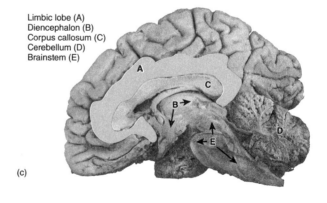

(c)

FIGURE 12-1 Major structures and directional terms of the brain. (a) Dorsal view of the brain's hemispheres. (b) Lateral view of the brain's left hemisphere. (c) Sagittal plane slice gives a medial view of the brain's right hemisphere.

Photos courtesy of Kirchgessner, A., PhD., and Capone Singleton, N., PhD, SLP-CCC.

etc. Reference to the brain using these directions and planes makes for easier reference to structural anatomy.

Gray Matter Versus White Matter

When you feel the brain, it is hard, dense, and compact. On the outside, it looks gray. This *gray matter* is densely packed with *cell bodies*. Pulling open the brain, teasing it apart, and separating it out a bit more help the *white matter tracts* become visible. White matter tracts are what connect the cell bodies to each other by their *axons*. What is being described here is a *neuron*. **FIGURE 12-2** illustrates the neuron. Parts of the neuron are:

- *Soma*—The cell body that integrates electrical signals
- *Dendrites*—Receive/collect information from other neurons at their synapses
- *Axon*—Conducts information away from the cell body
- *Axon terminals*—Transmit information to other neurons

Neurons transmit electrical (within the neuron) and chemical (between neurons) signals (Vanderah & Gould, 2016, p. 2). The transmission of electrical and chemical signals is how neurons communicate information. Many axons traveling together form a white matter tract. Information travels through the brain along white matter tracts and stops along the way at other cell body centers. Intermittent stopping between the cell body centers coordinates white matter and gray matter communication (Leonard, 2014).

The cerebral cortex is the exterior part of the brain you typically see in pictures, with its valleys or grooves—called *sulci*—and its hills—called *gyri*. (Singular forms are *sulcus* and *gyrus*, respectively). A very deep sulcus is a *fissure*. The cerebral cortex has a significant role in cognitive functioning, in addition to motor and sensory functioning. Cognitive functions include language, memory, problem solving, critical thinking, math, and more. The cellular structure that makes up the layers of the cortex is complex, and its details are well beyond the scope of this text. However, it is important to understand that white matter tracts course:

- Between cortical regions within a hemisphere
- Between cortical regions across hemispheres
- Between cortical and subcortical structures
- In and out of the brainstem and spinal column

This rich network of connections between neural areas allows children's experiences to be integrated. When experiences are integrated, they are perceived as meaningful.

Structures of the Brain

Harkening back to the start of this text, the brain is sectioned into large parts first—the cerebral cortex, the subcortical structures (including the *diencephalon*), the *cerebellum*, and the *brainstem*. Within each of these large sections, there are structures with specialized functions. Interconnections exist between the cerebral cortex and the subcortical brain as well as the cerebellum and the brain stem.

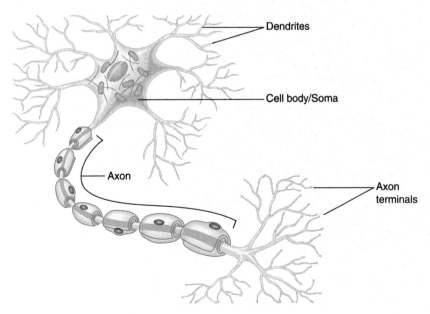

FIGURE 12-2 Parts of a neuron and communication pattern within and between neurons.

Cerebral Cortex

The cerebral cortex is the outermost layered surface of the brain that folds over the subcortical structures. "Sub" means the structures are "under" or "buried within" the cerebral cortex. The cerebral cortex has two subdivisions, or hemispheres, by the sagittal plane along the *longitudinal fissure*. The longitudinal fissure runs along the dorsal aspect of the brain. A lateral fissure runs along the side of each hemisphere. The *perisylvian language zone* abuts the lateral fissure (see **FIGURE 12-3**) on the left hemisphere. These structures are discussed again later. The *corpus callosum* connects the left and right hemispheres of the brain by crossing the midline between them. The corpus callosum is a substantial white matter tract. It is visualized on the medial surface of the brain (see Figure 12-1). From a sagittal cut along the longitudinal fissure, or along several coronal cuts, one can see the corpus callosum.

In addition to the left-right hemispheres division, the brain has boundaries attributed to lobes. There are four lobes visible from the outside of the brain (see Figure 12-1). These lobes are:

- Frontal lobe
- Parietal lobe
- Temporal lobe
- Occipital lobe

There is one lobe visible from the medial surface of the brain—the limbic lobe—and another that is a hidden lobe deep in the cerebral cortex of the frontal lobe—the insula. **TABLE 12-1** shows the most striking functions of each lobe, subcortical structure, and the cerebellum, although other functions may exist. Each

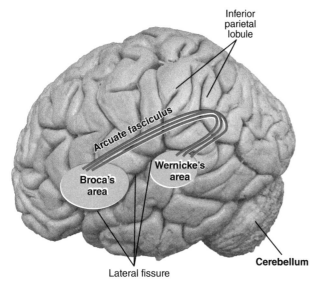

FIGURE 12-3 Select brain areas and landmarks involved in language processing.

Photos courtesy of Kirchgessner, A., PhD., and Capone Singleton, N., PhD, CCC-SLP.

of these lobes then has a left and a right hemisphere by division of the sagittal plane.

Brodmann Areas

Brodmann areas (BA) are regions of the cortex that were defined and numbered by neuroanatomist Korbinian Brodmann in the early 1900s. The BA were originally defined by cellular structure but have become more widely used to identify areas dedicated to sensory, motor, and cognitive functions. There are 52 BA across the cerebral cortex. For example, the left frontal lobe contains BA 44 and BA 45. These two BA together are referred to as *Broca's area*. The temporal lobe contains BA 22, which is a *primary auditory cortex*. *Wernicke's area* is located on BA 22. These Brodmann areas—BA 44 and BA 45—and BA 22 are well-established areas of the cerebral cortex known to be activated during language tasks. Contemporary research shows, however, that no brain area functions alone. Rather, neural areas network (much like people do!) to accomplish language functions. Some neural areas may bear the bulk of the work while other areas take on a supporting role (Stowe, Haverkort, & Zwarts, 2005).

Diencephalon

The diencephalon is a subcortical structure. It is found rostral to the brainstem. The diencephalon includes the thalamus and the hypothalamus. Fibers coursing to and from the cerebral cortex run through the thalamus (Kandel, 2013). The thalamus is implicated in certain areas of language discussed below. The hypothalamus regulates autonomic functions (e.g., blood pressure).

Cerebellum

The cerebellum fine-tunes motor movement. It abuts the dorsal surface of the brainstem and connects to the brainstem via white matter tracts (Kandel, 2013). The cerebellum regulates corrections in movement for coordination, posture, and motor movement learning. The cerebellum also activates learning verbs and retrieving verbs from memory (e.g., Yang, Wu, Weng, & Bandettini, 2014).

Brainstem

The brainstem includes three structures. Starting rostrally and moving caudally, these structures are the midbrain, the pons, and the medulla oblongata. The brainstem functions in maintaining arousal and awareness. These functions are critical for language

TABLE 12-1 Lobes and Cortical/Subcortical Structures Listed with Their Associated Behavioral Functions

Lobe	Cortical Area	General Function
Frontal	a. Primary motor cortex b. Premotor and supplementary motor c. Broca's (left hemisphere) d. Prefrontal cortex	a. Initiates voluntary motor movements b. Planning and initiating voluntary movements c. Production of written and spoken language d. Personality, insight, foresight
Parietal	a. Primary somatosensory cortex b. Inferior parietal lobule (left hemisphere) c. Remainder of lobe	a. Sensory processing of tactile and proprioception (senses location and position) b. Language comprehension; phonological storage c. Spatial orientation and directing attention
Temporal	a. Primary auditory cortex b. Wernicke's area (left hemisphere) c. Inferior surface d. Medial surface—as part of the limbic lobe (see below)	a. Processes sound b. Language comprehension c. Higher-order processing of visual information d. Learning and memory
Occipital	a. Primary visual cortex b. Visual association cortex	a. Processes visual information b. Higher order visual processing
Limbic	a. Medial surface of both hemispheres that follows a c-shape above the corpus callosum.	a. Emotional responses, drive-related behavior, memory
Cerebellum	a. Right hemisphere of cerebellum	a. Coordination and adjustment of voluntary movements b. Cognitive functions
Insula	a. Buried in the lateral sulcus	a. Fine motor coordination for articulation; singing
Thalamus Hypothalamus	a. Subcortical b. Subcortical	a. Most information between subcortical, limbic, and cerebellar brain to cortical areas passes here b. Autonomic function

Sources include Vanderah, T.W., & Gould, D.J. (2016); Stowe, Haverkort, & Zwarts (2005).

learning and use. Also, many cell nuclei for sensory and motor information from skin and muscles are present in the brainstem (Kandel, 2013). It contains an important nuclei center called the reticular formation.

▶ Sensory and Motor Information: From Body to Brain and Back

Children make sense of the world by moving through the world. By nature, children participate in the world around them with every sense they have, experiencing it hands-on. The body takes in sensory information via specialized cells for each sense—visual, auditory, olfactory, gustatory, vestibular, tactile, proprioceptive, and others related to temperature and maybe pain (Vanderah & Gould, 2016). The body receives sensory information from a variety of specialized sense cells. Information then travels across sensory white matter tracts to the brain for interpretation in *primary sensory areas* (e.g., primary visual cortex). Various senses are integrated into a meaningful experience in *sensory association areas*. Sensory association areas abut primary sensory cortex areas. Lexical-semantic networks build from hands-on, quality experiences. The meaningful integration of sensory experiences may elicit planning and programming of motor responses from motor areas of the brain. Any voluntary motor movement is transmitted from the brain down through the spinal cord via white matter tracts to the rest of the body for executed muscle movement. Muscle movements could include anything from a small facial flinch to a smile to full-body jump!

Language and the Left Hemisphere: A Traditional View

Language is largely lateralized to the left hemisphere. The brain's left hemisphere is dominant for language processes (Stowe et al., 2005). Put another way, the left hemisphere of the brain has many more areas dedicated to the learning and use of language. TABLE 12-2 lists traditional brain areas and their language functions. Asymmetry between right and left brain structures is usually present at birth (Vanderah & Gould, 2016). For example, the *planum temporale* is in the Sylvian fissure along the temporal lobe. The left planum temporale is longer than on the right hemisphere, thereby allotting more cortex to processing behind the primary auditory cortex (BA 22). While most people are left-hemisphere dominant for language, some brains are right-hemisphere dominant or even bilaterally represented for language.

Perisylvian Language Zone

The brain has lateral fissures demarcating the temporal lobes from the frontal and parietal lobes in both hemispheres. A notable landmark on the left hemisphere is the perisylvian language zone. The perisylvian language zone is the area surrounding the left lateral fissure. As introduced above, Broca's area and Wernicke's area are highly involved in language processing. Broca's area is active when we produce language (BA 44, BA 45), and Wernicke's area is engaged for language comprehension (BA 22). Broca's area is located rostral to the lateral fissure, and Wernicke's area is located caudally (Vanderah & Gould, 2016). Broca's area is officially on the "hill" of BA 44 and BA 45, located at the *left anterior frontal lobe*. Broca's area is involved in grammatical processing. BA 45, known as *pars triangularis*, activates syntactic processing, and BA 44, known as *pars opercularis*, is active for phonological processes involved in grammar.

Semantic processing happens in the left posterior brain at Wernicke's area (Neville & Mills, 1997; Stowe et al., 2005). These two areas of language processing—Broca's and Wernicke's areas, are connected by the white matter tract *arcuate fasciculus*, also known as the *superior longitudinal fasciculus*. Remember, information travels along the white matter tracts in the brain. The arcuate fasciculus allows information to be transferred between Broca's area and Wernicke's area. An additional area important in this language network is the *inferior parietal lobe*. The inferior parietal lobe stores phonological information related to words. Functionally, this means that syntactic, phonological, and lexical information is processed between these areas when understanding what is said or when formulating what to say.

There is a strong biological determination for left-hemisphere dominance of language representation (Neville & Mills, 1997). In fact, brain circuits for spoken language are "hard wired" (Neville & Mills, 1997, p. S10) in the brain and are under genetic influence (Rice, 2012). Spoken language develops despite impoverished economic and social conditions (Buchweitz, 2016).

TABLE 12-2 Neural Areas and Their Language-Specific Function	
Neural Area	**Function**
Primary auditory cortex	Process auditory information
Posterior temporal cortex	Systematic organization of word sounds
Inferior parietal cortex	Systematic organization of word sounds
Middle temporal cortex	Accessing word meaning
Inferior frontal cortex	Structure/syntax of language

Data from Buchweitz, A. Language and reading development in the brain today: neuromarkers and the case for prediction. *Journal De Pediatria 2016; 92* (3): 8-13.

Brain-Language Relationships Get their Start

The desire to understand brain-behavior relationships is not new. In the late 1800s, Francis Gall, an anatomist, founded the study of the brain, known as *phrenology*. Phrenology is a study of behavior and the brain. It maps abilities onto brain areas through the characteristics of the skull, such as the size of bulges. FIGURE 12-4 shows a modern phrenology skull map that a clinical scientist today might receive as a novelty gift. The pictures illustrate the gist of the phrenologist—certain areas of the skull

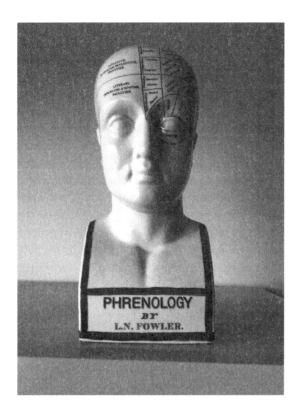

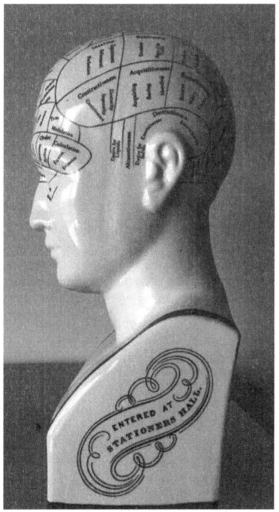

FIGURE 12-4 (a, b) Phrenology bust.

reflect behavior based on the physical structure of the skull. Phrenology was ultimately realized as invalid. However, Gall is recognized for two influences in neuroscience—first, for the broad idea that parts of the brain are localized for behavioral processes, and second (unrelated to phrenology), for an understanding that white matter is part of the neuron (Columbia University Press, 2017; Kandal, 2013).

Valid evidence about neurolinguistic relationships had some of its start in adult lesion studies and the study of adult language disorders (Kandel, 2013; Stowe et al., 2005). Paul Broca was a physician who started by reporting on a stroke patient with expressive language deficits but good comprehension (and later others). Later, Carl Wernicke reported on a patient with the opposite profile after a stroke—expressive language fluency, but poor comprehension of language. These language disorders were named after Paul Broca (Broca's aphasia) and Carl Wernicke (Wernicke's aphasia). These language profiles were linked to brain lesions of stroke, which were in the anterior brain and the posterior brain, respectively. The anterior brain site is now known as Broca's area. The posterior brain site is now known as Wernicke's area.

Clinical aphasiology practice today is not so cut-and-dry. As one example, adults with Broca's aphasia do not necessarily have spared comprehension as once thought. Instead, much like children who use heuristics to understand language early on, adults with Broca's aphasia also appear to use strategies to make it appear as if they understand some of the language spoken to them. Also, both Broca's and Wernicke's areas are found to be engaged in language comprehension and production tasks, not one or the other, as previously thought (Stowe et al., 2005).

▶ Capturing Brain Processing Events with Event-Related Brain Potentials (ERP) and Functional Magnetic Resonance Imaging (fMRI)

Methods of understanding brain-language relationships and development are growing more quickly and accurately in contemporary practice. Two modern technologies for studying the brain are *event-related brain potentials* (ERP) and *functional magnetic resonance imaging* (fMRI). Both ERP and fMRI have benefits and limitations, but together, they have moved the science of developmental neurolinguistics forward quite a bit. With the ERP technique, electrodes are placed on a participant's scalp. The electrodes read electrical activity from the brain out through the scalp. Electrical activity from neurons is then transmitted to the computer and drawn as a waveform trace over time. The timing of the waveform as well as the amplitude (i.e., size) and direction (i.e., positive, negative) of the waveform convey changes in activation. For example, processing word meaning (i.e., semantics) is linked to the N200 and N350 ERP component. The "N" indicates a negative direction to the amplitude of the wave, and the values "200" and "350" reference the number of milliseconds at which the negative amplitude of the wave occurred. The size of the amplitude is not indicated here. The P100 has a positive amplitude that occurs 100 milliseconds after the stimulus, and it indexes early auditory processing (Mills & Neville, 1997). These variables that change are compared to control variables to see whether the changes are significant. The control variables include a baseline amplitude before the stimulus is applied, the ERP of a control task, the ERPs between neural areas, or the ERPs between different types of children (e.g., children who are late talkers and children who are not late to talk).

The primary benefit of ERP is in detecting the timing of signals in relation to the administration of task stimuli. The limitation of ERP is in its spatial acuity (Neville & Mills, 1997). Spatial measurements are measurements of brain areas that the electrodes cover on the skull. Therefore, more errors occur in localizing neural areas involved in processing the stimuli being shown or heard while children are viewing them or hearing them.

In contrast, fMRI has better spatial resolution than timing measurement taken by ERP. Superior spatial acuity means fMRI is good with honing in on areas of the brain while children are viewing or hearing stimuli. With this technique, nothing is attached to the skull or body, but the participant must lie still in a tubelike scanner. The fMRI monitors the change in cell metabolism while processing stimuli. Oxygen levels in the blood change with neuronal activity as blood flow increases with task demand (Neville & Mills, 1997). The fMRI then yields a map of blood flow throughout regions of the brain (Stowe et al., 2005). A limitation of fMRI is that young children are often excluded due to their motor restlessness because this technique requires stillness. Also, from the author's personal experience, the scanner can give some participants a feeling of claustrophobia.

A Broader View of the Language Network

With the advent of neural processing and imaging techniques, additional brain regions have been recognized to network alongside traditional areas introduced above. The original functions assigned to BA have also been expanded. For example, in addition to grammatical processing, Broca's area appears to be involved in music! Broca's area may also play a role in working memory. When processing sentences, Broca's area may help with maintaining verbal information in temporary storage while it is being processed (Stowe et al., 2005).

Two language processing areas that have emerged relatively recently are:

- The cerebellum
- The right hemisphere

The cerebellum is active for motor learning, but it is also active when participants are asked to generate verbs over time and with practice (Yang, Wu, Weng, & Bandettini, 2014). In addition, the right hemisphere activates when a language task increases in complexity (Stowe et al., 2005). Right-hemisphere areas that activate tend to be homologues (or mirror images) of the left hemisphere. When language tasks become complex, additional neural resources are needed (e.g., when resolving semantically ambiguous sentences). The right hemisphere has also been implicated in paralinguistic processes such as the use of prosody.

Reading

Learning to read depends critically on (Buchweitz, 2016; Rueckl et al., 2015):

- The strength of oral language development
- Explicit instruction within a critical period of time in development

Put another way, strong oral language skills can support and bolster learning to read, but fragile spoken language development can very much constrain learning to read. The same language circuitry is shared between oral and written language. This is true cross-linguistically, for very different languages! Rueckl et al. (2015) compared four different languages and showed that even though Spanish, English, Hebrew, and Chinese differed in their transparency, the four languages used the same neural networks to process oral and written language. Transparency (opaque vs. transparent) between oral and written language refers to how straightforward it is to identify the sound to orthographic (written) symbol translation. Participants from these four languages were imaged on fMRI by Rueckl and colleagues. They completed a semantic judgment task while reading and then hearing words. The following areas of the brain were activated for speakers of all four languages, whether they were listening or reading words:

Cortical areas:
- Inferior frontal gyrus
- Middle temporal gyrus
- Inferior parietal lobule

Subcortical areas:
- Insula
- Putamen
- Thalamus

From studies such as this, we see that a common group of brain structures activate and engage for reading print and for hearing speech.

In addition to strong spoken language skills, reading depends on a critical period of language development that is genetically determined (Buchweitz, 2016). For example, in infancy, the border between the occipital and temporal lobes is initially an area that processes faces and objects. As a child learns to read, this occipito-temporal border reprograms to specialize in identifying word forms. The occipito-temporal border then activates more in adults who had learned to read as children versus adults who were only learning to read later in life. In addition, the area generates activation in literate adults over illiterate adults (for review see Buchweitz, 2016). Findings such as these indicate that a critical or sensitive neural period exists. The brain has a period of time when learning a task may be optimal but this time will pass. Once this time passes, learning to read, for example, will be more difficult. Disruption of a white matter tract in this occipito-temporal area is also associated with dyslexia.

▶ The Developing Brain: From Diffuse to Localized Processing of Words and Grammar

As with any aspect of development, children are not born with an adult functioning brain. When it comes to language:

- Children have innate characteristics they are born with.
- The brain is malleable to environmental influence.
- Some phenotypes are unfolding on a developmental timeline of sensitive periods set forth genetically.

Word Learning

Over the course of early development, there is a shift in how activation occurs in the brain when processing words. Initially, when infants listen to words, neural activation is diffuse. Diffuse activation means activation occurs across both hemispheres. Over time, activation becomes more focused or localized to the posterior left hemisphere. Neurolinguists consider the posterior-left brain to be the semantic processing area of the brain in adults. This shift toward localized posterior left activation occurs by 20 months of age after the word spurt (Mills, Plunkett, Prat, & Schafer, 2005; Mills & Neville, 1997; Neville & Mills, 1997). It is characterized by having had direct experience with words. Posterior brain regions of activation are on the temporal and parietal lobes. The posterior activation at left temporal and parietal lobes is not for just any word heard. Rather, this specific activation is dependent upon direct experience with words. The posterior left brain is the site for known words.

Mills et al. (2005) found that having individual experience with *objects* when learning words is key to establishing lexical-semantic representations. They compared two word-learning conditions—in one condition, objects were paired with words, and in a second condition, children just heard the word label repeated but saw no object referent. Children 17- to 21-months old showed larger negative amplitudes at the N200–N500 (semantic) component of the ERP response for the words paired with objects. They did not show this rich neural response for semantic processing in the repeated word condition. Mills et al. (2005) then compared ERP responding between the young toddlers with larger versus smaller vocabularies. It was not vocabulary size overall that led to localized activation. Rather, it was the object experience in particular that led to localized activation.

Grammar

Semantic stimuli elicit asymmetrical activation of the left hemisphere by 20 months. Toddlers do not respond this way to grammatical stimuli at that age. When it comes to processing grammatical function words at 20 months, children's ERP responses do not show the shift in processing to only the left hemisphere that content words do. By 3 years of age, when children are *producing* function words, only then are ERP responses lateralized to the left hemisphere upon hearing them (Neville & Mills, 1997). The period between 2 and 3 years of age, after the word spurt, has been hypothesized as one critical period for initiating grammar development (Rice, 2012).

Development in comprehending syntax parallels brain maturation of certain tracts of the arcuate fasciculus (Vissiennon, Friederici, Brauer, & Wu, 2017). The reader will remember that the arcuate fasciculus connects Broca's and Wernicke's areas. However, smaller tracts that course within the arcuate fasciculus are not fully formed at birth. Vissiennon et al. (2017) found that 6-year-old children had more robust activation when comprehending early developing sentences than 3-year-olds. Connectivity of the left arcuate fasciculus was specifically between posterior temporal gyrus and the pars operculus of the frontal lobe in the 6-year-olds. Even though the three neural structures were involved in sentence comprehension, with age, functional connectivity continued to grow from 3 to 6 years of age.

Genetics and Disruptions to Language Development

In clinical evaluations of speech and language, clinicians ask whether there is a history of speech-language disorders. We do this because language impairments are largely heritable (e.g., Zubrick, Taylor, Rice, & Slegers, 2007). Put another way, language disorders can be passed down or inherited from relatives. Genetics is the study of inheritance through genes. This is a biological concept. Genes have an impact on behavior. A phenotype is an observable behavior or symptom when a gene is expressed. For example, nonword repetition performance is a phenotype of language disorder (e.g., Leonard, 2014). Specifically, children with language disorder perform poorly on the nonword repetition task.

Five genes have been implicated in expression of language impairments in children:

- *FOXP2* is a gene that has been implicated in rare speech-language impairment associated with motor speech disorder (i.e., childhood apraxia of speech; MacDermot et al., 2005).
- *CNTNAP2* is a gene that is associated with the language-impairment component of disorders.
- *KIAA0319* is a gene that is thought to influence neuronal development, which can involve language areas, particularly reading and spoken language.

- ATP2C2 is a gene that is implicated in nonword repetition.
- CMIP is a gene that is implicated in nonword repetition.

Disruptions of the FOXP2 gene have been studied extensively in the British family tree of individuals known as KE. The KE family had a rare disorder of speech (e.g., Belton, Salmond, Watkins, Vargha-Khadem, & Gadian, 2003; MacDermot et al., 2005). The disruption of this gene has been associated with childhood apraxia of speech more than language. On MRI, FOXP2 gene mutation in this family was associated with reduced density of gray matter in the caudate nucleus for both left and right brain hemispheres. The caudate nuclei are lateral to the thalamus in each hemisphere of the brain. Other areas were also implicated but included areas of language processing—the left inferior frontal gyrus (BA 44/45), the angular gyrus, and the cerebellum.

FOXP2 is part of the neural pathway to the CNTNAP2 gene where FOXP2 regulates expression of the CNTNAP2 gene (for review Leonard, 2014; Rice, 2012). The CNTNAP2 gene is associated with neuronal development. Disruptions of the CNTNAP2 gene are associated with the language impairments in both autism and language disorder. It is important to understand that in children who have just an isolated language disorder, CNTNAP2 is likely at play. In autism, CNTNAP2 is only one of the genetic mechanisms responsible for the phenotypes observed (Vernes et al., 2008). Associations have been found between the genes CNTNAP2, ATP2C2, and CMIP, and performance on the nonword repetition task by children with a language disorder. Finally, KIAA0319 is a gene that is likely influencing neuronal development as well as being a regulatory gene that influences the functions of other genes. A region of K1AA0319 exerts an effect on reading and spoken language measures (Rice, Smith, & Gayan, 2009).

Growth Signaling Dysfunction

Rice (2012) proposed one genetic mechanism of language impairment is the neural signal for growth in toddlerhood. Growth in vocabulary is delayed at the word spurt in late talking toddlers. Children who have missed the word spurt have missed this critical neural period of word learning and they then embark on grammatical development late. Specifically, too few words in the late talker's vocabulary does not stimulate grammatical morpheme development. The brain lacks plasticity in this group of children, which fails to catch up once delayed growth is initiated.

Rice et al. have found that children later diagnosed with language disorder in elementary school will persist with morphological deficits. Morphological deficits are specific to verb tense and agreement. Children with language disorder also show a deceleration in grammatical knowledge that is reflected in making poor grammaticality judgments of sentences. This latter phenotype continues into adulthood.

Brain Morphologies of Children with Language Impairments

The brains of children with language disorders look different from the brain of children without language impairments. As Leonard (2014) states, children with language disorders have "…less typical neurological configuration" (p. 197). Differences in brain structure and functions can occur because:

- Children inherit a different-looking brain
- The brain children inherit processes differently resulting in brain growth differences

If a child's brain processes information differently, this can change the morphology of the brain's structure over time. For example, children with a language disorder have a smaller pars triangularis on the left hemisphere than is typically seen in children without language disorder. Children with a language disorder/SLI also have atypical asymmetries in perisylvian regions (Gauger, Lombardino, & Leonard, 1997; Plante, Swisher, Vance, & Rapcsak, 1991). Children with language disorder do not show the asymmetry in planum temporale that typically developing children show (Foster, Hynd, Morgan, & Hugdahl, 2002). Select autopsies of children and adults with history of specific language impairment have revealed *symmetrical* plana temporale instead of the typical asymmetrical left larger than right-hemisphere presentation. Hodge et al. (2010) found size differences in the cerebellum and inferior frontal gyrus (i.e., Broca's area) when comparing four groups of children:

- Children with autism but no language disorder
- Children with autism + language disorder
- Children with language disorder
- Typically developing children

Children with language disorder (isolated and with comorbid autism) showed smaller left- than right-hemisphere brain volumes in the cerebellum and inferior frontal gyrus. Children with autism only (no language

disorder) and typically developing children showed the expected larger left- than right-hemisphere volumes in the cerebellar and inferior frontal gyrus areas.

The reader may keep in mind that the period between 3 and 6 years of age is a period of brain development and growth in children. Chen, Tsao, and Liu (2016) followed toddlers who were late talkers until they were 6 years of age. A subgroup of late talkers persisted in language delay at 6 years of age, while others were late bloomers. Late bloomers showed language abilities in the low-average range, whereas the typical comparison group fell well within average to high-average range. From 3 to 5 years of age, late bloomers and persistent late talkers showed slow maturation of neural processing on ERP measures. The late bloomer and persistent late talker waveforms looked different from those typical peers. In addition, while the typical child showed a shift toward a higher proportion of ERP signals localizing to the frontal lobe, late bloomers and persistent later talkers did not. By 6 years of age, group differences in ERP responses disappeared, yet differences continued in language performance between persistent late talkers and late bloomers, when compared to typical peers. So, even though the three groups of children eventually processed simple speech stimuli comparably, the behavioral language performance of the three groups of children never aligned.

On fMRI, school-age children who had a history of being late talkers showed depressed neural activation in several brain areas, when compared to on-time talkers and early talkers (Preston et al., 2010). **TABLE 12-3** lists speech and language functions associated with each brain area identified. In contrast, the right superior parietal lobule shows the reverse pattern of activation. Activation of the superior parietal lobule indicates that children who used to be late talkers may be putting in greater effort for visual attention than other children. Despite the three categories of children having the same skill, on testing, neural processing in these regions are found to be significantly different.

Epigenetics

A subfield that has grown out of genetics is epigenetics, which includes environmental and experiential influences on development and behavior. Epigenetics is a relatively new area of science. To oversimplify, we now know that nature *and* nurture influence development and behavior. In fact, it is through the study of epigenetics that scientists have understood that experience, when repeatedly applied, can affect a genetic outcome. This is terrific news for clinical scientists!

TABLE 12-3 Neural Areas That Showed Significant Decrements in Neural Activation from Early Talkers to On-time Talkers and the Least in Late-Talkers

Neural Area	Function
Superior temporal gyrus—Left	Understand speech and print
Putamen/globus pallidus (extending into the head of the caudate)—Left/Right	A gateway to language production Potentially for rule-learning in language
Thalamus—Left/Right	Potentially for rule-learning in language
Insula—Left	Formation of the motor plan for expressing language

Data from Preston, J.L., Frost, S.J., Mencl, W.E., Fulbright, R.K., Landi, N., Grigorenko, E., Jacobsen, L., & Pugh, K.R. (2010). Early and Late Talkers: School-age language, literacy and neurolinguistic differences. Brain. 133, 2185–2195

A chemical change occurs at the level of the gene because of experience—negative (e.g., abuse) or positive (e.g., enriched social interactions).

Parent-implemented interventions for young children revolve around social interaction. Enriched social interactions with supportive caregivers are epigenetic mechanisms that can be life-long and have cross-generational effects (National Scientific Council on the Developing Child, 2007). We are looking toward early interventions to have a long-term impact, not only on a single child, but also on perhaps several generations of children.

▶ Summary

The brain is made up of gray (cell bodies) and white (axons) matter. It is divided into hemispheres along the sagittal plane by the longitudinal fissure and into lobes—frontal, parietal, temporal, occipital, and limbic. Cerebral cortex is the outermost area of the brain, which folds over sub-cortical structures. There are two additional structures involved in life functions as well as motor and language—the brain stem and the cerebellum. The Brodmann's areas further section the cerebral cortex into functional areas. The core language network reported in this text includes Broca's area, Wernicke's area, arcuate fasciculus, cerebellum, inferior parietal lobe, thalamus, and left hemisphere homologues in the right hemisphere.

Likely candidates for genetic influences in language delay and disorder are CNTNAP2, FOXP2 (by way of regulating CNTNAP2, K1AA0319, ATP2C2), and CMIP genes. Through epigenetic influence, environmental factors, when applied repeatedly, could modify genetic outcomes of language impairments over time.

Study Questions

- What are the key brain structures involved in language processing and their associate functions? Include processing centers for grammar, semantics, and phonology as well as the white matter tract that connects them.
- Compare-contrast traditional and contemporary views of brain-language relationships.
- How do both ERP and fMRI technologies provide a well-rounded picture of the brain?

- What are the key genetic markers associated with language impairments? What behavioral observations are made in connection with these genetic disruptions?
- How does the idea of diffuse versus localized brain activation relate to language performance in young children learning words and grammar?

References

Belton, E., Salmond, C. H., Watkins, K. E., Vargha-Khadem, F., & Gadian, D. G. (2003). Bilateral brain abnormalities associated with dominantly inherited verbal and orofacial dyspraxia. *Human Brain Mapping, 18,* 194–200.

Buchweitz, A. (2016). Language and reading development in the brain today: Neuromarkers and the case for prediction. *Journal De Pediatria, 92*(3), 8–13.

Chen, Y., Tsao, F., & Liu, H. (2016). Developmental changes in brain response to speech perception in late-talking children: A longitudinal MMR study. *Developmental Cognitive Neuroscience, 19,* 190–199.

Columbia University Press. (2017). *Columbia electronic encyclopedia* (6th ed., Q1, p. 1). New York, NY: Columbia University Press. Accession No. 39008158.

Foster, L. M., Hynd, G. W., Morgan, A. E., & Hugdahl, K. (2002). Planum temporale asymmetry and ear advantage in dichotic listening in developmental dyslexia and attention-deficit/hyperactivity disorder (ADHD). *Journal of International Neuropsycholog Soc, 8*, 22–36.

Gauger, L., Lombardino, L., & Leonard, C. (1997). Brain morphology in children with specific language impairment. *Journal of Speech, Language and Hearing Research, 40*, 1272–1284.

Hodge, S., Makris, N., Kennedy, D., Caviness, V., Howard, J., McGrath, L., … Harris, G. J. (2010). Cerebellum, language and cognition, in autism, and specific language impairment. *Journal of Autism and Developmental Disorders, 40*, 300–316.

Kandel, E. R. (2013). Brain and behavior. In E. R. Kandell, J. H. Schwartz, T. M. Jessell, S. A. Sieglebaum, & A. J. Hudspeth (Eds.), *Principles of neural science* (5th ed.). New York, NY: The McGraw-Hill Companies, Inc.

Leonard, L. B. (2014). *Children with specific language impairment* (2nd ed.). Cambridge, MA: MIT Press.

Logothetis, N. K., Pauls, J., Augath, M., Trinath, T., & Oeltermann, A. (2001). Neurophysiological investigation of the basis of the fMRI signal. *Nature, 412*, 150–157.

MacDermot, K. D., Bonora, E., Sykes, N., Coupe, A. M., Lai, C. S., Vernes, S. C., … Fisher, S. E. (2005). Identification of FOXP2 truncation as a novel cause of developmental speech and language deficits. *American Journal of Human Genetics, 76*(6), 1074–1080.

Mills, D. L., & Neville, H. J. (1997). Electrophysiological studies of language impairment (R. Nass & I. Rapin (Eds.)), *Special Issue Seminar in Child Neurology, 4*, 125–134.

Mills, D. L., Plunkett, K., Prat, C., & Schafer, G. (2005). Watching the infant brain learn words: Effects of vocabulary size and experience. *Cognitive Development, 20*, 18–31.

National Scientific Council on the Developing Child. (2007). *The timing and quality of early experiences combine to shape brain architecture* (Working Paper No. 5). Retrieved from http://www.developingchild.net

National Scientific Council on the Developing Child. (2010). Early experiences can alter gene expression and affect long-term development (Working Paper No. 10). Retrieved from http://www.developingchild.net

Neville, H. J., & Mills, D. L. (1997). Epigenesis of language. *Mental Retardation and Developmental Disabilities Research Reviews, 3*, 282–292.

Plante, E., Swisher, Vance, R., & Rapcsak, S. (1991). MRI findings in boys with specific language impairment. *Brain and Language, 41*, 52–66.

Poelmans, G., Buitelaar, J. K., Pauls, D. L., & Franke, B. (2011). A theoretical molecular network for dyslexia: Integrating available genetic findings. *Molecular Psychiatry, 16*, 365–382.

Preston, J. L., Frost, S. J., Mencl, W. E., Fulbright, R. K., Landi, N., Grigorenko, E., … Pugh, K. R. (2010). Early and late talkers: School-age language, literacy and neurolingustic differences. *Brain, 133*, 2185–2195.

Rice, M. L. (2012). Toward epigenetic and generegulation models of specific language impairment: Looking for links among growth, genes, and impairments. *Journal of Neurogevelopmental Disorders, 4*, 27.

Rice M. L. (2016). Children with specific language impairment and their families: A future view of nature plus nurture and new technologies for comprehensive language intervention strategies. *Seminars in Speech Language, 37*(4), 310–318.

Rice, M. L., Haney, K. R., & Wexler, K. (1998). Family histories of children with SLI who show extended optional infinitives. *JSLHR, 41*(2), 419–432.

Rice, M. L., Smith, S., & Gayan, J. (2009). Convergent genetic linkage and associations to language, speech, and reading measures in families of probands with specific language impairment. *Journal of Neurodevelopmental Disorder, 1*, 264–282.

Rueckl, J. G., Paz-Alonso, P. M., Molfese, P. J., Kuo, W.-J., Bick, A., Forst, S. J., … Frost, R. (2015). Universal brain signature of proficient reading: Evidence from four contrasting languages. *Proceedings of the National Academy of Sciences of the USA, 112*(50), 155510–155515. doi:10.1073/pnas.1509321112

Stowe, L. A., Haverkort, M., & Zwarts, F. (2005). Rethinking the neurological basis of language. *Lingua, 115*, 997–1042.

Vanderah, T. W., & Gould, D. J. (2016). *Nolte's the human brain: An introduction to its functional anatomy* (7th ed.). Philadelphia, PA: Elsevier.

Vernes, S. C., Newbury, D. F., Abrahams, B. S., Winchester, L., Nicod, J., Groszer, M., … Fisher, S. E. (2008). A functional genetic link between distinct developmental language disorders. *The New England Journal of Medicine, 359*(22), 2337–2345.

Vissiennon, K., Friederici, A. D., Brauer, J., & Wu, C. Y. (2017). Functional organization of the language network in three- and six-year-old children. *Neuropsychologia, 98*, 23–33.

Whitehouse, A. J. O., Bishop, D. V. M., Ang, Q. W., Pennell, C. E., & Fisher, S. E. (2011). CNTNAP2 variants affect early language development in the general population. *Genes Brain Behavior, 10*, 451–456.

Yang, Z., Wu, P., Weng, X., & Bandettini, P. A. (2014). Cerebellum engages in automation of verb-generation skill. *Journal of Integrative Neuroscience, 13*(1), 1–17.

Zubrick, S. R., Taylor, C. L., Rice, M. L., & Slegers, D. W. (2007). Late language emergence at 24 months: An epidemiological study of prevalence, predictors, and covariates. *Journal of Speech, Language and Hearing Research, 50*, 1562–1592.

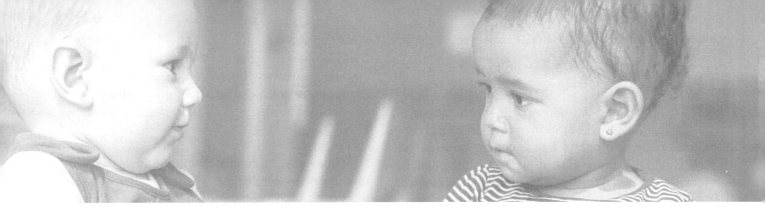

CHAPTER 13

Multicultural Perspectives: The Road to Cultural Competence

Luis F. Riquelme, PhD, CCC-SLP, BCS-S
Jason Rosas, MPhil, MS, CCC-SLP, TSSLD

OBJECTIVES

- Define culture and describe its impact on the assessment/treatment of communication disorders
- Outline best practices for least biased assessment of children with suspected communication disorders
- Outline procedures for the use of interpreters in the clinical practice of a speech-language pathologist

KEY TERMS

Acculturation
Assimilation
Code switching
Communicative competence
Criterion-referenced measures
Cultural bias
Cultural competence
Cultural diversity
Cultural humility
Cultural sensitivity
Cultural variables
Culture
Dialectal variance
Disability
Discourse competence
Dual-(differentiated-) language
    system hypothesis

Dynamic assessment
Ethnic diversity
Ethnicity
Ethnic majority
Ethnic minority
Ethnographic interviewing
Grammatical competence
Heritage
Illness
Interpreter
Language diversity
Language–ego permeability
Language loss
Language mixing
Language sampling
Language transfer
Language-use patterns

Linguistic bias
Nonverbal communication
Norm-referenced measures
Orientation
Race
Sequential-bilingual
Service delivery
Simultaneous-bilingual
Sociolinguistic/sociocultural
    competence
Sociological assessment model
Strategic competence
Traditional assessment model
Translator
Unitary language system view
Verbal communication

▶ Introduction

This chapter introduces the speech-language pathologist (SLP) to the provision of increasingly culturally sensitive clinical services for all children being evaluated or treated for possible communication disorders. The information presented here is also relevant to the researcher in the area of language development and/or disorders.

As population demographics change in the United States, a larger population of ethnic and culturally diverse, communicatively impaired persons obligates SLPs and audiologists to view service delivery with a fresh perspective (Payne, 1997). To deliver the highest quality of services and prevent misdiagnosis and/or mistreatment, every clinician must strive to become increasingly competent in providing services in a least-biased, nonjudgmental, and ethical manner. Today's clinical practice requires awareness of each person's customs, beliefs, and ethnicity. Moreover, cultural sensitivity is a requirement in the practice of speech-language pathology, as per the field's reliance on interpersonal communication. This chapter addresses issues of cultural and linguistic diversity, including a brief review of those related to bilingualism. It is important for all SLPs—whether monolingual or bilingual—to develop an understanding of the cultural and linguistic differences that may exist or emerge within the social communities they serve. Clinicians can provide high-quality services to all clients and their families by valuing and integrating a broad understanding of cultural practices, attitudes, and beliefs into the service delivery process. As the American Speech-Language-Hearing Association's (ASHA, 2004) document on providing culturally and linguistically appropriate services states:

> [B]eliefs and values unique to that individual clinician–client encounter must be understood, protected, and respected. Care must be taken not to make assumptions about individuals based upon their particular culture, ethnicity, language, or life experiences that could lead to misdiagnosis or improper treatment of the client/patient. Providers must enter into the relationship with awareness, knowledge, and skills about their own culture and cultural biases. To best address the unique, individual characteristics and cultural background of clients and their families, providers should be prepared to be open and flexible in the selection, administration, and interpretation of diagnostic and/or treatment regimens. When cultural or linguistic differences may negatively influence outcomes, referral to, or collaboration with, others with the needed knowledge, skill, and/or experience is indicated.

Differences in culture and ethno-biological factors are often overlooked when providing services to persons with communication and/or swallowing disorders. Ethnocentrism on the part of the service provider may be displayed during the assessment and/or treatment process. It is not uncommon for the service provider to focus solely on the language barrier issue and forget all other cultural factors involved in the communication process. To provide the best services possible, the SLP, or any of the members of the caregiving team, must take into account the person as a whole. This includes understanding the influence of assimilation and acculturation on the assessment and treatment process (Riquelme, 2007). Assimilation is the process in which someone in a new environment totally embraces the host culture (C2) (e.g., values, beliefs, behaviors). Acculturation, in contrast to assimilation, is viewed as positive for new immigrants. It allows individuals to identify with the primary community (C1) in which they have been socialized as well as with the broader majority community or host culture (C2) (Cabassa, 2003; Kohnert, 2008, p. 31).

The United States, as a country inhabited largely by immigrants, has a long history of struggles with assimilation and acculturation. These processes were mostly assimilatory until the middle of the twentieth century. Subsequent to that point, many immigrant groups began to acculturate—that is, balance their native cultures and beliefs with that of the host culture, or "mainstream America."

All service providers experience and practice the processes of assimilation and acculturation within the environments in which they exist (e.g., work, social, educational) (Dikeman & Riquelme, 2002). Think about your own first few weeks in a new job or a new academic setting: it was important to learn the "rules of the game" that were already established or the "culture" of the new setting. This notion further supports our need to expand the definition of culture to include more than the race/ethnicity of a particular person or group. Hence, it is suggested that any group of people with certain commonalities that abide by particular rules should be considered a culture onto itself. This translates into the notion of every individual being a part of many cultures—as suggested earlier, the culture of the workplace, the culture of the home, as well as the cultures and subcultures of those with particular lifestyles, religious beliefs, and so on.

Increased awareness about acculturation is needed to reduce the potential for stereotyping. Clinicians cannot assume that all persons from a particular group or culture are similar in every aspect of everyday life. It is extremely important for the clinician to obtain information about the person with whom they are working, as the client may not be able to provide all the details secondary to their communication impairment. It is important for clinicians to develop awareness of their own cultural notions in order to reduce errors in subjective observations, which are susceptible to bias and may restrict access to relevant clinical information. Understanding that the clinician encompasses many cultures, and that the client does as well, will provide a better balance and exchange between the two individuals. Creating an open communicative environment with the client may allow for this type of exchange (Riquelme, 2006b).

ASHA developed an ethics statement regarding cultural and linguistic competence within this scope of practice for the SLP (ASHA, 2017). There is also a set of tools for self-assessment of cultural competence for the SLP (ASHA, n.d.). The toolbox includes checklists on personal reflection, policies and procedures, and service delivery. In addition, there is a cultural competence awareness tool in an interactive web-based platform. These documents, tools, and many other articles written by respected colleagues in our field serve as a basis for arguing for achieving cultural competence to provide appropriate services to all our stakeholders. Most importantly, these documents and articles also support the notion that culture, multiculturalism, and diversity go beyond race and ethnicity (as reported in Riquelme, 2013, p. 43).

A few other points need to be made when considering the importance of perspective-taking in the incorporation of multicultural and multilingual aspects into our practice as specialists in the prevention, assessment, treatment, and management of communication and swallowing disorders. First, the concept first presented by Tervalon and Murray-García in 1998 espoused life-long learning and perspective-taking on the part of the practitioner, "cultural humility." According to them, "cultural humility incorporates a lifelong commitment to self-evaluation and critique, to redressing the power imbalances in the physician-patient dynamic, and to developing mutually beneficial and non-paternalistic partnerships with communities on behalf of individuals and defined populations" (p. 123). As mentioned in Riquelme, 2013, p. 44, the dynamic between provider and patient is often compromised by various sociocultural mismatches, including the providers' lack of knowledge regarding the patient's health beliefs and

life experiences and the provider's unintentional and intentional processes of racism, classism, homophobia, and sexism. Tervalon and Murray-Garcia's (1998) concept of cultural competence in clinical practice is best defined not by a discrete endpoint but as a commitment and active engagement in a lifelong process with patients, communities, colleagues, and within the professionals themselves.

Secondly, when discussing perspective-taking, the client/patient's view of the clinician-client interaction should be attended to. Some argue that cultural competence is a bilateral process, while others argue that it is not. Sánchez (2008) presents an argument against the bilaterality of cultural competence. He argues, based on the "difference principle" presented by Rawls (1971), that the patient receiving services is not necessarily empowered to expect culturally competent services. This power differential is in line with the concept of cultural humility presented above. He further states that, "Cultural expectations, which any member of an alien culture brings with him or her to the doctor–patient relationship, are barriers to proper medical care if and when these expectations are neither understood nor addressed" (p. 5). What the patient expects from their healthcare practitioner will vary by culture. It is relevant to note that a more comprehensive definition of culture, the patient's perspective, or expectation, will vary by ethnicity, socioeconomic status, prior experience, setting, or any other set of possible factors. Understanding each patient or client's unique perspective and expectation is of utmost importance, and we should not assume what these are based on stereotyping on the part of the practitioner. Take, for example, the clinician who, in the context of conducting an evaluation, meets the patient/client and caregivers for the first time and immediately begins to ask questions so as to complete the interview and take all necessary historical information. This clinician/examiner then goes on to test the patient and subsequently bids them farewell. Has this practitioner truly allowed the patient/client and caregivers to voice their concerns regarding communication and/or swallowing? Has this practitioner allowed for any insight into the patient's or family's perspective on the suspected problem? Has the practitioner gauged a sense of the impact this problem has on the patient/client's life, as stated by the informants and not assumed by the practitioner? Why would the clinician assume that the patient is aware of the diagnostic process? How did any stereotyping on the part of the clinician influence this session? The clinician must consider the patient and family/caregivers, perspective to be an asset to any clinical interaction. This means that clarifying any misperceptions is just as valid as concurring with the patient or family's suspicions of a disorder. All serve as an asset to this and future clinical interactions.

Terminology

Clinicians should become well versed in the socio-political vernacular denoting various social groups. To begin with, the terms *minority* and *majority* should be discussed. In efforts to categorize the general population, the U.S. Bureau of the Census (2000, 2010) defines all nonwhite persons as minorities. Payne (1997) has commented that lumping individuals together under the label of "minority" suggests inferiority, whereas the designation of "majority" connotes superiority. She argues that neither term is accurate for two reasons: (1) neither term accounts for the continuum of cultural experiences within the two categories and (2) neither term has saliency for the future. Payne also suggests that this classification system reinforces bias and stereotyping, further widening the cultural distance in cross-cultural communication.

Many individuals now use the term *racial/ethnic minority,* in keeping with the U.S. Census designations of minority groups: Hispanic Americans, African Americans, Native American Indians, Asian/Pacific Islanders, and Others. Of course, not all groups designated as such in this system are homo-racial—that is, of a single race/ethnicity. Hispanics, for example, may be of single or mixed race. In fact, many Hispanics self-identify as white, black, or mixed race, the latter being most common, as per the influence of Spain (white race), Africa (black race), and varied groups of native Indians (some other race, a new designation on the 2010 U.S. Census). For this reason, the U.S. Census Bureau added a question on ethnicity to the 2000 census so that persons (e.g., Hispanics) could self-identify based on country of origin (e.g., Mexico, Puerto Rico, Cuba, Colombia). Despite nonwhite groups being the majority in many towns and cities across the United States, the term *minority* is still applied broadly to these groups. Other common misconceptions are that all culturally and linguistically diverse groups are nonwhite or that ethnic diversity refers only to nonwhite persons. This is also true for the use of the terms *multicultural* and *diversity.* Following this logic, how would Russian immigrants be classified? These persons speak a non-English language, come to the United States from a different culture, and are considered racially Caucasian. Are Russians thought of as a culturally and linguistically diverse group? Are they ethnically diverse?

Another example of diversity arises when the patient or the clinician is gay/lesbian/bisexual/transgender (GLBT). While some people believe these are chosen lifestyles, many others disagree. Some believe that there is a "culture" associated with persons who are GLBT. Nevertheless, the clinician is expected to be sensitive to these aspects of culture/diversity and not make assumptions based on cultural misconceptions or heterosexism (Riquelme, 2006b). For example, why should the clinician assume that the child to be evaluated comes from a home with a mother and a father? The child may actually come from a home where both parents are of the same gender, or from a single-parent home.

In today's clinical practice, it is also relevant to be sensitive to families where a parent is transgender or where the child is transgender, or managing transitioning issues. Certainly, it should be clear to the SLP that a person who is actively working on gender identification issues may also face speech language delays/disorders that may have been concurrently identified and in need of attention.

These examples highlight the fact that cultural and linguistic diversity applies to all clinicians and their patients/clients regardless of ethnic background, lifestyle, religious beliefs, and other characteristics. The key point is that all individuals have many cultures and at least one language. To broaden perspectives on culture, clinicians need to define it at a personal level. This will then greatly impact all aspects of work in the discipline of communication disorders, which not only requires excellent interpersonal skills, but also a strong knowledge base of sociocultural factors so as to reduce the risk of misdiagnosis or mistreatment based on culturally based errors.

Culture

Before discussing culture and its relationship with assessment and intervention, we should develop a clear definition of *culture* and related terms. The definitions for *culture* vary as dramatically as the sciences that examine culture; the impact of culture on phenomena in the fields of psychology, anthropology, and sociology, among others, is widely documented. Carbaugh (1988) referred to ethnic culture as a system of interrelated behavior and belief patterns "that are (a) deeply felt, (b) commonly intelligible, and (c) widely accessible" and are used to create and share individual identity (p. 38). Clinicians must accept and fully incorporate the notion that everyone has a culture if they are to be able to provide culturally appropriate services. Furthermore, culture goes beyond race and ethnicity. It is up to the practitioner to define culture more broadly and include not only ethnicity, but also religious beliefs, lifestyles, special interests, and other factors (Riquelme, 2004, p. 1). As stated earlier in this chapter, if the clinician is to espouse the concept of "everyone is a part of many cultures," then this clinician also needs to include himself/herself. Including the perspective of sensitivity to the client/patient as well as understanding their perception of the clinician as a person and professional will only lead to better interpersonal communication and access to aspects of behavior that may ultimately influence impressions and treatment plans for the communication or swallowing complaints.

For our purposes, *culture* is defined as the behaviors, artifacts, and beliefs adopted by a person or group used to define their social identity. Culture comprises both explicit behaviors and artifacts and implicit beliefs (see **TABLE 13-1**). In other words, some behaviors are evident, external, and perceivable (explicit), whereas other behaviors are abstract and internal and must be inferred (implicit) (Chamberlain & Medinos-Landurand, 1991).

Culture gives shape to ethnicity and cultural heritage. *Ethnicity* is an ever-changing cultural construct that forms the basis for a sense of social cohesion. Those cultural variables that are shared and accepted help an ethnic group define itself. In other words, our ethnicity is determined by the cultural beliefs and practices we share with others. Deciding which traits are "common" to an ethnic group becomes very difficult because cultural behaviors shift according to historical

contexts. For example, an ethnic Neuyorican (New York–Puerto Rican) in the 1970s may have defined themselves very differently from a Neuyorican in the twenty-first century due to changes in the social, economic, and political climate.

Cultural behaviors, artifacts, and beliefs that are most valued and passed down from generation to generation constitute an ethnicity's *heritage*. For example, a family heirloom (artifact) that is passed down from mother to daughter over generations could represent a cultural artifact that has heritage value. Similarly, the language a family speaks (behavior) may have sufficient significance to be characterized as having heritage value. Because heritage is so intricately related to ethnicity, changes to cultural variables may influence which items or behaviors retain value and significance. For example, one generation of people may strongly value a native language and deem it essential to pass down to their children. In contrast, the next generation may devalue a native language in favor of another. The value of the native language may be diminished to the point where it no longer has significance in helping to define the ethnic group. Consequently, from one generation to the next, a once-prominent heritage variable such as language may be lost or replaced.

Race, a far more controversial construct and term, is widely used in sociopolitical circles when discussing individuals and social groups. Race, a construct used to classify humanity by arbitrary biological or anatomical features and/or nebulous geographical boundaries, is often misinterpreted and forms the basis for social blights, such as racism and discrimination.

TABLE 13-1 Explicit and Implicit Cultural Variables

Explicit Variables: Behaviors and Artifacts	Implicit Variables: Beliefs Inferred from Behaviors and Artifacts
Language	Language–Ego Permeability: degree to which language mixing or code switching is allowed/accepted
Religious practices	Child-rearing expectancies
Eating/feeding preferences	Role of parent/child/teacher in education
Manner of celebration	Role of parent/professional in the health profession
Music/dance	Role of males versus females
Homework, newspapers, paintings, crafts	Monotheistic versus polytheistic beliefs

Source: Adapted from Chamberlain, P., & Medinos-Landurand, P. (1991). Practical considerations for the assessment of LEP students with special needs. In E. Hamayan & J. Damico (Eds.), Limiting bias in the assessment of bilingual students (pp. 112–129, 131). Austin, TX: Pro Ed.

TABLE 13-2 Cultural Variables Affecting Language Development

Educational Level	Socioeconomic Status/Upward Class Mobility
Languages spoken	Religious beliefs/impact on activities of daily living (ADL)
Length of residence in an area	Neighborhood of residence/peer group
Country of birth	Degree of acculturation
Urban versus rural background	Generational membership
Individual choice within the intrapersonal realm	Age and gender

Source: Adapted from Roseberry-McKibbin, C. (1995). Multicultural students with special language needs: Practical strategies for assessment and intervention. Oceanside, CA: Academic Communication Associates.

Making decisions about a group or person based on appearance or place of origin leads to subjective interpretations of families or clients. This approach leaves little room for the development of interpersonal relationships based on cooperation, communication, and shared understanding—all of which are critical to successful clinical outcomes.

To better appreciate the key role played by the client and the family in the clinical process, SLPs should evaluate their own definitions of culture, ethnicity, heritage, and race. Put simply, a clinician who examines their own beliefs and behaviors will be better equipped to understand and interpret others' beliefs and behaviors. Roseberry-McKibbin (1995, 2002) has listed several cultural variables that may affect larger social groups and that may have unique effects on the individual lives of a family or client (see TABLE 13-2). Specifically, cultural factors that affect the collection of data from family members and the child's performance in assessment and treatment should be considered. Several of these cultural factors will be discussed in this chapter. A more thorough review of the literature discussing these variables should also be undertaken to better understand the complexity and depth of their effects on assessment and intervention.

▶ Cultural Competence/ Sensitivity

Cultural competence is not a skill that is acquired or learned but rather one that is developed over time. Hence, some argue that *cultural sensitivity* may be more appropriate term, as per the need to be sensitive to differences in all interactions and clinical decisions. The need for all SLPs to become culturally competent/sensitive—and not just those from ethnic minority backgrounds or those who are bilingual—is increasingly apparent. All across the United States, demographics show that more persons are from non-mainstream cultures and from homes where English may not be the first language. More clinicians are also seeing children that are English-dominant and come from bilingual/multilingual homes.

In 2004, ASHA approved a practice document entitled *Knowledge and Skills Needed by Speech-Language Pathologists and Audiologists to Provide Culturally and Linguistically Appropriate Services,* authored by members of its Multicultural Issues Board. This document outlines the knowledge and skills that clinicians must strive to develop so as to provide unbiased and culturally appropriate services. It also acknowledges the need for lifelong learning. The ASHA document lists a variety of competencies needed to achieve cultural competence, such as sensitivity to differences, understanding the influence of culture on service delivery, and the need to advocate for and empower consumers, families, and communities at risk for communication, swallowing, or balance disorders. Among the key cultural factors to understand when working with limited-English-speaking patients are increased respect for individual differences within and between groups (e.g., family structure and roles, approach to disability and rehabilitation); separation of the effects of culture from the effects of socioeconomic status; understanding the patient's sociocultural belief system; greater caution in interpreting and generalizing findings; greater caution in the use of formal tests; and awareness of differences in interpersonal relating (ASHA, 2004).

Learning to work effectively with individuals who are culturally or linguistically different from both the personal and professional experiences of the clinician presents formidable challenges as well as considerable opportunities for personal growth and professional excellence (Kohnert, 2008). Kohnert (2008, p. 35) describes four essential characteristics of the culturally competent SLP:

- To simultaneously appreciate cultural patterns and individual variation
- To engage in cultural self-scrutiny
- To embrace principles of evidence-based practice
- To seek to understand language disorders within the client's social context

She further states that a deep understanding that there are many different ways of seeing and being in the world is essential for cultural competence.

In discussing speech-language assessment issues within the multicultural context, differentiation must be made between cultural diversity, as discussed earlier, and language diversity. Embracing the concept that all persons have a culture, including the client and the clinician, requires using nonbiased assessment and treatment practices for all clients receiving speech-language services. Many of the tools utilized by the SLP for assessment and treatment are inherently culturally biased, hence nonbiased practices may be impossible. As part of the movement towards improved cultural sensitivity, in as much as possible, clinicians are encouraged to utilize *least-biased* clinical practices. In other words, every child—whether mainstream or not—must be treated in a culturally sensitive manner. In the case of language diversity, other clinical factors must be added to the picture. In this scenario, the clinician needs to be familiar with issues regarding second language acquisition and bilingualism. As demographics have changed in the United States, SLPs have begun to see more children who use English as the preferred language for communication but who are from bilingual homes and are often bilingual themselves. This presents many challenges to the clinician without experience in bilingualism, as testing such a child as a monolingual speaker of English would be inappropriate and may well result in the child being misdiagnosed with a communication disorder.

▶ Bilingualism: Perspectives in the United States

A review of the U.S. Census figures from 2013 indicates that over 60 million persons in the United States speak a language other than or in addition to English (just shy of 21% of the total U.S. population over age 5). Nearly 42% of that group reported speaking English less than "very well." 62% reported Spanish as the language they use other than or in addition to English. These figures, of course, include many school-aged children who are English language learners (ELLs), previously known as limited-English proficient (LEP) or non-English proficient (NEP). More recently, 2011 Census data reported that about 22% of children ages 5–19 (approximately 13.8 million) spoke a language other than English at home. Of these, more than 21% (or nearly 3 million) spoke English "less than very well" (Ryan, 2013). Several language groups have seen a relative increase in their home language use from 1980 to 2010, while others have seen a decline in the same period. Five languages have demonstrated a decline in home language use since 1980: Italian, Yiddish, German, Polish, and Greek. These changes may be attributed to declining immigration patterns by persons whose native country speaks these languages. Languages showing steady increase in home language use from 1980 to 2010 include Vietnamese, Russian, Chinese, Korean, Tagalog, Persian, and Spanish. Of these, Spanish has impacted the education landscape the greatest because of the size of the population involved (Vietnamese has the largest percentage change in home language use at 599% over the 40-year period; however, the ratio of Vietnamese to Spanish in the United States is 1:26) (Ryan, 2013).

It is also important to briefly discuss how bilingualism is viewed in this country. While bilingualism and multilingualism are viewed as assets in most countries around the world, that is not the case in the United States. According to Ruiz (1988, in Goldstein, 2004), the United States has had three main orientations to language planning:

- **Language as Problem.** In the 1950s, bilingualism was seen as a problem of modernization—that is, the need to deal with issues such as code selection, standardization, literacy, orthography, language stratification, and so forth. During this time, language issues were linked to the "disadvantaged," similar to other social issues such as poverty, low socioeconomic status, and lack of social mobility. Bilingualism, then, was perceived as a problem to be overcome and was viewed mostly as a deficit.
- **Language as Right.** In the 1960s, language was recognized as a civil right. This movement was manifested as government forms, ballots, instructional pamphlets, judicial proceedings, and civil service exams being printed in languages other than English.

■ **Language as Resource.** Historically, neither language diversity nor non-English language maintenance has been encouraged in the United States. There is, however, current support on some fronts for the "language as resource" perspective, which advocates the conservation of language abilities of non-English speakers and an increase in language requirements in universities (if for no other reason than the need for linguistic diversity for business purposes). There is, however, a contradiction, because most individuals support foreign-language instruction in schools but ask non-native English speakers to lose their first language.

The rapid growth of ELLs has greatly challenged the present support system for assessing and treating ELL children with communication disorders. As reported in the 23rd Annual Report to Congress on the Implementation of IDEA, "a significant number of LEP students also have a concomitant disability; those students are at even greater risk for negative educational outcomes" (U.S. Department of Education, 2007a). This is the same information reported in the 2001 annual report (pp. II–38). Significantly, no figures exist as to the exact number of ELLs who are mandated to receive special education programs and/or speech-language therapy. This underscores the need for improved professional training in this area. All SLPs, psychologists, and educators would benefit from cultural and linguistic diversity training. Failure to train and ensure cultural sensitivity may lead to misdiagnosis of ELLs. Efforts toward achieving cultural sensitivity and competence may help in ensuring reduced assessment bias for this population of children, and it may eliminate or greatly reduce the incidence of misdiagnosis.

▶ Case Studies

To better illustrate these factors, we will use the example of Josefina (previously Josephine), our "late-blooming" language learner. Relevant cultural and language developmental information has been added to her "significant history" so as to illustrate points mentioned previously. This example involves a girl of African-American/Puerto Rican culture and the Spanish language. The variables and factors presented here are not intended to be generalized for all African-American/Puerto Rican families and children. Instead, the cultural variables are used as exemplars of a broader set of variables that may be adapted by any family given their individual definitions of self and community.

▶ Cultural Variables Affecting the Assessment and Intervention Process

Orientation

Orientation describes the degree to which people orient themselves toward the considerations of a collective body (e.g., a family) or toward individual achievement and motivation. In some cultures, decisions are made for the greater good of the family rather than any one person's achievement. Support may be offered from a large network of relatives and friends. Also, success may be measured by the amount of prestige or honor that is brought to the family. In contrast, cultures that encourage individual performance may de-emphasize the importance of the larger social unit.

In Josefina's case, the extended family lives in the same residence as Josefina's immediate family. Exploring the parents' views and values of kinship and individual achievement may facilitate our clinical understanding of the support network available to Josefina and suggest how she may be encouraged to succeed in the clinical context.

Verbal and Nonverbal Communication

Verbal and nonverbal communication describes the beliefs governing communication between children and adults. Verbal communication, or discourse, rules may affect an SLP's interactions with parents and the child. Some cultures prefer succinct discourse exchanges and place unspoken limitations on the amount of talking children are allowed with adults. Other cultures allow children to be present in, but not participate in, adult conversations (Heath, 1983). Still other cultures place a high value on the direct role of family as the child's principal model for language form, content, and use. These cultures may emphasize the parent's role as facilitator and instructor in the parent-child dynamic and may encourage a child's increased responsiveness and openness with adults, both familiar and novel.

Nonverbal communication refers to the nonlinguistic behaviors that may accompany verbal interactions. Gestures, proximity, eye contact, and touch may have substantial meaning in social interactions (Chamberlain & Medinos-Landurand, 1991).

■ *Gestures*, such as head nods, head shakes, finger shaking, or other combined body movements, may have substantial meaning independent of the verbal utterances. They may also affect the

🔍 *CASE STUDY: JOSEPHINA: ADJUSTED RELEVANT HISTORY*

Josefina is a 5.5-years-old female child who was referred to this appointment due to teacher concerns about poor academic achievement. Josefina 's father, Mr. X, is African-American and her mother, Mrs. X, is Puerto Rican. Josefina's prenatal and birth histories were unremarkable. She was born at term, weighing 7 pounds, 2 ounces. Medical/health history was significant for pneumonia at 19 months and two bouts of otitis media (ear infections) since that time. She has known allergies to dust and mold. Josefina's hearing was recently evaluated and found to be within normal limits. Developmental milestones were reached in a timely manner (e.g., sat at 6 months, walked at 11 months). Josefina's speech-language development was remarkable for limited vocalizations during infancy, including little babbling. Her first words were delayed until 15 months, and her mother believed Josefina to have a small vocabulary for her age. Family history was remarkable for a paternal uncle who was described as "tartamudo"—that is, a stutterer.

Josefina lives with her parents and older twin siblings in a bilingual English–Spanish community in Brooklyn, New York. The family rents an apartment in a three-family home, which is also home to Josefina's godparents, paternal aunt, and grandmother. Mrs. X was originally from a rural district of Puerto Rico and moved to the United States 2 years ago. She completed high school and received vocational training in culinary arts. Mrs. X considered herself Spanish-dominant but used some English at home with her children. She suggested that her primary motivation for moving to the United States included better financial opportunities and educational advantage for her children. Mr. X was born in a small town in Georgia. Unlike his wife, Mr. X moved to New York at the age of five. He completed high school in Manhattan. Mr. X considered himself a conversational speaker of Spanish, who tries to use Spanish in the home when speaking to Josefina. The family seldom visits Puerto Rico but are exposed to Spanish reading and writing through their church bible study program. Mr. X works full-time at a small construction business and keeps long hours. Mrs. X works in a local neighborhood restaurant.

meaning of a verbal utterance. Consider the meaning transmitted when a mother says, "You are thinking of going outside now?" while shaking her head side-to-side. This could be interpreted as disapproval or a veiled comment suggesting to the child that going out is out of the question.

- *Proximity* is the degree of "personal space" used or shared during verbal interaction. Some cultures value distance between conversational partners, whereas others may embrace physical closeness. For example, a clinician who leans her body in to hear a speaker may be perceived as rude and aggressive or, conversely, give the impression that she is engaged and sympathetic.

- *Eye contact* (or eye gaze) is a variable that is used subjectively by clinicians to judge attentiveness and engagement. Averting direct eye contact when speaking may, in fact, be a sign of respect in some cultures. In other cultures, sustaining eye contact with adults when responding to or engaging in discourse demonstrates that the child has confidence, alertness, and honesty.

- *Touch* may be permitted as a sign of affection or to demonstrate communicative engagement. In some cases, touch is prohibited or restricted to specific persons or for specific meaning. These behaviors may have roots in religious beliefs and practices or may be governed by individual expectations regarding adult–child or adult–adult interaction.

In Josefina's case, it may prove useful to observe the nonverbal behaviors of the family during the interview process. Prolonged eye contact with adults may not be encouraged with adults or figures of authority. Distance and reduced contact with strangers may be promoted. Verbally, the child may be taught to "speak only when spoken to" as a show of respect to elders and proper "manners." Each of these factors could affect the child's interaction with the evaluator and, if not considered appropriately, could lead to erroneous judgments regarding the child's pragmatic capabilities.

Play Interactions

Play is often used in assessments of young children for evaluation of language skills in meaningful contexts. However, the manner in which a child plays is highly influenced by culture. Play dimensions, including self–other relations, symbolic play props, and thematic contexts, are all affected by cultural expectations (Westby, 1990) Some cultures may have finely defined expectations regarding which kinds of play or activities are permissible for a boy versus a girl. Play and gender role factors can influence how a child plays, which types of games are chosen, what level of prowess in play the child demonstrates, what the child plays with, and whom the child chooses or is allowed to play with (Farver, Kim, & Lee, 1995; Rubin & Coplan, 1998; Sutton-Smith, 1972). For example, Josefina's family may feel strongly about which kinds of toys she played with (i.e., dolls versus trucks). The parents may also engage her, to a limited degree, in adult–child play interactions. This may lead to a difference in play performance owing to lack of experience rather than underdeveloped symbolic (cognitive) play skills.

Illness and Disabilities

Another culturally influenced belief is the perception of disease, illness, and disability. *Disease* refers to the observable disruption of physical or mental processes, whereas *illness* refers to an individual's experience of that condition. (Kleinman, Eisenberg, & Good, 2006). In other words, *illness* is the term used to indicate when a change in physical or mental state is judged abnormal or deficient. This may result in a family's or client's change in social interaction and performance due to insecurities, shame, or other emotional reactions to the individual's condition. In a sociopolitical sense, nomenclature such as *disabled, handicapped,* and *impaired* also has stigmatizing effects for some groups.

Limited research has been conducted in the field of speech-language pathology with regard to cross-cultural beliefs of illness or disability (Bebout & Arthur, 1992; Maestas & Erickson, 1992; Salas-Provance, Erickson, & Reed, 2002). Remaining focused on the notion of individual differences in cultural beliefs may facilitate a clinician's understanding of the needs of the family or parent of a child with communication concerns. For example, Josefina's parents may have their own views on communication disabilities. These views should be examined, given the existence of an uncle with history of a fluency disorder.

Language–Ego Permeability

Adults may also have beliefs about how language should be used or produced. In other words, they develop a sense of "boundaries" for what is acceptable language use and what is not. They develop a sense for when language output is being degraded or changed and may have varying levels of tolerance for nonstandard forms of the language (e.g., language borrowing, code switching). These implicit beliefs are associated with language–ego permeability (Guiora & Acton, 1979; Schumann, 1986). The less flexible or closed the person is to allowing change to occur in the languages spoken, the greater the likelihood that the native language will persevere and be used actively in the home. This bears great significance for sustaining a non-mainstream language (Spanish, in Josefina's case). It may also affect the decision as to which language to intervene in and how active the non-mainstream

language remains after the child begins interacting with the mainstream language (for Josefina, English).

▶ Linguistic Variables Affecting the Assessment and Intervention Process

The societal manner in which language is used plays an important role in the development of language in a bilingual child. Chamberlain and Medinos-Landurand (1991) reviewed several linguistic factors that influence the assessment process—specifically, language-use patterns, language loss, code switching, and dialectal variance.

Language-use patterns refer to the way that language is used given the context of discourse. The pragmatics of language require that we pay attention to the participants, setting, functions, and topics involved in discourse (Fantini, 1985). In other words, who are the people involved in modeling language to the child? Where do these communicative acts take place? What reasons does the child have for communicating? What is spoken about and what are children expected to talk about? These questions must be answered from the point of view of both parent and child. How does the child seem to interpret the message of how language should be used given the input received from the environment?

Language loss refers to the apparent loss (attrition) of functional vocabulary and utterances in the nondominant language due to reduced exposure. This process may occur in children who undergo a change in the amount, frequency, or perceived relevance for a given language. If Josefina's parents were to stop using Spanish for some reason after months of providing that stimulation to Josefina, that decision may lead to a decrease in productive language in the child and ultimately a reduced ability to access the language that was learned without external, supporting input. Therefore, a history of inconsistent language input, where one language or the other is not supported, may lead to apparent delays in one or both languages. This assumption is a common diagnostic error leading to misdiagnosis of bilingual children.

Code switching is rule-governed socially and grammatically constrained communicative behavior, wherein a person alternates between two languages within the same communicative event. This behavior may be socially stigmatized as "improper" use of either language but may have functional and appropriate uses in a given speech community. Zentella (1997), for example, has provided a detailed account of code switching in an urban Puerto Rican community.

Understanding the cultural and societal role of code switching and the rules that govern permissible language alternations will reduce the likelihood of misdiagnosis.

Dialectal variance pertains to the sustainable changes in mainstream production of a language at the sound, word, or syntax level arising from consistent use in a speech community (Labov, 1972). These variations (also known as social dialects) may arise because of factors such as geographical location, social status, education level, and communicative contexts (Chamberlain & Medinos-Landurand, 1991). Josefina's parents, for example, may speak several dialectal variations of Spanish. Josefina's mother may speak a dialect specific to rural Puerto Rico, just as her father may speak varieties of Puerto Rican Spanish and urban New York English. Similarly, both parents may speak English and Spanish with differing accents. These language differences may be echoed in Josefina's productions. As long as her productions match the adult model(s) available to her, these language differences are not considered error patterns requiring therapeutic intervention.

An important final consideration: if the child demonstrates adequate language production in one of their languages, the child is not considered language impaired. Such a child may have mastered the linguistic elements of a language and, therefore, may communicate effectively in that language. In other words, a child who is born to bilingual parents, yet who grows up monolingual, is not considered a candidate for treatment. As long as the child's development in that language meets the standards of the linguistic community at some level, the child is judged communicatively within normal limits. However, if there is suspicion that the child is not meeting the communicative demands of their environment in one or either language, it becomes doubly essential that both languages be evaluated thoroughly.

▶ Language Development: Bilingual Perspectives

How does one define the type of language learner that the child is becoming, and, subsequently, how does one define the child's level of proficiency? Researchers have attempted to classify dual-language learners into those who have been exposed to two languages—say English and Spanish—from an early age (birth) and those who have become exposed to a second language later in their development (some time after birth). This distinction has led to the classifications known as simultaneous-bilingual and sequential-bilingual. The simultaneous-bilingual child has been exposed to two languages from an early age. The sequential-bilingual child is characterized by their exposure to a second language after developing a level of fluency in first language skills. Two additional subcategories within this type—classification as early versus late sequential bilingual—may also be used.

The age range suggested as a reasonable demarcation between simultaneous- and sequential-bilingual children has been the subject of some debate (Bhatia & Ritchie, 1999; de Houwer, 1995; McLaughlin, 1984). The age range for sequential-bilingual learners has been proposed as, at the earliest, 1-month old to approximately 3 years of age. Most experts agree that simultaneous-bilingualism requires a balanced input in each language from an early age. In reality, maintaining equal balance of both languages over the lifespan of the child is extremely difficult, if not unlikely (Fishman, 1966). In either case, it appears far more reasonable to define how the child has developed their

🔍 CASE STUDY: JOSEFINE: ADJUSTED RELEVANT ACADEMIC HISTORY

Josefina attended Pre-Kindergarten at age 4 after receiving childcare from the family. The neighborhood preschool program was reported to have two teachers, both of whom spoke Spanish fluently. The classroom comprised neighborhood children who were of diverse ethnic background. Most children spoke Spanish as a first language and this preschool was their first exposure to English. Josefina was exposed to English by her older siblings, who were 13 months older than her.

Josefina attended a general education kindergarten classroom. The class did not have any students from her pre-K program. Most children were classified as English-dominant speakers and Josefina was grouped with these students. Josefina was described as "shy," with "few friends," and "was not a disruption to the classroom." Josefina's teacher, Miss Z, indicated that she often needed to repeat instructions and that Josefina was slow to respond or complete assignments independently. She believed that Josefina's language skills were limited in vocabulary and ability to comprehend verbal questions and instructions consistently. Miss Z was planning to refer Josefina to a special education evaluation and would recommend a more restrictive educational environment with fewer students so Josefina could get more attention.

bilingualism by measuring quantity and quality of input rather than using a criterion based strictly on age. Josefina's background suggests primary exposure to Spanish from her parents and caregivers, but English-language input may come through siblings, classroom language exposure, television, and the neighborhood community. More detailed information would be useful regarding the communicative contexts in which Josefina has been engaged at school.

When addressing the critical period for second language (L2) acquisition, consensus has been reached on three points:

- Adults proceed more quickly through the very early stages of phonological, syntactical, and morphological development.
- When time and exposure are controlled, older children move through the stages of syntactical and morphological development in L2 faster than younger children do.
- Individuals who begin to acquire their L2 as young children usually achieve higher levels of oral proficiency in L2 phonology and syntax than individuals who begin to develop the L2 as adults. The prepubescent and postpubescent periods have been identified as major markers in this area.

An early theory proposed by Volterra and Taeschner (1978), the unitary language system view, suggested that children exposed to two languages simultaneously processed those languages through the same system, only to have the languages be separated over time before the age of three. This view was widely accepted until the dual- (differentiated-) language system hypothesis was proposed (Genesee, 1989; Pyke, 1986). According to this hypothesis, which is also referred to as a fractionated system view (Kohnert & Bates, 2002; Kohnert, Bates, & Hernández, 1999), a child processes each language through distinct language systems, thereby developing differentiated mental representations of the two languages from the onset of exposure. Modern research appears to support the dual-language system hypothesis given findings across linguistic domains. These studies support the notion that nascent dual-language learners process languages separately (Johnson & Lancaster, 1998; Nicoladis & Secco, 2000; Paradis, Nicoladis, & Genesee, 2000; Pearson, Fernández, & Oller, 1995; Quay, 1995).

It is important to note that the assessment of the child may be conducted at any time along the continuum of acquiring the second language. As a consequence, it becomes possible to see a child whose scores may be depressed in their native language, L1, because they have stopped developing in that area, so as to commence acquiring the second language, L2.

Thus, at the time of testing, this child may struggle with depressed scores for both L1 and L2. Does this imply a communication disorder? No, it does not. The clinician needs to be aware that this phase is part of the typical process of acquiring a second language.

▶ Confusing Language Impairment and Second Language Acquisition Processes

A significant outcome of poor cultural competence and misinformation about dual language development is the larger than expected numbers of ELLs and other culturally diverse students referred to and approved for special education programs. "Disproportionality" describes an over-representation of a demographic group in special education in comparison to the presence of the group in the overall student population (NEA Education Policy and Practice Department, 2008). The disproportionate referral of certain groups to special education has several effects: (1) it promotes stereotypes about the over-referred group; (2) it limits access to an appropriate general education by the group members; (3) it lowers student, teacher, and parent expectations about potential achievement; and (4) it places the blame of poor achievement on the results of the misidentification rather than critiquing the assessment and referral processes that created the problem. A memorandum from the Office of Special Education Programs in 2007 confirmed that "African-American children represented 14.8% of the population aged 6–21 [in 1998–1999 school year], yet comprised 20.2% of all children with disabilities" (U.S. Department of Education, 2007b).

Sequential bilinguals developing typically are often misidentified as having a language impairment because the normal processes of learning a second language in children share many patterns of behavior with that of monolingual students with speech-language impairments. For example, ELLs and monolingual SLI children both tend to have suppressed vocabularies and appear to make errors in acquisition of grammatical morphemes (Genesee, Paradis, & Crago, 2004). If a child is exposed to Spanish first and then to English in school, the uneven prestige and power of English in the United States may result in the child rejecting or suppressing their activities around Spanish language use in favor of the prestige language. When this occurs, some ELLs begin to lose access to the vocabulary and grammar they previously acquired, appearing as a sort of "language loss." Meanwhile, lack of experience with English will have the child appear limited in vocabulary and grammatical coherence in the L2. A child tested while in these stages of second language acquisition may appear delayed in both languages, a common referent used by practitioners to determine that a bilingual child has a communication impairment. Therefore, it is particularly important for evaluators to understand the historical language-learning context of the child in order to best frame the results of testing and avoid misdiagnosing the child.

Conversely, the challenging nature of assessment may also lead to "false negative" outcomes: evaluators incorrectly identifying a bilingual child with language impairment as "within normal limits." The misidentification of language-impaired bilingual students in either direction may come down to (1) the inexperience of the evaluator with typical dual language learners, (2) intrinsic differences between evaluators in how conservative they are in offering a diagnosis of "impaired" versus "unimpaired," and (3) intrinsic difference between evaluators with regard to cultural-linguistic competence.

▶ Developmental Similarities and Differences Between Simultaneous-Bilingual and Monolingual Children

Our case study, Josefina, provides an example of a simultaneous-bilingual language learner. Josefina receives Spanish-language input from her parents and caretakers and English from her siblings and school teachers. Researchers examining the development of simultaneous-bilingual children have found specific patterns of behavior across linguistic domains (phonology, morpho-syntax, semantics, and pragmatics). Let's consider some of the possible linguistic behaviors we could expect from Josefina compared to a monolingual child.

First, simultaneous-bilingual children generally produce the morpho-syntactic rules for each language to which they are exposed at approximately the same rate and order as a monolingual child producing each language separately (Meisel, 1989, 1994; Paradis & Genesee, 1996, 1997).

Second, language mixing is a common developmental process in simultaneous-bilingual children. Another term used to describe this phenomenon, *language transfer,* refers to the use of a linguistic structure from one language as a replacement for a structure in the other language for a period of time in development (Paradis, Crago, Genesee, & Rice, 2003). In this scenario, one morphological or syntactic system may be favored based on linguistic constraints (avoiding more difficult constructions), or the linguistic environment may shift in favor of one language versus the other.

Third, Vihman's (1985) research on bilingual phonological development suggests that the child's phonemic repertoire will consist of sounds from both languages given their relative salience and ease of production. Phonological transfers may occur just as they would for lexical or morpho-syntactic construction.

Fourth, lexical development is predominantly context-specific. That is, the child learns the vocabulary for specific items in a language through naturalistic interactions with the item or exposure to the concept. In some cases, this will lead to the child knowing only one term rather than two terms from each language for a concept. Research suggests that the child's vocabulary size in each language significantly correlates with the amount of vocabulary exposure or input they are given in each language (Marchman & Martinez-Sussmann, 2002; Pearson, Fernández, Lewedeg, & Oller, 1997).

Fifth, as the child approaches the age of 36 months (but perhaps earlier), the amount of language mixing/transfer decreases and the child develops greater awareness of the two languages. The use of the languages becomes more discrete, reflecting the environmental context, participants, topic, and other factors. Patterson (1998) suggests that the aggregate vocabulary of a bilingual child will equal that of a monolingual child. That is, if each language is measured separately, the child's total vocabulary in each language will seem deficient and will under-represent the bilingual child's true lexical development.

Sixth, if this behavior is sustained in the environment, simultaneous-bilingual children may demonstrate facility with code switching. Children may develop an understanding of the use constraints for this manner of communication and begin to apply them if supported. In assessing bilingual children, some clinicians look at communicative competence, which comprises the child's ability to communicate messages effectively. When adopting this perspective, the SLP should differentiate between the following types of competence:

- *Grammatical competence:* Phonological, syntactic, and lexical skills
- *Sociolinguistic/sociocultural competence:* The use of language and communication rules appropriate in one's language

- *Discourse competence:* The skills involved in the connection of a series of utterances to form a conversation and/or narrative
- *Strategic competence:* The strategies used by the bilingual person to compensate for breakdowns in communication that may result from imperfect knowledge of the rules or fatigue, memory lapses, distraction, and anxiety

Evaluating the child in a variety of communicative contexts may allow the clinician to observe competence in different areas (Riquelme, 2006a).

▶ Collaborating with Interpreters/Translators

Regulations on the use of interpreters/translators for speech-language assessment and intervention vary by state. In some states, every bilingual child referred for a speech-language evaluation is required to undergo an assessment that can be performed only by a clinician who is bilingual in the child's native language. Needless to say, this is sometimes quite difficult, as a match between the child's native language and the clinician's bilingual proficiency is not always possible. Indeed, approximately 5.1% of ASHA-certified SLPs identify themselves as bilingual or multilingual (ASHA, 2009).

An interpreter is a person who is specially trained to transpose oral or signed text from one language to another. A translator is a person who is trained to transpose written text from one language to another. SLPs most often require the services of an interpreter. Not every bilingual person has the ability to be an interpreter, of course. In addition to proficiency in two languages, other skills needed by the interpreter include (1) the ability to say the same things in different ways; (2) the ability to shift styles; (3) the ability to retain chunks of information while interpreting; and (4) familiarity with medical, educational, and professional terminology (Langdon, 2002). The interpreter should not be a friend or family member, as the information may be misunderstood, relayed inaccurately, or purposely omitted (Kayser, 1995).

Interpreters/translators are often used by the SLP for assessment and intervention purposes. Often, the interpreter/translator is hired as support personnel if the need is great (Kayser, 1995). This point underscores the need for all clinicians to become culturally competent, as even a monolingual/English SLP will likely have bilingual children in their caseload. Remember that the bilingual child may be dominant in English; thus, the clinician treating this child can be

a monolingual/English professional who will need to be sensitive to the cultural and linguistic differences of the child. In any event, it would be inappropriate to measure the bilingual child's communication skills and style against that of a monolingual/English language speaker. This understanding is particularly important with regard to the translation of testing material for assessment purposes. Translated tests are statistically invalid; the standardized norms associated with the original test are not representative of the translated version. Therefore, performance on the translated version must be evaluated by other measures (e.g., criterion-referenced measures) rather than by relying on the original norms. Likewise, the representation of developmental language milestones on translated tests can present challenges. Standardized tests assume a developmental progression of language skills across domains. However, this progression is language-specific. For example, aspects of English may not emerge in Spanish at an age-equivalent period of development. Therefore, a translated test should be adapted to address the developmental expectations for the target language used in the community. Establishing local norms for the translated, adapted test is critical. Also, using multiple measures (e.g., narratives, language samples) will support the clinical impressions derived from using translated, adapted material.

If a professional interpreter is used, training of that person by the SLP will be required. The clinician needs to introduce the interpreter to the goals of assessment and intervention, stressing the importance of accurate/direct interpretation as per the complexity of speech-language diagnostics. This training serves to highlight how the clinician reaches an impression based on what may be interpreted. If a professional interpreter is not available, then another professional may be trained to assist the SLP. As mentioned earlier, the SLP should avoid the use of a family member or friend as an interpreter.

During the session, it is important that the clinician direct their attention and communication attempts to the student/client—not to the interpreter. Other modifications to testing procedures may include the following measures:

- Reword instructions as needed.
- Allow additional response time.
- Record all responses for later analysis.
- Accept culturally appropriate responses.
- Repeat stimuli as needed.
- Use culturally appropriate pictures and themes.

Langdon (2002) has written a handbook that contains procedures and training exercises for the interpreter who is collaborating with the SLP. Additional guidelines and suggestions are offered by Wallace (1997) and Kayser (1995).

▶ Improving Cultural Sensitivity in Assessment

The most powerful weapon that SLPs have in their diagnostic repertoire is information. The more data one collects from colleagues, the community, family, and the child, the more likely one is to diagnose the child correctly. Cultural information may be obtained from several resources. Roseberry-McKibbin (1995) has provided a list of suggestions for improving cultural sensitivity and competence. Among these, three stand out as being essential: analyzing one's own assumptions and values, using cultural informants and interpreters, and considering the child's needs within their linguistic community. In addition to increasing cultural and linguistic knowledge, SLPs have other diagnostic tools at their disposal for data collection. Language sampling across naturalistic, communicative contexts is essential. In the case of the bilingual child, it is imperative to analyze both languages. The examiner has ethical and legal obligations to fulfill in determining the linguistic potential of a given child, and only by considering all aspects of a child's linguistic and cultural history will the strongest diagnosis take place.

Formal/Standardized Testing

Given the complexity of cultural and linguistic factors, strict use of standardized tests is not recommended with bilingual children. To appropriately validate an examination and deem its results to be reliable, the standardization sample must be well defined (McCauley, 1996). Unfortunately, the heterogeneity of bilingual populations makes standardization untenable for these groups. Although some sample characteristics are discrete (e.g., age, gender), the sample must also account for continuous variables (e.g., level of bilingualism, language proficiency, language-use patterns, dialect changes, acculturation) that are in a constant state of flux. This consideration is also relevant for children who may speak the language used by the examiner and the diagnostic tool but may differ in cultural terms. For example, vocabulary tests may present stimuli that are specific to a particular geographic region or cultural perspective. Looking at cultural relevance and the normative sample of a test battery should be a routine procedure for any examiner.

Nevertheless, any formal test battery employed inherently carries some sorts of linguistic and cultural biases (Anderson, 2002). Anderson describes linguistic bias as the language used during testing and/or the language expected in the child's responses. This decision is often quite subjective, as is the examiner's acceptance of responses from the child being tested. Anderson describes cultural bias as "the language used during testing and the language expected in the child's responses" (p. 146). She further defines cultural bias as referring to "the use of activities and items that do not correspond to the child's experiential base" (p. 146).

Another aspect to consider is that most children being tested are bilingual to differing degrees. Norm-referenced tests look at each language as a separate entity and do not assess the relationship between the two languages (Riquelme, 2006a). Research has shown that formal tests tend to over-identify Hispanic children as language learning disabled (Kayser, 1995; Peña, Quinn, & Iglesias, 1992). Unfortunately, in spite of these findings, many examiners and school districts continue to rely on the results of norm-referenced tests for the identification of children with communication disorders (Kayser, 1995).

Non-Standardized (Previously Informal) Testing

Many examiners consider informal testing to be an important part of the assessment process. The term *informal* often implies not as relevant as standardized testing. The authors suggest the SLP consider the term "non-standardized." For example, diagnostic observation/assessment of play skills is often reported as informal testing, and yet, the results of this play assessment may help differentially diagnose the child's communication delay/disorder. Hence, why devalue it by utilizing the term *informal*? It is important to note that often, when reporting results, this type of testing is presented/reported as if lacking in objectivity. Of greater validity are criterion-referenced procedures. These procedures provide the examiner with information that cannot be obtained from formal tests. They assess an individual's performance of a particular skill, structure, or concept. The fundamental purpose of criterion-referenced procedures is to distinguish between levels of performance (McCauley, 1996). Examples include measuring the percentage of syllables stuttered during a speech sample, maximum phonation time, percentage of correct consonants, and mean length of utterances (McCauley, 1996). Criterion-referenced measures are relatively narrow in focus, as they are used to differentiate among levels of performance. Anderson (2002) offers the following example:

> A criterion-referenced measure may be a child's ability to use episodic structure in a storytelling task. As such, it is developed so that the particular relevant aspects of the episodic structure during a retelling task can be scrutinized. The clinician may establish how many stories the child will retell, how many episodes each story contains, and the expected performance level, such as number of complete episodes produced.
>
> (p. 162)

An obvious advantage of these measures is that they can be tailored to the individual child. Use of familiar tasks and objects can reduce the effects of bias associated with reduced or limited experience and variations in culturally determined interaction styles. Another diagnostic alternative or adjunct is the use of *ethnographic observations*. This technique allows the examiner to observe the child in a variety of communicative contexts and determine their competence in those contexts. The examiner is cautioned, however, to observe a variety of settings (e.g., one or more classrooms, playground). Likewise, the examiner must understand that this type of observation is inevitably colored by the examiner's own view of the world. If the examiner interprets the child's behavior incorrectly, it may result in misdiagnosis of the child. To prevent examiner bias to the greatest extent possible, clear objectives/goals for the observation should be established in advance (Anderson, 2002; Kayser, 1995), and a cultural informant should review the results of the assessment.

Language sampling is another available technique for the assessment of bilingual children. This is a well-known technique in our field. For specific suggestions on conducting language sampling with Latino children, the reader is referred to works by Anderson (2002), Kayser (1995), and Restrepo (1997). Some of this material applies to any bilingual child being evaluated.

Another option for non standardized testing is *dynamic assessment*. This procedure assesses not only the child's current performance level, but also the child's potential to learn. Because dynamic assessment provides information on the child's ability to learn, it provides the examiner with great insight for both identifying a language disorder and planning intervention. Peña et al. (1992) and Ukrainetz, Harpell, Walsh, and Coyle (2000) have documented the benefits of using this procedure. They tested children in a particular task, then taught it to the children, and subsequently retested the children on the task without using cues or other supports.

Both studies documented that children who were language impaired failed to demonstrate learning in the same manner as children who had typical language skills. Dynamic assessment certainly appears to be a viable procedure for use by SLPs in assessing the communicative skills of bilingual and/or ELL children (Gutierrez-Clellen & Peña, 2001; Peña et al., 1992; Peña, Iglesias, & Lidz, 2001). Additional resources are provided at the end of this chapter to aid in better utilization of nonstandardized approaches to assessment and treatment of children with suspected communication disorders.

Background Information

For many SLPs, it is common practice to report a child's history as "background information" related to, but separate from, the linguistic data collected. A "traditional" assessment model imitates the psychological model of assessment. This view suggests that language is a self-contained domain that can be analyzed apart from other domains, namely the cognitive and emotional domains. In contrast, a sociological assessment model attempts to recognize the influences of other domains on language and observe language in the most authentic contexts possible while capturing the most naturally occurring form, content, and uses of the language as possible.

The cultural information that a family provides is not "background" but rather a central feature of the data needed to improve SLPs' diagnostic and therapeutic decision making. Many parent questionnaires and checklists have been developed to facilitate and streamline the collection of background information. Unfortunately, formal questionnaires or checklists may provide only a superficial understanding of the relevant cultural and linguistic behaviors specific to a family or social group. Although it may seem simple to generalize traits of a given social group to all members of that group, such action will obscure the individual behaviors of smaller units within the group—for example, the family unit. Because the behaviors of individual members of a cultural group can vary widely (Van Kleeck, 1994), it is especially important to hear the "story" of the family unit as unique and incomparable. Generalization may well lead to biases and misconceptions that endanger the diagnostic process and damage the relationship between the clinician and the family being served.

To strengthen the clinician–family relationship, an approach that focuses on the family's values and concerns from the onset of interaction may reduce inadvertent over-generalizations and biases. One such approach suggested by Westby (1990) includes *ethnographic interviewing*. Many parents and caregivers are accustomed to the traditional model of interviewing in which the clinician requests answers to a series of questions designed to obtain the most essential diagnostic information. In contrast, the clinician, when working as an ethnographic interviewer, attempts to gain a more intimate understanding of a family's dynamics and the child's role in that system. One can think of the ethnographic approach as a personalized method of exploration that provides the clinician with an opportunity to obtain a deep, true, and naturalistic understanding of the behavior or culture under study. Through this process, the clinician listens to the behaviors and beliefs reported by the parent or caregiver, as obtained through a systematic and guided dialogue with the caretaker. Essential elements of effective ethnographic interviewing required of the clinician include the following components (Wallace, 1997; Westby, 1990):

- Establishment of rapport
- Good listening skills
- A clear set of goals for information to be obtained
- Skill in selecting the appropriate types of questions (i.e., grand tour, mini-tour, example, experience, or native-language questions)
- Skill in framing questions, so that they are open-ended yet targeted to probe into key areas of interest
- Skill in looking for patterns and common theme expressions as an essential key to detecting critical concerns of interest to the client/patient and family

Ethnographic interviewing allows for the following outcomes:

- Conveys empathy/acceptance of the world as defined by the informant
- Collects information necessary for generating appropriate support and clinical practice
- Helps equalize the power differential between clinician and informant
- Provides a means for the professional to discover the culture of the family and their strengths and needs
- Provides a means for focusing on the perspective of the informant
- Helps reduce potential bias in assessment and intervention
- Allows the data to be collected in a more ecologically valid framework (Westby, 1990)

During ethnographic interviewing, the clinician has a general set of questions at the outset, but the flow of questioning is guided by the scope and depth of information obtained as the interview unfolds. The clinician is also advised to pay attention to how questions are worded: use open-ended rather than closed-ended questions, use presupposition questions effectively, ask one question at a time, make use of preliminary statements, and maintain control of the interview. Saville-Troike (1978) offered additional suggestions for asking questions that are geared to understanding the family's position on several cultural dimensions. In any case, the SLP conducting the interview must realize that their background will affect the kinds of questions to be presented, the way the questions are posed, and the way answers are interpreted.

Hammer (1998) notes the importance of using several resources to develop an understanding of a particular family's cultural beliefs and practices. In addition to interviews and questionnaires, Hammer suggests literature review, examination of written documents (e.g., medical records), and analysis of open observation systems (child interacting in naturalistic contexts) as a means to gather evidence. A correlation can then be determined between the anecdotal data of an ethnographic interview and the data collected from direct observations, prior research on that culture or language, and formal assessment procedures.

▶ Treatment Considerations

Choice of Language for Treatment

Deciding on the language of treatment for bilingual or non-English-speaking children has been a hotly debated issue in the bilingual education literature as well as in speech-language pathology. Many questions arise when deciding how to approach remediation of the bilingual child with a language disorder: will intervention in L1 retard the progression of L2? Should treatment be provided only in L2? Will treatment in both L1 and L2 be too "taxing" for the child? Gutierrez-Clellen (1999) provides an excellent review of these and other issues and their clinical implications. To date, no study has been able to support an "English only" (L2) approach. Instead, most studies have focused on bilingual or monolingual/L1 intervention. In reviewing the literature, researchers appear to emphasize that children's language learning can be maximized when the language of instruction/treatment matches the child's language(s), and L1 is used as an organizational language framework to facilitate second language learning (Gutierrez-Clellen, 1999). Language-impaired children who are learning a second language constitute a heterogeneous group. This diversity is evidenced by the various types of deficits presented (e.g., phonological, pragmatic, morpho-syntactic), the severity of the disorders, the modality of the disorders (e.g., receptive, expressive, both), the language experiences of the child in L1 and

L2, and the child's position along the second language acquisition continuum. All of these factors will influence the rate of learning each language as well as the child's progress in an intervention program.

Collaborations

Of great importance to the clinician working with bilingual children is the joint work with ESL teachers, classroom teachers, and parents. The SLP's success in treating a child with language impairment hinges on this collaboration and on their ability to develop culturally relevant strategies, tasks, and materials. Application of the previously mentioned culturally and linguistically sensitive considerations is as critical during treatment planning as it is during the assessment process.

Service Delivery

Another factor that influences the success of the child with language impairment is the type of service delivery models available for intervention. This factor is largely determined by the resources of the particular school district as well as by the school district's underlying philosophy in regard to bilingual and special education. Providing optimal treatment to a bilingual or non-English-speaking child is a multifaceted endeavor that requires commitment to working with families, students as individuals, and school team members to foster success for the child (Roseberry-McKibbin, 2002).

▶ Summary

As SLPs continue to practice in a multicultural world, and as they continue to provide services to culturally and linguistically diverse children, the need to become culturally sensitive becomes increasingly obvious. Cultural sensitivity, a lifelong process, will allow SLPs to provide services to children from all cultural and linguistic backgrounds with as little bias as is humanly and clinically possible.

Study Questions

- Define culture, and explain how it affects assessment and treatment practices with all children.
- Outline a protocol for least-biased assessment practices.
- Outline questions you might ask a parent during an evaluation, using ethnographic interviewing constructs.

The impact of language, as a cultural construct, has significance in our conception of children as dual-language learners. In the case study, Josefina's Spanish and English language use will be affected by the contexts of that exposure:

- Who will the participants in language input be?
- How does having the mother as a model of Spanish versus having the father as a model of English influence Josefina's development?
- Where will she obtain her language stimulation?
- Will she spend more time at home, where Spanish will abound, or will she spend more time in the community, where English is a more prominent fixture in daily activities?
- Will Josefina have contact with other caretakers? Will she have contact with other children?
- How will these individuals influence her language development?
- What do people talk to Josefina about?
- Is she privy to adult conversations, or will she be shielded from certain conversational topics?
- What are the contexts that drive Josefina's language use?
- Is she expected to remain a passive observer and listener, or will she be expected to produce language on par with peers or even adults?

The answers to these questions can be obtained by the SLP through observation and analysis of the culturally and linguistically significant behaviors unique to the family. The answers may not be readily accessible or easily learned in every case, but their discovery will result in improved outcomes for the families and children in SLPs' care.

SLPs face many challenges ahead, many of them linked to the notion of a culture that originally intended to be homogeneous (e.g., America as a "melting pot"). Providing culturally sensitive services to children of all cultural backgrounds should be a challenge that all clinicians approach with enthusiasm and passion. Until misdiagnosis because of cultural differences is a thing of the past, SLPs cannot stop learning and challenging their clinical practices.

- If formal tests currently in use (criterion-referenced) were normed on a population different from that which you are testing, how would you report the results of your assessment with these batteries? Why? Outline other options for assessment.
- Discuss the decision-making process for providing treatment to a child in L1, L2, or L1 + L2.

Advanced Study Questions

Consider the following scenarios as you did while using Josefina as our model client. Prepare responses to enrich your depth of understanding and for use with comparable situations:

1. A single parent from the Dominican Republic is told to speak only English to her 3-year-old monolingual Spanish-exposed daughter because that is the language everyone else will speak in school. Consider the factors leading the educator to make this recommendation and consider the ramifications of this recommendation on the language exposure and sociocultural development of this child. How would you counsel this parent if she were concerned about the child's language development?

2. A mother and father originally from Puerto Rico each attended college in the United States. Their 6-year-old son is now a fluent bilingual child but is having difficulty with development of reading skills in the first grade. The school is suggesting that the cause of the deficit might be the child's level of bilingualism. What information and observations might you need to provide guidance to the family and the staff working with this child?

3. A bilingual male raised in the United States is married to a monolingual English-speaking female and they have one son. Though Spanish is spoken by the boy's paternal grandmother while she cares for him 3 days a week, the child is not developing his Spanish language skills. His English language skills appear to be generally age appropriate at the time of an SLP consultation. What non developmental factors might be contributing to the child's limited second language development? Consider the ethnographic interviewing construct and the questions that might provide some context for the child's language development.

4. A 4-year-old Mexican female child is evaluated by a bilingual SLP. She engages the child in English and quickly establishes a rapport. When the evaluator switches to Spanish, she is responded to by the child only in English. The child's parent is told that the child is English-dominant and that the child's language skills are not functional in Spanish. The parent disagrees with this assessment and finds some flaws in the clinician's reasoning. What could the evaluator have done differently during the assessment that could have impacted the child's performance? Consider what kind of information and data the parent might have that the clinician could use to support or reject her initial conclusion.

References

American Speech-Language-Hearing Association (ASHA). (n.d.). Self-assessment for cultural competence (practice portal). Retrieved from https://www.asha.org/practice/multicultural/self/

American Speech-Language-Hearing Association (ASHA). (2004). Knowledge and skills needed by speech-language pathologists and audiologists to provide culturally and linguistically appropriate services. Retrieved from http://www.asha.org/policy/KS2004-00215.htm

American Speech-Language-Hearing Association (ASHA). (2009). Demographic profile of ASHA members providing bilingual and Spanish language services. Retrieved from www.asha.org/uploadedFiles/Demographic-Profile-Bilingual-Spanish-Service-Members.pdfASHA. (2011). Cult comp in prof service delivery.

American Speech-Language-Hearing Association. (2017). Issues in ethics: Cultural and linguistic competence. Retrieved from www.asha.org/Practice/ethics/Cultural-and-Linguistic-Competence/

Anderson, R. T. (2002). Practical assessment strategies with Hispanic students. In A. Brice (Ed.), *The Hispanic child*. Boston, MA: Allyn and Bacon.Bebout, L., & Arthur, B. (1992). Cross-cultural attitudes toward speech disorders. *Journal of Speech, Language, and Hearing Research, 35,* 45–52.

Bhatia T. K., & Ritchie, W. C. (Eds.). (1999). The bilingual child: Some issues and perspectives (pp. 457–491). *Handbook of child language acquisition*. San Diego, CA: Academic Press.

Cabassa, L. J. (2003). Measuring acculturation: Where we are and where we need to go. *Hispanic Journal of Behavioral Sciences, 25*(2), 127–146.

Carbaugh, D. (1988). Comments on "culture" in communication inquiry. *Communication Reports, 1,* 38–41.

Chamberlain, P., & Medinos-Landurand, P. (1991). Practical considerations for the assessment of LEP students with special needs. In E. Hamayan & J. Damico (Eds.), *Limiting bias in the assessment of bilingual students* (pp. 112–129, 131). Austin, TX: Pro Ed.

de Houwer, A. (1995). Bilingual language acquisition. In P. Fletcher & B. MacWhinney (Eds.), *Handbook of child language* (pp. 219–250). Oxford, UK: Basil Blackwell.

Dikeman, K. J., & Riquelme, L. F. (2002, October). Ethnocultural concerns in dysphagia. *Perspectives on Swallowing and Swallowing Disorders, 11*(3), 31–35.

Fantini, A. (1985). *Language acquisition of a bilingual child: A sociolinguistic perspective*. San Diego, CA: College Hill Press.

Farver, J. M., Kim, Y. K., & Lee, Y. (1995). Cultural differences in Korean- and Anglo-American preschoolers' social interaction and play behaviors. *Child Development, 66,* 1088–1099.

Fishman, J. A. (Ed.). (1966). *Language loyalty in the United States.* The Hague: Mouton.

Genesee, F. (1989). Early bilingual development: One language or two? *Journal of Child Language, 16,* 161–179.

Genesee, F., Paradis, J., & Crago, M. B. (2004). *Dual language development and disorders: A handbook on bilingualism and second language learning.* Baltimore, MD: Paul H. Brookes Publishing.

Goldstein, B. (2004). *Bilingual language development and disorders in Spanish–English speakers.* Baltimore, MD: Paul H. Brookes.

Guiora, A. Z., & Acton, W. R. (1979). Personality and language: A restatement. *Language Learning, 29,* 193–204.

Gutierrez-Clellan, V., & Pena, E. (2001). Dynamic assessment of diverse children: A tutorial. *Language, Speech, Hearing Services in Schools, 32,* 212–224.

Gutierrez-Clellen, V. F. (1999). Language choice in intervention with bilingual children. *American Journal of Speech-Language Pathology, 8,* 291–302.

Hammer, C. S. (1998). Toward a "thick description" of families: Using ethnography to overcome the obstacles to providing family-centered early intervention services. *American Journal of Speech-Language Pathology, 7,* 5–22.

Heath, S. (1983). *Ways with words: Language, life, and work in communities and classrooms.* New York, NY: Cambridge University Press.

Johnson, C., & Lancaster, P. (1998). The development of more than one phonology: A case study of a Norwegian–English bilingual child. *International Journal of Bilingualism, 2*(3), 265–300.

Kayser, H. (1995). *Bilingual speech-language pathology: An Hispanic focus.* San Diego, CA: Singular.

Kleinman, A., Eisenberg, L., & Good, B. (2006). Culture, illness, and care: Clinical lessons from anthropologic and cross-cultural research. *Focus, 4,* 140–149.

Kohnert, K. J. (2008). *Language disorders in bilingual children and adults.* San Diego, CA: Plural.

Kohnert, K. J., & Bates, E. (2002). Balancing bilinguals II: Lexical comprehension and cognitive processing in children learning Spanish and English. *Journal of Speech, Language, and Hearing Research, 45,* 347–359.

Kohnert, K. J., Bates, E., & Hernández, A. E. (1999). Balancing bilinguals: Lexical–semantic production and cognitive processing in children learning Spanish and English. *Journal of Speech, Language, and Hearing Research, 42,* 1400–1413.

Labov, W. (1972). *Sociolinguistic patterns.* Philadelphia, PA: University of Pennsylvania Press.

Langdon, H. W. (2002). *Interpreters and translators in communication disorders: A practitioner's handbook.* Eau Claire, WI: Thinking Publications.

Maestas, A. G., & Erickson, J. G. (1992). Mexican immigrant mothers' beliefs about disabilities. *American Journal of Speech-Language Pathology, 1,* 5–10.

Marchman, V. A., & Martínez-Sussmann, C. (2002). Concurrent validity of caregiver/parent report measures of language for children who are learning both English and Spanish. *Journal of Speech, Language, and Hearing Research, 45,* 983–997.

McCauley, R. J. (1996). Familiar strangers: Criterion-referenced measures in communications disorders. *Language, Speech, and Hearing Services in Schools, 29,* 3–10.

McLaughlin, B. (1984). Early bilingualism: Methodological and theoretical issues. In G. Duncan & J. Brooks-Gunn (Eds.), *Consequences of growing up poor* (pp. 35–48). New York, NY: Russell Sage Foundation.

Meisel, J. (1989). Early differentiation of languages in bilingual children. In K. Hyltenstam & L. Obler (Eds.), *Bilingualism across the lifespan: Aspects of acquisition, maturity and loss* (pp. 13–40). Cambridge, UK: Cambridge University Press.

Meisel, J. (1994). *Bilingual first language acquisition: French and German grammatical development.* Amsterdam, The Netherlands: John Benjamins.

Nicoladis, E., & Secco, G. (2000). Productive vocabulary and language choice. *First Language, 20*(58), 3–28.

Paradis, J., Crago, M., Genesee, F., & Rice, M. (2003). French–English bilingual children with SLI: How do they compare with their monolingual peers? *Journal of Speech, Language, and Hearing Research, 46,* 113–127.

Paradis, J., & Genesee, F. (1996). Syntactic acquisition of bilingual children: Autonomous or interdependent? *Studies in Second Language Acquisition, 18,* 1–15.

Paradis, J., & Genesee, F. (1997). On continuity and the emergence of functional categories in bilingual first language acquisition. *Language Acquisition, 6*(2), 91–124.

Paradis, J., Nicoladis, E., & Genesee, F. (2000). Early emergence of structural constraints on code-switching: Evidence from French–English bilingual children. *Bilingualism: Language and Cognition, 3*(3), 245–261.

Patterson, J. L. (1998). Expressive vocabulary development and word combinations of Spanish–English bilingual toddlers. *American Journal of Speech-Language Pathology, 7,* 46–56.

Payne, J. C. (1997). *Adult neurogenic language disorders: Assessment and treatment—A comprehensive ethnobiological approach.* San Diego, CA: Singular.

Pearson, B. Z., Fernández, S. C., Lewedeg, V., & Oller, D. K. (1997). The relation of input factors to lexical learning by bilingual infants. *Applied Psycholinguistics, 18,* 41–58.

Pearson, B. Z., Fernández, S. C., & Oller, D. K. (1995). Cross-language synonyms in the lexicons of bilingual infants: One language or two? *Journal of Child Language, 22,* 345–368.

Peña, E., Quinn, R., & Iglesias, A. (1992). The application of dynamic methods to language assessment: A non-biased procedure. *Journal of Special Education, 26,* 269–280.

Peña, E. D., Iglesias, A., & Lidz, C. S. (2001). Reducing test bias through dynamic assessment of children's word learning ability. *American Journal of Speech-Language Pathology, 10,* 138–154.

Pyke, C. (1986). One lexicon or two? An alternative interpretation of early bilingual speech. *Journal of Child Language, 13,* 591–593.

Quay, S. (1995). The bilingual lexicon: Implications for studies of language choice. *Journal of Child Language, 22,* 369–387.

Rawls, J. (1971). *A theory of justice.* Cambridge, MA: Belknap Press of Harvard University Press.

Restrepo, M. A. (1997). Guidelines for identifying primarily Spanish-speaking preschool children with language impairment. *Perspectives on Cultural and Linguistic Diverse Populations, ASHA Special Interest Division, 14*(3), 11–12.

Riquelme, L. F. (2004). Cultural competence in dysphagia. *The ASHA Leader, 9*(7), 8, 22.

Riquelme, L. F. (2006a). Working with Hispanic/Latino students. In E. H. Gravani & J. Meyer (Eds.), *Speech-language-hearing programs: A guide for students and practitioners,* (2nd ed., pp. 429–446). Austin, TX: Pro Ed.

Riquelme, L. F. (2006b). Working with limited-English speaking adults with neurological impairment. *Perspectives on Gerontology, ASHA SID 15, 11*(2), 3–8.

Riquelme, L. F. (2007). The role of cultural competence in providing services to persons with dysphagia. *Topics in Geriatric Rehabilitation, 25*(3), 228–239.

Riquelme, L. F. (2013). Cultural competence for everyone: A shift in perspectives. *Perspectives on Gerontology, 18*(2), 42–49.

Roseberry-McKibbin, C. (1995). *Multicultural students with special language needs: Practical strategies for assessment and intervention.* Oceanside, CA: Academic Communication Associates.

Roseberry-McKibbin, C. (2002). Principles and strategies in intervention. In A. Brice (Ed.), *The Hispanic child* (pp. 199–233). Boston, MA: Allyn and Bacon.

Rubin, K. H., & Coplan, R. J. (1998). Social and nonsocial play in childhood: An individual differences perspective. In S. N. Saracho & B. Spodek (Eds.), *Multiple perspectives on play in early childhood education* (pp. 144–170). Albany, NY: State University of New York Press.

Ruiz, R. (1988). Orientations in language planning. In S. L. McKay & S. C. Wong (Eds.), *Language diversity: Problem or resource? A social and educational perspective on language minorities in the United States* (pp. 3–25). Boston, MA: Heinle & Heinle Publishers.

Ryan, C. (2013). *Language use in the United States: 2011*, American Community Survey Reports, ACS-22. U.S. Census Bureau, Washington, DC.

Salas-Provance, M., Erickson, J. G., & Reed, J. (2002). Disabilities as viewed by four generations of one Hispanic family. *American Journal of Speech-Language Pathology, 11,* 151–162.

Sánchez, C. A. (2008). Cultural (in) competence, justice and expectations of care: An illustration. *Online Journal of Health Ethics, 5*(1), 1–6.

Saville-Troike, M. (1978). *A guide to culture in the classroom.* Rosslyn, VA: National Clearinghouse for Bilingual Education.

Schumann, J. H. (1986). Research on the acculturation model for second language acquisition. *Journal of Multicultural Development, 7*(5), 379–392.

Sutton-Smith, B. (1972). *The folkgames of children.* Austin, TX: University of Texas Press.

Tervalon, M., & Murray-Garcia, J. (1998). Cultural humility versus cultural competence: A critical distinction in defining physician training outcomes in multicultural education. *Journal of Health Care for the Poor and Underserved, 9*(2), 117–125.

Ukrainetz, T. A., Harpell, S., Walsh, C., & Coyle, C. (2000). A preliminary investigation of dynamic assessment with Native American kindergarteners. *Language, Speech and Hearing Services in Schools, 31,* 142–154.

U.S. Bureau of the Census. (2000). *Statistical abstract of the United States* (119th ed.). Washington, DC: U.S. Department of Commerce.

U.S. Census Bureau. (2010). 2010 census shows America's diversity. Retrieved from http://www.census.gov/newsroom/releases/archives/2010_census/cb11-cn125.html

U.S. Department of Education. (2007a). *Executive summary OSERS 23rd Annual Report to Congress on the Implementation of the IDEA.* Retrieved from www.ed.gov/about/reports/annual/osep/2001/execsumm.html

U.S. Department of Education (2007b). *Disproportionality of racial and ethnic groups in special education.* Retrieved from www2.ed.gov/policy/speced/guid/idea/memosdcltrs/osep07-09disproportionalityofracialandethnicgroupsinspecialeducation.pdf

Van Kleeck, A. (1994). Potential cultural bias in training parents as conversational partners with their children who have delays in language development. *American Journal of Speech-Language Pathology, 3,* 67–78.

Van Roekel, N. P. D. (2008). *English language learners face unique challenges.* An NEA Policy Brief. National Education Association.

Vihman, M. (1985). Language differentiation by the bilingual infant. *Journal of Child Language, 12,* 297–324.

Volterra, V., & Taeschner, T. (1978). The acquisition and development of language by bilingual children. *Journal of Child Language, 5,* 311–326.

Wallace, G. L. (1997). *Multicultural neurogenics: A resource for speech-language pathologists.* San Antonio, TX: Communication Skill Builders.

Westby, C. E. (1990). Ethnographic interviewing: Asking the right questions to the right people in the right ways. *Journal of Childhood Communication Disorders, 13*(1), 101–111.

Zentella, A. C. (1997). *Growing up bilingual: Puerto Rican children in New York.* Malden, MA: Blackwell.

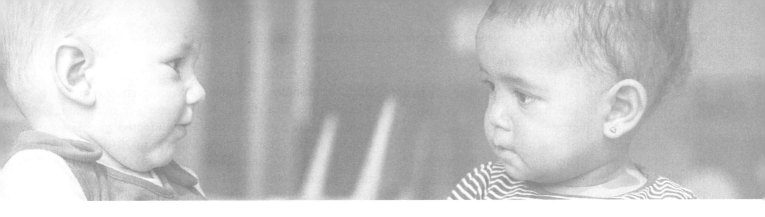

CHAPTER 14

Speech and Language Development of Children Who Were Adopted Internationally

Deborah A. Hwa-Froelich, PhD, CCC-SLP

Introduction

The process of international adoption results in a unique language acquisition trajectory in which children are born in one culture listening to and learning a language that is often different from the culture and language of their adoptive family. Children may have lived with their birth parents or other relatives prior to adoption, lived with foster parents, or they may have spent the majority of their life in an orphanage or hospital prior to being adopted. Some children may have experienced some or all of these environments before adoption (Hellerstedt et al., 2008). Thus, some of the children were exposed to loving, nurturing, socially interactive experiences, whereas others may have had few of these kinds of interactions, resulting in developmental differences in birth language development and socio-emotional communication development. Some of the children may have received adequate nutrition and medical care, whereas others did not (Leiden Conference on the Development and Care of Children without Permanent Parents, 2012). Following international adoption, children may not be exposed to or may be minimally exposed to their birth language or culture. Consequently, children do not always receive instructional or social support to continue their birth language development, often do not have enough birth language competence to be able to use their birth language to help them learn a second language, and may associate more positive feelings towards their adoptive language, which can result in rapid attrition of their birth language (Nicoladis & Grabois, 2002). They begin learning a second first language, but acquisition begins at a later age than monolingual children born and raised by their biological parents. Thus, children adopted internationally are often monolingual speakers who demonstrate a different timeline in their adopted language development. The purpose of this chapter is to describe the interrupted language development in children adopted internationally.

History

The history of international adoption (also known as intercountry adoption or transnational adoption) can be traced back to the 1950s, when children were adopted from Korea following the end of the Korean War (Holt International, 2017). The number of children who were adopted internationally increased significantly from 1950 to 2004, reaching more than 45,000 children adopted worldwide (Selman, 2009). However, since 2004–2014, the numbers of children

adopted internationally have declined 72%. In addition, the number of countries offering children for adoption has also declined over time. For example, in 2015, only 5,647 children were adopted internationally to the United States, whereas in 2010, there were 11,058 (U.S. State Department, 2015). In addition, children born in the United States are adopted by families from other countries. According to the State Department, more than 500 U.S. children were internationally adopted since 2008. Although international adoptions occur from more than 100 different countries, most of the international adoptions between 2004 and 2007 were from China, Russia, Guatemala, and Ethiopia (Selman, 2009). Currently China, Ethiopia, South Korea, Ukraine, and Uganda are the countries from which most of the children are adopted to the United States (U.S. State Department, 2015).

There are many reasons why international adoptions have declined over the years. Several countries have either changed their adoption laws or prioritized domestic adoption, which has influenced the rate of international adoption. Some countries have concerns regarding the quality of care children received from their adoptive parents and limited the agencies with whom they would work (Smolin, 2007). For example, China was concerned children would not be raised by heterosexual parents and stipulated that only dual-parent families could adopt. China also started to increase domestic adoptions, placing 20,000–30,000 children a year (U.S. State Department, 2015). Russia passed a law in 2013 prohibiting U.S. parents from adopting children from Russia largely due to political conflict between the two countries. Other countries began new processing procedures that slowed the adoption process (Haiti, Democratic Republic of the Congo), whereas others faced political strife that interrupted the adoption process (Ukraine, U.S. Department of State, 2015). Guatemala does not follow the Hague convention (issued by the international court for the Protection of Children and Co-operation in Respect of Intercountry Adoption), which resulted in the United States no longer accepting Guatemalan adoption applications since December 2007. Consequently, the number of children available for adoption has declined significantly, resulting in fewer infants available to adopt, children adopted at older ages, and more children with disabilities who are available for adoption.

Common Myths

There are several misconceptions about longitudinal outcomes for children who are internationally adopted

(Glennen, 2008). These misconceptions can influence how persons view or treat children who are adopted internationally. Thus, it is important to discuss these myths and the current evidence that exists. One misconception is that *children are placed in orphanages because they have no parents or relatives*. In many cases, the children's parents are alive but not able or willing to care for the child. In a study of 252 referrals for adoption from Eastern European countries, a reason for orphanage placement was provided in 75% of these cases. These included: (a) they were a foundling (5%), (b) the government removed them from the home for neglect (15%), (c) the parent(s) gave up their rights to care for the child due to imprisonment, social, and/or economic reasons (76%), and (d) 4% were in orphanages because their parents were deceased (Johnson, 2000). In China, the government initiated a one-child policy, limiting the number of children born to a family. China enforced this policy by forcing women to abort their unborn children if they had already given birth. Because of a cultural preference for male children and penalties for having more than one child, female infants were left in public places to be found and taken to orphanages (Miller, 2005).

It is also a myth that *after they are adopted by U.S. families, children are U.S. citizens*. Parents of children adopted from different countries must complete an application for citizenship before their child turns 18 years of age (N-600 USCIS). Several adults who were adopted internationally as infants are at risk of being unable to procure employment or being deported because their parents were either misinformed about citizenship requirements or did not complete the necessary paperwork to procure citizenship for their children.

Another myth is that *children adopted internationally are significantly delayed in all developmental areas*. There is much variability among children adopted internationally. Some children perform at or above average, whereas others demonstrate delays in one, some, or all developmental areas. Developmental catch-up is influenced by the duration of time spent in institutional care (a proxy for length of preadoptive care is adoption age) or the quality of preadoptive care: for example, the less time a child is exposed to adverse care or if the child receives adequate nutrition, medical care, and social interaction, the better the developmental outcomes. For example, researchers who conducted a meta-analysis of 62 studies found little to no difference in intelligence quotients between children adopted internationally and nonadopted peers (van IJzendoorn & Juffer, 2009). In contrast, children who spent less time in orphanages demonstrated more complete recovery in weight, although height and head circumference remained significantly lower than nonadopted peers (Ladage & Harris, 2012). However, many children demonstrated average growth over time (Loman, Wiik, Frenn, Pollak, & Gunner, 2009).

There is great variability in behavior and school achievement performance. In a meta-analysis, adolescents (grouped by age 12–13, 14–16, and 17–18 years) who were adopted (before 12 months, between 12–24 months, and older than 24 months old) demonstrated more externalizing behaviors such as impulsiveness and/or emotion regulation problems than internalizing behaviors such as withdrawal. Girls who were adopted had more behavior problems than girls who were not adopted. However, many adolescents were not significantly different from their peers who were not adopted or adopted domestically (Bimmel, Juffer, Van IJzendoorn, & Bakermans-Kranenburg, 2003). Researchers conducting a meta-analysis of studies on children adopted from abroad found that they had fewer behavior problems than children who were domestically adopted but more problems than children who were not adopted (Juffer & Van IJzendoorn, 2005, 2009). Now that more children are being adopted at older ages, a recent 3-year-longitudinal study reported on results of 48 children who were adopted internationally since 2010 (Helder, Brooker, Kapitula, Goalen, & Gunnoe, 2016). The authors found that an older adoption age, time spent in the adoptive home, and smaller family size correlated with more parent-reported inattentive and overactive behaviors. In other words, when children are exposed longer to institutional care, there is an increased risk of attention and hyperactive behavior problems that do not decline as they age. Although parents in larger families reported fewer of these behavior problems, the possible reasons for this finding remain unclear, ranging from different parental motivations for adoption that may have affected their behavioral expectations and increased their acceptance of behavior variability. However, their sample was small, adoption ages ranged between 6 months and 15 years of age, and the average amount of time the children had lived with their adoptive families was approximately 19 months with a standard deviation of 48 months. This wide variability in a small sample may have influenced their results.

In terms of school achievement, children adopted internationally are at higher risk of learning problems and poorer school achievement (Van IJzendoorn & Juffer, 2006; Van IJzendoorn, Juffer, & Poelhuis, 2005). However, variability may be based on the quality of preadoptive care. Since international adoptions began with South Korean children, South Korea had devoted more resources to provide high quality institutional and preadoptive care. Korean prenatal and post-partum care has been well-established. Orphanage staff includes psychologists, physicians, nurses, and college-educated counselors. South Korea also has a well-established foster care system. Vinnerljung, Lindblad, Hjern, Rasmussen, and Dalen (2010) and Odenstad et al. (2008) conducted a Swedish national cohort study of 16-year-old adolescents and adults who had been adopted as children before the age of 10 years. They compared academic performance based on country of origin that included subjects adopted from non-Western countries, with a large group from South Korea. Other countries included India, Thailand, Chile, Ethiopia, Columbia, and Sri Lanka (and Ecuador in the Vinnerljung et al. study). Odenstad et al. (2008) found that regardless of adoption age, if the participants had been adopted from South Korea, their cognitive performance was similar to adults who had not been adopted. They argued that adults who were adopted as children from South Korea received "good enough" care so that age of adoption was not a factor in intellectual capabilities (p. 1803). Vinnerljung et al. (2010) found that children adopted from South Korea had similar grades as nonadopted peers across academic courses but lower grades than their siblings who were not adopted. Thus, children who received *good enough* care prior to adoption had similar academic achievement and intellectual performance as their peers.

An additional myth is that *children adopted internationally are bilingual speakers, speaking their birth language and another language.* In most cases, children adopted internationally are adopted by parents who are monolingual in a different language than their children's birth languages. Consequently, young children adopted at 5 years of age or younger stop speaking their birth language within 3 months and demonstrate no interference or influence from their birth language on their adopted language (Glennen, Rosinsky-Grunhut, & Tracy, 2005; Nicoladis & Grabois, 2002).

Some children will be raised as bilingual speakers. For example, if children are adopted by parents who speak the child's birth language and another language such as English, the child will continue to be exposed to their birth language and begin learning a second language. In some cases, the adoptive parents hire a nanny or provide tutoring in the children's birth language to help the children maintain their birth language. Finally, children may be adopted by parents who are bilingual in languages different from the child's birth language. For example, at the Saint Louis University International Adoption Clinic, we have worked with children adopted by parents whose primary language is Spanish. Their children, who were born in an Eastern European country, lost their birth language and learned to speak Spanish initially. When the children were preschool age, they were exposed to English. In these cases, the child loses the birth language and is exposed to two adopted languages to become a bilingual speaker. We have also seen children who were adopted at older ages (6–15 years). In these clinical cases, the children demonstrated a plateau in first language development because they were no longer receiving input in their birth language. For younger adopted children, they demonstrate a progression of birth language attrition in that they stop expressing the language initially followed by loss of receptive language comprehension. When older adopted children were tested in their birth language, their performance was commensurate with their adoption age. Thus, birth language development stopped at the age when they no longer received input in that language. Although their English or adopted language was developing quickly, it was not yet at their chronological age level. Variables that are reported to influence language development include length of exposure to institutional environments, timing/length of foster care, and quality of care (Windsor et al., 2011; Tan & Marfo, 2006).

▶ Importance of Studying Interrupted Language Acquisition

Language learning depends on having consistent, nurturing, and stimulating social interactions with an adult. Some orphanages are able to provide this quality of care, whereas others are not. Some children spend more time in foster care prior to adoption, which in most cases would provide nurturing social interactions. When children receive adult mediation through social interaction, children develop adequate cognitive and communication skills (Vygotsky, 1986). However, the process of international adoption places children in an unusual position of exposure to two different languages at different times, with acquisition of one at a later age. This language acquisition process differs from monolingual language learners. The process of interrupted language acquisition is somewhat similar to children who are delayed in expressing themselves (late talkers) in that children adopted internationally rapidly learn and understand their adopted language but their expressive language abilities lag behind. However, children adopted internationally differ from late talkers in the amount of birth language input and social interaction as well as timing of adopted language input.

▶ Input Matters

Children who experience the international adoption process may demonstrate development similar to the development of monolingual children who were neglected or from low-income environments. Children living in orphanages that are not well-supported economically are often cared for in large groups of same-aged peers with a high child-to-adult ratio. Adult caregivers may not have received adequate education or training on how to appropriately interact with children to facilitate their growth and development. Thus, the children may not receive the kind or amount of social interaction they need to develop typical communication or social, emotional, or cognitive development, not to mention adequate nutrition and medical care (Johnson, 2000; Leiden Conference on the Development and Care of Children without Permanent Parents, 2012). This type of institutional care may negatively influence their language development in ways similar to children from neglected environments. Children exposed to abuse and/or neglect demonstrated early vocabulary and syntax delays compared to children from the same socio-economic background who were not abused or neglected (Eigsti & Cicchetti, 2004; for a review, refer to Hwa-Froelich, 2012a). More research is needed to compare developmental outcomes between children adopted internationally from countries with few resources to support children living in institutions and children exposed to abuse and/or neglect.

Children adopted internationally may resemble children who lived in families from low-income backgrounds who may not be able to receive as much linguistic input as children from middle and upper socioeconomic backgrounds. They may not have as many learning experiences such as vacations, summer camps, and other extra-curricular activities. As a result, children from low-income backgrounds had lower vocabulary and syntax performance than children who were from middle-income backgrounds (Fernald, Marchman, & Weisleder, 2013; Hoff, 2003; Huttenlocher, Haight, Bryk, Seltzer, & Lyons, 1991; Huttenlocher, Vasilyeva, Cymerman, & Levine, 2002; Vernon-Feagans, Garrett-Peters, Willoughby, Mills-Koonce, & Family Life Project Investigators, 2012). However, to determine whether these similarities exist, research is needed to compare children from low socioeconomic backgrounds and children adopted internationally.

If, however, children are adopted from foster care or countries that economically support and provide better quality institutional care, they demonstrate better developmental outcomes. Some countries have the economic resources to provide adequate care for children living in orphanages and these children demonstrate more positive academic achievement in adolescence and intellectual and verbal skills in adulthood than children who were adopted from countries who did not provide *good enough* care (Odenstad et al., 2008; Vinnerljung et al., 2010).

▶ Timing of Exposure Matters

The timing of increased nurturance, stimulation, and communication acquisition is also important in that the earlier the exposure to improved care, stimulation, social interaction, and a communication system, the better the developmental outcomes. For example, deaf adults who acquired their first language at school-age had poorer language competence than adults who acquired a first language prior to school-age (Boudreault & Mayberry, 2006; Mayberry, 1993; Mayberry & Lock, 2003). Adults who were taught sign language or lip-reading as a communication system prior to attending school performed better than adults who were not taught a communication system until they attended school. In other words, timing of first language exposure matters.

Timing of language exposure, increased social interactions, and more nurturing care had positive effects on language development. Children who are placed in foster care families receive better care and social interactions than what can be provided in orphanages. Children who received foster care at younger ages have better language development than children who do not receive foster care or who receive foster care at an older age (Miller, 2005; Windsor et al., 2011). For example, Windsor and colleagues conducted a randomized control-trial study with Romanian community children, children in Romanian orphanages, and children placed in Romanian foster care at (1) 15 months old, (2) 16–24 months old, (3) 25–29 months old, and (4) after 29 months old. They collected a parent report of receptive language and expressive language sample measures. The results indicated that children placed in foster care before 24 months-old performed as well as community children. In other words, as long as children receive more nurturance and social interaction by the age of 2 years, they demonstrate similar receptive and expressive monolingual language development.

After children are adopted into loving homes, they receive more social interaction, exposure to stimulating materials and experiences, improved nutrition, and medical care, which positively influences their growth and development. Adoption has been studied as an intervention for institutionalization. Children who are adopted clearly fare better than their peers who remain in institutional care (Windsor et al., 2011). However, the process of international adoption results in interrupted language acquisition that may affect language acquisition in the adopted language.

▶ Communication Development in Children Adopted Internationally

Children adopted internationally acquire their adopted language rapidly and fall within acceptable ranges of performance on standardized assessments within 2–3 years following adoption. There is some variability due to the adoption age, linguistic differences between the birth and adopted language, and in comparison to standardized test norms or nonadopted peers, but in general, children adopted internationally rapidly learn and acquire an adopted language. Hearing, vision, speech, language, and social language development are described in this section.

▶ Hearing and Vision Diagnoses

In a recent survey study by Eckerle et al. (2014), children adopted internationally were often not screened immediately following adoption. Only 61% had their vision screened and only 59% had their hearing screened. Of the children who had been screened, 25–31% had vision problems and 12–13% had hearing problems. In terms of vision problems, the most common diagnosis was strabismus, with 36% having multiple abnormalities. Hearing problems were mostly associated with temporary or correctable hearing loss. However, during the first year of adoption, 43.7% had ear infections, with 14.6% having four or more ear infections. What this study tells us is that children adopted internationally need to have their hearing and vision screened and followed consistently so that appropriate services and early intervention can be provided.

▶ Speech Development

Children adopted internationally show few delays or problems with articulation and little first language interference. Roberts et al. (2005) recruited 55 children adopted from China who were adopted between 6 and 25 months (mean age = 13.5 months) and were 3–6 years old (mean age = 4 years, 5 months) at the time of the study. Among several English standardized language measures, they administered an articulation test. Most of the children (93%) scored within 1.25 standard deviations of the mean. Several single case studies and studies with small sample sizes confirm this finding (for a review see Hwa-Froelich, 2012b). Pollock is also following a small group of children adopted from Haiti who demonstrate similar post-adoption outcomes (Hwa-Froelich & Pollock, 2013).

For children adopted from Eastern European countries, Glennen (2007) reported that most children demonstrate little to no birth language interference on English standardized articulation tests. In a study of 27 children adopted before the age of 2 years, 89% scored at or above a standard score of 80, which is considered to be within normal range of performance (±1.25 standard deviations). These findings were confirmed in a later longitudinal study of 56 children adopted from Eastern Europe at ages ranging from 1 to 4 years and 11 months (Glennen, 2014). After 9 months of English exposure, articulation scores ranged from 91.64 to 97.82 for children adopted at 2 years of age or older. Thus, children adopted at older than 2-years old were performing well above average in English articulation.

▶ Language Development

Although there has been much research documenting the development of children adopted internationally, not all researchers use the same methods of measurement or comparison. Some used parent- or teacher-report survey instruments, whereas others used norm-referenced or behavioral measures. Some researchers compared children to the test norms, whereas others compared children to different control groups such as children adopted domestically, children who lived with a foster family for the majority of their preadoptive life, or a control group of children who had not been adopted but lived in families with similar socioeconomic backgrounds. Some included children adopted from several different countries with different preadoption conditions, whereas others focused on a group of children from one country. Thus, it is challenging to determine which children are delayed because of these many different research variables. Scott, Roberts, and Glennen (2011) conducted a meta-analysis and reported that children's performance was higher on survey measures than on standardized tests and performance was better when compared to norms on a standardized test than when compared to a control group. They suggested that the research on children adopted internationally reflects a "lens problem" in that the research community has not established an agreement as to the standard of comparison for children with this kind of language experience. Children adopted internationally are not included in the sample of standardized tests and are adopted into families with a higher than average socioeconomic status. Thus, the children attend schools with peers from similar socioeconomic backgrounds and their parents tend to have higher academic expectations. Although children's performance may be within normal limits on standardized tests when compared to a larger population, their performance may be lower than their peers from similar socioeconomic backgrounds because their peers received more cognitive, social, and linguistic input and exposure.

Scott, Roberts, and Glennen also reported that performance measured at different ages varied. When children adopted internationally were measured at preschool ages, Scott et al. (2011) reported that they were not significantly different than children who were not adopted. However, in studies that measured performance at school-age in children adopted before the age of 2 years, children adopted internationally lagged behind their peers. What this may indicate is that children adopted internationally demonstrate rapid developmental recovery immediately following adoption, which may be slow or they may not develop at the same rate as their peers who are not adopted. Therefore, initially, when children are adopted, they may not have language delays requiring special services but as language demands increase in academic settings, they may demonstrate language difficulties for which services are needed. More longitudinal research is needed to determine whether children adopted internationally demonstrate slower developmental growth over time. For speech-language pathologists, it is important to follow these children's developmental progress through their academic lives to ensure appropriate identification of learning needs.

Adoption age or length of time prior to adoption has a short-term effect on language performance. Glennen (2014) found that adoption age was not related to articulation performance 2–3 months following adoption but it was related to English language performance. This effect remained significant up to 9 months postadoption, but adoption age was not significantly related to performance 1, 2, or 3 years later. What this means is that duration of institutional care may not have long-lasting negative impact on children's language learning.

Language development of children adopted internationally can be separated into adoption age categories, that is, children adopted by the age of 2 years and children adopted at older ages (2–5 years). Children adopted at younger ages up to the age of 2 years, 11 months demonstrate average receptive language within 1 year and average expressive language performance within 2 years compared to standardized test norms (Glennen, 2007; Hwa-Froelich & Matsuo, 2010). Children adopted at ages 3 and 4 years need at least 2 years of English exposure to reach average scores on standardized receptive language tests. The 3-year-olds need 2 years and the 4-year-olds at least 3 years to catch-up in expressive language performance (Glennen, 2014, 2015). However, mean length of utterance lagged behind all other measures and in comparison to population norms after 3 years in the adoptive home. In other words, the children were showing continued developmental gains but slower expressive language development.

▶ Social Language Development

As Carol Westby describes earlier in this text, developing social communication competence is dependent upon neurologically integrated development, which is influenced by intrinsic and extrinsic interactions. Infants are dependent upon and expect to receive nurturing care and social interaction while engaging with their environment. Consistent, developmentally appropriate experiences and nurturing interactions help the infant develop trusting attachments to adults who infants look to for guidance in their interactions with others and the world. It is within these social interactions that infants learn the foundational nonverbal, verbal, and cognitive skills for social communication competence. While some children receive this type of social interaction prior to adoption, many do not. For these reasons, it is important to consider the development of nonverbal skills such as interpreting facial expressions, verbal skills such as pragmatic language, and cognitive skills such as understanding false beliefs.

Children adopted internationally have more difficulty identifying emotions from facial expressions (Camras, Perlman, Wismer Fries, & Pollak, 2006; Glennen & Bright, 2005; Hwa-Froelich, Matsuo, & Becker, 2014; Wismer Fries & Pollak, 2004). Parents reported that children adopted from Eastern European countries have more difficulty with nonverbal communication, including reading facial expressions (Glennen & Bright, 2005). In the Camras et al. and Wismer Fries and Pollak studies, they compared children adopted from Eastern Europe and China with a nonadopted control group. They found that children adopted from Eastern Europe had more difficulty than the children adopted from China who were similar to the control group. Their samples, however, differed in terms of adoption age or chronological age and the investigators did not measure the children's language competence, which may have influenced their results. Hwa-Froelich, Matsuo, and Becker (2014) compared children adopted from Eastern Europe and Asia with a control group that was similar in chronological age, socioeconomic status, and parent education. In this study, country of origin differences in emotion identification were not found but differences between children who had experienced international adoption had more difficulty identifying emotions from photographs of facial expression. The children's language competence predicted their emotion identification performance.

There is emerging evidence that children adopted internationally have difficulty with pragmatic language (Hwa-Froelich, 2016; Petranovich, Walz, Staat, Chiu, & Wade, 2017). Petranovich and colleagues asked parents to rate their children's social communication behaviors and found that children adopted from Eastern European countries had poorer performance than children adopted from China and poorer pragmatic communication in comparison to a group of children who were not adopted. However, their sample consisted of children adopted from Eastern Europe who were adopted at older ages than the Chinese group, and several of the children had received speech or language treatment, which may have influenced their results. Hwa-Froelich reported lower pragmatic scores on a sample of children adopted from Eastern European and Asian countries similar in adoption age, chronological age, and their parents' socioeconomic status and education level. Although the Eastern European and Asian groups did not differ between each other and the U.S. group, the combined group of children adopted internationally had lower pragmatic language scores than a U.S. control group. Thus, children adopted internationally perform less well than their peers on an English pragmatic language measure. Again, language competence predicted pragmatic language performance.

Social language competence also involves the knowledge of one's mental states and emotions as well as how to compensate for one's and others' mental states and emotions. The ability to verbally explain these concepts is dependent upon language ability and social knowledge about one's own and others' mental states. This social cognition is often measured by administering false belief tasks. These kinds of tasks involve asking participants to identify that they or a fictional character had a mistaken belief about an

object's identity or location. Children who have both linguistic competence and diverse social experiences tend to perform better on these tasks. Research studies measuring social cognition in children adopted internationally have reported weaker performance on false belief tasks (Hwa-Froelich, Matsuo, & Jacobs, 2017; Tarullo, Bruce, & Gunnar, 2007). Tarullo and colleagues compared children who had spent most of their preadoptive lives living in institutions with children who had spent most of their preadoptive lives in foster care and children who were not adopted. Children who had received foster care scored between the other two groups, an indication that increased social interaction was important in social understanding. Hwa-Froelich and colleagues reported similar findings in that language competence and the number of older siblings in the adoptive family predicted better social understanding. In other words, increased opportunities for social interaction prior to or following adoption were important for social understanding development.

▶ Associated Development

Other developmental areas are important in language development, such as cognition, executive function, attention/activity, and attachment. Although children adopted internationally tend to demonstrate average to above-average intelligence quotients across time (Van IJzendoorn et al., 2005), specific cognitive abilities may not be as strong. Executive function and attention/activity are cognitive skills that are also important in learning. Children must learn to selectively attend and focus on a challenge or problem while inhibiting attention and energy on distractions. They must use their executive function to maintain their attention on the task while searching through their memories for solutions, select and organize behaviors to execute, and monitor the execution of these behaviors. In addition, attachment security in social communication development is particularly important in social communication development, as discussed in the chapter on social-emotional bases of pragmatic and communication development by Westby.

Children adopted internationally are at risk of weaker executive function (Hostinar, Stellern, Schaefer, Calrson, & Gunnar, 2012), inattention and overactivity (Helder et al., 2016), insecure attachment (Barcons et al., 2014), and poorer academic achievement (Van IJzendoorn et al., 2005). Van IJzendoorn et al. reported from their meta-analysis that children adopted domestically and internationally had more learning problems and received more special education services than nonadopted peers or siblings. Thus, children experiencing an adoption experience, especially those who were adopted after 12 months of age, may be at increased risk of developing learning problems.

▶ Assessment Considerations

Because of the complex developmental profiles of children adopted internationally, an interdisciplinary approach, with a team of professionals who have clinical experience with this population, is recommended. The primary professionals should include an adoption medical specialist, clinical psychologist, occupational therapist, audiologist, and speech language pathologist. The adoption medical specialist monitors general health and immunizations and can prescribe medications or order neurological tests if needed. The clinical psychologist can assess the attachment/attunement of the child and family and diagnose and treat behavioral, social emotional, or cognitive issues. The occupational therapist provides assessment and treatment for visual motor, sensory motor, or feeding problems. The audiologist provides hearing evaluations. The speech language pathologist completes the team by providing assessment and intervention in speech, language, social communication, speech and language processing, and executive function measures (attention, inhibition, short-term memory, and working memory). However, for this chapter, the focus will be on assessment and treatment of speech and language impairment.

Families and children vary significantly. In addition, because many orphanages do not assess or treat ear infections, hearing loss, visual impairment, respiratory infections, or immunize children routinely, hearing, vision, and health evaluations are imperative. Thus, it is important to conduct an ethnographic interview to gather information from the families about the adoption process, orphanage or foster care, previous health or educational assessments, and observed strengths and weaknesses to individualize the assessment.

No standardized measures have been normed on children adopted internationally. Since most children adopted internationally become monolingual speakers of their adopted language, it is logical to use standardized measures in their adopted language. To determine whether a particular child is demonstrating delayed or deviant postadoption development in their adopted language, it is important to compare them with other children who were adopted at the same approximate age and from the same country of origin. If no such data is available, speech language pathologists can compare children more generally to other children adopted internationally. As described earlier, children adopted internationally should score within normal limits on articulation and phonological measures. Expected language development for children adopted internationally is summarized in **TABLE 14-1**.

TABLE 14-1 Cut-off Scores by Measure, Adoption, and Postadoption Age		
Adoption Age	**Months Postadoption**	**Measure and Cut off**
11–23 months	1–8 months	MCDI-WC DQ 47
11–23 months	2–6 months	CSBS-DP Speech Subtest standard score ≥6
11–23 months	2–6 months	CSBS-DP Total standard score ≥80
11–23 months	12–15 months	GFTA-2 ≥80
11–23 months	12–15 months	PLS-3 or 4 RL and EL ≥80
24–35 months	2–3 months	PLS-3 or 4 RL/EL range 62.67–78.75 RL $M = 78.75$ ($SD = 14.17$) EL $M = 76.92$ ($SD = 8.05$)
36–47 months	2–3 months	PLS-4 RL/EL range 62.67–78.75 RL $M = 67.57$ ($SD = 6.72$) EL $M = 71.29$ ($SD = 3.09$)

(continues)

TABLE 14-1 Cut-off Scores by Measure, Adoption and Postadoption Age		(continued)
Adoption Age	**Months Postadoption**	**Measure and Cut off**
48–59 months	2–3 months	PLS-4 RL/EL range 62.67–78.75 RL $M = 67.67$ ($SD = 15.87$) EL $M = 62.67$ ($SD = 16.94$)
24–35 months	9 months	CELF-P2 $M = 94.31$ ($SD = 14.96$)
36–47 months	9 months	CELF-P2 $M = 89.58$ ($SD = 10.95$)
48–59 months	9 months	CELF-P2 $M = 79.24$ ($SD = 9.96$)
24–59 months	15 months or 1;3 years 27 months or 2;3 years	CELF-P2 ≥ 80
24–35 months	40 months or 3;4 years	CELF-P2 and CELF-4 ≥ 80
36–59 months	40 months or 3;4 years	CELF-4 ≥ 80

Note: MCDI-WG = MacArthur-Bates communication development inventory-words and gestures (Fenson et al., 2006); DQ = Developmental quotient (closest 50th percentile age equivalence/chronological age X 100, Glennen, 2007); CSBS-DP = Communication, symbolic behavior scales-developmental profile (Wetherby & Prizant, 2002); GFTA-2 = Goldman-Fristoe Test of Articulation, second edition (Goldman & Fristoe, 2000); PLS 3 and 4 = Preschool Language Scale, third and fourth edition (Zimmerman, Steiner, & Evatt-Pond, 2002; Zimmerman, Steiner, & Evatt-Pond, 1992); RL = Receptive Language, EL = Expressive Language; CELF-P2 = Clinical evaluation of language fundamentals, second preschool edition (Semel, Wiig, & Secord, 2004); CELF-4 = Clinical evaluation of language fundamentals, fourth edition (Semel, Wiig, & Secord, 2003).
Adapted from Glennen, 2007; 2014; Hwa-Froelich, 2012c; Hwa-Froelich & Matsuo, 2010.

Children who do not meet these performance levels demonstrate delayed or deviant speech and language development indicative of a communication disorder and should receive speech and language services. In some cases, children may perform at or above these cut-off scores but demonstrate specific weakness in short-term verbal memory, attention, and social communication (interpreting facial expressions, pragmatic language, false belief) and may also qualify for and benefit from speech language services.

▶ Treatment Considerations

Speech language pathologists need to consider children's preadoption and postadoption experiences and relationships when planning intervention services. Because children adopted internationally may have experienced adverse early experiences that may be similar to abuse and/or neglect that may affect their attachment relationships and their adoptive family's attunement, it is important to frame interventions around relationship-based interventions to build or strengthen family relationships. Relationship-based intervention focuses on the nonverbal and verbal communication knowledge and skills that form the foundation for social communication. Interventions

to facilitate positive primary and secondary inter-subjectivity are important for children's emotional processing of nonverbal communication and help promote emotion and self-regulation as well as emerging social understanding. During these interactions, speech-language pathologists can guide parental language input to include rare words, mental state verbs, and emotional states in complex sentences, including conjunctions and complements. This rich language input will help children develop a diverse vocabulary to enable them to communicate more effectively with others about their own internal mental states and emotions as well as describe others' mental states and emotions (See Hwa-Froelich, 2012d, 2015).

It is also recommended that speech-language pathologists use a play-based model of intervention to facilitate and strengthen attention, inhibition, and memory development. It is through play that children make sense of their world, demonstrate their memory of life events in context, and socially engage with others. Children learn how to share their emotions, reference others, coordinate their actions to do activities together, think flexibly and dynamically when faced with conflict or challenges, and eventually reflect upon past events to plan for future events. These developmental stages naturally interact with attention, inhibition, and memory development as children learn how to attend to their parents' faces, coordinate their actions in concert with another, and plan and carry out goal-directed play scenarios as well as when they reflect and modify their plans while inhibiting distractions to think dynamically and flexibly when plans do not go as intended.

For specific language needs, speech language pathologists may find it useful to follow a social communication intervention framework (Adams, 2015) because of the research indicating social communication as a weakness of children adopted internationally. Intervention should (1) strengthen individual language needs in processing and expression, (2) strengthen pragmatics and meta-pragmatics, and (3) provide language-mediated practice in social understanding. Language processing involves improving children's ability to listen to, process, and respond appropriately to language structures and functions. Pragmatics and meta-pragmatics involves learning how to interpret and inference nonverbal and verbal social communication as well as the social rules for language use associated with context to apply them in practice situations. Finally, language-mediated social understanding requires the speech language pathologist and client or clients to discuss and interpret a variety of social interactions to reach an understanding of what and why the interaction progressed as it did and how to plan what they would do differently in a similar situation. Planning and executing role plays while being videotaped are excellent methods to use in therapy. Videotapes can be replayed for group discussion to dynamically and flexibly think and talk about the interaction to reflect and plan for future interactions. Subsequent videotapes can then be compared to previous ones to refine social communication behaviors and determine the effectiveness of the intervention.

▶ Case Studies

Two case studies will be described to provide clinical examples of how to translate published research data to diagnose language impairment in children adopted internationally. Two boys were adopted from the same Russian orphanage by the same family. The boys were not biologically related and did not know each other prior to adoption. For the sake of confidentiality, the names Isaac and Jacob will be used to refer to the children and Mr. and Mrs. Meltzoff as the boys' parents. Isaac and Jacob had different preadoption experiences and were not the same age at the time of adoption. Mr. and Mrs. Meltzoff told the team that while they would share in parenting both sons, they had decided each of them would be primarily responsible for one of the boys. Mrs. Meltzoff was the primary parent for Isaac and Mr. Meltzoff was the primary parent for Jacob. Both children were evaluated at 6, 14, and 24 months postadoption. Refer to **TABLES 14-2** and **14-3** for test scores presented in order of the time they were assessed following adoption.

In addition to the measures listed in the tables, an interdisciplinary team of students in Counseling and Family Therapy and Communication Sciences and Disorders graduate programs conducted an ethnographic interview, hearing screenings, speech and language evaluations, and a transdisciplinary play-based assessment.

TABLE 14-2 Isaac Meltzoff Postadoption Language and Articulation Standard Scores			
Measure	**6 Months**	**14 Months**	**24 Months**
CELF-P2 expressive language	63	67	79
SD below published means (Glennen, 2014)		−0.56	−1.95
CELF-P2 receptive language	59	88	79
SD below published means		−2.44	−2.51
CELF-P2 Core Score	59	86	79
GFTA-2	–	106	–

Note: CELF-P2 = Clinical evaluation of language fundamentals, preschool version (Semel et al., 2004); SD = standard deviation; GFTA-2 = Goldman-Fristoe Test of Articulation, second edition (Goldman & Fristoe, 2000).

TABLE 14-3 Jacob Meltzoff Postadoption Language and Articulation Scores

Measure	6 Months	14 Months	24 Months
CELF-P2 expressive language	79	89	115
SD below published means (Glennen, 2014)		0.42	1.30
CELF-P2 receptive language	85	85	125
SD below published means		−0.72	1.75
CELF-P2 core score	71	86	106
GFTA-2	–	–	107

Note: CELF-P2 = Clinical evaluation of language fundamentals, preschool version (Semel et al., 2004); SD = standard deviation; GFTA-2 = Goldman-Fristoe Test of Articulation, second edition (Goldman & Fristoe, 2000).

🔍 CASE STUDY: ISAAC (LD)

Isaac had spent most of his life residing at the orphanage and was adopted at 2 years, 6 months of age. He demonstrated flat tympanograms at 6 and 12 months postadoption. He was referred to an otolaryngologist for further evaluation. By the 24-month postadoption evaluation, his middle ear issues had been resolved and he passed his hearing screening.

His language scores showed an unusual pattern of gradual improvement in expressive language but a decline in receptive language progress across time. Isaac was assessed at 6 months, 14 months, and 24 months postadoption. Isaac demonstrated significantly lower expressive and receptive language composite scores. Specifically, he consistently had problems understanding pronouns, noun-verb agreement, auxiliary and copula verbs, as well as concrete vocabulary. Most of his problems involved inattention as well as an inability to understand and follow directions. In addition, his play behaviors were less complex, more impulsive, and he was less flexible when solving problems. Socially, he did not appear to be closely attached to either parent. The team recommended that the parents and Isaac begin family counseling to work on developing a stronger relationship with Isaac. Family counseling would focus on helping the parents learn play-based strategies to facilitate bonding, trust, and positive interdependence as well as positive ways to deal with conflict and negative behaviors. The team also recommended beginning language intervention because Isaac was demonstrating inconsistent growth and delay in receptive language with slow expressive language development in comparison to other children adopted internationally from Eastern European countries at similar ages assessed at approximately the same time following adoption (Glennen, 2014).

Although Isaac may be a "late-bloomer," he may also have language impairment. With these low scores, he would most likely struggle with academic language. Because early intervention can have long-lasting effects on later performance, our team recommended language intervention in the context of relationship and play-based intervention frameworks to improve Isaac's language processing, expression, and social communication in the context of socially interacting with others.

🔍 *CASE STUDY: JACOB (TD)*

Jacob had spent approximately 1 year in a hospital, 1 year living with his grandmother, and 1.5 years in the orphanage. He was adopted at 3 years, 10 months of age. He appeared to be developing well, catching up on all measures across time.

Jacob demonstrated consistent growth and development across time. He passed hearing screenings at all assessment time points. His language scores were consistently above average or within one standard deviation below published performance of other children adopted at similar ages from Eastern European countries and measured at similar time points following adoption (Glennen, 2014). He appeared to be securely attached to his father, demonstrating adequate attention, inhibition, problem-solving, memory, language, and speech skills in comparison to standardized measures. For these reasons, no intervention was deemed necessary.

It is possible that the time Jacob spent with his biological grandmother had provided him with enough nurturance and social interaction to mediate the effect of his time in the orphanage. In addition, his secure relationship with his father was enough support to enable him to thrive and adjust to his new family.

▶ Summary

In summary, children adopted internationally represent a different kind of language learner. Their language learning is one that involves an interrupted process of receiving input in one language, which is often arrested and replaced by different linguistic input. Initially, children adopted at younger ages achieve average language comprehension skills quickly (≤2 years old = catch up in 1 year; ≥3 years catch up in 2 years), but achieving average expressive language performance takes longer (≤2 years old = catch up in 2 years; ≥3 years catch up in 3 years). However, conversational or narrative language development lags behind other expressive language development.

Children adopted internationally have different social experiences prior to being adopted. Exposure to adverse early experiences can affect cognitive, social-emotional, language, and social communication development. Consequently, children adopted internationally demonstrate more difficulty with understanding and expressing social communication, attention/overactivity, academic achievement, and attachment than children who received foster care or lived with their biological families. These potential areas of concern should be addressed in an interdisciplinary assessment and intervention program. Using a relationship-and play-based intervention model with parents and siblings is recommended for children adopted internationally.

Study Questions

1. Discuss the types of preadoption environment variability that exist among children adopted internationally.
2. Identify the kinds of misconceptions people have about children adopted internationally.
3. How do input and timing of input affect language learning?
4. What developmental areas and behaviors should be assessed in children adopted internationally?
5. What cognitive and communication developments are at risk of delays and problems in children adopted internationally?
6. Who are important members of the interdisciplinary team-serving children adopted internationally?
7. How should speech-language pathologists frame their intervention approaches?

References

Adams, C. (2015). Assessment and intervention for social (pragmatic) communication disorder. In D. A. Hwa-Froelich (Ed.), *Social communication development and disorders* (pp. 141–170). New York, NY: Psychology Press.

Barcons, N., Abrines, N., Brun, C., Sartini, C., Fumadó, V., & Marre, D. (2014). Attachment and adaptive skills in children of international adoption. *Child and Family Social Work, 19*, 89–98. doi:10.1111/j.1365-2206.2012.00883.x

Bimmel, N., Juffer, F., van IJzendoorn, M. H., & Bakermans-Kranenburg, M. J. (2003). Problem behavior of internationally adopted adolescents: A review and meta-analysis. *Harvard Review of Psychiatry, 11*(2), 64–77.

Boudreault, P., & Mayberry, R. I. (2006). Grammatical processing in American Sign Language: Age of first-language acquisition effects in relation to syntactic structure. *Language and Cognitive Processes, 21*, 608–635.

Camras, L. A., Perlman, S. B., Wismer Fries, A. B., & Pollak, S. D. (2006). Post-institutionalized Chinese and Eastern European children: Heterogeneity in the development of emotion understanding. *International Journal of Behavioral Development, 30*(3), 193–199. doi:10.1177/0165025406063608

Eckerle, J., Hill, L., Iverson, S., Hellerstedt, W., Gunnar, M., & Johnson, D. (2014). Vision and hearing deficits and associations with parent-reported behavioral and developmental problems in international adoptees. *Maternal & Child Health Journal, 18*(3), 575–583. doi:10.1007/s10995-013-1274-1

Eigsti, I.-M., & Cicchett, D. (2004). The impact of child maltreatment on expressive syntax at 60 months. *Developmental Science, 7*(1), 88–102.

Fenson, L., Marchman, V. A., Thal, D. J., Dale, P. S., Reznick, J. S., & Bates, E. (2006). *MacArthur-Bates communicative development inventories.* San Diego, CA: Singular.

Fernald, A., Marchman, V. A., & Weisleder, A. (2013). SES differences in language processing skill and vocabulary are evident at 18 months. *Developmental Science, 16*(2), 234–248. doi:10.1111/desc.12019

Glennen, S. (2007). Predicting language outcomes for internationally adopted children. *Journal of Speech, Language and Hearing Research, 50*, 529–548. doi:10.1044/1092-4388(2007/036)

Glennen, S. (2008). Speech and language "mythbusters" for internationally adopted children. *The ASHA Leader, 13*, 10–13. doi:10.1044/leader.FTR1.13172008.10

Glennen, S. (2014). A longitudinal study of language and speech in children who were internationally adopted at different ages. *Language, Speech, and Hearing Services in Schools, 45*, 185–203. doi:10.1044/2014_LSHSS-13-0035

Glennen, S. (2015). Internationally adopted children in the early school years: Relative strengths and weaknesses in language abilities. *Language, Speech, and Hearing Services in Schools, 46*, 1–13. doi:10.1044/2014_LSHSS-13-0042

Glennen, S., & Bright, B. J. (2005). Five years later: Language in school-age internationally adopted children. *Seminars in Speech and Language, 26*(1), 86–101.

Glennen, S., Rosinsky-Grunhut, A., & Tracy, R. (2005). Linguistic interference between L1 and L2 in internationally adopted children. *Seminars in Speech and Language, 26*, 64–75.

Goldman, R., & Fristoe, M. (2000). *Goldman-Fristoe test of articulation* (2nd ed.). Circle Pines, MN: AGS.

Helder, E. J., Brooker, B., Kapitula, L. R., Goalen, B., & Gunnoe, M. L. (2016). Predictors and correlates of inattentive/overactive behaviors in internationally adopted children. *Applied Neuropsychology: Child, 5*(4), 237–251. doi:10.1080/21622965.2015.1038207

Hellerstedt, W. L., Madsen, N. J., Gunnar, M. R., Grotevant, H. D., Lee, R. M., & Johnson, D. E. (2008). The international adoption project: Population-based surveillance of Minnesota parents who adopted children internationally. *Maternal Child Health Journal, 12*(2), 162–171. doi:10.1007/s10995-007-0237-9

Holt International. (2017). Holt has always been about the children. Retrieved from: http://www.holtinternational.org/about/historical.shtml

Hoff, E. (2003). The specificity of environmental influence: Socio-economic status affects early vocabulary development via maternal speech. *Child Development, 74*(5), 1368–1378.

Hostinar, C. E., Stellern, S. A., Schaefer, C., Carlson, S. M., & Gunnar, M. R. (2012). Associations between early life adversity and executive function in children adopted internationally from orphanages. *PNAS, 109*, 17208–17212.

Huttenlocher, J., Haight, W., Bryk, A., Seltzer, M., & Lyons, T. (1991). Early vocabulary growth relation to language input and gender. *Developmental Psychology, 27*(2), 236–248.

Huttenlocher, J., Vasilyeva, M., Cymerman, E., & Levine, S. (2002). Language input and child syntax. *Cognitive Psychology, 45*, 337–374.

Hwa-Froelich, D. A. (2012a). Childhood maltreatment and communication development. *Perspectives on School-Based Issues, 13*(1), 43–53.

Hwa-Froelich, D. A. (2012b). Hearing, speech, and feeding development. In D. A. Hwa-Froelich (Ed.), *Supporting development in internationally adopted children* (pp. 133–148). Baltimore, MD: Paul H. Brookes.

Hwa-Froelich, D. A. (2012c). Prelinguistic, receptive and expressive language development. In D. A. Hwa-Froelich (Ed.), *Supporting development in internationally adopted children* (pp. 149–176). Baltimore, MD: Paul H. Brookes.

Hwa-Froelich, D. A. (2012d). Intervention strategies. In D. A. Hwa-Froelich (Ed.), *Supporting development in internationally adopted children* (pp. 205–232). Baltimore, MD: Paul H. Brookes.

Hwa-Froelich, D. A. (2015). Assessment and intervention for children exposed to maltreatment. In D. A. Hwa-Froelich (Ed.), *Social communication development and disorders* (pp. 287–319). New York, NY: Psychology Press.

Hwa-Froelich, D. A. (2016, April). *Social communication performance in children adopted internationally.* Poster presentation at the Canadian speech-Language Pathology and Audiology Conference, Halifax, Nova Scotia, Canada. Published abstract at http://sac-oac.ca/sites/default/files/resources/2016_abstracts_en.pdf

Hwa-Froelich, D. A., & Matsuo, H. (2010). Communication development and differences in children adopted from China and Eastern Europe. *Language, Speech, and Hearing Services in Schools, 41*, 1–18. doi:10.1044/0161-1461(2009/08-0085)

Hwa-Froelich, D. A., Matsuo, H., & Becker, J. C. (2014). Emotion identification from facial expressions in children adopted internationally. *American Journal of Speech-Language Pathology, 23*, 641–654. doi:10.1044/2014_AJSLP-14-0009

Hwa-Froelich, D. A., Matsuo, H., & Jacobs, K. (2017). False belief performance of children adopted internationally. *American Journal of Speech-Language Pathology, 26*, 29–43. doi:10.1044/2016_AJSLP-15-0152

Hwa-Froelich, D. A., & Pollock, K. E. (2013, November). *Speech, language, and social communication development of children adopted internationally.* Short Course presentation at the American Speech-Language-Hearing Association, Chicago, IL.

Johnson, D. E. (2000). Medical and developmental sequelae of early childhood institutionalization in Eastern European adoptees. In C. A. Nelson (Ed.), *The Minnesota Symposia on child psychology: The effects of early adversity on neurobiological development: Vol. 31. Minnesota Symposium on Child Psychology* (pp. 113–162). Minneapolis, MN: University of Minnesota Press.

Juffer, F., & Van IJzendoorn, M. H. (2005). Behavior problems and mental health referrals of international adoptees. *JAMA, 293*, 2501–2515.

Juffer, F., & Van IJzendoorn, M. H. (2009). International adoption comes of age: Development of international adoptees from a longitudinal and meta-analytic perspective. In. G. M. Wroebel & G. Neil (Eds.), *International advances in adoption research for practice* (pp. 169–192). London, UK: John Wiley & Sons.

Ladage, J. S., & Harris, S. (2012). Physical growth, health, and motor development. In D. A. Hwa-Froelich (Ed.), *Supporting development in internationally adopted children* (pp. 21–57). Baltimore, MD: Paul H. Brookes.

Leiden Conference on the Development and Care of Children without Permanent Parents. (2012). The development and care of institutionally reared children. *Child Development Perspectives, 6*, 174–180. doi:10.1111/j.1750-8606.2011.00231.x

Loman, M. M., Wiik, K. L., Frenn, K. A., Pollak, S. D., & Gunnar, M. R. (2009). Postinstitutionalized children's development: Growth, cognitive, and language outcomes. *Journal of Developmental & Behavioral Pediatrics, 26*(5), 426–434.

Mayberry, R. I. (1993). First-language acquisition after childhood differs from second-language acquisition: The case of American Sign Language. *Journal of Speech and Hearing Research, 36*, 1258–1270.

Mayberry, R. I., & Lock, E. (2003). Age constraints on first versus second language acquisition: Evidence for linguistic plasticity and epigenesist. *Brain and Language, 87*, 369–384.

Miller, L. C. (2005). *The handbook of international adoption medicine. A guide for physicians, parents, and providers.* Oxford: Oxford University Press.

Nicoladis, E., & Grabois, H. (2002). Learning English and losing Chinese: A case study of a child adopted from China. *The International Journal of Bilingualism, 6*(4), 441–454. doi:10.1177/13670069020060040401

Odenstad, A., Hjern, A., Linblad, F., Rasmussen, F., Vinnerljung, B., & Dalen, M. (2008). Does age at adoption and geographic origin matter? A national cohort study of cognitive test performance in adult inter-country adoptees. *Psychological Medicine, 38*, 1803–1814. doi:10.1017/S0033291708002766

Petranovich, C. L., Walz, N. C., Staat, M. A., Chiu, C-Y. P., & Wade, S. L. (2017). Structural language, pragmatic communication, behavior, and social competence in children adopted internationally: A pilot study. *Applied Neuropsychology: Child*, 1–12. doi:10.1080/21622965.2016.1182433

Roberts, J. A., Pollock, K. E., Krakow, R., Price, J., Fulmer, K. C., & Wang, P. P. (2005). Language development in preschool-age children adopted from China. *Journal of Speech, Language, and Hearing Research, 48*(1), 93–107. doi:10.1044/1092-4388(2005/008)

Scott, K. A., Roberts, J. A., & Glennen, S. (2011). How well do children who are internationally adopted acquire language? A meta-analysis. *Journal of Speech, Language, and Hearing Research, 54*, 1153–1169. doi:10.1044/1092-4388(2010/10-0075)

Selman, P. (2009). The rise and fall of intercountry adoption in the 21st century. *International Social Work, 52*(5), 575–594. doi:10.1177/0020872809337681

Semel, E., Wiig, E., & Secord, W. (2003). *Clinical evaluation of language fundamentals, fourth edition.* San Antonio, TX: Psychological *Corporation.*

Semel, E., Wiig, E., & Secord, W. (2004). *Clinical evaluation of language fundamentals, second preschool edition.* San Antonio, TX: Psychological *Corporation.*

Smolin, D. (2007). Child laundering as exploitation: Applying anti-trafficking norms to intercountry adoption under the coming Hague regime, ExpressO. Retrieved from www.childtrafficking.com/Docs/child_laundering_exploitation_270407.doc.

Tan, T. X., & Marfo, K. (2005). Parental ratings of behavioral adjustment in two samples of adopted Chinese girls: Age-related versus socio-emotional correlates and predictors. *Applied Developmental Psychology, 27*, 14–30.

Tarullo, A. R., Bruce, J., & Gunnar, M. R. (2007). False belief and emotion understanding in post-institutionalized children. *Social Development, 16*(1), 57–78. doi:10.1111/j.1467-9507.2007.00372.x

U.S. State Department. (2015). *Annual report on intercountry adoptions narrative.* Retrieved from https://travel.state.gov/content/dam/aa/pdfs/2015NarrativeAnnualReportonIntercountryAdoptions.pdf

Van IJzendoorn, M. H., & Juffer, F. (2006). The Emanuel Miller Memorial Lecture 2006: Adoption as intervention. Meta-analytic evidence for massive catch-up and plasticity in physical, socio-emotional, and cognitive development. *Journal of Child Psychology and Psychiatry, 47*(12), 1228–1245. doi:10.1111/j.1469-7610.2006.01675.x

Van IJzendoorn, M. H., & Juffer, F. (2009). International adoption comes of age: Development of international adoptees from a longitudinal and meta-analytical perspective. In B. M. Wrobel & E. Neil (Eds.)., *International advances in adoption research for practice* (pp. 169–192). Chichester, West Sussex, UK: John Wiley & Sons.

Van IJzendoorn, M. H., Juffer, F., & Klein Poelhuis, C. W. (2005). Adoption and cognitive development: A meta-analytic comparison of adopted and nonadopted children's IQ and school performance. *Psychological Bulletin, 131*(2), 301–316. doi:10.1037/0033-2909.1312.301

Vernon-Feagans, L., Garrett-Peters, P., Willoughby, M., Mills-Koonce, R., & The Family Life Project Key Investigators. (2012). Chaos, poverty, and parenting: Predictors of early language development. *Early Childhood Research Quarterly, 27*, 339–351. doi:10.1016/j.ecresq.2011.11.00

Vinnerljung, B., Lindblad, F., Hjern, A., Rasmussen, F., & Dalen, M. (2010). School performance at age 16 among international adoptees: A Swedish national cohort study. *International Social Work, 53*(4), 510–527. doi:10.1177/0020872809360037

Vygotsky, L. (1986). *Thought and language* (A. Kozulin, Trans.). London, UK: MIT Press.

Wetherby, A. M., & Prizant, B. M. (2002). *Communication and symbolic behavior scales-developmental profile.* Chicago, IL: Paul H. Brookes Publishing Co.

Windsor, J., Wing, C. A., Koga, S. F., Fox, N. A., Benigno, J. P., Carroll, P. J., … Zeanah, C. H. (2011). Effect of foster care on young children's language learning. *Child Development, 82*(4), 1040–1046. doi:10.1111/j.1467-8624.2011.01604.x

Wismer Fries, A. B., & Pollak, S. D. (2004). Emotion understanding in post-institutionalized Eastern European children. *Development and Psychopathology, 16*, 355–369.

Zimmerman, I., Steiner, V., & Evatt-Pond, R. (1992). *Preschool Language Scale* (3rd ed.). San Antonio, TX: Psychological *Corporation.*

Zimmerman, I., Steiner, V., & Evatt-Pond, R. (2002). *Preschool Language Scale* (4th ed.). San Antonio, TX: Psychological *Corporation.*

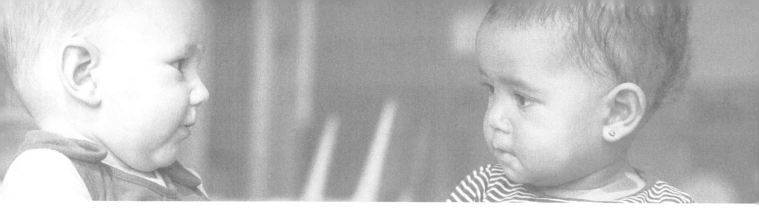

CHAPTER 15

Children with Language Impairment

Liat Seiger-Gardner, PhD, CCC-SLP

OBJECTIVES

- Differentiate between the various terms (e.g., *language impairment, language difference, language delay*) used to describe language abilities in children
- Understand the difference between primary and secondary language impairments
- Explain how language form (phonology, syntax, and morphology), content (semantics), and use (pragmatics) affect children with primary language impairments
- Describe the hallmark characteristics of late talkers, late bloomers, children with specific language impairment (SLI), and children with language learning disability (LLD)
- Differentiate between a language delay and a language disorder (late bloomers versus late talkers)
- Describe the language characteristics of children with autism spectrum disorder (ASD) and children with intellectual disability
- Explore the most commonly used methods for assessing the language abilities of infants, toddlers, preschoolers, and school-age children with primary and secondary language impairments
- Review commonly used facilitative intervention techniques for children with language deficits

KEY TERMS

Applied behavior analysis (ABA)
Autism spectrum disorder (ASD)
Criterion-referenced tests
Curriculum-based language assessment
Dynamic approach to assessment
Expansion

Facilitative play (indirect language stimulation)
Focused stimulation
Imitation
Incidental teaching procedure
Individual family service plan (IFSP)
Individualized education plan (IEP)

Individuals with Disabilities Education Act (IDEA)
Intellectual disability (ID)
Language delay
Language deviance
Language difference
Language disability

▸ Introduction

A variety of terms are used to describe the language difficulties seen in children whose ages range from infancy to school age. *Language impairment/disorder, language disability, language delay, language deviance*, and even *childhood aphasia* are often used interchangeably by non-professionals to refer to the same deficits; however, these terms are used to distinguish between and characterize different conditions or states.

Language Disorder/Impairment

According to the American Speech-Language-Hearing Association (ASHA), *language disorder* is defined as "an impairment in comprehension and/or use of spoken language, written, and/or other symbol system. The disorder may involve (1) the form of language (phonologic, morphologic, and syntactic systems), (2) the content of language (semantic system), and/or (3) the function of language in communication (pragmatic system), in any combination" (ASHA, 1993, p. 40). Paul adds that children exhibit a language disorder if they have a significant deficit in learning to talk, understand, or use any aspect of language appropriately, relative to both environmental and norm referenced expectations for age-matched typically developing children (Paul & Norbury, 2012). Thus, in addition to being noticeably impaired in the ability to use language to communicate, the child has to score significantly below age-expected norms on standardized or norm-referenced tests to be identified as having language impairment and be eligible for speech and language services. A score of one to two standard deviations below the mean for the child's age is typically the criterion used to diagnose a child as having language impairment and qualifies him for services. Fey (1986) has suggested a standard score of 1.25 as a criterion, which places the child below the 10th percentile for their expected level of language performance.

Primary Versus Secondary Language Impairment

Language impairments can be classified as primary or secondary. A *primary language impairment* is present when a language delay cannot be accounted for by a peripheral sensory deficit such as hearing loss; a motor deficit, such as cerebral palsy; a cognitive deficit, such as intellectual disability; a social or emotional impairment, such as autism spectrum disorder (ASD); harmful environmental conditions, such as lead poisoning or drug abuse; or a gross neurological deficit, such as that associated with traumatic brain injury (TBI) or lesions. This type of delay is often presumed to be due to impaired development or dysfunction of the central nervous system (Leonard, 1998, 2014). In research, it is referred to as *specific language impairment (SLI)*. Paul and Norbury (2012), use the term *primary developmental language disorders (primary DLD)* when describing children who do not develop language typically compared to their age-matched peers. *Secondary language impairment* refers to a language disorder that is associated with and presumed to be caused by factors such as sensory (hearing loss) or cognitive impairments (intellectual disability). This type of language disorder may also be part of a syndrome—that is, the presence of multiple abnormalities in the same individual that are all caused by or originated from the same source. For example, in fragile X syndrome or Down syndrome, language impairment is one of many other anomalies present; others may include intellectual disability or specific facial characteristics. This group is referred to as having secondary developmental language disorders (secondary DLD).

The importance of a language disorder diagnosis was recently acknowledged by the American Psychiatric Association (APA), which put forth a proposal to include its definition in the revised fifth edition of the DSM-5 (*Diagnostic and Statistical Manual of Mental Disorders*) (2013). According to the DSM-5 (2013), a language disorder is defined as

A. Persistent difficulties in the acquisition and use of language across modalities (i.e., spoken, written, sign language, or other) due to deficits in comprehension or production that include the following:
  1. Reduced vocabulary (word knowledge and use).
  2. Limited sentence structure (ability to put words and word endings together to form sentences based on the rules of grammar and morphology).
  3. Impairments in discourse (ability to use vocabulary and connect sentences to explain or describe a topic or series of events or have a conversation).
B. Language abilities are substantially and quantifiably below those expected for age, resulting in functional limitations in effective communication, social participation, academic achievement, or occupational performance, individually or in any combination.
C. Onset of symptoms is in the early developmental period.
D. The difficulties are not attributable to hearing or other sensory impairment, motor dysfunction, or another medical or neurological condition and are not better explained by intellectual disability (intellectual developmental disorder) or global developmental delay" (DSM-5, p. 42).

The language difficulties can be manifested in both comprehension and production of spoken language (i.e., receptive and expressive language disorders) or solely in the production of language (i.e., expressive language disorder). Children who exhibit expressive language deficits in the presence of age-appropriate receptive skills have a better prognosis than those with expressive-receptive language disorder (DSM-5, 2013).

Language and Learning Disorders/Disabilities

The term *language disability* refers to the consequences language impairment may have on a child's ability to function in the real world, and especially in school. The term *language disability* is often used hand in hand with the term *learning disability*, suggesting limitations in the ability to perform certain tasks such as reading, writing, listening, reasoning, spelling, and word recognition. Difficulties in learning how to perform these tasks are often attributed to deficits in language abilities and they affect individuals who

otherwise demonstrate average abilities essential for thinking or reasoning.

The reader may be familiar with terms such as Dyslexia or Dyscalculia which refer to difficulties that may be associated with reading and math, respectively.

The prevalence of specific learning disorder among school-age children is 5–15%.

Language Delay

A child is considered to have a *language delay* if they exhibit typical development in all other areas except for language. Language development in a child with a language delay is believed to follow the same patterns seen in children with typical language development; however, the development of language is protracted, with the child reaching the same milestones at a slower pace. Leonard (1998) has noted that the term *delay* suggests a late start and the possibility of making up for lost time (i.e., late bloomers). For many children with language impairment, the early delay involves not only the late emergence of first words and two-word combinations, but also the slow development of linguistic features until the point of mastery (Rescorla, 2005). This slow development can persist until adulthood, opening a gap that widens as children get older, and in turn making it more difficult to make up for lost time. At this point the language delay can be viewed as language impairment. A more extended overview of the characteristics that distinguish language delay (i.e., late bloomers) from language impairment (i.e., late talkers) is presented later in this text.

Language Deviance

The term *language deviance* suggests that the child's language development is not just slower than the typical but actually different in some qualitative way. This definition does not fit most children with primary language impairments, who tend to follow the same developmental patterns as typical but younger developing children (i.e., those presenting with a language delay). The language profiles of children exhibiting concomitant conditions such as ASD and intellectual disability may reveal some idiosyncratic patterns that deviate from typicality.

Language Difference

Paul and Norbury (2012) defines *language difference* as a rule-governed language form (i.e., dialect) that deviates in some ways from the standard language used by the mainstream culture. Some children from culturally diverse backgrounds who are speaking a dialect may also exhibit language impairment. In such cases, distinguishing between a language difference and true language impairment is one of the challenges faced by the speech-language pathologist. Language remediation by a speech-language pathologist for children exhibiting language differences is not warranted, although it may be offered through educational programs to facilitate communication in the mainstream culture (Paul & Norbury, 2012). The DSM-5 (2013), highlights the importance of a differential diagnosis (language disorder versus language difference) and the consideration of regional, social, or cultural/ethnic influence on language, when assessing children whose language differs qualitatively or quantitatively from their age-matched peers. Unfortunately, overreliance on standardized tests, which are biased toward Standard American English (SAE), results in an overidentification of children from culturally and linguistically diverse backgrounds as having language disorders (Paul & Norbury, 2012). The incidence of communication disorders in culturally and linguistically diverse children should be similar to what is reported for mainstream English-speaking children (ASHA, 2006).

This text focuses on the characteristics of primary and secondary language impairments/disorders in children spanning in age from toddlerhood to school age. It reviews the linguistic characteristics of primary language deficits in late bloomers and late talkers, preschool children with language disorder, and school-age children with specific language disorder, as well as the linguistic characteristics of secondary language deficits as in ASD and intellectual disability. In addition, key assessment methods and facilitative intervention techniques will be discussed in this text.

▶ Primary Language Impairment

Late Talkers

Whereas most children acquire language naturally and for the most part without formal instruction, for some children the acquisition of language poses a challenge. The majority of children with primary language impairments are not identified until they reach 24 months of age. In the absence of other significant sensory, cognitive, or motor disabilities, the first evidence for a language delay is the late onset of first-word production and a slow development of vocabulary growth (Ellis & Thal, 2008; Leonard, 1998, 2014; Thal, 2000; Weismer & Evans, 2002). Typically

in the first two years of life, toddlers developing language with no difficulties go through a developmental stage called the *emerging language stage* (Paul & Norbury, 2012). During this stage they acquire their first words, typically between 12 and 18 months of age; they then produce two-word combinations, typically between 18 and 24 months of age, after they have at least 50 words in their productive lexicon (Nelson, 1973). Children who fail to reach these lexical milestones at the specified ages are referred to as *late talkers* (Ellis, Borovsky, Elman, & Evans, 2015; Rescorla, 1989; Rescorla & Schwartz, 1990).

Delays in phonological development are also characteristic of late talkers (Paul, 1991; Paul & Jennings, 1992; Rescorla & Ratner, 1996; Roberts, Rescorla, Giroux, & Stevens, 1998). They are overall less vocal and verbal compared to their typically developing peers; they exhibit proportionally smaller consonantal and vowel inventories, with their consonantal inventory consisting of primarily voiced stops (/b/, /d/, /g/), nasals (/m/, /n/), and glides (/j/, /w/). They also exhibit a more restricted and less complex array of syllable structures, using predominantly single vowels (V) and consonant-vowel (CV) syllable shapes. The babbling stage in late talkers tends to extend over time, as does the use of phonological processes—that is, strategies children with and without language impairment use to simplify adults' speech (e.g., reduplication: /wawa/ for 'water'; unstressed syllable deletion: /ephant/ for 'elephant'). Late talkers are also slower and less accurate in recognizing familiar words (Fernald & Marchman, 2012), have difficulty linking novel labels to novel objects (Weismer, Venker, Evans, & Moyle, 2013), are less sensitive to phonological characteristics of novel words during word learning tasks, and are less able to use phonological knowledge stored in their lexicons to aid in novel word learning (MacRoy-Higgins, Schwartz, Shafer, & Marton, 2013; Weismer et al., 2013).

Delays in morpho-syntactic development are also characteristic of late talkers at age 3;0, 4;0, and 5;0 (Rescorla & Roberts, 1997; Rescorla & Turner, 2015). It is during the second and third years of life that new morphological forms such as grammatical morphemes and basic sentence forms (e.g., subject–verb–object as in *She drinks milk* and subject-copula-complement as in *She is pretty*) are evident in typically developing children (Brown, 1973). The difficulties late talkers exhibit in morpho-syntax are apparent in both noun and verb morphology (Paul & Alforde, 1993; Rescorla & Roberts, 2002), with nominal morphemes such as articles (*the, a*) and pronouns (*she, his*) and verbal morphemes such as contractible copulas (*he's a painter*) and auxiliaries (*she is dancing*) being the most difficult. Later pragmatic difficulties are also evidenced in late talkers at age 4 years (Paul & Smith, 1993); their narratives reflect their difficulties in encoding, organizing, and linking schemes, as well as retrieving precise and diverse words from their lexicons.

Some 75–85% of late talkers, who are identified at age 2;0, seem to catch up to their typically developing peers in their expressive language skills by age 5;0 (Paul, 1996; Rescorla, 2002; Rescorla & Lee, 2001; Rescorla, Mirak, & Singh, 2000; Whitehurst & Fischel, 1994). These children are referred to as *late bloomers* (Thal & Tobias, 1992; Thal, Tobias, & Morrison, 1991); although they may be slow in developing their productive lexicon in the first 2 years of life, they make tremendous progress after their second birthday, and by their third birthday they are very similar to their typically developing peers in terms of their language capabilities (Rescorla et al., 2000). Unfortunately, many toddlers never really catch up to their peers and continue to show persistent language difficulties even after the age of 3;0. These children are often identified at age 4;0 as having SLI. Children with SLI typically have performance IQs within normal limits, normal hearing acuity, no behavioral or emotional disorders, and no gross neurological deficits. Nevertheless, they present significant deficits in language production and/or comprehension (Leonard, 1998, 2014). The language characteristics of children with SLI are reviewed later in this text.

Two clinical markers can be used to distinguish transient language difficulties (i.e., late bloomers) from persistent language impairments (i.e., late talkers). Specifically, a delay in the development of receptive language (Thal, Reilly, Seibert, Jeffries, & Fenson, 2004; Thal & Tobias, 1992; Thal et al., 1991) and a delay in the use of conventional gestures (e.g., pointing, showing) and symbolic gestures (e.g., panting like a dog, sniffing to indicate a flower) (Thal & Tobias, 1992; Thal et al., 1991) are potential predictors of persisting language delays. Comprehension at 13 months of age has been shown to predict the development of receptive vocabulary and grammatical complexity (i.e., mean length of utterance [MLU]) at 28 months of age in typically developing children (Bates, Bretherton, & Snyder, 1988) and is suggested to play an important role throughout the second year of life in both receptive and expressive language acquisition (Watt, Wetherby, & Shumway, 2006). Similarly, the use of gestures early in the second year of life has been shown to correlate closely with total vocal production at 20 months (Capirci, Iverson, Pizzuto, & Volterra, 1996)

and with the development of receptive language at age 3 years (Watt et al., 2006). Early use of gestures was found to predict the onset of two-word combinations (Iverson & Goldin-Meadow, 2005) and children's ability to produce complex sentences, and later vocabulary competence (Rowe & Goldin-Meadow, 2009). Typically developing children use conventional and symbolic gestures prior to the use of words to communicate with others (Acredolo & Goodwyn, 1988; Caselli, 1990; see Capone & McGregor, 2004, for a full review and tutorial by Crais, Watson, & Baranek, 2009). Late bloomers appear to use more communicative gestures compared to their typically developing peers in an effort to compensate for their lack of words, whereas late talkers fail to show an increase in communicative gestures as a compensation for their verbal delay (Thal & Tobias, 1992). Thus compensatory use of communicative gestures is a positive prognostic sign for later typical language development.

The two case studies of Josephine and Robert presented in this text clearly demonstrate the two clinical markers that distinguish between transient language difficulties (i.e., late bloomers) and persistent language difficulties (i.e., late talkers). Josephine exhibited expressive language delays in the presence of age-appropriate receptive skills. For example, she was able to choose one object from a group of five and follow novel and two-step directions. Josephine compensated for her expressive language delay by using prelinguistic gestures (e.g., showing, pointing) and iconic gestures (e.g., hand under cheek to indicate sleeping). Her age-appropriate receptive skills and use of gestures suggest a good prognosis for outgrowing the expressive language delays.

Robert, by contrast, exhibited both expressive and receptive language delays. His receptive skills were appropriate for a 9- to 12-month-old child; hence, those skills are delayed in development by more than a year. Although he was able to respond to requests to say words and to choose two objects from an array of objects, Robert was inconsistent in responding to his name and had difficulty following commands involving two actions with an object. His gesture use was typical of a 9- to 12-month-old child, again reflecting a delay of more than a year. He used prelinguistic gestures such as showing and pointing, and he tended to use them to satisfy basic needs rather than for socialization. Considering the delays in both receptive and expressive language domains and the limited use of gestures, as well as the attention difficulties and the delay in play skills, Robert's prognosis for outgrowing his language delays is poor, suggesting persisting language impairments.

Preschool SLI

Late talkers who are identified at age 2 as having a language delay, as in the case of Robert, may continue to exhibit language deficits during the preschool years. These children are referred to as having SLI. SLI affects approximately 7% of all children (Leonard, 2014). It often runs in families and is suggested to have a genetic component (Newbury, Bishop, & Monaco, 2005), although a clear inheritance pattern or specific genes have not yet been identified. In Robert's case, his family history was remarkable, with an uncle diagnosed with SLI as a child. The appearance of subtle irregularities in brain structure suggests some neurological involvement in the disorder. For example, atypical left-right perisylvian area configurations, with a larger-than-usual right perisylvian area that is equal to or exceeding the size of the left perisylvian area, is associated with SLI (Leonard, 2014).

The language deficits exhibited by children with SLI can be manifested solely in language production or in both language production and comprehension; they can affect one or more areas of language (i.e., form-phonology, syntax, morphology, content-semantics, and use-pragmatics). Considering his prognosis, it is suspected that Robert, our 27-month-old late talker, will continue to exhibit language difficulties during the preschool years. His linguistic profile as a toddler suggests persisting language impairments in both receptive and expressive language domains.

Limitations in Language Content: Semantics

Children with SLI exhibit a slower rate of vocabulary growth (Windfuhr, Faragher, & Conti-Ramsden, 2002) and have a less diverse and more restricted lexicon (Watkins, Kelly, Harbers, & Hollis, 1995). Word learning deficits are frequently observed in children with SLI (Alt & Plante, 2006; Alt, Plante, & Creusere, 2004; Chen & Liu, 2014; Dollaghan, 1987; Gathercole & Baddeley, 1990; Gray, 2003, 2004, 2005). Children with SLI require two to three times as many exposures, compared to their typical language developing peers, to learn a new word (Gray, 2003). In language production, their semantic difficulties are apparent in the speech errors they produce, which tend to be semantic in nature—for example, saying *dog* to refer to a *horse* or *clown* to refer to a *circus*. They reveal low performance on lexical comprehension tests (Lahey & Edwards, 1999; McGregor, 1997) and on tasks focusing on multiple levels of noun hierarchy such as super-ordinate nouns (e.g., *furniture*), coordinate nouns (e.g., *chair*), and subordinate nouns (e.g., *rocking chair*) (McGregor & Waxman, 1998; see review of lexical-semantic deficits by Brackenbury & Pye, 2005). In addition, preschoolers with SLI may exhibit *word-finding difficulties*—that is, difficulties in generating a specific word for any given situation (Rapin & Wilson, 1978). Their difficulties are manifested in single-word naming tasks as well as in conversational discourse (German & Simon, 1991). Their language is characterized by repetitions, substitutions, reformulations, pauses, and use of nonspecific words such as *stuff* or *thing* (Faust, Dimitrovsky, & Davidi, 1997; German, 1987; McGregor & Leonard, 1989; also see review by Messer and Dockrell, 2006).

Difficulties in lexical comprehension are apparent in the understanding and use of basic concepts that mark spatial relations (e.g., *on, in, above, behind*), temporal relations (e.g., *tomorrow, before, after*), kinship relations (e.g., *grandmother, sister, daughter*), causal relations (e.g., *because, why*), sequential relations (e.g., *first, next, finally*), and physical relations (e.g., *hard/soft, wide/narrow, shallow/deep*).

The difficulties preschoolers with SLI exhibit in semantics are not limited to concepts or nouns; they also extend to verb learning. The verb lexicon of such children is characterized as small and less diverse with heavy reliance on "general all-purpose" (GAP) verbs such as *go, make, do*, and *look* (Conti-Ramsden & Jones, 1997; Rice & Bode, 1993; Thordardottir & Weismer, 2001).

Limitations in Language Form: Phonology, Morphology, and Syntax

Phonology. Children with SLI follow similar patterns of phonological development as typically developing children; however, their development is protracted over time. As a result, they show many of the phonological characteristics seen in younger, typically developing children. Preschoolers with SLI exhibit difficulties in the acquisition of the sound system of the language, which is apparent in activities that involve phonological awareness (Gillon, 2018). *Phonological awareness* refers to the explicit awareness that words in the language are composed of syllables and phonemes (i.e., consonants and vowels) (Catts, 1991), and that words can rhyme or begin with the same sound. Children demonstrate phonological awareness by tapping syllables (i.e., segmenting multisyllabic words into their syllable components), recognizing and producing rhymes, segmenting words into their phonemic components, blending and manipulating sounds within words, and understanding letter-sound correspondence. Phonological awareness is a predictor and prognostic marker for early reading success (Carroll & Snowling, 2004; Catts, Fey, Tomblin, & Zhang, 2002; Catts, Fey, Zhang, & Tomblin, 2001). Early difficulties in acquiring phonological awareness skills are linked to later difficulties in reading skills (Torgesen, Wagner, & Rashotte, 1994). Compared to their typically developing peers, preschoolers with SLI perform more poorly on phonological awareness tasks (Bishop, McDonald, Bird, & Hayiou-Thomas, 2009; Catts, Adlof, Hogan, & Weismer, 2005; Fazio, 1997; Vandewalle, Boets, Ghesquière, & Zink, 2012).

Morphology. Preschoolers with SLI display extraordinary difficulty with nominal (e.g., noun plural *-s* inflection) and verbal morphology (e.g., third singular *-s*, regular past tense *-ed*, copula *be* forms), with the latter being more challenging for these children (Bedore & Leonard, 1998; Norbury, Bishop, & Briscoe, 2001; Rice, Wexler, & Cleave, 1995). In fact, a delay in acquiring verb morphology is considered to be a clinical marker for language impairment (Conti-Ramsden, Botting, & Faragher, 2001; Gladfelter & Leonard, 2013). Similar to the path seen with development of phonology, preschoolers with SLI follow the same morphological patterns as their typically developing peers, but their development is protracted, occurring over a longer period of time (Rice & Wexler, 1996; Rice et al., 1995). Compared to language- and age-matched peers, children with SLI produce verb and noun morphological markers less consistently and with a lower percentage of use in sentence completion tasks and in spontaneous speech (Leonard, Eyer, Bedore, & Grela, 1997; Rice & Wexler, 1996; Rice et al., 1995). For example, they are likely to omit the "be" verb form (i.e., auxiliary) or the present progressive *-ing* form, producing sentences such as *I playing with these dolls* (omitting the auxiliary) or *look, I play* (omitting auxiliary and the present progressive). Similarly, they are likely to misuse the "be" verb form, as in the sentence *She were driving the car* (misuse of auxiliary "be" form) or in the sentence *The boy and the girl is sad* (misuse of copula "be" form). In addition, preschoolers with SLI are likely to misuse pronouns in discourse. For example, sentences such as <u>*Him*</u> *not nice,* <u>*Me*</u> *play with the doll,* and *This is not my book, it is* <u>*her*</u> may be apparent in the language of a child with SLI.

Syntax. The limitations children with SLI exhibit in syntactic development are manifested in the reduced length and complexity of the syntactic forms they use. Specifically, they produce shorter sentences (Scott & Windsor, 2000), do not elaborate on noun and verb phrases within sentences, and use simple conjunctions (e.g., *and*) to produce compound sentences. Most often, preschoolers with SLI fail to use prepositional phrases, as in the sentence *The house* <u>*on the corner*</u> *is mine*, or embedded phrases, as in the sentences

He fought <u>*with courage*</u> and *The man* <u>*in the green suit*</u> *is my father* (Schuele & Dykes, 2005; Schuele & Tolbert, 2001).

Limitations in Language Use: Pragmatics

Many conversational skills are acquired during the preschool years. Preschoolers who are developing language typically exhibit gradual improvement in their ability to respond to their conversational partners, to engage in short dialogues, to adjust their language style to the listener, to self-monitor and self-correct errors produced during conversation, to provide clarifications to their conversational partner, and to introduce or shift to a new topic of conversation. By comparison, preschoolers with SLI exhibit difficulties in the acquisition and implementation of many of these conversational skills. They display difficulties initiating and sustaining conversation beyond a few exchanges (Hadley & Rice, 1991). Their difficulties in auditory comprehension and short-term memory impede their ability to maintain the flow of conversation and follow through with directions. Preschoolers with SLI avoid asking for clarifications or providing clarifications in cases where communication breakdowns occur (Fujiki, Brinton, & Sonnenberg, 1990). They also show difficulty in adapting their speech and language to their listener (Leonard, 2014). Preschoolers with SLI not only engage in fewer peer interactions (Rice, Sell, & Hadley, 1991), but also are less likely to be picked by typically developing peers as potential conversational partners. They engage less in active interactions, are less sensitive to the initiations offered by others, and manifest situationally inappropriate verbal responses (Craig & Washington, 1993; Fujiki, Brinton, Isaacson, & Summers, 2001; McCormack, Harrison, McLeod, & McAllister, 2011). Their overall language difficulties prevent them from being able to resolve conflicts in a verbal manner, resulting in their withdrawal or expression of aggression (Leonard, 2014). Experiencing pragmatic difficulties during childhood means that many children with SLI enter adolescence less equipped with the much-needed pragmatic skills to develop adult relationships.

School-Age Language and Learning Disability

Language learning disability (*LLD*), like SLI and late talkers, is an impairment that does not stem from a cognitive deficit, a sensory impairment, a social deficit, or a gross neurological deficit (Paul & Norbury, 2012). School-age children with LLD experience difficulties not only in speaking and listening, but also in reading and writing. In particular, they exhibit difficulties in reading comprehension, identifying and distinguishing between salient and extraneous information in a story, connecting and sequencing ideas in stories, and using visual and contextual cues to understand the story lines. These difficulties affect the child's ability to acquire knowledge about the world from reading books, magazines, and newspapers, leading to increased gaps in their knowledge base. School-age children with LLD exhibit difficulties writing well-formed and grammatically correct sentences. They have difficulty spelling and perform poorly on tasks that tap into letter-sound correspondence and phonological awareness. Like children with SLI, their difficulties may be manifested in one or more of the areas of language (i.e., content, form, or use). Let's reflect on our two case studies, Robert and Josephine. If Robert, our 27-month-old late talker, were to continue exhibiting language impairments in the preschool years—as suggested by his prognosis—these deficits may persist into his school years, ultimately affecting other skills such as reading and writing. Although Josephine, our 22-month-old late bloomer, has a good prognosis for outgrowing her language delays, research suggests that slow development of language in the first few years of life may place children at risk for slower acquisition of a wide range of language-related skills (e.g., vocabulary, grammar, verbal memory, and reading comprehension) during the middle school years and even into adolescence (Rescorla, 2002, 2005). Despite performance within the normal range on most language measures during the school-age years, late bloomers tend to score on the lower end of the distribution compared to their typically developing peers (Paul, 1996; Rescorla, 2002, 2005). Thus, it is important to continue monitoring the development of language and literacy skills during the school-age years of children, who were identified early on as late bloomers. Rescorla (2005) suggested that delivery of services to these children may improve their language processing, phonological discrimination, verbal memory, and word retrieval, thereby preventing later, more advanced language limitations.

Limitations in Language Form: Phonology, Morphology, and Syntax

Phonology. Children with LLD, although usually intelligible, may have experienced phonological deficits as preschoolers. These subtle but often persistent phonological deficits may, in fact, underlie the reading difficulties exhibited during the school years. Such deficits are manifested in these children's poor performance on tasks that require phonological awareness. Phonological awareness is found to be a good predictor of reading ability and is an essential skill for the development of print literacy.

Morphology and Syntax. The language output of students with LLD can be characterized as syntactically simple and immature. These children produce fewer complex sentence structures and fewer embedded clauses than their typically developing peers (Marinellie, 2004). They use fewer modifiers (e.g., *Look at the tall, funny-looking clown*), prepositional phrases (e.g., *The car in the driveway is my father's*), embedded clauses (e.g., *The dress I bought last year does not fit me anymore*), and adverbs (e.g., *She ate her hamburger very quickly*). School-age children with LLD interpret passive structures based on the order of appearance of the subject and object in the sentence instead of relying on the meaning of passive forms. For example, children with LLD will interpret the sentence *The cat was chased by the dog* to mean "The cat chased the dog," instead of the other way around. They also exhibit difficulty with grammatical morphemes that are typically acquired later in development, such as comparatives (*small-smaller*) and superlatives (*smallest*), and advanced prefixes and suffixes (*unrelated, rewrite, disinterested, accomplishment*, and *madness*).

Limitation in Language Content: Semantics

The semantic difficulties exhibited by school-age children with LLD are apparent at the word level as well as at the sentence level. At the word level, these children present with a small vocabulary size that is restricted to high-frequency or short words with low phonological complexity. Their knowledge of word meanings is often restricted, revealing limited associations between words and poor categorization skills (Lahey & Edwards, 1999; McGregor, 1997; McGregor & Waxman, 1998; McGregor & Windsor, 1996). They also have difficulty in understanding the meaning of abstract words (e.g., *wonder, thought, postulate, ponder*) and using words that mark temporal relations (e.g., *next week, while, before*), spatial relations (e.g., *behind* and *above*), quantity (e.g., *more* and *a lot*), and order (e.g., *first* and *next*). Finally, school-age children with LLD may exhibit word-finding difficulties (Faust et al., 1997; German, 1987; McGregor & Leonard, 1989)—that is, the momentary inability to retrieve already known words from the lexicon. Their language is characterized by repetitions, substitutions, pauses, and the use of nonspecific words such as *thing* (Faust et al., 1997).

At the sentence level, school-age children with LLD exhibit difficulty in understanding complex verbal directions and explanations. They struggle to integrate meaning across sentences and paragraphs, revealing their limited ability to process semantic information. Children with LLD also reveal difficulty in understanding and producing figurative language and tend to interpret language literally. For example, a child with LLD may interpret a sentence such as *Break a leg* as an insult, assuming that someone really wants them to get hurt instead of wishing them good luck (Seidenberg & Bernstein, 1986).

Limitations in Language Use: Pragmatics

The limitations that school-age children with LLD exhibit are manifested in their use of language for communication, social development, peer relations, and classroom learning. In most cases, children with LLD have difficulty learning the rules of classroom discourse. They exhibit difficulties initiating conversations with their peers (Liiva & Cleave, 2005), clarifying miscommunications, maintaining the topic of conversation, noticing a shift in the topic of conversation and adjusting accordingly, and contributing relevant information to conversations (Paul & Norbury, 2012). Due to their language and social difficulties, school-age children with language impairment are less likely to be addressed by their classroom peers and are more likely to have their initiations ignored (Hadley & Rice, 1991; Rice et al., 1991). They tend to experience fewer reciprocal relationships (Conti-Ramsden & Botting, 2004; Fujiki, Brinton, Hart, & Fitzgerald, 1999) and describe themselves as lonelier and less satisfied with their peer relationships compared to their typically developing classmates (Fujiki, Brinton, & Todd, 1996).

Presupposition and other conversational skills, such as the ability to initiate conversation, contribute to ongoing conversation, and ask appropriate questions, were found to be highly related to peer acceptance (Gallagher, 1993; Kemple, Speranza, & Hazen, 1992). This suggests that children with social-pragmatic deficits are at a disadvantage in developing peer relations.

The concept of a pragmatic language impairment (PLI) was suggested by several researchers (Adams, 2008; Bishop, 1997; Rapin & Allen, 1983), describing a population who does not meet the criteria for autism but may exhibit some features of ASD in a subtle form (Adams, 2008; Bishop & Norbury, 2002; Conti-Ramsden, Simkin, & Botting, 2006). Rapin and Allen (1983) described these children as having fluent expressive language that is phonologically intact and contains well-formed syntactic structures in the presence of difficulty encoding contextually relevant information, difficulty engaging in communicative discourse, difficulty comprehending ongoing discourse, and difficulty answering questions providing

relevant information. According to Bishop (2000), PLI is an intermediate condition between autism and language impairment. Children exhibiting PLI show some of the language characteristics apparent in SLI (e.g., grammatical and word finding difficulties) as well as mild social difficulties similar to those exhibited by children with high functioning autism or children who used to be diagnosed with Asperger's syndrome (Norbury, Tomblin, & Bishop, 2008). Children with PLI also exhibit difficulties with inference, nonliteral comprehension, and social skills.

In response the DSM-5 (2013) has included a new diagnosis – ***Social (Pragmatic) Communication Disorder***. A Social (Pragmatic) Communication Disorder affects verbal and nonverbal communication behavior within the domain of pragmatic language. This diagnostic category excludes Autism as a diagnosis because children with Social (Pragmatic) Communication Disorder do not show other behaviors associated with Autism (e.g., restricted behavior patterns; see below).

Limitations in Narrative Production

The limitations children with LLD exhibit in language form, content, and use are manifested in their narrative productions. They use fewer cohesive ties (e.g., *after, because, while*) and often use them incorrectly (Liles, 1985a,b, 1987; Ripich & Griffith, 1988). They use a less diverse vocabulary in narration (Paul & Smith, 1993), and their narratives are less informative, lack details, and are short with less overall organization (Scott & Windsor, 2000). In addition, these children have poor understanding of temporal and causal relations and have difficulty answering inferential questions that assess the relationships between the story parts (Merritt & Liles, 1987; Purcell & Liles, 1992).

Expository texts or textbooks present an even greater challenge for children with LLD (Bernstein & Levey, 2002). Expository texts usually contain information that is new to the reader, making it difficult or impossible for the reader to use prior knowledge to comprehend the text. Compared to narratives, textbooks provide very limited contextual support, have no known structure (i.e., the settings, the characters, the main event, and the consequences) to facilitate interpretation, and rely most heavily on children's ability to process linguistic information.

▶ Secondary Language Impairment

In this section we will review two common conditions, ASD and intellectual developmental disorder

(IDD), where the language impairments are secondary to another notable condition, such as intellectual disability or social-pragmatic deficit. While there are many other conditions associated with secondary language impairments, we chose to review ASD and IDD as they are prevalent in the population, and children with these disorders are commonly treated by speech-language pathologists.

Autism Spectrum Disorder

ASD is a childhood disorder involving deficits in social, communication, play, and verbal behavior that was first identified in 1943 by Leo Kanner, an American psychiatrist. Its prevalence in the United States, according to the Centers for Disease Control and Prevention (CDC), is that 1 out of 68 children has been reported to exhibit ASD. ASD is about 4.5 times more prevalent in boys than in girls (Christensen et al., 2016). According to the DSM-5 (2013), the reported frequency of ASD both in and outside the United States, across both child and adult populations, has approached 1%. The increased prevalence was speculated to be attributed to the broad diagnostic criteria delineated in the DSM-5 versus the DSM-4, increased awareness, or a true increase in the frequency of ASD. The onset of autism usually occurs prior to age 3, during the second year of life. Twin and familial studies suggest a genetic component as the etiological basis for autism.

The diagnostic criteria based on the DSM-5 require a child to manifest the following:

A. Persistent deficits in social communication and social interaction across contexts, as manifested by the following:
1. Deficits in social-emotional reciprocity; ranging from abnormal social approach and failure of normal back and forth conversation to reduced sharing of interests, emotions, or affect to failure to initiate or respond to social interactions.
2. Deficits in nonverbal communicative behaviors used for social interaction, ranging from poorly integrated verbal and nonverbal communication to abnormalities in eye contact and body language, or deficits in understanding and use of gestures, to a total lack of facial expression and nonverbal communication.
3. Deficits in developing, maintaining, and understanding relationships, ranging from difficulties adjusting behavior to suit various social contexts to difficulties in sharing imaginative play and in making friends to absence of interest in peers.

B. Restricted, repetitive patterns of behavior, interests, or activities as manifested by at least two of the following:
1. Stereotyped or repetitive motor movements, use of objects, or speech (e.g., simple motor stereotypes, lining up toys or flipping objects, echolalia, idiosyncratic phrases).
2. Insistence on sameness, inflexible adherence to routines, or ritualized patterns of verbal or nonverbal behavior (e.g., extreme distress at small changes, difficulties with transitions, rigid thinking patterns, greeting rituals, needing to take same route or eat same food every day).
3. Highly restricted, fixated interests that are abnormal in intensity or focus (e.g., strong attachment to or preoccupation with unusual objects, excessively circumscribed or perseverative interests).
4. Hyper- or hyporeactivity to sensory input or unusual interest in sensory aspects of the environment (e.g., apparent indifference to pain/temperature, adverse response to specific sounds or textures, excessive smelling or touching of objects, visual fascination with lights or movement).

C. Symptoms must be present in the early developmental period (but may not become fully manifest until social demands exceed limited capacities, or may be masked by learned strategies in later life).

D. Symptoms cause clinically significant impairment in social, occupational, or other important areas of current functioning.

E. These disturbances are not better explained by intellectual disability or global developmental delay. Intellectual disability and autism spectrum disorder frequently co-occur; to make comorbid diagnoses of autism spectrum disorder and intellectual disability, social communication should be below that expected for general developmental level.

Some children with autism may demonstrate over- or undersensitivity to sensory input; they may also exhibit behaviors such as sensitivities to sounds, tastes, textures, and touch, or visual avoidance or tactile defensiveness. In addition to the atypical motor behaviors of hand flapping, spinning, and jumping, children with autism may experience difficulties in motor planning, manipulation, balance, and coordination. These difficulties are apparent in activities such as speaking, writing, dressing, playing with toys, toilet training, and adapting to changes in routine or environments (Prelock, Dennis, & Edelman, 2006).

The language deficits exhibited by children with autism are not limited to pragmatics. Children with autism may also show evidence of deficits in semantics. Their language is very concrete, lacking abstract thinking. They tend to interpret language literally and lack the understanding of figurative language. These children also exhibit difficulties with verbal reasoning and problem solving as well. Nonmeaningful, *echolalic speech*—that is, the immediate or delayed imitation of others' speech—occurs very frequently in children with autism disorder.

Despite the existence of tools and checklists to diagnose autism, accurate diagnosis of the disorder remains challenging and relies heavily on clinical experience. Prelock and Contompasis (2006) have summarized some of the early indicators (i.e., "red flags") that can be used by clinicians to diagnose children with autism:

- Poor social visual orientation and attention
- Failure to point so as to express interest
- The use of hand leading or another's body as a tool
- Mouthing of objects excessively
- Talking stops after using three or more meaningful words
- Use of fewer than five meaningful words on a daily basis at age 2 years or lack of vocalizations with consonants
- Failure to look at others or abnormal/inappropriate eye contact
- Failure to show interest in other children, ignoring people, and a preference to be alone
- Failure to orient to name or a delayed response to name, or lack of attention to voice
- Lack of symbolic play and conventional play with a variety of toys
- Unusual hand and finger mannerisms or repetitive movements
- Aversion to social touch
- Lack of expressive behaviors and gestures or the presentation of unusual behaviors
- Failure to share enjoyment or interest

- Failure to show objects, interest, or joint attention to games for pleasure or connection with others
- Failure to spontaneously direct another's attention
- Failure to show warm, joyful expressions with gaze; lack of emotional facial expression and social smile
- Production of repetitive movements with objects
- Unusual prosody
- Failure to respond to contextual cues (pp. 23–24)

Early identification of autism is key to the development of appropriate and effective intervention programs. Some toddlers, later diagnosed with ASD, exhibit a developmental plateau with gradual decline in social development and language use in the second year of life, which is rare in other disorders and can serve as a "red flag" for ASD (DSM-5, 2013).

Because communication deficits are the central feature of the disorder, speech-language pathologists are primarily the professionals treating children with autism. Nevertheless, a variety of other professionals—such as occupational therapists, psychologists, and *applied behavior analysis (ABA)* therapists—provide important services to children with autism to facilitate their difficulties in other areas of development.

Intellectual Developmental Disorder

The term *mental retardation* (MR) previously described a condition that is characterized by a significantly lower than average level of intellectual functioning and adaptive behavior. It is no longer in use internationally or in the United States. The term *intellectual developmental disorder* is now a widely used term to describe deficits in cognitive capacity that begin in the developmental period.

IDD is diagnosed by measuring the individual's intellectual capacity or functioning on an IQ test, or by clinical judgment in the case of individuals who cannot take an IQ test. The Individuals with Disabilities Education Act (IDEA) defines intellectual disability as "significantly subaverage general intellectual functioning, existing concurrently with deficits in adaptive behavior and manifested during the developmental period, that adversely affects a child's educational performance" [34 *Code of Federal Regulations* §300.7(c)(6)].

The DSM-5 proposed to remove the IQ scores and standard deviations from the criteria for IDD as it is delineated in the DSM-IV. It continues to specify that standardized psychological testing must be included in the assessment of individuals, but that psychological testing should accompany clinical assessment. It suggests that assessment and diagnosis should take into account factors that may limit one's performance (e.g., socio-cultural background, native language, associated communication/language disorder, motor or sensory handicap) and advocates for the use of cognitive profiles for describing intellectual abilities as opposed to a single IQ score.

Many of the language characteristics of children with intellectual disability are similar to those seen in children with primary language impairments. In particular, children with IDD present with deficits in both language comprehension and production, and they show delays in language form, content, and use. Their acquisition of words is much slower, and they exhibit a tendency to rely on concrete word meanings. They use shorter, less complex syntactic structures, with the acquisition of the sound system being protracted over time. The speech intelligibility of children with intellectual disability may also be affected due to involvement of facial traits, such small oral cavity and low muscle tone, as in Down syndrome. For some children with intellectual disability, the acquisition of speech and language poses such a challenge that the use of alternative and augmentative communication may be needed.

Among the most common causes of intellectual disability are the following:

- Genetic conditions. Intellectual disability can be the result of abnormal genes inherited from parents, as in Fragile X syndrome, or chromosomal changes, as in Down syndrome.
- Problems in fetus development during pregnancy. Intellectual disability can be the result of maternal infections during pregnancy, such as rubella or cytomegalovirus (CMV), or the consumption of toxins or chemicals that are hazardous to the fetus, as in the case of fetal alcohol syndrome (FAS).
- Complications during pregnancy or delivery. Intellectual disability can be the result of the fetus not receiving enough oxygen (i.e., anoxia), as in the case of cerebral palsy, or the fetus being born prematurely.
- Exposure to diseases such as measles and meningitis or to toxins and poisons such as lead and mercury.
- Environmental factors such as neglect, malnutrition, and sensory deprivation (as in the case of prolonged isolation or institutionalization). All of these factors can negatively affect the child's development and result in mental disability.

As in the case of primary language impairments, it is vital to provide remedial programs to children with secondary language deficits as early as possible to help them in overcoming difficulties related to their speech, language, and communication disorders.

Whereas primary language deficits are usually not identified until the second year of life, secondary language deficits are often identified very early in the first year of life, as soon as the primary deficit (e.g., hearing loss, intellectual disability) is recognized. Thus, children with secondary language deficits tend to receive speech and language services much earlier compared to children with primary language impairments. Assessment and intervention in these children need to take into account the primary deficit the child exhibits. For example, in the case of a child with intellectual disability, the child's mental age, rather than the chronological age, may guide decisions about the appropriate assessment tools and intervention strategies that should be used in the clinic. Similarly, in the case of a child with a hearing loss, other modes of communication (e.g., sign language, alternative and augmentative communication devices) may be used to target the child's language deficits.

The remainder of this text reviews the procedures most commonly used to assess the language of children with primary and secondary language deficits from toddlerhood to the school-age years. A short review of the most common intervention strategies used by speech-language pathologists for treating children with language deficits follows.

▶ Assessment Procedures for Children with Language Impairments

Early identification of children, who present with language deficits, is vital. A language evaluation, performed by a certified speech-language pathologist (SLP), should be the assessment method of choice when early signs of language impairment are present. The purpose of this kind of language evaluation is twofold: identification and diagnosis.

First, the SLP must either confirm or rule out the existence of language impairment. During the evaluation process, the child's language abilities are compared to age-expected speech, language, and communication milestones or norms gathered from age-matched children, who are developing language in a typical fashion. This process is typically used to determine the eligibility of a child for speech and language services.

Next, following the identification process, the SLP diagnoses the child to understand the nature of the language difficulty, and confirms the presence of a specific language disorder. The SLP needs to determine whether the language deficit is (1) primary, as in late talkers, preschoolers with SLI, and school-age children with LLD, or (2) secondary, resulting from other deficits (e.g., cognitive deficit, autism, hearing loss). During the course of making a diagnosis, the SLP gathers information about the child's strengths and weaknesses, their needs, the family's concerns and priorities, and the resources available to the child and their parents. Especially in the case of infants and toddlers, it is important to incorporate the caregivers in the evaluation process. It is also important to gather information from multiple sources—for example, pediatricians and other professionals working with the child, as well as other family members, who frequently interact with the child and can provide information about their abilities. This information will eventually guide the selection of an intervention plan and ensure that the intervention is carried out effectively.

Evaluation of Infants and Toddlers

In infants, language assessment and intervention are inseparable processes due to the rapid rate of development that occurs during the first months of life. The two most commonly used models of communication assessment for very young children are the *traditional (developmental) approach* and the *dynamic approach.* The traditional or developmental approach to assessment relies almost exclusively on age expectations and normative data. It includes checklists of age-expected behaviors to which infants and toddlers are compared or measured against. The dynamic approach advocates for a more naturalistic approach to assessment, in which the SLP examines a child's language and communication skills in natural contexts. It involves the observation of the child in routine activities—for example, interacting with familiar people, manipulating objects, and playing with different toys alone and with others. Play-based assessment is an important component of the dynamic approach. It allows the SLP to collect information about a child's language and communication skills in play-oriented activities. In addition, it allows the SLP to determine the strategies that may optimally stimulate the child to communicate at higher developmental levels.

Evaluation of Preschool and School-Age Children

The evaluation of a preschooler or a school-age child with language deficits involves the use of standardized tests, criterion-referenced measures, or performance assessment procedures.

Standardized tests (also called *norm-referenced measures*) rank the child's abilities against the performance of age-matched children with typical language development. Norms, which summarize the average performance of children in a specific age group, are used to compare a child's score to the scores of their age-matched peers. This comparison allows the SLP to determine whether a child's score falls within the age-expected range or below it, suggesting the presence of language impairment. Obtaining scores on standardized tests is usually necessary to determine the child's eligibility for services. Most standardized tests consist of a set of subtests that are designed to measure various aspects of receptive and expressive language in one or more areas of language (i.e., phonology, syntax, morphology, semantics, and pragmatics). Subtests that require the child to manipulate objects or point to pictures usually measure receptive language skills, whereas subtests that require the child to imitate, complete, or formulate sentences, or provide descriptions, usually measure expressive language skills.

Although standardized tests are the most commonly used method for evaluating a child's language abilities and are often mandated by the board of education as well as other agencies to determine eligibility for speech and language services, they have several limitations. These tests are limited in the content and scope of what is being examined, usually devoting only a few items to assessment of each linguistic form. They provide a cursory overview of the child's linguistic abilities, which minimizes the SLP's ability to use the results to determine the appropriate intervention goals. Furthermore, most standardized tests do not focus on language use, social communicative skills, and play skills.

Criterion-referenced measures are nonstandardized tools that measure the child's language skills in terms of absolute level of mastery instead of comparing the child's skills to those of their age-matched peers to determine whether the child differs significantly from the norm. These measures provide more in-depth information about the child's performance in specific domains and, as such, are more appropriate for formulating intervention goals. The results of a child's performance on criterion-referenced measures are summarized as pass/fail scores, percentages correct, or performance rates; these scores indicate the child's level of mastery of a specific linguistic form.

Performance assessment procedures are methods by which the SLP evaluates a child's language knowledge, abilities, and achievements in a more naturalistic manner. One of the most common procedures is *language sampling.* Language sampling can be used to assess a child's strengths and weaknesses in all language areas: syntax and morpho-syntax (e.g., calculating MLU, examining the length and complexity of utterances), phonology (e.g., phonetic inventory, syllable structure complexity, and phonological processes), semantics (e.g., vocabulary size), and pragmatics (e.g., conversational skills, the use of gestures, maintenance of eye contact). Language sampling can also be used to establish treatment goals and to monitor progress in therapy or assess the effects of intervention by comparing the language samples pre- and post-intervention. Language sampling is performed while the child is engaged in free play with the SLP or the child's caregiver. Alternatively, it can be carried out in more structured situations using predictable contexts (i.e., scripts), which employ familiar toys/activities.

For school-age children, the assessment of *narratives* is a more commonly used sampling procedure in the evaluation of their language abilities (Paul & Smith, 1993). In a narrative, all language components come together to form a cohesive, well-formulated, meaningful story. The analysis of narratives provides information about the child's morphological and syntactic abilities (Scott & Windsor, 2000), the child's ability to use cohesive devices (e.g., *because, after, if*) to relate meanings across sentences (Hesketh, 2004; Liles, 1985a, 1985b, 1987; Liles, Duffy, Merritt, & Purcell, 1995) and the ability to organize and sequence the story's content in a meaningful way (Liles et al., 1995; Merritt & Liles, 1989; Scott & Windsor, 2000). Similar to the case with language sampling, the analysis of narratives provides a lot of information about a child's language. Narratives can be elicited from children by using sequencing cards, using wordless books, or having children describe routine events and personal experiences.

Another type of assessment that can be used to assess the language skills of preschoolers and school-age children is the *transdisciplinary play-based assessment* (Linder, 2005). This approach to assessment is advantageous in that it allows the assessment of not only language and communication skills, but also social-emotional, cognitive, and sensory-motor abilities. The context of the assessment is play activities that vary depending on the child and the areas being evaluated. This approach is natural and follows the child's attentional needs. It is less stressful and demanding compared to other assessment tools (e.g., standardized tests), which makes it very useful when assessing the language abilities of children, who demonstrate language impairments secondary to other disorders, such as ASD or intellectual disability. Information gathered during play-based assessment is very useful in developing treatment goals and assessing treatment progress, especially in the areas of pragmatics and discourse, which standardized measures often neglect to assess.

School-age children with language impairments can also be evaluated using *curriculum-based language assessment*. These tools assess a child's ability to use language to learn classroom material (Paul & Norbury, 2012) and include evaluations of a child's written work

for the level of narrative development, grammaticality and complexity, use of diverse vocabulary, and use of figurative language.

Systematic observations may also be used to assess a child's pragmatic skills and ability to adhere to classroom discourse rules and expectations. The SLP can observe the child during classes to assess the demands that classroom activities place on the student and, in turn, the child's ability to handle and manage these demands.

▶ Intervention in Children with Language Impairments

Federal law (Part C of Disabilities Education Act [IDEA], 1997) requires that states must provide services to children younger than 3 years of age if they experience developmental delays, as measured by appropriate diagnostic instruments and procedures, in five areas of development: cognitive, physical, communication, social or emotional, and adaptive behavior. Such services must also be provided if the child has a diagnosed physical or mental condition that has a high probability of resulting in a developmental delay (Sec. 632 (5)). Early language intervention often provides a means for toddlers with language delays to catch up to their typical language-developing peers (Leonard, 1998). Conversely, delayed intervention may lead to adverse academic outcomes later in a child's life. Continuing difficulties in reading comprehension, verbal memory, grammar, and vocabulary have been reported in late bloomers during adolescence (Rescorla, 2005).

Part H of the Education of the Handicapped Act (1990) requires the development of an *individual family service plan* (*IFSP*) for each family with an eligible child younger than the age of 3 years. IDEA requires states to provide all children with a free, appropriate public education. When a school-age child is diagnosed with an LLD, the school personnel and the child's parents meet to develop an *individualized education plan* (IEP) that describes the child's strengths and weaknesses, the goals and objectives for therapy, the type of services the child needs, and the amount of time each week that services will be provided.

Many techniques that facilitate language learning and use can be incorporated into therapy for children who exhibit language difficulties. These techniques can be used with children spanning in age from infancy to school age and can be modified according to the child's language abilities, their age, and the focus of the therapy.

Regardless of the strategy chosen for the therapy session, the SLP should (1) use slow speech, (2) emphasize specific linguistic structures by placing

CLINICAL APPLICATION EXERCISES

Jack, a 2;10-year-old child was referred to your clinic for assessment and treatment. According to Jack's parents, Jack uses only 15 words to communicate his wants and needs and does not string words together. His speech is often unintelligible and he uses his pointer frequently to identify his wants. Jack has difficulty following simple one-step directions but responds to his name. He is able to engage in play activities, exhibiting appropriate turn-taking skills and eye contact. He is described by his parents as a happy child who seeks the company of other kids, but does not have the age-appropriate speech and language skills to communicate with them effectively.

1. Based on the description above, which of the following initial diagnosis describes Jack best? Explain why he would not fit into any of the other diagnoses.
    a. Based on the description by Jack's parent, Jack seems to present with autism spectrum disorder
    b. Based on the description by Jack's parent, Jack seems to present with a language delay
    c. Based on the description by Jack's parent, Jack seems to present with language learning disorder
    d. Based on the description by Jack's parent, Jack seems to present with intellectual disability
2. As the treating clinician, what guidelines will you follow to collect more information and make appropriate intervention decisions for Jack?
3. Describe three treatment strategies that might be utilized in your treatment protocol with Jack.

Name of Technique	Description
Enhanced milieu teaching:	
1. Modeling	The targeted linguistic form/behavior is modeled to the child by the SLP in a naturalistic context.
2. Mand-model procedure	The SLP mands (explicitly directs the child, "Tell me what this is"), or provides the child with a choice ("Is the ball red or blue?") and then provides the child with the model.
3. Time delay procedure	The SLP anticipates the child's needs or desires and intentionally waits for the child to initiate.
4. Incidental teaching procedure	Toys are strategically placed to elicit specific linguistic or communicative forms.
Expansion and recasting	SLP reinforces correct production of an erroneous linguistic form by repeating the child's utterance while adding the missing grammatical markers or lexical items.
Imitation	The SLP provides a verbal model and asks the child to imitate the target
Facilitative play/indirect language stimulation	■ Language is facilitated by using toys or objects that draw the child's interest. ■ The SLP arranges the environment such that opportunities for the child to provide target responses occur as a natural part of the play. ■ The SLP may hold back items, hide them, use objects inappropriately or in a funny way, or place objects out of reach to force the child to initiate a request.
Self-talk and parallel talk	In self-talk, the SLP describes their own actions; in parallel talk, the SLP describes the child's actions.
Scripted play	The child and the SLP enact a play routine based on common scripts the child is familiar with such as daily routines of waking up, brushing teeth, eating breakfast, or special-occasion scripts such as planning a birthday party.
Focused stimulation	The child is bombarded with the target form in a variety of contexts. Following exposure, the child is provided with opportunities to spontaneously produce the targeted linguistic form.

stress or emphasis or positioning them at the end or the beginning of an utterance, (3) reduce sentence length and complexity while maintaining the grammaticality of the utterance, (4) repeat information presented to the child multiple times, either by imitating the same structure presented previously or by modifying, rephrasing, or restating the information in a more simplistic way, (5) utilize visual, tactile, and any other cues to support learning, especially through the auditory route, and (6) modify the environment to create optimal conditions for learning, that is, eliminate auditory or visually distracting stimuli.

▶ Summary

A child's language abilities are the foundation for social and communication success as well as school achievement. Therefore, early identification of children with language impairments and early implementation of language services are vital. The speech-language pathologist plays an important role in the identification of these children and the delivery of remedial programs to them. This text discussed the characteristics of primary language impairments in toddlers (i.e., late bloomers and late talkers), preschoolers (i.e., SLI) and school-age children (i.e., LLD), as well as the characteristics of secondary language deficits characteristic of children with intellectual disability and ASD. Speech-language pathologists use a variety of assessment methods to evaluate the language of children with

primary and secondary language deficits. The information gathered by the speech-language pathologist using the assessment tools is then used to devise intervention plans for supporting communication in infants, toddlers, preschoolers, and school-age children.

Study Questions

- Define the following terms and discuss the differences between them: language impairment, language delay, language deviance, and language difference.
- What are the two clinical markers that can help differentiate between late bloomers and late talkers? How do they come into play in the two case studies of Josephine and Robert?
- Describe some of the limitations preschool children with primary language impairments exhibit in language form, content, and use.
- Our late talker, Robert, is now in first grade and his language skills need to be reevaluated to devise more appropriate school-related intervention goals. What are some of the assessment tools/methods you might use to evaluate his language?
- Describe some of the characteristics of children with ASD and explain how they may guide your decision regarding the most appropriate assessment and intervention tools/strategies for use with these children.

References

Acredolo, L., & Goodwyn, S. (1988). Symbolic gesturing in normal infants. *Human Development, 28*, 40–49.

Adams, C. (2008). *Intervention for children with pragmatic language impairment.* In C. F. Nobury, B. J. Tomblin, & D. V. M. Bishop (Eds.), *Understanding developmental language disorders: From theory to practice* (pp. 189–204). New York, NY: Psychology Press.

Alt, M., & Plante, E. (2006). Factors that influence lexical and semantic fast mapping of young children with specific language impairment. *Journal of Speech, Language, and Hearing Sciences, 49*(5), 941–954.

Alt, M., Plante, E., & Creusere, M. (2004). Semantic features in fast-mapping: Performance of preschoolers with specific language impairment versus preschoolers with normal language. *Journal of Speech, Language, and Hearing Sciences, 47*(2), 407–420.

American Psychiatric Association (APA). (2013). *Diagnostic and statistical manual of mental disorders* (5th ed.). Washington, DC: Author.

American Speech-Language-Hearing Association (ASHA). (1993). *Definitions of communication disorders and variations.* Rockville, MD: American Speech-Language-Hearing Association.

American Speech-Language-Hearing Association (ASHA). (2006). *Issues brief for CLD students.* Retrieved from www.asha.org.

Bates, E., Bretherton, I., & Snyder, L. (1988). *From first words to grammar: Individual differences and dissociable mechanisms.* Cambridge, UK: Cambridge University Press.

Bedore, L., & Leonard, L. (1998). Specific language impairment and grammatical morphology: A discriminant function analysis. *Journal of Speech, Language, and Hearing Research, 41*, 1185–1192.

Bernstein, D., & Levey, S. (2002). Language development: A review. In D. K. Bernstein & E. Tiegerman-Farber (Eds.), *Language and communication disorders in children* (5th ed., pp. 28–94). Boston, MA: Allyn & Bacon/Pearson Education.

Bishop, D. V. M. (1997). *Uncommon understanding: Development and disorders of language comprehension in children.* Cambridge, UK: Psychology Press.

Bishop, D. V. M. (2000). Pragmatic language impairment: A correlate of SLI, a distinct subgroup, or part of the autistic continuum? In D. V. M. Bishop & L. Leonard (Eds.), *Speech and language impairments in children: causes, characteristics, intervention, and outcome* (pp. 99–113). Hove, UK: Psychology Press.

Bishop, D. V. M., McDonald, D., Bird, S., & Hayiou-Thomas, M. E. (2009). Children who read words accurately despite language impairment: Who are they and how do they do it? *Child Development, 80*, 593–605.

Bishop, D. V. M., & Norbury, C. F. (2002). Exploring the borderlands of autistic disorder and specific language impairment: A study using standardized diagnostic instruments. *Journal of Child Psychology and Psychiatry, 43*, 917–929.

Brackenbury, T., & Pye, C. (2005). Semantic deficits in children with language impairments: Issues for clinical assessment. *Language, Speech, and Hearing Services in Schools, 36*, 5–16.

Brown, R. (1973). *A first language, the early stages*. Cambridge, MA: Harvard University Press.

Capirci, O., Iverson, J., Pizzuto, E., & Volterra, V. (1996). Gestures and words during the transition to two-word speech. *Journal of Child Language, 23*, 645–673.

Capone, N., & McGregor, K. (2004). Gesture development: A review for clinical and research practices. *Journal of Speech, Language, and Hearing Research, 47*, 173–186.

Carroll, J. M., & Snowling, M. J. (2004). Language and phonological skills in children at high risk of reading difficulties. *The Journal of Child Psychology and Psychiatry, 45*(3), 631–640.

Caselli, M. (1990). Communicative gestures and first words. In V. Volterra & C. Erting (Eds.), *From gesture to sign in hearing and deaf children* (pp. 56–67). New York, NY: Springer-Verlag.

Catts, H. W. (1991). Facilitating phonological awareness: Role of speech-language pathologists. *Language, Speech, and Hearing Services in Schools, 22*, 196–203.

Catts, H. W., Adlof, S. M., Hogan, T. P., & Weismer, S. E. (2005). Are specific language impairment and dyslexia distinct disorders? *Journal of Speech, Language, and Hearing Research, 48*, 1378–1396.

Catts, H. W., Fey, M. E., Tomblin, J. B., & Zhang, X. (2002). A longitudinal investigation of reading outcomes in children with language impairments. *Journal of Speech, Language, and Hearing Research, 45*, 1142–1157.

Catts, H. W., Fey, M. E., Zhang, X., & Tomblin, J. B. (2001). A longitudinal investigation of reading outcomes in children with language impairments. *Language, Speech, and Hearing Services in Schools, 32*, 38–50.

Chen, Y., & Liu, H. M. (2014). Novel-word learning deficits in Mandarin-speaking preschool children with specific language impairments. *Research in Developmental Disabilities, 35*, 10–20.

Christensen, D. L., Baio, J., Van Naarden Braun, K., Bilder, D., Charles, J., Constantino, J. N., … Centers for Disease Control and Prevention (CDC). (2016). Prevalence and characteristics of autism spectrum disorder among children aged 8 years— Autism and developmental disabilities monitoring network, 11 Sites, United States, 2012. *MMWR Surveillance Summaries, 65*(No. SS-3)(No. SS-3), 1–23. doi:10.15585/mmwr.ss6503a1

Conti-Ramsden, G., & Botting, N. (2004). Social difficulties and victimization in children with SLI at 11 years of age. *Journal of Speech, Language, and Hearing Research, 47*, 145–161.

Conti-Ramsden G., Botting N., & Faragher B. (2001). Psycholinguistic markers for specific language impairment (SLI). *Journal of Child Psychology and Psychiatry, 42*(6), 741–748.

Conti-Ramsden, G., & Jones, M. (1997). Verb use in specific language impairment. *Journal of Speech, Language, and Hearing Research, 40*, 1298–1313.

Conti-Ramsden, G., Simkin, Z., & Botting, N. (2006). The prevalence of autism spectrum conditions in adolescents with a history of specific language impairment. *Journal of Child Psychology and Psychiatry, 47*, 621–628.

Craig, H. K., & Washington, J. A. (1993). Access behaviors of children with specific language impairment. *Journal of Speech and Hearing Research, 36*, 322–337.

Crais, E. R., Watson, L. R., & Baranek, G. T. (2009). Use of gesture development in profiling children's prelinguistic communication skills. *American Journal of Speech Language Pathology, 18*, 95–108.

Dollaghan, C. A. (1987). Fast mapping in normal and language-impaired children. *Journal of Speech and Hearing Disorders, 52*(3), 218–222.

Education of the Handicapped Act of 1990, PL 101–476.

Ellis, E. M., Borovsky, A., Elman, J. L., & Evans, J. L. (2015). Novel word learning: An eye-tracking study. Are 18-month-old late talkers really different from their typical peers? *Journal of Communication Disorders, 58*, 143–157.

Ellis, E. M., & Thal, D. J. (2008). Early language delay and risk for language impairment. *Perspectives on Language Learning and Education, 15*, 93–100.

Faust, M., Dimitrovsky, L., & Davidi, S. (1997). Naming difficulties in language-disabled children: Preliminary findings with the application of the tip-of-the-tongue paradigm. *Journal of Speech, Language, and Hearing Research, 40*, 1037–1047.

Fazio, B. B. (1997). Learning a new poem: Memory for connected speech and phonological awareness in low-income children with and without specific language impairment. *Journal of Speech, Language, and Hearing Research, 40*, 1285–1297.

Fernald, A., & Marchman, V. A. (2012). Individual differences in lexical processing at 18 months predict vocabulary growth in typically developing and late-talking toddlers. *Child Development, 83*(1), 203–222.

Fey, M. (1986). *Language intervention with young children*. San Diego, CA: College-Hill Press.

Fujiki, M., Brinton, B., Hart, C. H., & Fitzgerald, A. H. (1999). Peer acceptance and friendship in children with specific language impairment. *Topics in Language Disorders, 19*(2), 49–69.

Fujiki, M., Brinton, B., Isaacson, T., & Summers, C. (2001). Social behaviors of children with language impairment on the playground: A pilot study. *Language, Speech, and Hearing Services in Schools, 32*, 101–113.

Fujiki, M., Brinton, B., & Sonnenberg, E. A. (1990). Repair of overlapping speech in the conversations of specifically language-impaired and normally developing children. *Applied Psycholinguistics, 11*, 201–215.

Fujiki, M., Brinton, B., & Todd, C. M. (1996). Social skills of children with specific language impairment. *Language, Speech, and Hearing Services in Schools, 27*, 195–201.

Gallagher, T. M. (1993). Language skill and the development of social competence in school-age children. *Language, Speech, and Hearing Services in Schools, 24*, 199–205.

Gathercole, S. E., & Baddeley, A. D. (1990). Phonological memory deficits in language disordered children: Is there a causal connection? *Journal of Memory and Language, 29*, 336–360.

German, D. J. (1987). Spontaneous language profiles of children with word-finding problems. *Language, Speech, and Hearing Services in Schools, 18*, 217–230.

German, D. J., & Simon, E. (1991). Analysis of children's word-finding skills in discourse. *Journal of Speech and Hearing Research, 34*, 309–316.

Gillon, G. T. (2018). *Phonological awareness: From research to practice*. London, UK: Guilford Publications.

Gladfelter, A., & Leonard, L. (2013). Alternative tense and agreement morpheme measures for assessing grammatical deficits during the preschool period. *Journal of Speech, Language, and Hearing Research, 56,* 542–552.

Gray, S. (2003). Word-learning by preschoolers with specific language impairment: What predicts success? *Journal of Speech, Language, and Hearing Research, 46,* 56–67.

Gray, S. (2004). Word learning by preschoolers with specific language impairment: Predictors and poor learners. *Journal of Speech, Language, and Hearing Research, 47,* 1117–1132.

Gray, S. (2005). Word learning by preschoolers with specific language impairment: Effect of phonological or semantic cues. *Journal of Speech, Language, and Hearing Research, 48,* 1452–1467.

Hadley, P. A., & Rice, M. L. (1991). Conversational responsiveness of speech- and language-impaired preschoolers. *Journal of Speech and Hearing Research, 34,* 1308–1317.

Hesketh, A. (2004). Grammatical performance of children with language disorder on structured elicitation and narrative tasks. *Clinical Linguistics and Phonetics, 18,* 161–182.

Individuals with Disabilities Education Act [IDEA] of 1997, PL 101–336.

Iverson, J. M., & Goldin-Meadow, S. (2005). Gesture paves the way for language development. *Psychological Science, 16*(5), 367–371.

Kemple, K., Speranza, H., & Hazen, N. (1992). Cohesive discourse and peer acceptance: Longitudinal relation in the preschool years. *Merrill-Palmer Quarterly, 38,* 364–381.

Lahey, M., & Edwards, J. (1999). Naming errors of children with specific language impairment. *Journal of Speech, Language, and Hearing Research, 42,* 195–205.

Leonard, L. (1998). *Children with specific language impairment.* Cambridge, MA: MIT Press.

Leonard, L. (2014). *Children with specific language impairment* (2nd ed.). Cambridge, MA: MIT Press.

Leonard, L., Eyer, J., Bedore, L., & Grela, B. (1997). Three accounts of the grammatical morpheme difficulties of English-speaking children with specific language impairment. *Journal of Speech, Language, and Hearing Research, 40,* 741–753.

Liiva, C. A., & Cleave, P. (2005). Roles of initiation and responsiveness in access and participation for children with specific language impairment. *Journal of Speech, Language, and Hearing Research, 48,* 868–883.

Liles, B. Z. (1985a). Narrative ability in normal and language disordered children. *Journal of Speech and Hearing Research, 28,* 123–133.

Liles, B. Z. (1985b). Production and comprehension of narrative discourse in normal and language disordered children. *Journal of Communication Disorders, 18,* 409–427.

Liles, B. Z. (1987). Episode organization and cohesive conjunctives in narratives of children with and without language disorders. *Journal of Speech and Hearing Research, 30,* 185–196.

Liles, B. Z., Duffy, R. J., Merritt, D. D., & Purcell, S. L. (1995). Measurement of narrative discourse ability in children with language disorders. *Journal of Speech and Hearing Research, 38,* 415–425.

Linder, T. W. (2005). *Transdisciplinary play-based assessment: A functional approach to working with young children* (revised). Baltimore, MD: Brookes.

MacRoy-Higgins, M., Schwartz, R. G., Shafer, V. L., & Marton, K. (2013). Influence of phonotactic probability/neighbourhood density on lexical learning in late talkers. *International Journal of Language and Communication Disorders, 8*(2), 188–199.

Marinellie, S. A. (2004). Complex syntax used by school-age children with specific language impairment (SLI) in child-adult conversation. *Journal of Communication Disorders, 37*(6), 517–533.

McCormack, J., Harrison, L. J., McLeod, S., & McAllister, L. (2011). A nationally representative study of the association between communication impairment at 4–5 years and children's life activities at 7–9 years. *Journal of Speech, Language, and Hearing Research, 54,* 1328–1348.

McGregor, K. K. (1997). The nature of word-finding errors of preschoolers with and without word finding deficits. *Journal of Speech and Hearing Research, 40,* 1232–1244.

McGregor, K. K., & Leonard, L. B. (1989). Facilitating word-finding skills of language-impaired children. *Journal of Speech and Hearing Disorders, 54,* 141–147.

McGregor, K. K., & Waxman, S. R. (1998). Object naming at multiple hierarchical levels: A comparison of preschoolers with and without word-finding deficits. *Journal of Child Language, 25,* 419–430.

McGregor, K. K., & Windsor, J. (1996). Effects of priming on the naming accuracy of preschoolers with word-finding deficits. *Journal of Speech and Hearing Research, 39,* 1048–1058.

Merritt, D. D., & Liles, B. Z. (1987). Story grammar ability in children with and without language disorder: Story generation, story retelling, and story comprehension. *Journal of Speech and Hearing Research, 30,* 539–552.

Merritt, D. D., & Liles, B. Z. (1989). Narrative analysis: Clinical applications of story generation and story retelling. *Journal of Speech and Hearing Disorders, 54,* 429–438.

Messer, D., & Dockrell, J. E. (2006). Children's naming and word-finding difficulties: Descriptions and explanations. *Journal of Speech, Language, and Hearing Research, 49*(2), 309–324.

Nelson, K. (1973). Structure and strategy in learning to talk. *Monographs of the Society for Research in Child Development, 38,* 1–2.

Newbury, D. F., Bishop, D. V. M., & Monaco, A. P. (2005). Genetic influences on language impairment and phonological short-term memory. *Trends in Cognitive Sciences, 9,* 528–534.

Norbury, C. F., Bishop, D. V. M., & Briscoe, J. (2001). Production of English finite verb morphology: A comparison of SLI and mild–moderate hearing impairment. *Journal of Speech Language and Hearing Research, 44,* 165–178.

Norbury, C. F., Tomblin, J. B., & Bishop, D. V. M. (2008). *Understanding Developmental Language Disorders: From Theory to Practice.* New York, NY: Psychology Press.

Paul, R. (1991). Profiles of toddlers with slow expressive language growth. *Topics in Language Disorders, 11,* 1–13.

Paul, R. (1996). Clinical implications of the natural history of slow expressive language development. *American Journal of Speech-Language Pathology, 5,* 5–21.

Paul, R., & Alforde, S. (1993). Grammatical morpheme acquisition in 4-year-olds with normal, impaired, and late developing language. *Journal of Speech and Hearing Research, 36,* 1271–1275.

Paul, R., & Jennings, P. (1992). Phonological behavior in toddlers with slow expressive language development. *Journal of Speech and Hearing Research, 35,* 99–107.

Paul, R., & Norbury, C. (2012). *Language disorders from infancy through adolescence: Assessment and intervention* (4th ed.). St. Louis, MO: Mosby-Year Book.

Paul, R., & Smith, R. L. (1993). Narrative skills in 4-year-olds with normal, impaired, and late-developing language. *Journal of Speech and Hearing Research, 36,* 592–598.

Prelock, P. A., & Contompasis, S. H. (2006). Autism and related disorders: Trends in diagnosis and neurobiologic considerations. In Prelock, P. (Ed.), *Autism spectrum disorders:*

Issues in assessment and intervention (pp. 3–63). Austin, TX: Pro-Ed.

Prelock, P. A., Dennis, R. E., & Edelman, S. (2006). Sensory and motor considerations in the assessment of children with ASD. In Prelock, P. (Ed.), *Autism spectrum disorders: Issues in assessment and intervention* (pp. 303–339). Austin, TX: Pro-Ed.

Purcell, S., & Liles, B. Z. (1992). Cohesion repairs in the narratives of normal-language and language-disordered school-age children. *Journal of Speech and Hearing Research, 35*, 354–362.

Rapin, I., & Allen, D. (1983). Developmental language disorders: Nosologic considerations. In U. Kirk (Ed.), *Neuropsychology of language, reading, and spelling.* New York, NY: Academic Press.

Rapin, I., & Wilson, B. (1978). Children with developmental language disability. Neurological aspects and assessment. In M. Wyke (Ed.), *Developmental dysphasia* (pp. 13–41). New York, NY: Academic Press.

Rescorla, L. (1989). The language development survey: A screening tool for delayed language in toddlers. *Journal of Speech and Hearing Disorders, 54*, 587–599.

Rescorla, L. (2002). Language and reading outcomes to age 9 in late-talking toddlers. *Journal of Speech, Language, and Hearing Research, 45*, 360–371.

Rescorla, L. (2005). Age 13 language and reading outcomes in late-talking toddlers. *Journal of Speech, Language, and Hearing Research, 48*, 459–472.

Rescorla, L., & Lee, E. C. (2001). Language impairments in young children. In T. Layton & L. Watson (Eds.), *Handbook of early language impairment in children: Volume I: Nature* (pp. 1–55). Albany, NY: Delmar.

Rescorla, L., Mirak, J., & Singh, L. (2000). Vocabulary growth in late talkers: Lexical development from 2;0 to 3;0. *Journal of Child Language, 27*, 293–311.

Rescorla, L., & Ratner, N. B. (1996). Phonetic profiles of typically developing and language-delayed toddlers. *Journal of Speech and Hearing Research, 39*, 153–165.

Rescorla, L., & Roberts, J. (1997). Late-talkers at 2: Outcomes at age 3. *Journal of Speech and Hearing Research, 40*, 556–566.

Rescorla, L., & Roberts, J. (2002). Nominal versus verbal morpheme use in late talkers at ages 3 and 4. *Journal of Speech, Language, and Hearing Research, 45*, 1219–1231.

Rescorla, L., & Schwartz, E. (1990). Outcome of toddlers with expressive language delay. *Applied Psycholinguistics, 11*, 393–407.

Rescorla, L., & Turner, H. L. (2015). Morphology and syntax in late talkers at age 5. *Journal of Speech, Language, and Hearing Research, 58*(2), 434–444. doi:10.1044/2015_JSLHR-L-14-0042

Rice, M. L., & Bode, J. (1993). GAPs in the lexicon of children with specific language impairment. *First Language, 13*, 113–132.

Rice, M. L., Sell, M. A., & Hadley, P. A. (1991). Social interactions of speech and language impaired children. *Journal of Speech and Hearing Research, 34*, 1299–1307.

Rice, M. L., & Wexler, K. (1996). Toward tense as a clinical marker of specific language impairment in English-speaking children. *Journal of Speech and Hearing Research, 39*, 1239–1257.

Rice, M. L., Wexler, K., & Cleave, P. L. (1995). Specific language impairment as a period of extended optional infinitive. *Journal of Speech and Hearing Research, 38*, 850–863.

Ripich, D. N., & Griffith, P. L. (1988). Narrative abilities of children with learning disabilities and nondisabled children: Story structure, cohesion, and propositions. *Journal of Learning Disabilities, 21*(3), 165–173.

Roberts, J., Rescorla, L., Giroux, J., & Stevens, L. (1998). Phonological skills of children with specific expressive language impairment (SLI-E): Outcome at age 3. *Journal of Speech, Language, and Hearing Research, 41*, 374–384.

Rowe, M. L., & Goldin-Meadow, S. (2009). Differences in early gesture explain SES disparities in child vocabulary size at school entry. *Science, 323*(5916), 951–953.

Schuele, C. M., & Dykes, J. (2005). A longitudinal study of complex syntax development in a child with specific language impairment. *Clinical Linguistics and Phonetics, 19*, 295–318.

Schuele, C. M., & Tolbert, L. (2001). Omissions of obligatory relative markers in children with specific language impairment. *Clinical Linguistics and Phonetics, 15*, 257–274.

Scott, C. M., & Windsor, J. (2000). General language performance measures in spoken and written narrative and expository discourse of school-age children with language learning disabilities. *Journal of Speech, Language, and Hearing Research, 43*, 324–339.

Seidenberg, P., & Bernstein, D. (1986). The comprehension of similes and metaphors by learning disabled and non-learning disabled children. *Language, Speech, and Hearing Services in Schools, 17*, 219–229.

Thal, D. (2000). *Late talking toddlers: Are they at risk?* San Diego, CA: San Diego State University Press.

Thal, D. J., Reilly, J., Seibert, L., Jeffries, R., & Fenson, J. (2004). Language development in children at risk for language impairment: Cross-population comparisons. *Brain & Language, 88*, 167–179.

Thal, D., & Tobias, S. (1992). Communicative gestures in children with delayed onset of oral expressive vocabulary. *Journal of Speech and Hearing Research, 35*, 1281–1289.

Thal, D., Tobias, S., & Morrison, D. (1991). Language and gesture in late talkers: A 1-year follow-up. *Journal of Speech and Hearing Research, 34*, 604–612.

Thordardottir, E. T., & Weismer, S. E. (2001). High frequency verbs and verb diversity in the spontaneous speech of school-age children with specific language impairment. *International Journal of Language and Communication Disorders, 36*, 221–244.

Torgesen, J. K., Wagner, R. K., & Rashotte, C. A. (1994). Longitudinal studies of phonological processing and reading. *Journal of Learning Disabilities, 27*(5), 276–286.

Vandewalle, E., Boets, B., Ghesquière, P., & Zink, I. (2012). Development of phonological processing skills in children with specific language impairment with and without literacy delay: a 3-year longitudinal study. *Journal of Speech, Language, and Hearing Research, 55*(4), 1053–1067.

Watkins, R. V., Kelly, D. J., Harbers, H. M., & Hollis, W. (1995). Measuring children's lexical diversity: Differentiating typical and atypical learners. *Journal of Speech and Hearing Research, 39*, 1349–1355.

Watt, N., Wetherby, A., & Shumway, S. (2006). Prelinguistic predictors of language outcome at 3 years of age. *Journal of Speech, Language, and Hearing Research, 49*, 1224–1237.

Weismer, S. E., & Evans, J. L. (2002). The role of processing limitations in early identification of specific language impairment. *Topics in Language Disorders, 22*(3), 15–29.

Weismer, S. E., Venker, C. E., Evans, J. L., & Moyle, M. J. (2013). Fast mapping in late-talking toddlers. *Applied Psycholinguist, 34*(1), 69–89.

Whitehurst, G., & Fischel, J. (1994). Practitioner review: Early developmental language delay: What, if anything, should the clinician do about it? *Journal of Child Psychology and Psychiatry, 35*, 613–648.

Windfuhr, K., Faragher, B., & Conti-Ramsden, G. (2002). Lexical learning skills in young children with specific language impairment (SLI). *International Journal of Language and Communication Disorders, 37*, 415–432.

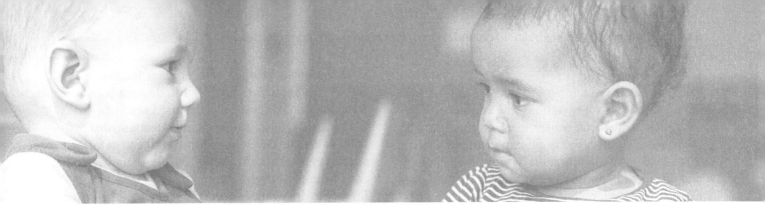

CHAPTER 16

Listening, Language, and Literacy for Children with Auditory Devices: From Hearing Aids to Cochlear Implants

Patricia Chute, EdD
Mary Ellen Nevins, EdD

OBJECTIVES

- Review basic information regarding the anatomy and physiology of the auditory mechanism
- Describe the acoustical analysis required to understand spoken language and how it is affected by competing noise
- Review the types of hearing technologies (such as traditional hearing aids and cochlear implants) used to ameliorate hearing loss
- Outline principles and strategies for intervention that underscore the concepts of auditory-based instruction
- Identify the developmental factors that contribute to literacy learning of children who are deaf or hard of hearing
- Discuss the role of the speech-language pathologist in addressing the effects of hearing loss on executive function, cultural identity, and educational achievement overall

KEY TERMS

Auditory-based intervention
Auditory skills

Deaf/hard of hearing
Hearing technologies

Listening and spoken language

▶ Introduction

In less than two generations, the educational, linguistic, and social achievement of children with hearing loss has increased exponentially. This is a result of early identification, improved technology, and advances in approaches to therapy that embrace a focus on developmental principles to drive intervention and education. That said, it is still crucial to provide concentrated efforts to guide, shape, and fine-tune the acquisition of linguistic skills to support the levels of success that are now possible for greater numbers of children who are deaf and hard of hearing. With the advent of universal newborn hearing screening (UNHS), the age for identification of children with hearing loss has decreased markedly from an average of 2.5 years of age to 2–3 months of age (Ching et al., 2017). This permits the fitting of auditory devices at early stages of development and allows access to spoken language that would have eluded the infant who was not diagnosed until much later. Early intervention has now become the entry point from which families and professionals work in partnership to launch all learning, especially emphasizing listening, delivered by today's sophisticated hearing devices. Because babies who are deaf or hard of hearing are being identified earlier, new paradigms of practice have evolved. Of necessity, professionals have retooled to consider developmentally appropriate interactions with infants and toddlers and coaching and guiding families to drive the child's listening and language acquisition. As this occurred, it created a cadre of children who entered the educational system with abilities that exceeded the prior generation of deaf children. Syntactically based drill and practice intervention and laborious articulation practice for deaf children was no longer appropriate.

Today's early identification of hearing loss and early technology fitting have been the drivers of a marked change in the manner in which we approach intervention with children who are deaf or hard of hearing. For all families, especially those whose goals include a child's learning the language of the home (and of the heart), the power of families/caregivers as the first and most effective teachers is recognized. This belief is operationalized when models of family-centered intervention or family-professional partnerships are implemented (JCIH, 2013). Assisting families in negotiating the often-complex maze of service provision is foundational to working with a newly identified child with hearing loss. The majority of these same families are envisioning listening and spoken language outcomes for their child's future (BEGINNINGS, 2014); the need for highly competent early interventionists charged with guiding families along the journey to their desired goal attainment is critical. Research would indicate that the first 3 years of a child's life are crucial to launching the early learning that contributes to brain development and sets the stage for later success in school (Zauche et al., 2017). An understanding of the path from listening to spoken language to literacy to drive this success may serve as the backdrop for identifying the dispositions, skills, and knowledge that will be required of the speech-language pathologist who provides services to children who are deaf or hard of hearing and their families. Despite incredible attainment, children who are deaf or hard of hearing present with learning challenges that must be accommodated. It is no longer possible to make sweeping categorical pronouncements about what deaf children need. Presumption of performance based on an audiologic metric alone may limit educational outcomes. Attention must be paid to the nature of the hearing loss in order to provide the most appropriate intervention, both from the standpoint of the sensory aid as well as the approach to developing spoken-language skills. An overview of audiologic issues follows.

▶ The Auditory System

For a child to learn spoken language, there is a presumption that an intact auditory system exists upon which all other assumptions rest. The fine structure of the ear with its outer, middle, inner, and central components is the ultimate analyzer that filters, refines, and interprets messages that can be environmental, musical, and, most importantly, linguistic in nature. This analysis occurs in milliseconds despite the fact that the complexity of the spoken word incorporates acoustical aspects that convey meaning via suprasegmental (tonal/quality information) as well as segmental (frequency/timing) cues. For the speech-language pathologist (SLP), an understanding of the basics of hearing is required to support interventions that use auditory-based instruction. These fundamental tenets include knowledge of anatomy, physiology, and acoustics of the auditory mechanism. Without this consideration, the outcome for a child learning spoken language will be limited, and, in some cases, be a failure. With this in mind, the reader is provided with a concise presentation of the auditory system.

The Anatomy

As noted previously, the auditory mechanism consists of the outer, middle, and inner ear with a central component that sends signals to the brain. The *outer* portion includes the pinna, external auditory meatus (ear canal), and tympanic membrane (eardrum). After sound leaves the eardrum, it enters the *middle* ear, which contains the three bones known as the malleus (hammer), the incus (anvil), and the stapes (stirrup). In addition to the three middle ear bones, also known as ossicles, there are several muscles as well as the entrance to the Eustachian tube within the middle ear space. The final middle ear bone, the stapes, connects to the *inner* ear, known as the cochlea. This snail-shaped part of the anatomy contains both a bony portion and a membranous portion filled with fluid. Additionally, the vestibular mechanism (known as the semicircular canals) dovetails off the cochlea into three separate channels that control balance.

Because a great deal of the acoustical analysis that occurs in the inner ear transpires in the cochlea, it is important to have an understanding of the other anatomical features that make up this important piece of the ear's composition. As noted previously, the two portions of the cochlea include both a bony and membranous portion. The membranous portion includes a structure known as the basilar membrane, which supports 30,000 hair cells (also known as cilia) along its length. These 30,000 hair cells, which are imbedded in other supporting structures, are specifically arranged in precisely tuned rows. These rows are tuned to frequencies that are high in pitch at the base of the cochlea to those that are lower in pitch at its apex or top. Sounds are analyzed via a complex system within the cilia and basilar membrane and are forwarded to the auditory nerve (which is the eighth cranial nerve in the human body). The auditory nerve has two subdivisions, one for acoustical analysis and one for vestibular analysis. Signals from the eighth cranial nerve are delivered to the brain for final processing and comprehension. Needless to say, this is but a cursory review of the major anatomical portions of the cochlea. For more in-depth information, the reader is directed to Gelfand (2001).

Physiology

The physiology of the auditory mechanism is one whose complexities continue to elude researchers today. However, there are some basic functions that have been well known since the early days of physiological acoustics, when Bekesy performed his early experiments (Bekesy & Rosenblith, 1958). The beauty of the auditory system is that each of its portions has both a specific and redundant role in the delivery of sound to the brain. To begin, the outer ear's major function is one of collection of the signal for ultimate delivery into the inner ear. The pinna is constructed in such a way that sounds coming from the front of a listener will be louder, while those from behind will be reduced in intensity. The fact that there are two ears instead of one provides additional filtering to reduce background noise. Sound itself is composed of different pitches or frequencies, some of which can be overshadowed by noise or even reduced loudness from the source. High frequency sounds (those that are found in the consonants of speech) are often the weakest in volume and so the pinna attempts very early on to enhance them through the various undulations of its shape. After they are "collected," sounds are then funneled through the ear canal, which again enhances some sounds while decreasing the intensity of others so as not to have the eardrum become stressed and then break.

As an SLP, it is important to observe a child's outer ear for any malformations that will inhibit sound from entering the ear. Malformations of the outer ear are often indicative of anatomical deformities in structures further along in the system. The size of the pinna will vary and may also be an ethnic variant, but should not be of concern unless it is extremely small. Very narrow ear canals will also block sound from getting into the system, as will impacted cerumen (wax), which may not be observable without an otoscope. The tympanic membrane (TM) sits at the end of the ear canal and its role is to further enhance sound and deliver it to the middle ear. If there is a hole in the TM either due to trauma or infections that cause it to burst, sounds will be affected. When there is scarring on the TM (normally due to recurrent ear infections that result in the TM bursting and then closing on its own), sound transmission will be compromised. Although this examination requires the use of an otoscope, there may be information provided by the family during history intake that might require medical follow-up recommendations. Of note, for children with pressure equalizing (PE) tubes, a small hole has been made in the TM to place the PE tube; it is located in a position that does not affect hearing in a negative manner. In fact, for children with recurrent ear infections, the placement of a PE tube restores hearing to appropriate levels.

As sound enters the middle ear through the TM, acoustical changes occur to augment and decrease both the frequency and the intensity of the incoming signal. Attached to the TM is the malleus, which sends the signal to the incus and finally the stapes. Because the three ossicles are the smallest bones in the body and are the same size throughout life, the relative size of the TM to that of the stapes is so different that without this frequency/intensity transformation, the incoming signal would destroy the inner ear with a single sound.

Musculature in the middle ear prevents the sound from getting so loud as to cause damage to the inner ear. The Eustachian tube (ET) provides the middle ear with a method of equalizing pressures that can otherwise build up and create hearing and medical problems. Hearing loss that occurs either at the level of the outer or middle ear is classified as *conductive* in nature and is generally amenable to medical intervention with great success and only temporary loss of hearing.

After sound reaches the stapes, the vibrations are transmitted to the fluid-filled portion of the cochlear, which creates a "travelling wave" based on the frequency content of the signal. The movement of the basilar membrane causes the cilia in the areas tuned to the incoming signal to bend and transforms the signal from a mechanical to an electrical one. These electrical signals are analyzed by frequency and intensity along the basilar membrane and sent to the cochlear nerve, which carries it ultimately to the brain. Sensorineural hearing loss (commonly but erroneously known as "nerve" deafness) occurs when there is damage to any portion of the cochlea. Damage or absence of cilia is permanent in nature and can be a function of genetics, neo-natal events, medical conditions, infections, and/or acoustic trauma. In some cases, the hearing loss may be sudden, whereas in other circumstances, it may progress over time. Regardless, the damage is irreversible and requires (re)habilitative intervention in the form of hearing aids or cochlear implants.

It is most important to understand that signals from the cochlea, whether a normal or abnormal structure, still require significant processing in the brain in order for it to recognize and respond to incoming information. The challenges faced by the child with hearing loss are exacerbated by the fact that the incoming signal to the brain is one that will not carry the same information to which a normal cochlea would have access. The question of what each child might access given the hearing loss will depend on a multiplicity of factors that include the signal itself, the type and degree of hearing loss, and the presence of any other confounding variables. Understanding the nature of the incoming signal, therefore, becomes an important factor in the overall approach to (re)habilitation protocols for a child with language delays associated with hearing loss.

Speech Acoustics

The speech signal is composed of various frequencies and intensities that interplay with each other depending upon placement in a sequence within a word, phrase, or sentence. When added to the fact that certain dialects confound the production of particular vowels or consonants, one has to wonder how any of us actually understands what is being said. When listeners have hearing loss, problems abound as an individual attempts to piece together information that is at best distorted and at worst absent. The role the SLP plays in facilitating strategy development that builds language competence is paramount to the outcomes of the child with hearing loss. Because this text addresses spoken language acquisition only, approaches to building a linguistic foundation for children using hearing technologies is fundamental to auditory-based intervention. Whether a child enters the process with no language or with some linguistic abilities already acquired, knowledge of the speech signal becomes critical to practitioners providing a comprehensive, evidence-based approach to language intervention. It should be evident, then, that a child's access to any speech signal is predicated upon the pairing of the most appropriate listening device to the level of hearing impairment.

Listening Devices

Hearing technologies run the gamut of traditional hearing aids, implantable devices, and cochlear implants. The magnitude and type of hearing loss will influence the proper selection of the sensory aid relative to the medical history of the child. For children with mild or moderate levels of hearing loss, standard hearing aids are the device of choice. In some cases, implantable bone-anchored hearing systems may be an option. Most often, bone-anchored devices are utilized in children with external malformations of the ear. Because aural malformations are usually conductive in nature, the auditory capability of an activated device brings the child's hearing to near-normal limits. Generally, these children demonstrate relatively good language abilities, but still benefit from interventions that hone fine listening, language, and literacy skills. Regardless of whether the devices are bone anchored or traditional in nature, they work in a similar manner. These instruments consist of a microphone that detects the signal, which is then delivered acoustically (either through the bones of the skull or the ear canal) to be processed in the cochlea. Prior to reaching the cochlea, sounds are further processed and filtered to emphasize certain frequencies depending upon the degree and type of hearing loss.

Hearing loss is categorized in degree and is identified by levels labeled very mild, mild, moderate, moderately severe, severe, and profound. Depending upon the degree and frequency configuration of the hearing loss, traditional amplification can provide substantial benefit so that the listener can access most of the acoustical features of speech. For the child with severe to profound hearing loss, when hearing aids are not providing enough sound access, a cochlear implant is considered best practice since it delivers sound in a different manner from conventional hearing aids. A cochlear implant utilizes electrical stimulation, whereas a traditional hearing aid is acoustic in nature. Cochlear implants consist of several components, some of which are similar to traditional hearing aids. There is a microphone that detects sounds, filters them through an external speech processor, and delivers them instead to an electrode array that is inserted by a surgeon into the cochlea. These electrodes are tuned to certain frequencies to mimic those in the normal inner ear, but are not matched on a one-to-one basis because the array does not extend throughout the entire cochlea. The process in which an audiologist adjusts the electrical levels to each of the electrodes is known as *mapping* and requires specific equipment. Adjustments in these electrical levels will often change over time, especially during the initial stages of cochlear implant use. It is important for the SLP to communicate with the audiologist in order to provide feedback regarding a child's performance so that map adjustments can be made. Any problems with implant equipment or function should be communicated as well.

Regardless of whether the child with hearing loss uses an implant or a hearing aid, there is no guarantee that each child will receive the same type of benefit. It behooves the SLP to understand the device, when the child received it, the duration of use, and the impression of the audiologist as to the effectiveness of the device for that child. Collaboration with other professionals is key to understanding each child's potential for auditory learning.

The Speech Signal

The vowels and consonants that make up the speech signal (and in this case spoken English) combine in a manner that brings frequencies and intensities together in a precise fashion. No utterance in English is composed of a single frequency or intensity. Vowels are produced by movements of the articulators that enhance a series of frequencies—some in the lower range and others in a higher range. These are known as *formants,* and the ability to distinguish vowels and consonants will depend on the relationship between the first formant (F1) and second formant (F2). There are also transitions between F1 and F2 that contribute to discrimination. First formant information occurs below 1,000 Hz and is often more discriminable for a child with hearing loss because there is often access

to low frequency information either with or without hearing aids and/or cochlear implants. The challenges of providing high frequency information to the damaged cochlea has always been the logjam in those with hearing loss as the acoustics of delivering the signal coupled with the lack of receptors in the inner ear that are tuned to those frequencies is not easily resolved. For this reason, it is important for the SLP to have a basic understanding of these frequency relationships (see **FIGURE 16-1**). However, one must understand that *detection* of a particular frequency does not translate into *discrimination* of frequencies due to the damaged cochlea. As a starting point, every session should always begin with a rudimentary sound "test" to ensure that the sensory aid is in proper working order. The Ling 6 sound test (ah, ee, oo, sh, s, m) is one that has been used consistently throughout decades of rehabilitation paradigms as it tests perception (or in some cases merely detection) across the speech frequency range. At the beginning of each session, the SLP should provide an opportunity for the child to respond to the six sounds presented in an auditory-only condition with either a mere yes/no response or with an acknowledgment of the exact sound being presented.

Acoustic Environment

The need for a clear signal without background interference becomes critical for professionals engaged in habilitative strategies to ensure that the listener has access to the frequency and intensity information of the spoken word. For the individual with hearing loss, there is already a deficit in the fine structure of speech, and even with hearing aids or a cochlear implant an exact replication of the signal output to the device will not be available. In school environments where there is precious little space, it is not unusual to find the SLP providing services in less than optimal areas of the school building. This will create challenging listening experiences in addition to those challenges that are already a result of the hearing loss. It stands to reason, therefore, that any student/clinician interaction should take place in a quiet setting to maximize attention as well as the acoustical signal. Additionally, if there is any physical barrier (e.g., placing the hand over the mouth), this too will not deliver sufficient intensity or frequency information and will create additional challenges to the listener. Often, the SLP may sit off to the side out of the line of sight to the listener to hone the auditory skill, but it is important that access to the microphone on the device is on the side of the speech output and is capable of detecting the signal from the distance and angle of delivery.

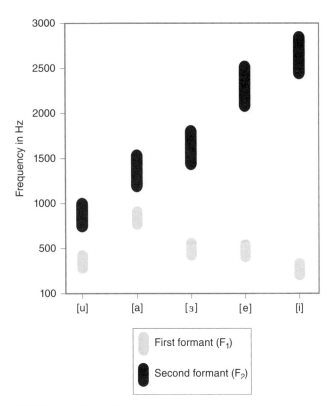

FIGURE 16-1 Vowel formant chart.

In many cases, children may utilize frequency-modulation (FM) systems that link directly to the device being used. These systems require the SLP to utilize a transmitting microphone that links to the receiver worn by the child. Because each of these devices has special settings and adaptations for input, it is important that the SLP communicate with the audiologist (who likely is not part of the school staff) to ensure proper usage. When an audiologist is unavailable, contacting the FM manufacturer is recommended. All FM manufacturers have audiologists on staff to assist in answering any questions regarding the system. Because these assistive devices often have additional settings and different transmitters, it is critical that the SLP be familiar with the equipment.

Care and maintenance of equipment is generally the responsibility of the parent; however, the SLP needs to understand those portions that might be more vulnerable to damage or malfunction. In most cases, the SLP will have a baseline of performance from which to proceed and any deviation from that should raise a red flag to inspect and check the equipment. In some cases, a return to the audiologist may be required. If the child has been implanted for a long period of time and there is a sudden change, it is most probably due to equipment and not mapping issues (in cases of the child using a cochlear implant). For the child who recently got a hearing aid or cochlear implant, a referral back to the audiologist is necessary.

The most difficult part of any SLP's assessment is determining if the outcome that is being observed is appropriate, timely, and consistent. Any deviation from those three aspects of performance requires further investigation on the part of the SLP. An *appropriate* response is one that takes into account the age of onset of the hearing loss, the duration of hearing loss, the duration of sensory aid use, and the skillset that the child brought to the therapeutic setting. A *timely* response is one that considers the child's language abilities and whether there has been progress over time that is consistent with some of the factors listed above in the realm of the appropriateness of the response. Finally, *consistency* in the development of the acquired skill (spoken language/auditory perception) provides the SLP with a roadmap directing the therapist to plan and deliver intervention that guides the child to the next developmental level.

Customized Intervention for Children with Hearing Loss

Beyond providing services with an understanding of the auditory system and the device/s in use by the child, what is it that differentiates intervention for a child who is deaf or hard of hearing and another child presenting with a specific language impairment? Many children with hearing loss are capable of *developmentally driven* acquisition of listening and spoken language skills, albeit slightly delayed. Therefore, a *remedial* effort appropriate for children with language disorders may be inappropriate for a child with hearing loss. After children have early access to appropriately fit, well-maintained listening devices that they wear all waking hours (McCreery, 2015), their learning trajectory will likely follow that of a child with typical hearing. It is important to remember, however, that in the same manner as typically developing hearing children, a child who is deaf or hard of hearing may present with additional language and reading difficulties that are unrelated to hearing loss. Regardless, providing a rich listening and language environment with "embellished" interactions (Cole & Flexer, 2016) is preferred to a bottom up, corrective approach to intervention. In other words, when a child with hearing loss has the advantage of early identification, early fitting of appropriate hearing technologies, and early intervention by a highly qualified service provider, there is a greater chance for developmental synchrony. This suggests that milestones of development across all domains (including language acquisition) can occur at or near the biologically pre-programmed period (Robbins, Koch, Osberger-Phillips, & Kishon-Rabin, 2004).

Attention to the Purposeful Development of Auditory Skills

Perigoe and Patterson (2015) have suggested that "spoken language happens for the typically developing child in such an integrated, progressive manner that how the child *receives, perceives, and processes the auditory sensory input* from his or her environment may be taken for granted." These authors would suggest that there is a unique knowledge base and skill set, as well as a set of attitudes and values, required by practitioners who are qualified to do the "heavy lifting" for the timely development of listening and spoken language acquisition. Across the country, a number of graduate programs in speech-language pathology have created specialty tracks for aspiring professionals interested in a course of study in listening and spoken language (LSL) for the population of children who are deaf or hard of hearing. The AG Bell Association for Deaf/Hard of Hearing has supported the development of the post-graduate LSLS Certificate through its Academy (http://www.agbell.org/Academy.aspx?id=555). Because of this program, SLPs who find children with hearing loss on their caseload may access numerous resources that will support delivering the best intervention possible despite limited experience with this population. More specific recommendations, in the form of strategies and techniques for the population of children who are deaf or hard of hearing (Fickenscher, Gaffney, & Dickinson, 2016), may support the practicing SLP in planning and delivering therapy that sustains the developmental momentum of auditory learning that has been directed by an LSL specialist in early intervention. The following broad principles of LSL intervention for the novice professional are presented as a starting point for the SLP to customize intervention specifically for a child with hearing loss. As a bonus, the SLP should also consider their application, when appropriate, to the broader population of children for whom services are provided.

Recommendations and Reminders to Drive Intervention for a Child with Hearing Loss

1. Establish appropriate listening and spoken language goals as the foundation of the therapy session; choose tasks and experiences that provide functional opportunities to advance listening skill.

    As with any therapy client, good intervention begins with comprehensive assessment. Based on case history, current age, and presenting problem, the SLP chooses and administers appropriate assessments in the area of functional auditory skills, spoken language, and vocal development/speech. (See Bradham & Houston, 2014, for a detailed description of assessment instruments especially designed for children with hearing loss.) It is only after administering a comprehensive battery of tests that an SLP is ready to plan intervention for the child who is deaf or hard of hearing. Keeping in mind that there is a complex relationship between listening and spoken language, SLPs must have a broad understanding of the hierarchy of listening skill development and a child's exact and current level of auditory and linguistic ability in order to develop purposeful intervention experiences (Perigoe & Patterson, 2015, provide a comprehensive discussion of auditory skills development and the child with hearing loss). Disconnected drill and practice tasks will likely result in little real-life application to listening and spoken language demands at home or in the classroom. Fortunately, when books become the centerpiece of a therapy session, and listening and language goals are advanced through their use, there is an economy of effort that contributes to listening, language, AND literacy outcomes.

2. Begin every session with a check of listening device function.

    The importance of assuring auditory access in order to maximize a child's intervention time with an SLP cannot be overstated. This is done by completing a listening check of the child's hearing technology that is both visual and functional. Virtually every hearing technology manufacturer has a website with links to device check routines. Additionally, performing the "Ling 6 Sound Check" at the start of every session establishes the functionality of the listening device for children who cannot (or do not) indicate that they are not hearing properly. See http://www.audiologyonline.com/articles/using-ling-6-sound-test-1087 for more information about completing a comprehensive listening device check. Without this check, a child may bring limited auditory capacity to the session; without full access, scheduled intervention may be virtually meaningless.

3. Use "positioning" to limit visual cues to ensure that tasks are auditory.

While never explicitly stated, traditional models of therapy call for the SLP to be seated at an appropriately sized table in a position across from the child/children receiving the intervention. In order to place emphasis on auditory input, however, it is recommended that the SLP sit beside and slightly behind the child using hearing technology (ensuring that this happens on the side of the "better hearing ear"). This seating arrangement also supports joint attention and following the child's lead. Side by side positioning makes it natural for the SLP and child to attend to a shared book in an auditory-only condition; in addition to building auditory skills, building new vocabulary, expanding language, and promoting general knowledge growth are also effectively addressed through literacy.

4. Regardless of the task, consider an "auditory first" presentation of listening stimuli; add clues and supports as necessary before providing visual assistance.

Especially when introducing materials or a book that is to be used in the session, the "tell, don't show" recommendation asks the child to listen and make sense of what is heard before the physical presentation of the item. The child may be able to respond using a key word or phrase that allows the SLP to act as a diagnostician and learn more about the type of intervention that will be selected. In so doing, the clinician has more information about what part of the message was not received or was misunderstood (Fickenscher, Gaffney, & Dickson, 2016). The clinician could repeat the opening statement exactly, or repeat with a strategy called "acoustic highlighting." In acoustic highlighting, a word (or sound) is emphasized auditorily in any one of a number of ways: perhaps by making it a little longer in duration (e.g., a balloooon), or slightly emphasizing (highlighting) or pausing before and after the target word (e.g., the little girl got a big, red—pause—balloon—pause—at the circus). If these prompts do not provide sufficient assistance to the child, the clinician may then give a visual clue, perhaps showing the materials or the cover of the book, and continue with some additional "auditory first" commentary. The SLP can further probe after the child has the context

revealed, but before actually beginning the activity or sharing/reading the book. Keep in mind, however, that the use of this technique requires a sufficient level of linguistic sophistication to ensure that the child can be successful with the task.

5. Consider that a student who is deaf or hard of hearing may need additional time for processing what has been heard; embed sufficient "wait time" into the stimulus-response exchange.

A good clinician is always prepared to assist a child in completing a task successfully by providing a clue, additional prompt, or other support. In the case of children with hearing loss, it is recommended that extra time be given for the auditory stimuli to be interpreted and an appropriate response to be formulated before providing the hint or clue. Although this may feel immeasurably long at first, extending the wait time may result in an independent response from the child. It may be helpful to consider that we want to "go slow" (as in providing extra wait time) to "go fast" (to promote accelerated language development).

6. The sabotage strategy is particularly appropriate for eliciting a language turn from the child.

There are many ways to use sabotage to elicit language. Physical sabotage makes it impossible for the child to participate in an assigned task (e.g., a child cannot reach or open a container to access something that is needed for activity participation). This obligates communication by the child. The therapist must be prepared to be steadfast in withholding assistance until the child communicates the need. According to Garber (2012), saying one thing and doing another can also be categorized as a type of sabotage. This visual/verbal sabotage presents the child with a mismatch between what is seen and what is heard. The child is expected to comment upon or correct the intentional difference between the two. This might call for the SLP to state a fact from the story, but deliberately misspeak: "After the caterpillar ate through the apple he was...full" (rather than still hungry). When faced with this obvious error, the child corrects the clinician... "No! He was still hungry." Thus, sabotage is a successful strategy to make communication moments happen.

7. Make any listening task practical and meaningful; targeting listening and spoken language intervention through the use of classroom content (from preschool onward) is an ideal way to make intervention meaningful and fun.

   Pinterest has become the SLP's greatest ally in the quest to add value to the classroom teacher's unit or theme and to overlay listening and language tasks to topics already under discussion. Language sessions that provide a language experience story connected to similar language experiences found in the story (Moog, Stein, Biedenstein, & Gustus, 2003) provide opportunities to reinforce or enrich lessons in the classroom. When active engagement, listening, and linguistic participation are required, therapy becomes multidimensional; events and language are paired, giving rise to opportunities to make language "stick." This further supports the application of practiced auditory and language skills to the classroom, resulting in a child's becoming a more confident participant in group discussions with their classmates.

8. Be on the lookout for "linguistic hazards" that challenge even the most successful children with hearing loss.

   Any child's achievement in reading and academics is dependent upon a rich vocabulary that sustains early linguistic gains during more challenging subject matter and literary selections. Advanced Tier Two vocabulary words (Beck, McKeown, & Kucan, 2002) are especially elusive for a child with hearing loss who has limited opportunity to access and determine the meanings of words overheard in conversations. For example, knowing the meaning of the word *reluctant* will assist a child in understanding a character's behavior in a given story. This is a highly valuable word to have in the lexicon, especially when considering preteen behavior in stories written with this age group in mind. Similarly, receptive understanding of figurative language, similes, and metaphors will be challenging for a child who is deaf or hard of hearing to understand in face-to-face conversation as well as in reading materials.

Consider a character who has an idea that "comes to him in a flash." What does this figurative expression suggest to you as a mature user of language? How might a misunderstanding of this phrase preclude a child from answering a teacher's question correctly? For many of us, the meaning of figurative language is virtually transparent because the expression is also in the speaking/listening repertoire. But imagine what other (incorrect) interpretations may be made if one did not already know this expression. The vigilant SLP who uses classroom content to drive intervention may be able to anticipate difficulty with vocabulary and language in advance of its appearance in lessons. With intervention customized by a knowledgeable SLP, the student will be equipped with the friendly definitions and linguistic interpretations that will allow full participation in classroom instruction.

9. Consider the development of social language and pragmatic skills as appropriate goals for children with hearing loss.

   Research has suggested that children who are deaf or hard of hearing lag behind their hearing peers in the mastery of pragmatic skills (Goberis et al., 2012). Using a pragmatic skills checklist (Goberis, 1984) that included items from "making polite requests" to "asking questions to problem solve," Goberis and her colleagues found that 95% of items were mastered by children with normal hearing by 4 years of age. Conversely, only 69% of items were mastered by 7 years of age in children with hearing loss. Because pragmatic language difficulties increase risk for social and emotional deficits, attention to this important element of linguistic skills is warranted. Unorthodox though it may seem, additional attention to the language of email and texting, providing interpretation and instruction as needed, may assist a child who is deaf or hard of hearing in appropriately identifying the structure and use of sarcasm in electronic formats. In an age in which cyberbullying has become rampant, the deaf or hard of hearing student must be aware of some of the more subtle meanings cloaked in what might otherwise be interpreted as an innocent use of words and phrases. Conversely, innocent remarks might be over-interpreted, with the receiver becoming offended when this was not the intent of the sender.

10. As a long-term and ancillary goal, include objectives for building self-advocacy skills and independence for managing hearing technologies regardless of the age of the student with whom you work. It's never too early to help a child "be the boss of the hearing loss" (Kroll, 2004).

Because language skills are essential for becoming a good self-advocate, it is reasonable to include practicing the language of advocacy as goals for children enrolled in intervention. Whether signaling that a hearing device is not functioning properly, requesting that other students use the pass-around microphone, or asking the teacher to repeat a question, having the language and vocabulary to be clear in communicating advocacy needs is crucial. There are a number of resources particularly suitable for the SLP wishing to learn more about advocacy objectives as a function of age, most notably the website Supporting Success for Children with Hearing Loss, developed by Karen Anderson, which will also direct the clinician to other available resources. Visit http://successforkidswithhearingloss.com /self-advocacy/ to take advantage of the wealth of materials that have been compiled to assist professionals (and parents) in navigating systems from birth to the school-aged population and to "improve the futures of children with hearing loss."

Destination Literacy

When Diane McGuinness (2004) wrote "The skills that produce an expert reader are exactly the same skills that make an expert listener" (p. 9), she was not writing about children with hearing loss, but rather all children on their path to literacy. Her perceptive text, *Growing a Reader from Birth*, reminds us of our ultimate goal in today's literacy-based society. Whether text is traditional print or digital, the ability to independently build meaning from text is a highly desirable skill. For all children who have the requisite cognitive ability, reading comprehension is a measurable outcome of the educational experiences that begin at home and are supported through schools; children must receive the instruction that leads to this goal. If this journey does indeed begin at birth as McGuinness suggests, then listening and language competence

are precursors to literacy for the vast majority of the populace. Recent reports identify the "reading" brain (Wolf, 2013) as one that is primed to break the code efficiently as well as comprehend what is read through understanding the syntactic and semantic components of the language that is decoded. When children with hearing loss receive hearing technologies matched to their auditory profile at the earliest possible age, it is more likely that their path to literacy will eventually mirror that of typically hearing children.

Whether a child is typically hearing or deaf or hard of hearing, it would be naïve to assume that this path to literacy is simply sequential. There are obvious developmental factors at play and one cannot deny the complex interconnectedness of listening, language, and literacy skill acquisition throughout the early, middle, and later ages and stages of a child's life. The following graphic (**FIGURE 16-2**) may be helpful in conceptualizing the "big picture" for what is at stake and the various listening, language, experiential, and thinking milestones in the journey. The seminal work of van Kleeck and Schuele (1987) regarding precursors to literacy was influential in developing the following graphic, especially with regard to the journey from listening to reading comprehension for the child who is deaf or hard of hearing.

As the speech-language pathologist contemplates the conceptualization that this figure represents, it may be prudent to consider the key experiences that occur during the precursor period, which will ultimately contribute to becoming an independent reader. Some may be obvious; others may not. Keep in mind that there are also a number of learning activities that will flow directly from the precursor stage to the stage of decoding; this too is a vital step in the journey to reading with comprehension. The following behaviors (although not exhaustive by any means) are suggested to detail some of the outcomes of the learning that takes place in the multi-year precursor stage of a developing child that contribute to later reading achievement; the majority of these occur before "formal" reading and code-breaking instruction commences.

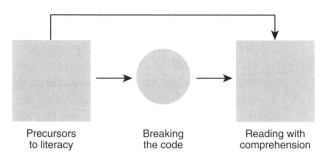

FIGURE 16-2 The path to literacy.

Behaviors indicative of auditory development:

- Enjoys listening; responds to auditory stimuli
- Associates voices with emotions
- Responds to auditory-only stimuli
- Understands simple auditory directions
- Appreciates music and singing
- Comprehends through listening alone (at increasingly complex linguistic levels)
- Develops appreciation for rhyming words in books selected for this purpose
- Demonstrates auditory closure in listening-only tasks

Behaviors indicative of linguistic development:

- Enjoys sound-making, especially associated with animals and common objects
- Demonstrates receptive language understanding
- Builds Tier One vocabulary
- Displays expressive language expansion
- Demonstrates an increasingly sophisticated speech repertoire and appropriate speech intelligibility
- Asks/answers questions
- Associates letters with sounds

Behaviors indicative of critical thinking skill development:

- Makes predictions
- Relates stories/events to own experiences
- Draws basic conclusions
- Categorizes and classifies
- Makes connections across experiences/stories
- Makes basic inferences
- Retells stories; gets the "main idea"

Behaviors indicative of experiential learning:

- Participates in book sharing/dialogic reading
- Begins to identify feelings in self and then in others
- Follows routines
- Develops schema/world knowledge
- Learns time sequence
- Learns character traits
- Tells stories about shared experiences

Breaking the Code of Reading

The child with hearing loss who has a history of early identification, early fitting of appropriate listening devices with full-time wear, and early access to competent service providers is poised to experience success with the "on time" development of phonological awareness. When auditory skill development has been nurtured, tasks associated with phonological awareness such as syllable segmentation, identifying initial consonants, and rhyme recognition may be well within the reach of children with hearing loss. In fact, Miller, Lederberg, and Easterbrooks (2013) used their balanced literacy program, Foundations for Literacy (Lederberg, Miller, Easterbrooks, & Connor, 2011) to explore the ability of preschool deaf or hard of hearing children with "functional" hearing to benefit from specific instruction to advance these aspects of phonological awareness. They concluded that children with hearing loss benefitted from direct phonological awareness instruction and practice. This suggests that SLPs with children with hearing loss (preschool aged or older) on their caseload may successfully target these skills in therapy after ensuring the child's hearing device(s) has proven to be in working order.

Nonlinguistic Factors That Affect the Deaf or Hard of Hearing Child When Learning

In all communication exchanges, especially instructional, the role that attention plays cannot be overstated. Research shows that listeners can "tune out" a speaker after 10 minutes of a presentation (McKeachie & Sviinicki, 2006). These data are based on typically hearing individuals and underscore the role that attention plays in communication events. For those with hearing loss, the problem is exacerbated. Despite the tremendous advances of listening technologies, recent publications regarding speech-processing fatigue of children with hearing loss in educational settings (Bess & Hornsby, 2014; Hornsby, Davis, McGarrigle, Camarata, & Bess, 2017) have shed light on the challenging task of attention during instruction. Bess and colleagues found that children with hearing loss on average report fatigue across "multiple domains" including general, sleep/rest, and cognitive issues. It behooves the SLP to design the intervention session with several short learning experiences that are timed to match these attention parameters. In addition, children with hearing loss can be more easily distracted due to noise or lack of understanding of the topic. Because attention and distraction control are essential elements of executive function (see discussion in the next section), identifying this physiological contributor to possible attention drift is noteworthy. In fact, Peters (2012) has suggested that the increased effort for a child who is deaf or hard of hearing to listen and comprehend may lead to reduced cognitive control and impulsivity.

Executive Function

Students in classrooms require the ability to comprehend and subsequently execute assignments as prescribed by the teacher. Executive function is the capacity of an individual to attend, integrate, and plan accordingly. This important cognitive capacity remains one of the key components for children with hearing loss to be successful across the educational lifespan. This set of mental skills and abilities is controlled by the frontal lobe, and includes inhibition, shift, emotional control, initiation, working memory, planning and organization, organization of materials and self-monitoring. Regardless of the physiology, executive function is amenable to improvement through targeted intervention.

More than 90% of children with hearing loss have hearing parents (Mitchell & Karchmer, 2004) and these children are especially at risk for deficits in executive function. More importantly, this demographic is the one most commonly seen in local school districts. Among the possible reasons for challenges with executive function in the population of children who are deaf or hard of hearing may be a lag in auditory access, atypical early parent–child interactions, and a skill set that does not include sophisticated language to manage executive function development. Peters (2012, citing Gioia, Isquith, & Guy, 2001) recommends that in order to assist in the development of executive function, the SLP with deaf or hard of hearing children on the caseload may wish to consider novel learning experiences and activities, rather than repetitive and overly simplistic tasks. It is recommended that the SLP consider how language can be the infrastructure upon which executive function is accomplished. For example, planning and organization is reliant upon clauses that are temporal in nature, such as understanding the adverbial conjunctions before, after, and while. As a case in point in literacy class, the teacher may direct the students, "*After* you finish reading the chapter, summarize the main theme." Another assignment might call for students to "identify and record new vocabulary *while* reading the chapter." Receptive and expressive control of these linguistic features contributes to building a foundation upon which executive function depends.

Because the raw material of working memory is often provided auditorily, building capacity for retaining units of instruction may be warranted. SLPs may find the concept of critical elements one that parallels that of strengthening auditory memory. One practical and academic application of auditory memory takes place in the math classroom. Understanding, writing, and reading aloud four, five, and six-digit figures is part of any lesson associated with expanded notation and understanding place value to create large numbers. For example, a teacher might provide the number 146,382. Not only does a student need to *hear* the numbers, but must also *attend* to them in order, *hold* them in short-term memory, and finally *write* them in the precise place value location to arrive at the correct figure. SLPs strengthening tasks such as these as part of an intervention plan for the child who is deaf or hard of hearing are providing functional practice in academic support as well as pinpointing the component thinking skills associated with executive function. This intervention can be highly productive.

Long-term projects that require future planning to meet ultimate due dates become more common as students move through the educational system. Managing and assisting the student in successful organization of tasks and due dates can serve as a template for future projects such as these. SLPs may wish to explore activities that are used to help facilitate the development of executive function with a special eye toward the linguistic elements related to time management and self-monitoring behaviors needed by the student. Executive function transcends every aspect of everyday life. In fact, executive function is not merely a classroom phenomenon; it is one that reaches beyond the traditional auditory/linguistic activities that SLPs often address.

Considerations Beyond Intervention

Changes in the healthcare landscape have resulted in a more cross-disciplinary, interprofessional practice (IPP) approach to management that transects all aspects of health and well-being. Although relatively new to general medicine, this multi-disciplinary team style has been foundational in the treatment and education of the child with hearing loss (Nevins & Chute, 1996). Today, the only difference in the execution of IPP is the number of professionals that have been added to the team over the years as the complex needs of children who are deaf or hard of hearing have received more attention. Current standards of IPP require the school SLP to ensure that every attribute of the child is fully evaluated and addressed as part of the (re)habilitative process. In order for this approach to be maximally successful, however, there must be a cohesive plan that begins with the initial diagnosis/identification of hearing loss and continues with regular assessment of capabilities and outcomes as the child moves through the school system.

Without good management from the start, delays, reduced effectiveness, and, in some cases, limited outcomes for the child are observed. But, even under the best circumstances, there must be continuity of care and persistence to evaluating the *whole* child. Of the total population of children with hearing loss, 40% will present with additional disabilities (Guardino & Cannon, 2015). Depending on the etiology of the hearing loss, it is possible that these may be significant issues that can include cognitive deficits, sensory-motor delays, and psychosocial issues that are a result of underlying neurological problems. Challenges may develop over time and may appear in subtleties that might elude the professional who is not attuned to changes in student performance. It is imperative that the SLP remain vigilant with regard to all aspects of the deaf or hard of hearing child's capacity to learn, respond, and adjust to everyday life, whether it be inside or outside the classroom.

Most importantly, communication among professionals that are involved in the habilitation of the deaf or hard of hearing child is key to ensuring that changes in behaviors, abilities, and outcomes are addressed in the most expeditious manner. The difficulties of monitoring any child's performance over time is complicated by the fact that they may change schools, or the professionals addressing the child's needs may rotate to other positions. The challenge of case management, therefore, often becomes the responsibility of the parents or the children themselves.

Cultural Identity

Beyond the role of SLP as language infuser, literacy supporter, and auditory instructor, this professional may also find the need to address the cultural aspects of the deaf or hard of hearing child in a proactive manner. For children who are deaf, who communicate with spoken language and have limited or no knowledge of sign language, there may be a need to provide a social and political context so that they understand their position within the deaf and hearing worlds. Discussion of the rift that has separated members of the deaf community who use American Sign Language (ASL) from those who have selected spoken language requires sensitivity and respect. Often, family choice is the basis for the selection of communication methodology. In youngsters who are born deaf to hearing parents, there is neither family history nor a linguistic role model from which the child can experience ASL. In many cases, hearing parents are reluctant to expose their child to ASL for fear that it will limit their ability to develop spoken language skills. Regardless, it is crucial that children who are deaf or hard of hearing have an appreciation of their unique character and their potential contribution to the larger society. Some children have very limited exposure to members of the deaf community and, as such, have questions about the similarities and differences between deaf persons who sign and those who communicate through spoken language. The SLP may wish to provide information, insight, and support for students as they make inquiries regarding the auditory/linguistic differences of their growing awareness of distinct groups and their curiosity for social exploration. However, for minor children, the consent of families must be obtained before embarking on any in-depth discussion of these issues. It is here where the SLP's role as a family counselor becomes especially important. Resources are available for the SLP who has limited knowledge of deaf culture through www.nad.org.

▶ Summary

The use of the spoken word to convey meaning and thought should not be overshadowed by a focus on developing semantic and syntactic expertise. In order to address the "whole" child who is deaf or hard of hearing, it is important to emphasize language as a social, educational, and economic means to an end. The challenges that face student learners whether they have hearing loss or not require attention to preparation, motivation, time management, and access to resources. Recent focus on purposeful learning has been the catalyst for new strategies of instruction. Transparency in teaching is now a fundamental pedagogical process that should not only occur in the classroom but in the therapy room as well. The student who is deaf or hard of hearing deserves to understand the functional implications of *why* they are learning something as opposed to just being told to learn it. Therapeutic interventions that merely present information to the student who is then expected to passively hear as opposed to actively listen do little to build learning capacity that challenges many children regardless of hearing status. Additionally, in the age of social media and internet access, the manner in which students learn and engage has evolved and continues to evolve. Building upon these new paradigms is an aspect of intervention that requires focused attention on the part of the speech and hearing professional. If it is ignored, students may feel marginalized by the generational cohort which identifies them as "immature communicators." Despite the fact that the educational, social, and linguistic achievement of children with hearing loss has surpassed expectations from those set only two generations ago, it is the responsibility of today's speech and language professional to plan and implement interventions that maximize the potential of current learners who are deaf and hard of hearing.

Study Questions

1. How does the degree of a child's hearing loss influence selection of appropriate hearing technology?
2. What is the role of the SLP or educator in ensuring auditory access for a child who is deaf or hard of hearing?
3. What is developmental synchrony and how does that concept intersect with the age of identification of hearing loss?
4. Name three precursors to literacy that may be found in the domain of experiential learning.
5. Why is executive function/auditory memory especially important for academic learning?

References

AG Bell Association for the Deaf/Hard of Hearing. Retrieved from http://www.agbell.org/Academy.aspx?id=555

Anderson, K. (2014). Retrieved from http://successforkidswithhearingloss.com/self-advocacy/

Beck, I. L., McKeown, M. G., & Kucan, L. (2002). *Bringing words to life*. New York, NY: Guilford Press.

Beginnings. (2014). Retrieved from www.ncbegin.org

Bekesy, G., & Rosenblith, W. A. (1958). *The mechanical properties of the ear*. In S. S. Stevens (Ed.), *Handbook of experimental psychology* (pp. 1075–1115). New York, NY: John Wiley & Sons.

Bess, F., & Hornsby, B. (2014). The complexities of fatigue in children with hearing loss. *SIG 9 Perspectives on Hearing and Hearing Disorders in Childhood, 24*(2), 25–39.

Bradham, T., & Houston, K. T. (2014). *Assessing listening and spoken language in children with hearing loss*. San Diego, CA: Plural Publishing, Inc.

Ching, T. C., Dillon, H., Button, L., Seeto, M., Van Buynder, P., Marnane, V., … Leigh, G. (2017, September). Age at intervention for permanent hearing loss and 5-year language outcomes. *Pediatrics, 140*(3).

Cole, E., & Flexer, C. (2016). *Children with hearing loss: Developing listening and talking, birth to six* (3rd ed.). San Diego, CA: Plural Publishing.

Fickenscher, S., Gaffney, E., & Dickson, C. (2016). *Auditory verbal strategies to build listening and spoken language*. Licensed under a Creative Commons Attribution-Non-Commercial-No Derivatives 4.0 International License.

Garber, A. (2012). *Listening and spoken language strategies in the classroom*. Retrieved from http://www.audiologyonline.com/articles/listening-and-spoken-language-strategies-11245-11245

Gelfand, S. (2001). *Anatomy and physiology of the auditory system in essentials of audiology* (2nd ed., pp. 37–90). New York, NY: Thieme.

Gioia, G. A., Isquith, P. K., & Guy, S. C. (2001). Assessment of executive function in children with neurological impairments. In R. Simeonsson & S. Rosenthal (Eds.), *Psychological and developmental assessment* (pp. 317–356). New York, NY: Guilford Press.

Goberis, D. (1984). Pragmatics Checklist (adapted from Simon, C. S., 1984).

Goberis, D., Beams, D., Dalpes, M., Abrisch, A., Baca, R., & Yoshinaga-Itano, C. (2012). The missing link in language development of deaf and hard of hearing children: Pragmatic language development. *Seminars in Speech and Language, 33*(04), 297–309. doi:10.1055/s-0032-1326916

Guardino, C. A., & Cannon, J. E. (Eds.). (2015). Theory, research, and practice for students who are deaf and hard of hearing with disabilities [Special Issue]. *American Annals of the Deaf, 160*(4), 347–355.

Head, L., Zauche, L. H., Mahoney, A. E., Thul, T. A., Zauche, M. S., Weldon, A. B., & Stapel-Wax, J. L. (2017). The power of language nutrition for children's brain development, health, and future academic achievement—Continuing education posttest. *Journal of Pediatric Health Care, 31*(4), 504–505. doi:10.1016/j.pedhc.2017.02.003

Hornsby, B. Y. W., Davis, H., McGarrigle, R., Camarata, S., & Bess, F. H. (2017). *Measuring fatigue in school-age children with hearing loss*. Indiana, IN: Academy Research Conference (ARC).

JCIH. (2013). Supplement to the JCIH 2007 position statement: principles and guidelines for early intervention after confirmation that a child is deaf or hard of hearing. *Pediatrics, 131*(4), e1324–1349.

Kroll, A. (2004). *I'm the Boss of my Hearing Loss*. Tampa, FL: Cool Gal LLC.

Lederberg, A. R., Miller, E. M., Easterbrooks, S. R., & Connor, C. M. (2011). *Foundations for literacy*. Atlanta, GA: Distributed through Georgia State University.

McCreery, R. (2015). *Maximizing auditory development outcomes in children with hearing loss*. Rochester, MN: Mayo Clinic Audiology Conference.

McGuinness, D. (2004). *Growing a reader from birth; Your child's path from language to literacy*. New York, NY: W.W. Norton & Co., Inc.

McKeachie W. J., & Svinicki, M. (2006). *McKeachie's teaching tips: Strategies, research, and theory for college and university teachers*. Boston, MA: Houghton-Mifflin.

Miller, E. M., Lederberg, A. R., & Easterbrooks, S. R. (2013). Phonological awareness: Explicit instruction for young deaf and hard-of-hearing children. *Journal of Deaf Studies and Deaf Education, 18*, 206–227.

Mitchell, R., & Karchmer, M. (2004) Chasing the mythical ten percent: Parental hearing status of deaf and hard of hearing students in the United States. *Sign Language Studies, 4*(2), 138–163.

Moog, J. S., Stein, K. K., Biedenstein, J., & Gustus, C. (2003). *Teaching activities for children who are deaf and hard of hearing*. St. Louis, MO: The Moog Center for Deaf Education National Association of the Deaf.

Nevins, M. E., & Chute, P. M. (1996). *Children with cochlear implants in educational settings*. San Diego, CA: Singular Publications.

Perigoe, C., & Patterson, M. (2015). Understanding auditory development and the child with hearing loss. In D. R. Welling & C. A. Ukstins (Eds.), *Fundamentals of audiology for the speech-language pathologist*. Burlington, MA: Jones & Bartlett Learning.

Peters, K. (2012). *Executive functions in children who are deaf/hard of hearing*. Presentation at the Childhood Communication Center. Seattle, WA: Seattle Children's Hospital.

Robbins, A. M., Koch, D. B., Osberger, M. J., Phillips, S., & Kishon-Rabin, L. (2004). Effect of age of cochlear implantation on auditory skills development in infants and toddlers. *Archives of Otolaryngology Head & Neck Surgery, 130*, 570–574.

Van Kleeck, A., & Schuele, M. (1987). Precursors to literacy: Normal development. *Topics in Language Disorders, 7*(2), 13–31.

Wolf, M. (2013). *How the reading brain resolves the reading wars; A Literate Nation White Paper*. Retrieved from www.literatenation

Zauche, L. H., Mahoney, A., Thul, T., Zauche, M., Weldon, A., & Stapel-Wax, J. (2017). The power of language nutrition for children's brain development, health, and future academic achievement. *Journal of Pediatric Health Care, 31*, 493–503.

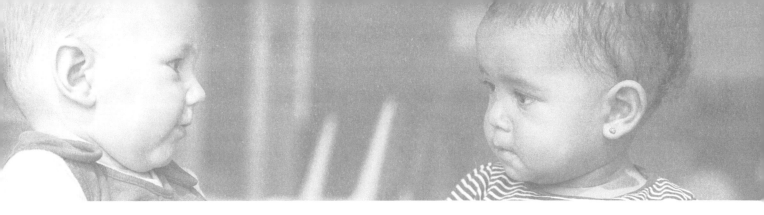

CHAPTER 17

Communication Development in Children with Multiple Disabilities: The Role of Augmentative and Alternative Communication

Andrea Barton-Hulsey, PhD, CCC-SLP
Melissa A. Cheslock, MS, CCC-SLP
Rose A. Sevcik, PhD
Mary Ann Romski, PhD, CCC-SLP

OBJECTIVES

- Describe factors contributing to communicative profiles of children with multiple disabilities
- Describe the roles that augmentative and alternative communication (AAC) plays in overall development of children with multiple disabilities
- Describe the components of an AAC system
- Discuss challenges that children with multiple disabilities face when using AAC
- Discuss foundations of augmented language intervention and assessment that address challenges

KEY TERMS

AAC assessment
AAC strategy
AAC system
AAC technique
Aided language stimulation
Augmentative and alternative
  communication (AAC)

Augmented communication
  input
Communication
Communication aid
Communication partners
Communicative profile
Diagnostic intervention

Environmental controls
Language comprehension
Language production
Multiple disabilities
Speech-generating device (SGD)
Symbols

▶ Introduction

The inability to speak, or the inability to communicate one's own words fluently, is the greatest disability a person can have in the social circle of life …

—**Tony Diamanti**, "Get to Know Me" (2000)

Communication is the very essence of human life. It forms the foundation for everyday learning, social relationships with friends and family, and participation in familial and societal events. Put simply, it affects quality of life for all individuals. Children with multiple disabilities who have difficulty learning to communicate effectively often lack the same opportunities for participation that same-aged children without disabilities are offered. They also face challenges in the form of social and educational isolation and significant frustration because they are unable to adequately convey their necessities, desires, knowledge, and emotions to their parents, siblings, extended family members, peers, friends, and teachers (Romski & Sevcik, 2005).

It is the philosophy of the National Joint Committee (NJC) for the Communication Needs of Persons with Severe Disabilities (Brady et al., 2016), as well as the authors of this chapter, that all children can and do communicate. Speech-language pathologists (SLPs) who interact with children with significant communication disabilities recognize these children's natural communication behaviors and seek ways to promote the functionality and effectiveness of their communication (Brady et al., 2016). Augmentative and alternative communication (AAC) is a multimodal intervention approach (Romski, Sevcik, Cheslock, & Barton-Hulsey, 2016) that uses forms of communication such as manual sign language, picture communication boards, and computerized/electronic devices that produce speech called speech-generating devices (SGDs), with the goal of maximizing the functional language and communication abilities of individuals who have severe communication impairments and little to no speech (ASHA, 2002). It incorporates their full communication abilities, including any existing

vocalizations, gestures, sign language, pictures, and/ or SGDs.

In this chapter, we describe the communicative development of children with multiple disabilities, and more specifically the role AAC can play in that development. The many challenges these children face on a daily basis are discussed, followed by a description of foundational principles necessary for the successful implementation of AAC as a means to navigate those challenges.

Multiple disabilities is a general term that indicates a combination of two or more impairments occurring at the same time and can apply to children with a broad range of impairment in cognitive development, expressive and receptive communication, and physical ability. Children with multiple disabilities may be born with a complex congenital disorder that hinders their development, or they may experience an acquired injury or illness early in life that substantially affects their development. While some children with multiple disabilities may need little to no support, most will require extensive supports to fully participate in daily life activities (e.g., social, educational, and personal). Primary diagnoses for these children may include cerebral palsy, a specific genetic syndrome, intellectual disability, autism, or even a stroke at or near birth (Romski, Sevcik, & Forrest, 2001). Other concomitant impairments may include diagnoses such as seizure disorder, scoliosis, speech and language disorders, or sensory impairment. It is important to recognize that each child with multiple disabilities is unique in their individual communication patterns, motor ability, and cognitive ability.

Multiple factors must be considered when describing, assessing, or intervening in the communication development of children with multiple disabilities. *Communication* is defined as "any act by which one person gives to or receives from another person information about that person's needs, desires, perceptions, knowledge, or affective states" (NJC, 1992, p. 2). It includes speech as well as other forms of expression such as body gestures, eye gaze, symbols, and the printed word. Children with multiple disabilities may demonstrate one or any combination of difficulties with communication.

This chapter introduces three children with multiple disabilities—Sam, Amber, and Oscar—each of whom requires individualized and specific communication intervention and supports for their development. You will see that all of these children with multiple disabilities, regardless of the type and level of their individual impairment, can develop language and communication skills.

▶ Communication Profiles of Children with Multiple Disabilities

Sam

Sam is an 8-year-old boy whose multiple diagnoses include spastic quadriplegia cerebral palsy, cleft lip/palate, severe intellectual disability, and severe receptive and expressive language delay. He enjoys playing with toys and reading books, just like any other 8-year-old boy. Sam is severely physically limited. He is unable to walk and uses a wheelchair. He has difficulty initiating and terminating muscle activity throughout his body, including his legs, torso, arms, and facial muscles, due to his diagnosis of cerebral palsy.

Receptively, Sam is able to eye-gaze to familiar named objects to show his comprehension of specific words and is reported to understand some words from a variety of categories, including words for animals, body parts, clothing, and food and drink; action words; descriptive words; words about time; and question words. His receptive language is difficult to characterize accurately using standardized assessments partially owing to his significant physical limitations; however, his abilities in this area have been estimated to be scattered across a developmental range of 16–32 months.

Although his receptive language skills are delayed, Sam is able to understand more than he is able to speak. He primarily communicates by pointing or reaching toward an item or picture of interest. He also uses focused eye gaze to communicate specific interest in one item over another when interacting with someone. Sam produces vocalizations consisting of mostly vowel sounds and few consonants to approximate fewer than 10 words for verbal communication.

Given Sam's limitations in terms of his current expressive and receptive communication skills, his learning and social development are at risk for being affected by his disabilities. Without effective communication skills, a child with multiple disabilities is unable to have a reciprocal conversation, share their knowledge, and improve upon their comprehension by asking further questions. (See **APPENDIX 17-A**: Case Study 1 for more detailed information on Sam.)

Amber

Amber is a 12-year-old girl with moderate intellectual disability and delays in receptive and expressive language development with extreme word-finding difficulties. In addition to her intellectual disability and subsequent language deficits, Amber exhibits speech production deficits characterized by low oral motor tone, frequent drooling, articulation errors, and low volume. She uses vocalizations, limited single-word and two- to three-word phrases, gestures, facial expression, and pictures to communicate. Amber's immediate family understands her when she uses these communicative forms, but unfamiliar people and other communication partners rarely understand her.

Amber often has behavioral problems when at school. When she does not want to participate in classroom activities, she will often cry, vocalize strongly to protest the activity, or refuse to comply with activities presented to her by pushing away or throwing items she is given. Unlike Sam, Amber is able to walk and communicate through limited speech. Similar to Sam, Amber comprehends much more than she is able to expressively produce. (See **APPENDIX 17-B**: Case Study 2 for more information on Amber.)

Oscar

Oscar is a 3-year, 10-month-old little boy who has a diagnosis of schizencephaly, a rare neurological disorder characterized by abnormal clefts in the cerebral hemispheres of the brain. His gross and fine motor development has been delayed as a result of his condition. Oscar is unable to walk independently and uses a wheelchair.

Oscar's play skills, social skills, and overall receptive language skills appear to be age-appropriate as assessed through standardized language and vocabulary assessments and observations during play with his family. His cognitive, receptive language, and social abilities are areas of strength. In contrast, his motor limitations in producing expressive speech appear to be his greatest barrier to communication. Oscar uses mostly vowel sounds and some consonants to approximate short words that only close family members who are very familiar with him understand. He is rarely understood by anyone unfamiliar to him.

He often uses focused eye-gaze and pointing combined with vocalizations to expressively communicate. (See **APPENDIX 17-C**: Case Study 3 for more information on Oscar.)

Identifying a Communicative Profile

For children like Sam, Amber, and Oscar, the identification of a thorough communicative profile is essential to fully understanding the child's language development thus far, and to perceive how the child may continue to develop further communication skills. A *communicative profile* is a complete description of a child's strengths and needs in a variety of settings as related to the child's language comprehension and expression (e.g., vocabulary, grammar, and social use of language), speech, oral-motor skills, and ability to communicate using nonconventional forms of communication such as gestures or sign language. Factors that contribute to a child's unique communicative profile are the child's cognitive development, communicative experiences, vocal and gestural production skills, and comprehension skills (Romski, Sevcik, Hyatt, & Cheslock, 2002).

Cognitive Development

The cognitive skills of a child with multiple disabilities can vary from no evidence of intellectual and developmental disabilities to significant intellectual and developmental disabilities. A child who exhibits an intellectual disability will have limitations in both intelligence and adaptive behavior skills. The *intelligence* of a child refers to their general mental capability and involves their ability to reason, plan, problem-solve, think abstractly, understand complex ideas, learn quickly, and generalize information from one context to another. *Adaptive behavior* refers to a child's conceptual (e.g., language understanding and use, money concepts), social (e.g., interpersonal skills and following community rules), and practical (e.g., eating and dressing) skills (Schalock et al., 2010). Significant limitations in these skills affect the child's ability to fully function in everyday activities and routines.

Knowledge of where a child falls within this range of development affects where a child will begin along the continuum of communication intervention strategies. Nevertheless, cognitive development should never be the sole factor that determines whether a child actually receives intervention services (Brady et al., 2016). For example, Sam was diagnosed as having a severe intellectual disability, whereas Oscar was assessed as having no intellectual disability. Regardless of their differences in cognitive ability, both Sam and Oscar achieve success in improving in their communication development.

Communicative Experiences

The communicative experiences of a child with multiple disabilities are highly variable and will ultimately depend on factors such as the age of the child and their communication partners. Ideally, an older child will have had a greater number of opportunities for successful communication, which may in turn positively affect their comprehension and production skills. For example, Amber, who is 12 years of age, is reported to make herself understood by her immediate family using limited verbal expression, facial expressions, and gestures. Through intervention, her family has learned to give Amber multiple opportunities to communicate in a variety of familial situations and then allow her the time needed to successfully respond communicatively. In contrast, Amber is rarely understood by unfamiliar communication partners, who typically limit their interactions with her owing to her unintelligibility. Amber's limited expressive communication ability reduces her opportunity to interact with new people and, therefore, constrains her ability to develop further communication skills in a variety of contexts.

Amber demonstrates how others' communicative interaction styles may ultimately affect a child's communicative experiences and profile. Among typically developing children, children whose parents are more responsive to their communication attempts have better language outcomes than children whose parents are less responsive (Tamis-LeMonda, Bornstein, & Baumwell, 2001; Tamis-LeMonda, Kuchirko, & Song, 2014; Snow, 1991). For children with disabilities, the literature suggests that a communication partner's communicative input tends to be different in quality and quantity than the input received by their typically developing peers. Specifically, input to children with disabilities may be more adult-directed (Davis, Stroud, & Green, 1988; Girolametto, Weitzman, Wiigs, & Pearce, 1999; Warren et al., 2010) and less frequent in nature (Blackstone, 1997; Calculator, 1997; Fey, Warren, Bredin-Oja, & Yoder, 2017). For children with multiple disabilities, their interaction with a variety of communication partners and in a variety of settings should be taken into consideration when identifying their strengths and areas of needed intervention for developing their communication.

Vocal and Gesture Ability

Children with multiple disabilities may have a wide range of vocalizations and gestures they use for producing communication. Many children with multiple disabilities are described as having extensive natural vocal skills, albeit being unintelligible, prior to the onset of intervention (Romski, Sevcik, Reumann, & Pate, 1989). Abbeduto (2003) reports that most children with multiple disabilities will develop functional spoken communication skills. The amount of functional spoken communication they develop will vary, however, based on factors such as cognitive development and/or underlying oral motor weakness or dysfunction. Some children with multiple disabilities will not develop functional spoken communication skills.

Sam, Amber, and Oscar provide examples of different levels of functional speech. Sam uses gross vowel sounds for vocalizations combined with occasional consonant sounds and focused eye gaze, and some gestures. The vowel sounds he uses are not easily discriminated and are not used to refer to a set of specific items. By comparison, Oscar uses mostly vowel sounds, with changes in intonation that refer to specific items. Amber uses two- to three-word short phrases combined with facial expression and gestures to communicate.

The differences in communication patterns across each individual child also vary greatly, such that not every child who lacks functional communication skills as a toddler will be nonspeaking into adolescence and adulthood. Amber, for example, did not begin speaking real words and word approximations until she was 3 years of age, and at age 12 uses two- to three-word phrases. It is important to remember that a child with multiple disabilities may have a changing vocal or gestural profile over the course of their development. This change over time should be monitored so that the intervention directed at that child's communication development can evolve accordingly.

Language Comprehension

Speech and language comprehension skills are also incorporated into the communicative profiles of children with multiple disabilities. Their comprehension may range from no or minimal comprehension to comprehension skills that are appropriate to their chronological age (Nelson, 1992). Children who do comprehend some speech show that they have knowledge about the relationship between words and their referents in the environment (Sevcik & Romski, 2002). Children who do not understand spoken words must establish conditional relationships between words or symbols to be learned and their real-world referents.

As mentioned earlier, each child with multiple disabilities presents with a unique pattern of development and experiences that contribute to their overall communicative profile. There is no one specific course

of communication development that children with multiple disabilities will follow. Each child's communication development reflects their stage of cognitive development, communication experiences, ability to vocalize and gesture, and language comprehension skills. Many of these children will be able to use functional speech for communication; however, for children who are unable to develop functional expressive speech, or who have difficulty using or understanding language, *augmentative and alternative communication (AAC)* may be used to successfully enhance their communication development (Beukelman & Mirenda, 2013; Goossens, 1989; Romski & Sevcik, 1996; Romski et al., 2010; Smith, Barker, Barton-Hulsey, Romski, & Sevcik, 2016).

▶ The Role of Augmentative and Alternative Communication in Language and Communication Development

What Is AAC?

AAC is a multimodal intervention approach (Romski et al., 2017) that uses forms of communication such as manual sign language, communication boards, computerized/electronic devices that produce speech called *speech-generating devices (SGDs)*, or apps that are downloaded on mobile devices that produce speech, with the goal of maximizing the functional language and communication abilities of individuals who have severe communication impairments and little to no speech (ASHA, 2002). Communication boards and SGDs typically display pictures that represent what the child wants to say or express. When a specific picture is pressed on an SGD, it generates speech in a digitized (recorded) or synthesized (computerized) form for the communication partner to hear. AAC intervention approaches take into account a child's total communication abilities, including more conventional forms such as existing speech, vocalizations, gestures, facial expressions, body language, eye gazing, and/or posturing.

What Are the Components of an AAC System?

AAC does not comprise one single component, but rather is an integrated system of components, working in concert to provide the maximum amount of support needed for a child to fully communicate in all situations. The four primary components of an *AAC system* are aids, symbols, strategies, and techniques. A child's unique communicative profile, skills, preferences, and learning characteristics, along with the family's preferences, concerns, resources and learning styles, should all be taken into account when developing an AAC system and intervention program (Hurth, Shaw, Izeman, Whaley, & Rogers, 1999; Paul, 2001). The following paragraphs describe the components of an AAC system for a child with multiple disabilities.

Aids or Modes of Communication

The first component of an AAC system is the mode of communication or the way in which an individual communicates. As previously defined, AAC is a multimodal intervention approach, encompassing all available communicative methods including behaviors, gestures, eye gaze, pictures, SGDs, written communication, or extant vocalizations or speech. The term *communication aid* itself is defined as "a device, whether electronic or non-electronic, that is used to transmit or receive messages" (ASHA, 2004). Aids can range from simple devices, such as a choice board with objects or pictures or a single-message SGD, to very high technology, such as a dedicated SGD or AAC-based applications for use with non-dedicated personal computer tablet devices that include multiple pictures and text capabilities (Transpose "and": the web sites http://www.augcominc.com, https://www.atia.org, and http://www.closingthegap.com/solutions/search/ provide extensive information on a variety of communication aids and vendors). The modes or aids that a child uses to communicate with others at any given point in time will vary depending on a variety of factors and circumstances, such as the child's developmental abilities, child/family preference, and communication partners. For example, a child such as Sam with cerebral palsy and significant physical involvement may benefit from use of a SGD by directly pressing the pictures during morning activities, but due to physical fatigue, may benefit from use of a communication board via eye gaze for afternoon activities.

Romski, Sevcik, Cheslock, and Barton-Hulsey (2017) contend that the use of a SGD as a mode for communication may be more beneficial for children with multiple disabilities than are other modes such as sign language and picture boards alone because the "voice" of a SGD allows a child to immediately be understood by communication partners. This aspect of SGDs is particularly important when children are integrated within the general community and need to interact with unfamiliar communication partners (Lilienfeld & Alant, 2002). Research with individuals

with severe disabilities who use SGDs (Schlosser, Belfiore, Nigam, Blischak, & Hetzroni, 1995) has also suggested that the synthetic speech of the SGD can contribute to more efficient learning of the pictures used to represent concepts and ideas.

Vocabulary and Symbols

The vocabulary available on an AAC system plays a vital role: It provides the foundation on which communicative interaction is built (Romski et al., 2017). Regardless of the aid or mode of communication used, the child's communication partners identify what the child needs to say to achieve functional communication during daily activities and routines and then select appropriate vocabulary words to target in intervention. This vocabulary includes core words that are used frequently across contexts and environments (e.g., go, up, my, in, out, help, bye), but may also include less used, fringe vocabulary (e.g., shoe, juice, blue). When possible, the child should be given opportunities to indicate preferred vocabulary.

After the vocabulary targets are chosen, *symbols* are selected to represent the vocabulary. A variety of symbol types may be used with children with multiple disabilities, not limited to the modality of an SGD alone. Symbols can be unaided (e.g., signs, manual gestures, and facial expressions) when there is no need for any extrinsic support, or aided (e.g., actual objects, pictures, line drawings, multiple meaning icons, and printed words) when the individual must rely on supports beyond those that are available naturally (ASHA, 2004). For example, when sign language is used as the mode of communication, vocabulary is represented through the use of manual signs (unaided). When a non-electronic communication board or an electronic SGD or app is used as the mode of communication, vocabulary is typically represented on the board, SGD, or app in the form of visual-graphic symbols (aided). Children with visual impairments may benefit from the use of auditory symbols (aided) or tactile/textured symbols (aided).

A number of symbol sets are available for use, ranging from arbitrary to transparent (refer to the following website for extensive examples of symbols and available symbol sets: http://www.closingthegap.com/solutions/search/). *Arbitrary symbols* do not resemble the vocabulary they represent (e.g., printed words, Blissymbols), whereas *transparent symbols* do resemble, in varying degrees, what they represent (e.g., a photograph of a concrete object). Often, in clinical practice, easily depicted fringe vocabulary items (e.g., nouns) are chosen for children with cognitive and/or multiple disabilities, limiting their available vocabulary for communication interactions. The rationale underlying this decision is that these words are concrete and more easily learned than less easily depicted abstract words (e.g., core words such as verbs, adjectives, social-regulatives; Romski, et al., 2017). Research, however, has shown that when social-regulative symbols are placed on an SGD, children with cognitive disabilities can readily use them appropriately in context (Adamson, Romski, Deffebach, & Sevcik, 1992). Children do not necessarily have to readily understand vocabulary words or their corresponding symbol in order for them to be placed on the SGD. Through implementation of appropriate strategies, such as augmented communication input and teaching through natural contexts, children with multiple disabilities are able to learn and use new vocabulary and symbols (Romski et al., 2010). In recent years, the options for the organization of symbols on the SGD display have expanded from traditional grid-based layouts where symbols are organized in rows and columns, to options of visual scene displays, where a photograph or line drawing of the communication context (e.g., birthday party) is depicted, and objects within that scene provide a spoken message when pressed (Light & McNaughton, 2012; Olin, Reichle, Johnson, & Monn, 2010). SGD symbol vocabulary, organization, and display design are features important to consider when making decisions about the features unique to support a particular child's language and communication development. Further discussion regarding issues surrounding symbol representation, symbol set selection, and symbol display organization are provided by Barton-Hulsey, Wegner, Brady, Bunce, and Sevcik (2017), Fuller and Lloyd (1997), Reichle and Drager (2010), Sevcik, Romski, and Wilkinson (1991), Wilkinson and Snell (2011).

For use of the AAC system to be successful, the targeted vocabulary should be meaningful, motivating, functional, and individualized (Fried-Oken & More, 1992). Individualized factors to consider include the child's age, gender, and experiences; developmental appropriateness of vocabulary; and child/family preferences. Vocabulary is identified by using various selection techniques (e.g., environmental inventories, standard word lists, and communication diaries) and involving multiple communication partners (Fallon, Light, & Paige, 2001; Morrow, Mirenda, Beukelman, & Yorkston, 1993).

Techniques

An *AAC technique* consists of the various ways in which messages can be transmitted (ASHA, 2004).

Selection techniques can be classified into two broad categories: direct selection and scanning.

Direct selection allows the AAC user to communicate specific messages from a large set of options and includes techniques such as pointing, signing, gesturing, and touching. Some children with significant physical disabilities may benefit from the use of a head pointer or eye pointing (eye gaze) to select pictures or objects.

Scanning is a technique in which the messages are presented to the AAC user in a sequence by either a person or an SGD. The individual specifies their choice by responding "yes" or "no" to the person presenting the messages or by pressing a switch that is connected to the SGD. Scanning techniques include linear scanning, group-item scanning, directed scanning, and encoding (ASHA, 2004).

Strategies

The last and perhaps the most important component of an AAC system comprises the strategies used to implement the system. Strategies are specific ways in which AAC aids, symbols, and techniques are used to develop and/or enhance communication efficiency and effectiveness (e.g., language stimulation strategies, augmented input, aided language stimulation, communication-partner instruction, peer modeling, and rate of communication enhancement strategies). A strategy includes the intervention plan for facilitating a child's ability to actively participate and communicate in all environments (ASHA, 2004).

How Does AAC Facilitate the Development of Children with Multiple Disabilities?

AAC can play many important roles in the language, communication, and social development of a child with multiple and severe disabilities that may not be as obvious as simply providing an outlet for expressive communication. The roles will vary depending on each individual child's unique communicative strengths and needs. AAC intervention can augment existing natural speech, provide a primary output mode for communication (i.e., expressive use), provide input and output modes for language and communication (i.e., understanding and expressive use), serve as a language intervention strategy (Romski & Sevcik, 2005; Romski et al., 2010), and enhance social communicative development and participation.

The most well-known AAC role is to provide an expressive output mode for communication. For example, Oscar's attempts at speech are somewhat unintelligible to family members and highly unintelligible to communication partners other than his family members owing to his diagnosis of schizencephaly and his oral-motor limitations for expressive communication. Oscar understands everything spoken to him—his understanding of language and cognitive abilities are within normal limits for his age. Oscar could use AAC as a primary expressive output mode with less familiar communication partners (e.g., teachers, community) or to augment his existing speech in his interactions with family and friends in a variety of settings.

The other roles of AAC interventions are also important, especially for a child who is just beginning to develop communication skills. Consider Amber, who is 12 years old and has cognitive and language delays. She also has some challenging behaviors (i.e., tantrums, throwing) related to her communicative profile. Amber understands concrete words and concepts and has approximately 200 words in her expressive vocabulary. She is learning to use AAC in the form of activity-specific picture boards to indicate her wants and needs and to comment during daily activities and routines. AAC provides Amber with a visual system that (1) allows her to express what she already comprehends but may not be able to readily recall for communication, and (2) facilitates her comprehension and learning of new vocabulary words. Amber's family and teachers also use the picture board and spoken words when communicating with her (aided language stimulation) to demonstrate an acceptable means of communication and to help Amber increase her understanding of unknown words by pairing them with pictures. In Amber's case, AAC serves very different roles than it did for Oscar, functioning as an input-output mode and a language intervention strategy. In this context, AAC interventions can be viewed as tools that foster the development of early language skills and set the stage for later vocabulary development regardless of whether the child eventually talks.

In addition to facilitation of language and communication development, AAC plays an important role in the social development and well-being of a child. The ability to communicate is paramount to being able to interact with others and to establish friendships and social closeness. In some cases, the social interaction itself is more important than the precise grammar and vocabulary used for the message (Beukelman & Mirenda, 2013). Sam, for example, has diagnoses of severe intellectual disability and spastic quadriplegia cerebral palsy. He attends regular education classes for portions of his school day. At school, Sam's teachers programmed his Step-by-Step SGD (Ablenet Company, 2008), one of the aids in his AAC system, so that Sam can tell age-appropriate jokes to his peers before class starts in the mornings. Although Sam has

difficulty fully understanding the complex language involved in telling jokes, the social interaction that ensues by making his peers laugh may facilitate further social initiation by Sam and his peers as well as further develop Sam's overall communication ability.

Continual advances in AAC technology provide new opportunities for facilitating language, communication, reading skills, and social learning for children with multiple disabilities. A young child does not need to have age-appropriate language comprehension abilities in place before initiating the use of speech generating AAC devices. Furthermore, access to printed words and keyboards on SGDs can provide experience with letters and printed words that may encourage the development of reading skills and provide a mode of output for communication during activities of reading instruction. In social situations, AAC becomes the means to increase communicative participation and interactions during daily activities and routines and to enhance intellectual credibility as perceived during social interactions with peers, friends, and family (Cheslock, Barton-Hulsey, Romski, & Sevcik, 2008).

▶ Challenges for Successful AAC Communication in Developing Language

Children with multiple disabilities face many challenges in successfully accessing communication on a daily basis, whether it be natural or augmented communication. These challenges may be internal to the child and their disability characteristics, or they may be externally oriented, deriving from the child's environment and those providing communication supports. The challenges children with multiple disabilities face are often rooted in myths about the roles that AAC can play in their communication and language development instead of in empirical research. This section discusses these factors as they relate to communicative success, and particularly as they apply to AAC.

Internal Challenges
Medical Needs

Sustaining health and nutrition often do, and naturally should, take priority early on for children with multiple disabilities. Medical complications during infancy, surgeries during the toddler years, and chronic feeding difficulties often take precedence over communicative development and intervention and may be some reasons why there are delays in providing access to

AAC for very young children. After intervention with AAC is initiated, children with multiple disabilities may continue to have chronic medical needs requiring recurring hospitalizations and/or surgeries that interfere with consistent experience and practice with augmented communication. Progress may be slowed, but intervention should be continued.

Physical Ability

A wide variety of motoric difficulties present significant challenges for some children with multiple disabilities in physically accessing an AAC system. Motoric difficulties are often caused by injury to the parts of the brain that control our ability to use our muscles and bodies, as in the case of cerebral palsy; they can be mild, moderate, or severe. Their effects may be seen in one part of the body, such as the right arm, or they may be more widespread, affecting the arms, legs, torso, and facial muscles. Other diagnoses that may contribute to children's impairments in motor difficulty include Rett's syndrome, mitochondrial disorder, stroke, and traumatic brain injury.

Regardless of the etiology, motor function in a child is dependent on and influenced by multiple factors, including emotional state, level of arousal, comfort, motivation or attitude, attention, and understanding (Treviranus & Roberts, 2003). Certainly, these motor challenges can contribute to a child's ability to directly or indirectly access symbols on an AAC system. Nevertheless, these challenges should not be used as an excuse for failing to provide AAC to the child with physical disabilities. The NJC for the Communication Needs of Persons with Severe Disabilities (Brady et al., 2016) asserts that everyone has the right to access AAC technology (electronic or non-electronic) and states that physical ability or the lack thereof should not be used as a prerequisite to the implementation of AAC intervention. Accommodations using switches for scanning, head pointers, keyguards, eye tracking, and other specific modifications can all be used to ensure a child's most appropriate access to an AAC system (Campbell, Milbourne, & Wilcox, 2008).

When working with children who have motor difficulties, it is important to remember that complex interactions are involved in learning motor control for access to an AAC system. Continued practice with a consistent mode of access is often necessary for a child with significant motoric challenges to achieve their fullest ability in accessing AAC (Treviranus & Roberts, 2003).

Learned Helplessness

Some older children with multiple disabilities have a long history of being unable to successfully control their environment independently either physically or through communication (Beukelman & Mirenda, 2013). This lack of control over one's environment may lead to what is known as *learned helplessness*, an attitude of dependence on others to speak for the person and to make decisions for the individual.

Support teams working with children with multiple disabilities can provide an intervention plan to establish multiple opportunities for children and their caregivers or other communication partners to successfully communicate and participate in natural daily activities and routines. Technology such as adapted toys and adapted controls called *environmental controls* can be utilized to help the child interact with their environment where they were previously unable to interact (Beukelman & Mirenda, 2013; Campbell et al., 2008). Children with multiple disabilities can be taught early that they have a voice, and that their voice can influence their environment and the people around them. This understanding is important to their ability to advocate for themselves throughout their lives.

Challenging Behavior

Some children with multiple disabilities engage in *challenging behaviors*, such as biting, tantrums, screaming, task refusal, or self-injurious behaviors that constitute barriers to their receiving appropriate communication services, including AAC. For example, the child's behavior may present a barrier to her access of an appropriate AAC system if her service providers cannot resolve or do not know how to resolve the behaviors. In the case study, Amber's challenging behaviors have been cited in the past as a barrier to her access of an AAC system. Because Amber has some functional speech, her need for an AAC system to enhance her communication has been overlooked as her behaviors have escalated.

Many researchers view these challenging behaviors as a form of unconventional communication (Carr & Durand, 1985; Carr et al., 1994; Durand & Merges, 2001) in which the child attempts to express wants and needs related to objects and activities (Sigafoos & Mirenda, 2002) or social interaction (Hunt, Alwell, & Goetz, 1988), to refuse objects/activities (Sigafoos, O'Reilly, Drasgow, & Reichle, 2002), or to indicate pain and discomfort. It is quite difficult and frustrating for clinicians, parents, and caregivers to interpret and manage such socially inappropriate behaviors. It is, therefore, important to determine and understand the underlying message or function that the problem behavior is serving. This goal can be achieved through a process known as *functional behavior assessment*

(Bopp, Brown, & Mirenda, 2004), which should be conducted prior to determining appropriate intervention strategies. A behavior intervention plan (BIP) can be put in place so that all members of the child's intervention team are aware of how to consistently support positive behavior throughout the child's daily routines (Drasgow, Yell, Bradley, & Shriner, 1999). AAC is often included as an intervention strategy for children with challenging behaviors as it can replace their unacceptable forms of communication with more conventional forms (Romski & Sevcik, 2005).

Amber's behavior was determined to be caused partially by her difficulty in understanding verbal communication. AAC was then implemented as an input strategy to assist her in comprehending communication; it was successful in reducing the amount of challenging behaviors she exhibited. Amber has also used AAC expressively to replace some of her challenging behaviors and better communicate her needs.

External Challenges

Attitudes and Lack of Knowledge

A number of negative attitudes influence the access of AAC to children with disabilities, most often resulting in low expectations and limited opportunities for these children's participation in activities in which children without disabilities readily participate (Beukelman & Mirenda, 2013). Professional and familial attitudes, philosophy, and beliefs about the use of AAC during the early childhood years continue to evolve, however. The literature supports the idea that even very young children with severe disabilities can use and benefit from AAC, specifically SGDs. Nevertheless, some SLPs continue to believe that AAC is a "last resort" measure, to be used only after intensive spoken language intervention has failed. Others believe that the use of an SGD will hinder the child's development of spoken language. Still others think that children must have a certain set of skills—such as the ability to point, identify pictures, or understand causal relationships—to use AAC. TABLE 17-1 details a list of common myths and the reality behind each one as it relates to the use of AAC in language intervention.

The lack of knowledge about available AAC technology and the roles AAC can play in the life of a young child with severe communication difficulties poses great barriers to the child's participation and enhanced communication development.

Environmental Barriers

Environmental barriers may be locations in the community, school, and/or home that create physical segregation between the child and their ability to communicate using the AAC system effectively. Beukelman and Mirenda (2013) discuss space/location adaptations and physical structure adaptations of the environment that can be made to eliminate barriers. For example, Sam, who has an SGD mounted on his wheelchair, wants to participate in an art class activity but cannot because there is no accessible route for him to navigate his chair through the aisles of tables and chairs within the classroom while taking his SGD with him. A simple modification—rearranging the furniture—can allow Sam to easily enter the classroom with his SGD so that he can communicate during art class activities.

Opportunities for Participation

Beukelman and Mirenda (2013) indicate that the first step to increasing communication is to increase children's meaningful participation in natural activities and routines. Unfortunately, many children with multiple disabilities lack the same participation opportunities as their typically developing peers, both in school and through community activities. Because of motor and/or intellectual impairments, these children may be segregated from participation in activities such as baseball, dance classes, physical education at school, cooking activities, and art lessons. This lack of participation in natural activities is primarily attributable to lack of effort or knowledge on the part of these children's teachers, SLPs, or caregivers, who all too often do not find ways to engage them.

Sam, for example, is engaged in many activities at school, including music, art, computer time, lunch, and speech, physical, and occupational therapies. He is also involved in private therapies, frequently attends doctor appointments, and participates in church activities. One of his favorite daily activities is riding the bus to and from school. Because of his multiple diagnoses involving severe motor impairment and limited speech ability, Sam's participation and communication interaction with others would be significantly limited without the use of AAC technology. Sam requires others to acknowledge the need for him to continue participation in activities he enjoys and to successfully use and learn to use his AAC system. Without responsive communication partners in real environments at home, in school, and in the community, Sam would have no opportunity to communicate and thus learn communication.

Like Sam, many children with multiple disabilities encounter participation barriers in daily activities when those around them do not allow the appropriate modifications for their participation. To achieve full

TABLE 17-1 Myths and Realities in AAC Intervention	
Myth	**Reality**
AAC is a last resort in speech-language intervention.	AAC can play many roles in early communication development including the development of natural speech (Cress & Marvin, 2003; Reichle, Buekelman, & Light, 2002; Romski et al., 2010).
AAC hinders or stops further speech development.	A number of empirical studies suggest that AAC actually improves speech skills and provides for greater gains in verbal speech development than does spoken intervention alone (Beukelman & Mirenda, 2013; Romski & Sevcik, 1996; Romski et al., 2010).
Children must have a certain set of skills to benefit from AAC.	There is a continuum of AAC systems that can be used to develop language skills (Brady et al., 2016; NJC, 1992). Access to these systems is critical if the individual is expected to make cognitive gains. Early communication behaviors including spontaneous and nonintentional behaviors support the development of later symbolic communication (Siegel & Cress, 2002).
Speech-generating devices are only for children with intact cognition.	A broad range of speech-generating devices are available to use with children along the continuum of communication development. Children as young as two years of age with cognitive delays have been taught to use basic speech-generating devices for communication (Romski et al., 2010).
Children have to be a certain age to benefit from AAC.	There is no evidence to support this myth. Infants, toddlers, and preschoolers with a variety of disabilities have benefited from the use of AAC (Cress, 2003; Romski, Sevcik, & Forrest, 2001; Romski et al., 2009, 2010).
There is a representational hierarchy of symbols from objects to written words that children must master in sequence.	Namy, Campbell, and Tomasello (2004) have found that children as young as 13–18 months have been able to learn symbol-referent relationships regardless of the iconicity of the symbol. Preschool-age children with developmental disabilities have been able to learn symbol-referent relationships regardless of symbol iconicity (Barton, Sevcik, & Romski, 2006).

Source: Adapted from Romski, M. A., & Sevcik, R. A. (2005). Augmentative communication and early intervention: Myths and realities. *Infants & Young Children, 18*(3), 174–185.

and optimal participation for children with disabilities, their natural environments and the communication opportunities within those environments should first be addressed through comprehensive AAC assessment or diagnostic intervention. Then intervention strategies, such as increasing opportunities for communication and using adaptive toys, SGDs, and environmental controls, can be implemented.

▶ Navigating the Challenges: Foundations for Implementation of Augmented Language Intervention

Several foundational principles that address the previously discussed challenges must be acknowledged for the successful implementation of AAC with children

with multiple disabilities. These principles are based on research, values and perspectives, policy, clinical knowledge of early language and communication development, and clinical expertise and can be used as guides in providing effective services and supports. **TABLE 17-2** summarizes the research base and provides a broad overview of practical strategies for implementation of foundational principles in using AAC to facilitate the communication and language development of children with multiple disabilities.

Philosophical Beliefs

Central to the SLP's ability to facilitate a child's ability to communicate within their environment is the philosophical belief that all children can and do communicate (Brady et al., 2016). While the effectiveness and efficiency of that communication may vary from child to child, communication inevitably begins at birth, starting with non-symbolic forms such as crying,

TABLE 17-2 Practical Strategies for Implementation of AAC

Foundations	Research Bases	Strategies for Implementation
Philosophical beliefs	All children can and do communicate (www.asha.org/njc). Intervention with young children with multiple disabilities requires a collaborative service-delivery model (ASHA, 2008).	Read more information about these philosophies and working with children with multiple disabilities on the NJC website.
AAC assessment	Assessment is a critical component of AAC service delivery and provides the foundation for basing intervention decisions (Romski et al., 2002). AAC assessment focuses on the AAC user, various communication partners, environments, and the AAC system (Beukelman & Mirenda, 2013; NJC, 1992; Brady et al., 2016; Peck, 1989; Siegel-Causey & Bashinski, 1997; Wasson, Arvidson, & Lloyd, 1997).	Conduct a comprehensive, team-based assessment to determine child's strengths and needs. Conduct diagnostic AAC intervention when needed.
Begin AAC intervention early	Children are likely to make the greatest gains when services begin early in development (Girolametto, Wiigs, Smyth, Weitzman, & Pearce, 2001). A number of empirical studies report increases in speech skills following AAC intervention (Romski et al., 2010; Beukelman & Mirenda, 2013).	Supplement early language and communication intervention with AAC strategies, as opposed to using AAC as a last resort.
Knowledge of language comprehension and production	For young children to develop functional language and communication skills, they must be able to comprehend and produce language so that they can take on the roles of both listener and speaker in conversational exchanges (Sevcik & Romski, 2002).	Integrate goals focused on language development, including comprehension, production, and literacy, into AAC intervention plans.
Systematic language-based instruction	Research has indicated successful outcomes for young children in AAC intervention integrated with existing naturalistic language interventions (Romski, et al., 2010; Schepis, Reid, Behrmann, & Sutton, 1998; Yoder & Stone, 2006).	Systematically and consistently implement AAC strategies within existing language intervention. Establish functional, language-based goals.
Teaching through natural communicative activities and routines	Implementation of AAC in home and community (e.g., daycare center, local park) settings emphasizes functional language, facilitates generalization, and increases spontaneous communication (Romski et al., 2002, 2010).	Implement AAC into the child and family's existing routines and activities. Use the child's own toys, books, and personal items.
Communication-partner instruction and education	Education and training is a dynamic process of joint discoveries, problem-solving, and guided practice (Buysse & Wesley, 2005). Training of AAC systems is essential to its long-term use; conversely, lack of training is associated with abandonment (Johnson, Inglebret, Jones, & Ray, 2006; Smith, 2002).	Acknowledge the family's pre-existing knowledge, values, beliefs, perspectives, and experiences. Consider adult learning styles and provide materials and/or feedback appropriately (e.g., video feedback, Internet, books, articles, written instructions).

| Ongoing monitoring | AAC intervention is a dynamic process; abilities change over time, albeit sometimes very slowly. The system for use at one age may need to be modified as a young child grows and develops (Beukelman & Mirenda, 2013). Continuous updating of AAC systems has been identified as a factor contributing to long-term use (Smith, 2002). | Regularly observe the child's participation in targeted daily routines and document abilities and needs. Establish formal and informal ways of gaining information from family members, such as journals, emails, and teleconferencing. |

Source: Adapted from Cheslock, M. A., Romski, M. A., Sevcik, R. A., & Barton-Hulsey, A. (2007). Providing quality AAC intervention services to young children and their families. Poster session presented at the annual meeting of the American Speech-Language Hearing Association, Boston, MA.

vocalizations, facial expressions, eye-gazing, or natural gestures, and then, as the child grows and develops, evolves into more symbolic forms, such as words, pictures, or sign language. In addition, some children with severe disabilities develop unconventional and socially inappropriate means to communicate, including aggressive behaviors toward themselves or others. SLPs who interact with individuals with severe disabilities must develop skills in recognizing all communication behaviors produced by those children and diligently seek ways to promote the effectiveness of their communication (Brady et al., 2016). The NJC also provides a series of frequently asked questions highlighting the fact that all children can and do communicate, indicating how to look for signs of that communication regardless of level and type of disability, and ultimately answering questions about the multiple issues revolving around AAC intervention (see www.asha.org/njc).

Successful implementation of AAC for children with multiple disabilities also requires a philosophical focus on collaborative service delivery models that embrace inclusive practices and services delivered in natural environments and focus on functional communication during the child and family's natural daily activities and routines (ASHA, 2008). Consistent and positive communicative interaction among the child's family, caregivers, teachers, and the SLP is an important factor in the provision of collaborative service delivery. This model is critical to the belief that children can learn language and communication skills in the natural environment with communication supports to bolster achievement (Romski et al., 2017).

AAC Assessment

Assessment is a critical component of AAC service delivery and provides the foundation for making intervention decisions for all individuals who require AAC intervention. The focus of *AAC assessment* is typically not to determine the need for AAC but rather to explore the range of appropriate AAC strategies, adaptations, devices, and services that may help children fully participate in their environment and enhance their functional communication with a variety of communication partners within multiple environments (Romski et al., 2002).

AAC assessment is conducted within a comprehensive, team-based assessment framework, often in a variety of environments and with several team members providing essential information. A comprehensive AAC assessment includes assessment of the AAC user's communicative strengths and needs, various communication partners, environments, and the AAC system or selection of appropriate communication apps (Beukelman & Mirenda, 2013; Brady et al., 2016; Peck, 1989; Siegel-Causey & Bashinski, 1997; Wasson et al., 1997). **TABLE 17-3** outlines these assessment areas in more detail. Gosnell, Costello, and Shane (2011) discuss a clinical framework for selecting an appropriate app for communication based on key features for comparison to other apps. Because SLPs have specialized knowledge of typical and atypical language, communication, cognitive, and early literacy development, they usually lead AAC assessment teams. Because of the depth of knowledge needed in so many developmental areas pertaining to the child, other team members also play crucial roles in the assessment, including the child, family, and other caregivers or family friends, as well as the physical therapist, occupational therapist, psychologist, teacher(s) and/or educational specialist, and medical doctor.

Because of the various motor, behavioral, or other developmental factors involved, making a valid determination of the developmental abilities of a child with multiple disabilities can be quite challenging. Information, however, is obtained using multiple methods, including standardized and nonstandardized tests, informal observations during authentic activities and routines (e.g., playtime, meals, story reading, diaper changing/toileting) with multiple communication partners (e.g., parents, grandparents, childcare workers, friends) within the child and family's natural environments, and family/caregiver questionnaires.

TABLE 17-3 Comprehensive AAC Assessment Areas

I. Person Using AAC	II. Communication Partners
Language comprehension Language production Cognitive abilities Play behaviors Motor functioning, including oral-motor development Literacy skills Sensory acuity and processing ability, including vision, hearing, and tactile skills Motivation to communicate Present communication needs Future communication needs	Identify critical partners in each of the child's daily environments Measure communication opportunities and other acts that may or may not facilitate the communicative development of the child provided by identified partners Assess the child's responses to the communication partners

III. Environments	IV. AAC System
Identify multiple locations and activities the child attends Identify opportunities for participation in those environments Identify barriers or challenges to participation Identify communication opportunities and needs within the environments Identify communicative functions that may be useful in the identified environments	Device(s) or aid(s) Vocabulary Symbols Techniques used to access the system Strategies for effective and efficient use Ability of system to meet multiple communication needs of child Cultural appropriateness of the system

Sources: National Joint Committee for the Communication Needs of Persons with Severe Disabilities (NJC). (1992). Guidelines for meeting the communication needs of persons with severe disabilities. Retrieved from www.asha.org/policy; www.asha.org/njc; Brady, N. C., Bruce, S., Goldman, A., Erickson, K., Mineo, B., Ogletree, B. T., ... Wilkinson, K. (2016). Communication services and supports for individuals with severe disabilities: Guidance for assessment and intervention. *American Journal on Intellectual and Developmental Disabilities, 121*(2), 121–138; and Wasson, C. A., Arvidson, H. H., & Lloyd, L. L. (1997). AAC assessment process. In L. L. Lloyd, D. R. Fuller, & H. H. Arvidson (Eds.), *Augmentative and alternative communication: A handbook of principles and practices* (pp. 169–198). Needham Heights, MA: Allyn & Bacon.

Standardized and nonstandardized tests can be useful for identifying specific developmental abilities, communicative strengths, and areas of need in a structured manner. Some children may benefit from standard-assessment adaptations, where permissible, to enhance their ability to understand and respond to test directives. When adapting a standardized assessment, the validity of norm-referenced scoring is reduced; even so, valuable information may be gained about the child's language ability in the process.

TABLE 17-4 lists some adaptation needs and methods that are often used with children who have multiple disabilities so that a standardized assessment may be administered. Wasson et al. (1997) provide further details on test adaptation. Beukelman and Mirenda (2013) describe specific assessment tests that may be easily adapted for use with children with multiple and severe disabilities. See *The Communication Complexity Scale* (Brady et al., 2012) and *The Communication Matrix* (www.communicationmatrix.org; Rowland, 2011)

for tools that provide a systematic evaluation of communication ability in children who are at the earliest stages of communication where even adapted standardized assessments may not provide sufficient information. Because the goal of AAC is to enhance an individual's functional communication and language abilities within their natural environment, observations and family/caregiver interviews may also provide more valuable information than administration of tests (Blackstone, 1994). This information may, for example, support standardized and nonstandardized test information; provide qualitative information regarding everyday communicative strengths, opportunities, and needs; identify critical communication partners; and help determine internal and external challenges that affect the child's participation in play, cognitive, communication, physical, and self-help activities.

Although the assessment provides a rationale for AAC service delivery to the specific child, it should not delay the beginning of intervention services in its

TABLE 17-4 Adapting Standardized Assessments	
Adaptation Need	**Method**
Simplification of lengthy test instructions	Paraphrase the test instructions by using less complex directions that the child understands
Child needs consistent feedback to sustain performance	Give positive feedback instead of only neutral feedback, as most tests instruct
Physical adaptation: The child cannot physically point to a picture choice	Read the test question and then ask the child to give a yes/no response while you scan through the picture choices Picture choices may be placed in four corners of an eye-gaze board for the child to use eye gaze to make a choice
Testing material is too small	Enlarge the test materials manually and/or with color to meet the child's visual needs

Source: Adapted from Lloyd, L., Fuller, D. R., & Arvidson, H. H. (1997). Augmentative and alternative communication: A handbook of principles and practices. Needham Heights, MA: Allyn & Bacon.

absence. Some children may be on long waiting lists to receive an AAC assessment. For others, the extent of their disability and, therefore, their ability to participate in assessment activities may preclude the full completion of valid assessment in a more timely fashion. In these cases, *diagnostic intervention* may be warranted. Goossens (1989), for example, described a 6-year-old child with cerebral palsy who participated in naturalistic augmented language intervention utilizing spoken language stimulation coupled with pictures, referred to as *aided language stimulation*. Because of the child's physical limitations and lack of spoken communication, cognitive skills of the child were originally estimated to be at a 16- to 20-month age level. After 7 months of intervention, the child developed a viable method of communication using AAC (i.e., eye-gaze to pictures) and the cognitive abilities were found to be within normal limits. Goossens's study demonstrates the need for diagnostic AAC intervention with some children and reinforces the idea that AAC assessment should be viewed as a continual process.

Beginning AAC Intervention as Early as Possible

Beginning intervention as early as possible not only improves the life and functioning of a child, but also reduces the stress on the family, which in turn improves the family environment (Guralnick, 2000). Over the past 30 years, research with children from birth to 6 years of age has shown that AAC intervention enhances speech and language development, and has been successful in teaching parents to support the use of AAC with their children (see Romski, Sevcik, Barton-Hulsey, & Whitmore, 2015 for a review). Despite the trend toward early intervention, many young children with multiple disabilities are not introduced to AAC until they are 3 or 4 years of age, or even older. One reason for this delay, as previously discussed, may be the medical challenges faced by the child. However, the justification most commonly cited by interventionists and parents for not using AAC is that it may hinder speech development. In reality, a modest number of empirical studies have actually reported improvement in natural speech skills after AAC intervention (see Beukelman & Mirenda, 2013, for a review; Romski et al., 2010; Sigafoos, Didden, & O'Reilly, 2003). Just as important, there are no studies that support the idea that AAC hinders speech development (Romski, Sevcik, Adamson, Cheslock, & Smith, 2007; Romski et al., 2017; Smith et al., 2016).

AAC is a multimodal communication intervention strategy that is incorporated into a child's program to enhance both expressive and receptive communication skills and should incorporate a child's full communication abilities, including any existing vocalizations, gestures, manual signs, and aided communication (ASHA, 2002). For young children for whom AAC may function to facilitate speech, monitoring and encouraging the emergence of intelligible speech are integral parts of the AAC intervention process (Paul, 1997; Romski et al., 2002). While children are likely to make the greatest gains when services begin during the early stages of development (Girolametto et al., 2001), AAC can be successfully implemented beginning at any age.

Knowledge of Language Comprehension and Production

Implementation of AAC requires a belief that language and communication development focuses on a child's comprehension and production skills. *Language comprehension* is the ability to understand what is said so that one can function as a listener in conversational exchanges. *Language production* is the ability to express information so that one can function as a speaker in conversational exchanges. For young children to develop functional language and communication skills, they must be able to comprehend and produce language so that they can take on the roles of both listener and speaker in conversational exchanges (Sevcik & Romski, 2002).

To function as a listener, an individual must be able to understand the information that is conveyed to them by a variety of communication partners. In practice, children with multiple disabilities are often asked to produce communication with the assumption that they have an adequate foundation of understanding on which to build AAC productions. This may have occurred for a variety of reasons—for example, lack of knowledge of the importance of language comprehension in AAC interventions, incorrect assumptions about the child's communication abilities, or even a lack of methods for adequately assessing comprehension in children with significant disabilities (Cheslock, 2004). For children with multiple disabilities, including cognitive and/or comprehension difficulties, this sole focus on production may make learning to communicate via an AAC system a slow or extremely difficult process.

The language comprehension skills of children with multiple disabilities vary widely, and this individual variance may determine how a child will respond to a particular AAC device or intervention strategy. If a symbols-based AAC system (e.g., a communication board or SGD) is used, a child must heavily rely on the visual modality to understand the symbolic relationship between words and their picture referents (Romski & Sevcik, 1996; Romski et al., 2002).

For example, Sam was provided with an eight-picture, level-based SGD at the age of 3 years while he was continuing to develop language comprehension skills. He learned the meaning of visual-graphic symbols and their object referents or actions to expressively communicate. His development of language comprehension relied heavily on visual symbols at an early age.

In contrast, Amber developed language comprehension primarily through spoken words (no visual-graphic symbols) until the age of 12, when she was first provided with picture communication boards for multiple activities. She understood that a visual-graphic symbol had meaning for communication of basic wants and needs, just as a spoken word did. In her case, AAC was used to further enhance her expressive language ability.

It is critical to understand where children fall along the continuum of language comprehension if

SLPs are to adequately identify their communication profiles and intervene in their communication development using developmentally appropriate AAC devices or intervention strategies. SLPs must, therefore, incorporate their knowledge of early language development, both comprehension and production, into AAC intervention practices so that the end goal of enhanced and functional language and communication can be achieved for each child.

Systematic Language-Based Intervention

AAC intervention should be integrated within a framework of individualized language interventions. Research has indicated successful communication outcomes for young children with multiple disabilities in AAC intervention integrated with existing evidence-based naturalistic language interventions and strategies (Schepis et al., 1998; Yoder & Stone, 2006; see Romski et al., 2002, 2015; Smith et al., 2016, for a review), such as milieu teaching, functional communication training, and prompting. Intervention approaches are carefully planned and systematically implemented by identifying valid goals, outlining procedures for teaching skills to children and caregivers, consistently implementing the procedures, and evaluating effectiveness of the intervention based on data (Gresham, Beebe-Frankenberger, & MacMillan, 1999).

Language and communication goals and objectives for AAC intervention should be functional in nature and derived from knowledge obtained as part of the comprehensive, team-based AAC assessment, as described earlier. Siegel-Causey and Bashinski (1997) describe a tri-focus framework, in which intervention goals focus not only on the child's communicative development (e.g., language, literacy, and natural speech), but also on the communication environment and communication partners. For example, at an early age Oscar was provided with an SGD to use in his natural communication environments at home. When he was first introduced to an SGD, his goals focused on providing increased opportunities for communication in multiple environments and teaching communication enhancement strategies to multiple communication partners. One strategy his mother was taught to use was *augmented communication input* to teach Oscar how the symbols on his SGD were to be used for communication. His mother modeled the use of the SGD during natural communication interactions with him, and Oscar ultimately used the SGD himself to communicate to her.

With some children, it may also be necessary to establish goals and objectives related to their use and access of the AAC system. It is important to remember though that AAC systems are tools to achieve functional language and communication goals and not the goal in and of itself (Romski et al., 2002).

▶ Teaching Through Natural Communicative Activities and Routines

The literature strongly advocates the use of natural, integrated settings as the preferred environments for intervention for children with multiple disabilities (Beukelman & Mirenda, 2013; Roberts & Kaiser, 2011; Romski et al., 2002). The implementation of AAC interventions within these natural settings maximizes teaching and learning opportunities throughout the day (Wilcox & Woods, 2011; Woods & Wetherby, 2003), emphasizes the functional nature of language, facilitates the generalization of communicative routines to diverse contexts, increases the spontaneity of communication interactions (Bruder, 1998; Romski et al., 2002), and provides for increased social opportunities with peers. Natural environments for consideration include home and community settings (e.g., a neighborhood park, church or synagogue, library story time, grocery store, or a local school) in which typically developing children of the same age would participate. However, the provision of AAC intervention in natural environments goes beyond the consideration of location alone to also integrate intervention within natural and authentic activities and routines of the child within those locations (e.g., feeding, washing hands, and dressing at home; art/music class, field trip, and taking morning papers to the office at school). For example, during his morning dressing routine, Oscar's mother gives him choices of what color shirt to wear. Oscar then uses his SGD to answer his mother. For Sam, his SLP consulted with future field trip sight personnel to determine messages Sam might need to say during those scheduled activities. The SLP was able to ensure that Sam had access to the appropriate vocabulary needed to respond accordingly on his SGD. Sam was then able to communicatively participate in role play activities using those messages on his SGD while on the field trip.

Communication-Partner Instruction and Education in Language Intervention

Family members are the most stable, influential, and valuable people in a child's life (Iovannone, Dunlap, Huber, & Kincaid, 2003) and are the young child's primary *communication partners*. Immediate family members include parents, siblings, and perhaps

grandparents. Extended family members might include aunts, uncles, or cousins. As a child becomes older and is involved in more activities, other communication partners become influential as well; they could potentially include teachers (e.g., child care, preschool, Sunday school), child and family friends, peers, people in the community (e.g., librarians, athletic coaches, dance/art instructors), and other caregivers.

Family members and other caregivers in a child's life have unique expertise and insight to offer relative to that child that cannot be obtained through assessment by professionals. For the SLP, it is important to consider their perspectives because they can positively or negatively affect AAC outcomes. In recent years, many researchers and practitioners have explicitly acknowledged the importance of family/caregiver participation in AAC service delivery (Bruno & Dribbon, 1998; Culp, 2003; Culp & Carlisle, 1988; Kent-Walsh, Murza, Malani, & Binger, 2015; Romski & Sevcik, 1996; Romski et al., 2017). Research has indicated that the inclusion of instructing caregivers in the use of AAC systems in the intervention process is essential to its long-term use and that lack of instruction is associated with abandonment of the use of AAC (Johnson et al., 2006). Research has also demonstrated that interventions implemented by parents are just as effective at facilitating expressive language as clinician-implemented interventions (Law, Garrett, & Nye, 2004; Romski et al., 2007). Communication partner instruction and education can be viewed as a dynamic process of problem-solving and reflective-learning opportunities that can involve a variety of activities ranging from ongoing hands-on support and coaching for implementing AAC intervention devices and strategies, sharing resources, and advocacy training (Culp, 2003; Romski et al., 2007, 2017).

Professionals may first work with families and communication partners by providing educational information and support. McWilliams and Scott (2001) have described three types of support necessary to offer to communication partners: informational support, material support, and emotional support. Provision of informational support focuses on child development, disabilities, research-based interventions and strategies, and area resources. Material support may involve helping the family to find requested resources, an SGD, or picture symbols for a communication board; adapt toys or books for enhanced participation and communication; or locate funding for purchase of equipment. Emotional support can be provided by listening to and talking with families and communication partners in a positive and friendly manner, and by acknowledging their concerns. Throughout the communication partner instruction and education process, it is important to respect each child's and family's values, beliefs, customs, cultural identification, and preferences. SLPs should also consider the various adult learning styles and provide materials and/or feedback appropriately (e.g., video feedback; information via the Internet, books, or journal articles; written instructions).

SLPs also work with communication partners to identify and implement AAC techniques and strategies that can be easily integrated into the child's natural activities and routines. For example, the SLP may teach strategies such as modeling language, augmented input, environmental arrangement, or pausing by providing the partner with in-depth and multiple examples of targeted strategies during hands-on activities; the SLP may then provide feedback to the partner as they implement those strategies with the child. Peers without communication difficulties are often overlooked as valuable communication partners within the classroom environment who can also learn these basic strategies. Trottier, Kamp, and Mirenda (2011) found that peers were successful in using intervention strategies during routine games at school to increase communication with their classmates who used AAC. Peers were taught to use pause time and simple verbal prompting and models to interact with students using AAC. Students using AAC made positive gains in communication when given this opportunity for peer-mediated instruction.

Ongoing Monitoring

AAC intervention is a dynamic and ongoing process, reflecting the fact that children's abilities change over time, albeit sometimes very slowly. The system that is appropriate at one age may need to be modified as a young child grows and develops (Beukelman & Mirenda, 2013). Given this potential for flux, it is important to consider the child's success as falling along a continuum rather than as being an all-or-nothing phenomenon (Romski et al., 2017).

Systematic plans for periodic assessment of intervention progress along the continuum should be in place to monitor intervention successes or challenges. Wolery (2004) has suggested that such monitoring serves three broad functions:

- To validate the conclusions from the initial assessment
- To develop a record of progress over time
- To determine whether and how to modify or revise intervention plans

For AAC service delivery, ongoing monitoring should focus on the effectiveness and efficiency of the communication mode(s), vocabulary development

and use, communication interactions with all partners, developmental abilities of the child including understanding and use of language, use of strategies in multiple environments, challenges that may impede communication, and, if appropriate, development of speech (ASHA, 2004). This continuous updating of an AAC system has been identified as a factor contributing to long-term successful use (Johnson et al., 2006).

The SLP, in conjunction with family and other team members, monitors the child's progress toward goals and outcomes on a regular basis, revising and establishing new goals and outcomes as appropriate to meet the changing needs of the child. Various options are available for monitoring progress, including structured and informal observations during targeted daily routines and activities, caregiver/parent perception surveys (Romski et al., 2007), questionnaires, and traditional progress reports tracking behavior for a set period of time. SLPs can establish multiple methods to obtain information from family members and other caregivers, such as journals, periodic face-to-face meetings, e-mail, and teleconferencing.

▶ Summary

First and foremost, children with multiple disabilities are children who enjoy similar activities as children without disabilities, such as social interaction games with caregivers, playing with toys, and listening to stories. Children with multiple disabilities, however, have unique impairments in two or more developmental areas, including communication, physical, or cognitive skills, that typically affect their ability to fully participate in daily activities.

This chapter focused on the communicative development of children with multiple disabilities and, more specifically, on the role AAC can play in that development. There is no one pattern of development that leads to certain communication strengths and needs. Instead, each child presents with a unique pattern, regardless of their diagnoses, that becomes their own personal communicative profile. Important factors to consider include a child's cognitive development, communication experiences, ability to vocalize and gesture, and ability to understand the world around himself.

Most children with multiple disabilities will be able to functionally communicate, to varying degrees, via spoken language (Abbeduto, 2003). For other children, the severity of their disability may preclude their ability to expressively communicate with speech, despite intensive spoken language intervention. For these children, AAC intervention approaches have proved successful in enhancing their overall ability to communicate with family, friends, and other communication partners. The roles AAC can play in communicative language intervention for children with multiple disabilities are broader than just providing an expressive means of communication, however: AAC can also be used to supplement existing natural speech, enhance understanding and use of speech, serve as a language intervention strategy, replace unacceptable behaviors that are being used as communication, and facilitate the social development of friendships and closeness with others through communication.

Children with multiple disabilities face many challenges in accessing successful communication to convey their wants and needs, knowledge, and emotions. These challenges are often rooted in philosophical beliefs about what children with multiple disabilities can and cannot achieve and in myths about how an intervention approach such as AAC can facilitate communicative development. When implemented using sound research and principles, values, stakeholder perspectives, policy, and clinical knowledge, AAC can be a means to navigating the many challenges that children with multiple disabilities face on a daily basis.

Study Questions

- Describe the primary components of an augmentative communication system.
- Discuss three roles that AAC can play in the language development of children with multiple disabilities.
- There are at least six myths associated with introducing AAC to children younger than the age of 3 years. List three of these myths and discuss the evidence against them.
- Name four factors that contribute to a child's individual communicative profile. Why are these factors important to consider when planning an appropriate AAC intervention?
- Discuss two adaptations of a standardized assessment that would make it accessible for children with multiple disabilities. What scoring outcomes should be considered when making these adaptations?
- Discuss in detail the areas that should be addressed when conducting a comprehensive AAC assessment.
- What does it mean to provide ongoing monitoring of a child's use of an AAC system? Why

should a child's use of AAC be continually monitored?
- Discuss the role of AAC as a language intervention strategy rather than an external means of communication alone.
- Describe the role of the communication partner in AAC intervention with children with multiple disabilities. Why are they so important?

CLINICAL APPLICATION EXERCISE

1. Name four factors that contribute to a child's individual communicative profile. Why are these factors important to consider when planning an appropriate AAC intervention?
2. Explain two internal and two external challenges that children with multiple disabilities may face when using an AAC system. How could these challenges be navigated with their families', teachers', or SLP's help?

Recommended Readings

Beukelman, D., & Mirenda, P. (Eds.). (2013). *Augmentative and Alternative Communication: Supporting Children & Adults with Complex Communication Needs* (4th ed.). Baltimore, MD: Brookes Publishing.
Pistorius, M. (2013). *Ghost boy: The miraculous escape of a misdiagnosed boy trapped inside his own body.* Nashville, TN: Thomas Nelson Books.

Sevcik, R., & Romski, M. A. (Eds.). (2016). *Communication interventions for individuals with severe disabilities: Exploring research challenges and opportunities.* Baltimore, MD: Brookes Publishing.

References

Abbeduto, L. (2003). *International review of research in mental retardation: Language and communication.* New York, NY: Academic Press.
Ablenet. (2008). Step-by-step communicator. Retrieved from http://www.ablenetinc.com

Adamson, L. B., Romski, M. A., Deffebach, K., & Sevcik, R. A. (1992). Symbol vocabulary and the focus of conversations: Augmenting language development for youth with mental retardation. *Journal of Speech and Hearing Research, 35,* 1333–1343.

American Speech-Language-Hearing Association (ASHA). (2002). Augmentative and alternative communication: Knowledge and skills for service delivery. *ASHA Supplement, 22,* 97–106.

American Speech-Language-Hearing Association (ASHA). (2004). *Roles and responsibilities of speech-language pathologists with respect to augmentative and alternative communication: Technical report.* Retrieved from www.asha.org/policy

American Speech-Language-Hearing Association (ASHA). (2008). *Roles and responsibilities of speech-language pathologists in early intervention: Guidelines.* Retrieved from www.asha.org/policy

Barton, A., Sevcik, R., & Romski, M. A. (2006). Exploring visual-graphic symbol acquisition by pre-school age children with developmental and language delays. *Augmentative and Alternative Communication, 22,* 10–20.

Barton-Hulsey, A., Wegner, J., Brady, N. C., Bunce, B. H., & Sevcik, R. A. (2017). Comparing the effects of speech-generating device display organization on symbol comprehension and use by three children with developmental delays. *American Journal of Speech-language Pathology, 26,* 227–240.

Beukelman, D. R., & Mirenda, P. (Eds.). (2013). *Augmentative and alternative communication: Supporting children & adults with complex communication needs* (4th ed.). Baltimore, MD: Brookes Publishing.

Blackstone, S. (1994). The purpose of AAC assessment *Augmentative Communication News, 7*(1), 2–3.

Blackstone, S. (1997). The intake's connected to the input. *Augmentative Communication News, 10*(1), 1–6.

Bopp, K. D., Brown, K. E., & Mirenda, P. (2004). Speech-language pathologists' roles in the delivery of positive behavior support for individuals with developmental disabilities. *American Journal of Speech-Language Pathology, 13,* 5–19.

Brady, N. C., Bruce, S., Goldman, A., Erickson, K., Mineo, B., Ogletree, B. T., … Wilkinson, K. (2016). Communication services and supports for individuals with severe disabilities: Guidance for assessment and intervention. *American Journal on Intellectual and Developmental Disabilities, 121*(2), 121–138.

Brady, N. C., Fleming, K., Thiemann-Borque, K., Olswang, L., Dowden, P., Saunders, M. D., & Marquis, J. (2012). Development of the communication complexity scale. *American Journal of Speech-Language Pathology, 21,* 16–28.

Bruder, M. B. (1998). A collaborative model to increase the capacity of childcare providers to include young children with disabilities. *Journal of Early Intervention, 21*(2), 177–186.

Bruno, J., & Dribbon, M. (1998). Outcomes in AAC: Evaluating the effectiveness of a parent training program. *Augmentative and Alternative Communication, 14,* 59–70.

Buysse, V., & Wesley, P. W. (2005). *Consultation in early childhood settings.* Baltimore, MD: Paul H. Brookes.

Calculator, S. (1997). Fostering early language acquisition and AAC use: Exploring reciprocal influences between children and their environments. *Augmentative and Alternative Communication, 13,* 149–157.

Campbell, P. H., Milbourne, S., & Wilcox, M. J. (2008). Adaptation interventions to promote participation in natural settings. *Infants & Young Children, 21,* 94–106.

Carr, E. G., & Durand, V. M. (1985). Reducing behavior problems through functional communication training. *Journal of Applied Behavior Analysis, 18,* 111–126.

Carr, E. G., Levin, L., McConnachie, G., Carlson, J. I., Kemp, D. C., & Smith, C. E. (1994). *Communication-based intervention for problem behavior: A user's guide for producing positive change.* Baltimore, MD: Paul H. Brookes.

Cheslock, M. A. (2004). Issues of language input and output in AAC with young children. *Perspectives on Augmentative and Alternative Communication, 13,* 3.

Cheslock, M. A., Barton-Hulsey, A., Romski, M. A., & Sevcik, R. A. (2008). Using a speech-generating device to enhance communicative abilities for an adult with moderate intellectual disability. *Intellectual and Developmental Disabilities, 46,* 376–386.

Cress, C. (2003). Responding to a common early AAC question: "Will my child talk?". *Perspectives on Augmentative and Alternative Communication, 12,* 10–11.

Cress, C., & Marvin, C. (2003). Common questions about AAC services in early intervention. *Augmentative and Alternative Communication, 19,* 254–272.

Culp, D. (2003). "If mama ain't happy, ain't nobody happy": Collaborating with families in AAC interventions with infants and toddlers. *Perspectives on Augmentative and Alternative Communication, 12,* 5.

Culp, D. M., & Carlisle, M. (1988). *Partners in augmentative communication training: A resource guide for interaction facilitation training for children.* Tucson, AZ: Communication Skill Builders.

Davis, H., Stroud, A., & Green, L. (1988). Maternal language environment of children with mental retardation. *American Journal of Mental Retardation, 93,* 144–153.

Diamanti, T. (2000). Get to know me. In M. B. Williams & C. J. Krezman (Eds.), *Beneath the surface: Creative expressions of augmented communicators* (p. 98). Toronto, ON: International Society for Augmentative and Alternative Communication.

Dragsow, E., Yell, M. L., Bradley, R., Shriner, J. G. (1999). The IDEA amendments of 1997: A school-wide model for conducting functional behavioral assessments and developing behavioral intervention plans. *Education and Treatment of Children, 22,* 244–266.

Durand, V. M., & Merges, E. (2001). Functional communication training: A contemporary behavior analytic technique for problem behavior. *Focus on Autism and Other Developmental Disabilities, 16,* 110–119.

Fallon, K. A., Light, J. C., & Paige, T. K. (2001). Enhancing vocabulary selection for preschoolers who require augmentative and alternative communication (AAC). *American Journal of Speech-Language Pathology, 10,* 81–94.

Fey, M. E., Warren, S. F., Bredin-Oja, S. L., & Yoder, P. (2017). Responsivity education/Prelinguistic milieu teaching. In R. McCauley, M. Fey, & R. Gillam (Eds.), *Treatment of language disorders in children* (2nd ed., pp. 57–85). Baltimore, MD: Paul H. Brookes.

Fried-Oken, M., & More, L. (1992). An initial vocabulary for nonspeaking preschool children based on developmental and environmental language sources. *Augmentative and Alternative Communication, 8,* 41–56.

Fuller, D. R., & Lloyd, L. L. (1997). AAC model and taxonomy. In L. Lloyd, D. R. Fuller, & H. H. Arvidson (Eds.), *Augmentative and alternative communication: A handbook of principles and practices* (pp. 27–37). Needham Heights, MA: Allyn & Bacon.

Girolametto, L., Weitzman, E., Wiigs, M., & Pearce, P. (1999). The relationship between maternal language measures and language development in toddlers with expressive vocabulary delays. *American Journal of Speech-Language Pathology, 8,* 364–374.

Girolametto, L., Wiigs, M., Smyth, R., Weitzman, E., & Pearce, P. S. (2001). Children with a history of expressive vocabulary delay: Outcomes at 5 years of age. *American Journal of Speech-Language Pathology, 10,* 358–369.

Goossens, C. (1989). Aided communication intervention before assessment: A case study of a child with cerebral palsy. *Augmentative and Alternative Communication, 5,* 14–26.

Gosnell, J., Costello, J., & Shane, H. (2011). Using a clinical approach to answer "What communication apps should we use?" *SIG 12 Perspectives on Augmentative and Alternative Communication, 20*(3), 87–96.

Gresham, F. M., Beebe-Frankenberger, M. E., & MacMillan, D. L. (1999). A selective review of treatments for children with autism: Description and methodological considerations. *School Psychology Review, 28,* 559–575.

Guralnick, M. J. (2000). Early childhood intervention: Evolution of a system. *Focus on Autism and Other Developmental Disabilities, 15*(2), 68–79.

Hunt, P., Alwell, M., & Goetz, L. (1988). Acquisition of conversation skills and the reduction of inappropriate social interaction behaviors. *Journal of the Association for Persons with Severe Handicaps, 13,* 20–27.

Hurth, J., Shaw, E., Izeman, S. G., Whaley, K., & Rogers, S. J. (1999). Areas of agreement about effective practices among programs serving young children with autism spectrum disorders. *Infants and Young Children, 12,* 17–26.

Individuals with Disabilities Education Improvement Act of 2004, 20 U.S.C. §1400 *et seq.*

Iovannone, R., Dunlap, G., Huber, H., & Kincaid, D. (2003). Effective educational practices for students with autism spectrum disorders. *Focus on Autism and Other Developmental Disabilities, 18*(3), 150–165.

Johnson, J. M., Inglebret, E., Jones, C., & Ray, J. (2006). Perspectives of speech language pathologists regarding success versus abandonment of AAC. *Augmentative and Alternative Communication, 22*(2), 85–99.

Kent-Walsh, J., Murza, K. A., Malani, M. D., & Binger, C. (2015). Effects of communication partner instruction on the communication of individuals using AAC: A meta-analysis. Augmentative and Alternative Communication, 31(4), 271–284.

Law, J., Garrett, Z., & Nye, C. (2004). The efficacy of treatment for children with developmental speech and language delay/disorder: A meta-analysis. *Journal of Speech, Language, and Hearing Research, 47,* 924–943.

Light, J., & McNaughton, D. (2012). Supporting the communication, language, and literacy development of children with complex communication needs: State of the science and future research priorities. *Assistive Technology, 24*(1), 34–44.

Lilienfeld, M., & Alant, E. (2002). Attitudes of children toward an unfamiliar peer using an AAC device with and without voice output. *Augmentative and Alternative Communication, 18,* 91–101.

McWilliams, P. A., & Scott, S. (2001). A support approach to early intervention: A three-part framework. *Infants and Young Children,* 13, 55–66.

Morrow, D., Mirenda, P., Beukelman, D., & Yorkston, K. (1993). Vocabulary selection for augmentative communication systems: A comparison of three techniques. *American Journal of Speech-Language Pathology, 2*(2), 19–30.

Namy, L., Campbell, A., & Tomasello, M. (2004). The changing role of iconicity in non-verbal symbol learning: A u-shaped trajectory in the acquisition of arbitrary gestures. *Journal of Cognition and Development, 5,* 37–56.

National Joint Committee for the Communication Needs of Persons with Severe Disabilities (NJC). (1992, March). Guidelines for meeting the communication needs of persons with severe disabilities. *ASHA, 34* (Suppl. #7), 1–8.

Nelson, N. (1992). Performance is the prize: Language competence and performance among AAC users. *Augmentative and Alternative Communication, 8,* 3–18.

Olin, A. R., Reichle, J., Johnson, L., & Monn, E. (2010). Examining dynamic visual scene displays: Implications for arranging and teaching symbol selection. *American Journal of Speech-Language Pathology, 19,* 284–297.

Paul, R. (1997). Facilitating transitions in language development for children using AAC. *Augmentative and Alternative Communication, 13,* 141–148.

Paul, R. (Ed.). (2001). *Language disorders from infancy through adolescence* (2nd ed.). St. Louis, MO: Mosby.

Peck, C. A. (1989). Assessment of social competence: Evaluating environments. *Seminars in Speech and Language, 10,* 1–16.

Reichle, J., Beukelman, D. R., & Light, J. C. (Eds.). (2002). *Exemplary practices for beginning communicators: Implications for AAC.* Baltimore, MD: Paul H. Brookes.

Reichle, J., & Drager, K. D. R. (2010). Examining issues of aided communication display and navigational strategies for young children with developmental disabilities. *Journal of Developmental and Physical Disabilities, 22,* 289–311.

Roberts, M. Y., & Kaiser, A. P. (2011). The effectiveness of parent-implemented language interventions: A meta-analysis. *American Journal of Speech-Language Pathology, 20,* 180–199.

Romski, M. A., & Sevcik, R. A. (1996). *Breaking the speech barrier: Language development through augmented means.* Baltimore, MD: Paul H. Brookes.

Romski, M. A., & Sevcik, R. A. (2005). Augmentative communication and early intervention: Myths and realities. *Infants & Young Children, 18*(3), 174–185.

Romski, M. A., Sevcik, R. A., Adamson, L. B., Cheslock, M., & Smith, A. (2007). Parents can implement AAC interventions: Ratings of treatment implementation across early language interventions. *Early Childhood Services, 1*(4), 249–259.

Romski, M. A., Sevcik, R. A., Adamson, L. B., Cheslock, M. A., Smith, A., Barker, R. M., & Bakeman, R. (2010). Randomized comparison of parent-implemented augmented and non-augmented language intervention on vocabulary development of toddlers with developmental delays. *Journal of Speech, Language, and Hearing Research, 53,* 350–364.

Romski, M. A., Sevcik, R. A., Barton-Hulsey, A., & Whitmore, A. S. (2015). Early Intervention and AAC: What a Difference 30 Years Makes. *Augmentative and Alternative Communication, 31,* 180–202.

Romski, M. A., Sevcik, R. A., Cheslock, M. A., & Barton-Hulsey, A. (2017). The system for augmenting language: AAC and emerging language intervention. In R. McCauley, M. Fey, & R. Gillam (Eds.), *Treatment of language disorders in children* (2nd ed., pp. 155–186). Baltimore, MD: Paul H. Brookes.

Romski, M. A., Sevcik, R. A., & Forrest, S. (2001). Assistive technology and augmentative communication in early childhood inclusion. In M. J. Guralnick (Ed.), *Early childhood inclusion: Focus on change* (pp. 465–479). Baltimore, MD: Paul H. Brookes.

Romski, M. A., Sevcik, R. A., Hyatt, A. M., & Cheslock, M. A. (2002). A continuum of AAC language intervention strategies for beginning communicators. In J. Reichle, D. R. Beukelman, & J. C. Light (Eds.), *Exemplary practices for beginning communicators: Implications for AAC* (pp. 1–23). Baltimore, MD: Paul H. Brookes.

Romski, M. A., Sevcik, R. A., Smith, A., Barker, R. M., Folan, S., & Barton-Hulsey, A. (2009). The system for augmenting language: Implications for young children with autism spectrum disorders. In P. Mirenda & T. Iacono (Eds.), *Autism spectrum disorders and AAC* (pp. 219–245). Baltimore, MD: Paul H. Brookes.

Romski, M. A., Sevcik, R. A., Reumann, R., & Pate, J. L. (1989). Youngsters with moderate or severe spoken language impairments I: Extant communicative patterns. *Journal of Speech and Hearing Disorders, 54*, 366–373.

Rowland, C. (2011). Using the communication matrix to assess expressive skills in early communicators. *Communication Disorders Quarterly, 32*, 190–201.

Schalock, R. L., Borthwick-Duffy, S. A., Bradley, V. J., Buntinx, W. H. E., Coulter, D. L., … Yeager, M. H. (2010). *Intellectual disability: definition, classification, and systems of supports* (11th ed.). Washington, DC: American Association on Intellectual and Developmental Disabilities.

Schepis, M., Reid, D., Behrmann, M., & Sutton, K. (1998). Increasing communicative interactions of young children with autism using a voice output communication aid and naturalistic teaching. *Journal of Applied Behavioral Analysis, 31*, 561–578.

Schlosser, R., Belfiore, P. J., Nigam, R., Blischak, D., & Hetzroni, O. (1995). The effects of speech output technology in the learning of graphic symbols. *Journal of Applied Behavior Analysis, 28*, 537–549.

Siegel, A., & Cress, C. (2002). Overview of the emergence of early AAC behaviors. In J. Riechle, D. Beukelman, & J. Light (Eds.), *Exemplary practices for beginning communicators: Implications for AAC* (pp. 25–57). Baltimore, MD: Paul H. Brookes.

Siegel-Causey, E., & Bashinski, S. M. (1997). Enhancing initial communication and responsiveness of learners with multiple disabilities: A tri-focus framework for partners. *Focus on Autism and Other Developmental Disabilities, 12*(2), 105–120.

Sevcik, R. A., & Romski, M. A. (2002). The role of language comprehension in establishing early augmented conversations. In J. Reichle, D. R. Beukelman, & J. C. Light (Eds.), *Exemplary practices for beginning communicators: Implications for AAC* (pp. 453–474). Baltimore, MD: Paul H. Brookes.

Sevcik, R. A., Romski, M. A., & Wilkinson, K. (1991). Roles of graphic symbols in the language acquisition process for persons with severe cognitive disabilities. *Augmentative and Alternative Communication, 7*, 161–170.

Sigafoos, J., Didden, R., & O'Reilly, M. (2003). Effects of speech output on maintenance of requesting and frequency of vocalizations in three children with developmental disabilities. *Augmentative and Alternative Communication, 19*(1), 37–47.

Sigafoos, J., & Mirenda, P. (2002). Strengthening communicative behaviors for gaining access to desired items and activities. In J. Reichle, D. Beukelman, & J. Light (Eds.), *Exemplary practices for beginning communicators: Implications for AAC* (pp. 123–156). Baltimore, MD: Paul H. Brookes.

Sigafoos, J., O'Reilly, M., Drasgow, E., & Reichle, J. (2002). Strategies to achieve socially acceptable escape and avoidance. In J. Reichle, D. Beukelman, & J. Light (Eds.), *Exemplary practices for beginning communicators: Implications for AAC* (pp. 157–186). Baltimore, MD: Paul H. Brookes.

Smith, A., Barker, R. M., Barton-Hulsey, A., Romski, M. A., & Sevcik, R. (2016). Augmented language interventions for children with severe disabilities. In R. Sevcik & M. A. Romski (Eds.), *Communication interventions for individuals with severe disabilities: Exploring research challenges and opportunities* (pp. 123–146). Baltimore, MD: Paul H. Brookes.

Smith, G. (2002). *Users' perspectives of factors related to long-term use or abandonment of augmentative and alternative communication systems.* Unpublished master's research project. Spokane, WA: Washington State University.

Snow, C. E. (1991). The language of the mother-child relationship. In M. Woodhead, R. Carr, & P. Light (Eds.), *Becoming a person* (pp. 195–210). New York, NY: Routledge.

Tamis-LeMonda, C. S., Bornstein, M. H., & Baumwell, L. (2001). Maternal responsiveness and children's achievement of language milestones. *Child Development, 72*, 748–767.

Tamis-LeMonda, C. S., Kuchirko, Y., & Song, L. (2014). Why is infant language learning facilitated by parental responsiveness? *Current Directions in Psychological Science, 23*, 121–126.

Treviranus, J., & Roberts, V. (2003). Supporting competent motor control of AAC systems. In J. C. Light, D. R. Beukelman, & J. Reichle (Eds.), *Communicative competence for individuals who use AAC: From research to effective practice* (pp. 199–240). Baltimore, MD: Paul H. Brookes.

Trottier, N., Kamp, L., & Mirenda, P. (2011). Effects of peer-mediated instruction to teach use of speech-generating devices to students with autism in social game routines. *Augmentative and Alternative Communication, 27*, 26–39.

Warren, S. F., Gilkerson, J., Richards, J. A., Oller, D. K., Xu, D., Yapanel, U., & Gray, S. (2010). What automated vocal analysis reveals about the vocal production and language learning environment of young children with autism. *Journal of Autism and Developmental Disorders, 40*, 555–569.

Wasson, C. A., Arvidson, H. H., & Lloyd, L. L. (1997). AAC assessment process. In L. L. Lloyd, D. R. Fuller, & H. H. Arvidson (Eds.), *Augmentative and alternative communication: A handbook of principles and practices* (pp. 169–198). Needham Heights, MA: Allyn & Bacon.

Wilcox, J. M., & Woods, J. (2011). Participation as a basis for developing early intervention outcomes. *Language, Speech, and Hearing Services in Schools, 42*, 365–378.

Wilkinson, K. M., & Snell, J. (2011). Facilitating children's ability to distinguish symbols for emotions: The effects of background color cues and spatial arrangement of symbols on accuracy and speed of search. *American Journal of Speech-Language Pathology, 20*, 288–301.

Wolery, M. (2004). Monitoring children's progress and intervention implementation. In M. McLean, M. Wolery, & D. Bailey (Eds.), *Assessing infants and preschoolers with special needs* (pp. 545–584). Baltimore, MD: Paul H. Brookes.

Woods, J. J., & Wetherby, A. M. (2003). Early identification of and intervention for infants and toddlers who are at risk for autism spectrum disorders. *Language, Speech and Hearing Services in Schools, 34*, 180–193.

Yoder, P., & Stone, W. (2006). A randomized comparison of the effect of two prelinguistic communication interventions on the acquisition of spoken communication in preschoolers with ASD. *Journal of Speech, Language, and Hearing Research, 49*, 698–711.

Appendix 17-A

Case Study 1: Speech-Language Evaluation

Name: Sam
Sex: Male
Age: 8 years

▶ Significant History

Sam is an 8-year-old boy whose mother requested this assessment to receive recommendations regarding his use of a recently acquired dynamic display speech-generating augmentative communication device (SGD) that could enhance Sam's overall communication abilities throughout his functional daily routines and activities.

Sam's prenatal and birth histories were unremarkable. He was born at full term weighing 7 pounds, 6 ounces.

Sam's medical/health history *is* remarkable. Sam is diagnosed as having spastic quadriplegia cerebral palsy, a cleft lip and palate, and severe intellectual disability. He is able to eat some foods, but also has a G-tube to support adequate nutrition intake.

Hearing and vision are reportedly within normal limits.

Developmental milestones are delayed for motor, speech-language, and cognitive development. His physical abilities are a direct result of his diagnoses, as Sam is unable to walk and uses a wheelchair. He has difficulty initiating and terminating muscle activity throughout his body, including his legs, torso, arms, and facial muscles, as a result of his cerebral palsy. He is unable to communicate functionally using verbal speech.

Sam's expressive speech-language development is significantly delayed. He also has difficulty learning language, generalizing language concepts to a new context, and problem-solving. Nevertheless, his receptive language and cognitive skills have bypassed his ability to expressively communicate. Sam has received speech/language therapy since infancy to improve his oral motor skills, with gains being noted in his increased ability to chew and swallow foods and produce some consonants.

Sam began receiving weekly speech/language intervention using an eight-location voice output augmentative communication system at the age of 3 years through his state's early intervention program. He transitioned to services through his local public school system and also receives private speech/language therapy.

Family history for Sam is negative for speech disorders.

▶ Clinical Procedures

Assessment Tests

Peabody Picture Vocabulary Test—IV (PPVT-IV, Form B)

MacArthur-Bates Communicative Development Inventory Words and Gestures

Sequenced Inventory of Communication Development, Revised (SICD-R)

Other

Informal observations at home

▶ Clinical Findings

General Observations

Sam is an 8-year-old boy who enjoys music, playing ball, and reading books. Sam's mother reported that one of Sam's favorite daily activities is riding the bus to and from school. He enjoys interactions with friends, family, and teachers; however, his ability to interact with others is significantly limited as a result of his lack of verbal communication ability.

Nonverbal Communication

Sam has successfully used an eight-location speech-generating device to communicate in multiple environments, including home and private speech/language therapy. Vocabulary has been represented using Boardmaker Picture Communication Symbols (Mayer-Johnson), and Sam uses his hand to directly access the device. He typically has had six to eight pictures available per activity overlay (playtime, book reading, snack time). Although Sam fully understands the concept of using this communication device, his functional communication has been somewhat limited owing to his inconsistent ability to access it given his physical limitations and the limited vocabulary/memory capabilities of the augmentative communication device. By report and observation, Sam is able to directly hit the appropriate picture for voice output with no difficulties. At other times—and especially later in the day as the result of fatigue—Sam has many mis-hits or accidental hits to inappropriate pictures as he attempts to directly access the appropriate pictures. Sam primarily communicates nonverbally by pointing/reaching, focused eye-gaze, laughing, and vocalizations. His family has recently purchased a dynamic display SGD. This device has the capability for Sam to use an external switch to access the device using his head when his hand becomes fatigued.

Receptive Language

Sam's understanding of vocabulary was formally assessed using the PPVT-IV. Adaptations were made by cutting out the four pictures per test item and mounting them farther apart onto a rectangular-shaped, clear Lexan board. Sam responded accurately to test items by looking at his selected picture and then looking back to the examiner. In addition, he often reached for the correct picture with his hand. Incorrect items were noted when there was a much shorter eye-gaze time to a particular picture accompanied with random looks to other pictures. Sam received a raw score of 12, a standard score of 40, a percentile rank of less than 1, and an age equivalent of less than 21 months. Sam was quite accurate in identifying familiar pictured objects but had more difficulty with conceptual pictured vocabulary such as shapes and body parts and pictured actions.

To get a broader picture of Sam's understanding of vocabulary in typical daily routines, his mother was asked to fill out the *MacArthur-Bates Communicative Development Inventory: Words and Gestures*, a parent questionnaire of vocabulary comprehension and use. Out of a possible 396 words, Sam's mother indicated that he understands 311 words and uses 0. Sam was reported to functionally understand vocabulary in a variety of categories, including words for animals, body parts, clothing, food and drink; action words; descriptive words; words about time; and question words.

On the Receptive Language Portion of the SICD-R, Sam received 100% accuracy at the 16- and 20-month age levels. He readily identified some color-pictured body parts, identified color-pictured objects, and responded to the question type "where" by looking toward the person. He achieved 25% accuracy at the 28-month age level, primarily due to his physical limitations. Accuracy at the 32-month age level increased to 75%, as Sam was able to discriminate noise-makers, demonstrate function of objects through pictures, and understand turn-taking.

Expressive Language

Sam's expressive language skills were formally assessed using the SICD-R. Item administration was achieved through parent report, direct child participation, and informal clinical observations. As Sam's chronological age is outside the limits of this test, any scores reported should be used with great caution. Sam received an expressive language age equivalent of 8 months of age. He was reported to produce vowel sounds, consonant sounds, consonant-vowel (C-V) combinations, and C-V combinations that sound like words, and to inconsistently imitate sounds. He was unable to imitate motor acts because of his physical skills. During informal activities, Sam was observed to vocalize with intent, reach and eye-gaze toward desired objects, and laugh often.

Oral-Motor Examination

Sam has received speech/language therapy since infancy to improve his oral motor skills, with gains being noted in the form of his increased ability to chew and swallow foods and produce some consonants. However, his oral-motor deficits related to his medical diagnosis of cerebral palsy are such that there will most likely be no improvement for effective and functional speech production purposes, despite intervention. His lack of speech production has, and will continue to have, a significant impact on his ability to communicate his wants and needs, to tell if and how he may be hurt, to comment on his environment, and to socially interact with peers, teachers, doctors, and family.

▶ Diagnosis and Prognosis

Sam's prognosis for functional communication is good given the use of an appropriate augmentative communication system using an SGD along with adequate and consistent assistive technology services and supports.

▶ Recommendations

It is recommended that Sam be seen for a minimum of one time per week for approximately 8–12 weeks to facilitate his communications skills and use of the dynamic display speech-generating augmentative communication device. Intervention services should focus on customizations of vocabulary within activity-based pages; helping Sam to use the device throughout his functional communication environments, routines, and activities (e.g., home, school, community activities); helping Sam to communicate with a variety of communications partners (e.g. family, friends, therapists); and conducting communication partner training on a variety of communication enhancement techniques. The SGD should be used in all environments and during all parts of the day with Sam. Sam's need for additional services will also be monitored on a quarterly basis, as his vocabulary and communication needs will most likely change over time. Sam's mother will primarily be responsible for the care, programming, and troubleshooting of the SGD.

It will be very important for Sam's family and other communication partners to receive training for the SGD so that they may become proficient in its usage. Sam's family and communication partners should consistently and systematically utilize a variety of communication enhancement strategies, including aided input, modeling, expansion, and environmental arrangement, to teach Sam to independently use features of the SGD and to provide multiple opportunities for communication during natural everyday activities and routines.

Sam should continue his school- and private-based speech/language interventions. The goals of these interventions should focus on functional communication skills, understanding and use of language, oral-motor skills, and early literacy skills. It will be important for current therapies to be coordinated and to address use of the SGD in Sam's natural and functional activities and routines.

Given that Sam will most likely need to rely on technology throughout his lifetime, it is recommended that he have consistent access to technology that will allow him control over his environment. Most notably, the dynamic display communication device will allow Sam to control his environment through communication. The device also features a universal remote control so that Sam can learn to control common household appliances and develop his play/social/language/cognitive skills through play with infrared toys. After they are set up, all of these devices can be controlled with the communication device. Environmental controls are also commercially available to allow Sam to independently participate in other daily activities, such as cooking, playing, music, and art.

Appendix 17-B

Case Study 2: Speech-Language Evaluation

Name: Amber
Sex: Female
Age: 12 years

▶ Significant History

Amber's prenatal and birth histories were unremarkable. She weighed 8 pounds and was the product of a full-term pregnancy.

Amber's medical/health history was significant for ear infections and having her adenoids removed at age 3 years. Amber also experienced a seizure at the age of 6 years.

Amber's hearing was evaluated in school and found to be within normal limits.

Her developmental milestones have generally been slow. Amber walked unassisted at 19 months and began speaking when she was 3 years old. Her mother reported that she had problems coordinating the oral-motor movements required for breastfeeding, bottle feeding, and chewing and swallowing food until she was 2.5 years old, which resulted in frequent choking and drooling.

Amber's speech-language development is severely delayed, as evidenced by receptive language scores indicating a 6.5-year delay and an expressive language delay of 4–5 years. Her speech, although within normal limits for sounds in words, is moderately unintelligible in conversation. Her mother reported that she and Amber's immediate family understand Amber about half the time, but unfamiliar people and other communication partners rarely understand her.

In terms of early intervention, Amber attended a preschool readiness program from age 4 through 5 and has received language therapy, physical therapy, and sensory integration therapy.

Family history was negative for speech-language disorders.

▶ Clinical Procedures

Assessment Tests

Expressive Vocabulary Test-2nd edition (EVT-2)
Peabody Picture Vocabulary Test–IV (PPVT-IV)
Sequenced Inventory of Communication Development (SICD) for Adolescents and Adults

Other

Educational placement and intervention history, informal observations at home

▶ Clinical Findings

General Observations

Amber is a female, 12 years old, who has a medical diagnosis of moderate intellectual disability. Amber experiences expressive and receptive language deficits and has received speech/language therapy since she was 4 years old. Her mother reported that Amber shows overall delays in cognitive and language development. She expressed the belief that Amber receptively understands much more than she is able to communicate.

Amber is observed and reported to have extreme word-finding difficulties. In addition to her intellectual disability and subsequent language deficits, Amber exhibits speech production deficits characterized by low oral-motor tone, frequent drooling, articulation errors, and low volume. She uses vocalizations, limited speech, gestures, facial expression, and pictures to communicate. Her mother reported that she and Amber's immediate family understand Amber about half the time when she uses the previously mentioned communicative forms, but unfamiliar people and other communication partners rarely understand her.

Amber's teachers reported that she often has behavioral problems when at school and she does not want to participate in classroom activities. She often cries, vocalizes strongly to protest the activity, or refuses to comply with activities presented to her by pushing away or throwing items she is given.

Amber has received only spoken communication language intervention until now. She has recently been introduced to an activity-based static display picture communication board by her speech-language pathologist. The SLP has noted a reduction in her negative behaviors and an increase in verbal and symbolic expressive communication since the introduction of this form of AAC.

Nonverbal Communication

As reported by her mother, Amber most often uses facial expression, gestures, and telegraphic speech to communicate. Her ability to spontaneously express her wants and needs is extremely limited by her word-finding difficulties. Amber's mother reported that she understands Amber using these forms of communication approximately 50% of the time, and others understand Amber about 20% of the time they are communicating with her.

Receptive Language

On the PPVT-IV test, an assessment of Amber's receptive vocabulary requiring her to point to the picture named from an array of four, Amber's score fell below the first percentile. The age-equivalent score given to her performance was 6 years, 0 months (6;0).

The SICD for adolescents and adults was given to Amber to further assess her receptive and expressive language. The SICD is an assessment with items on it that require the individual to process multiple directions, descriptive vocabulary, and numbers. During this assessment, Amber was able to follow two-step directions and identify coins (penny, dime, nickel). She had difficulty, though, following three-step directions, often doing only the last step in the sequence.

Expressive Language

On the EVT-2, Amber's scores fell below the first percentile; in other words, less than 1% of peers her age scored below her. Amber's standard score was 40, and she was assessed as having an age equivalent of 4 years, 1 month. She demonstrated the ability to speak the labels of highly familiar pictures such as colors, animals, and body parts. However, she often took

in excess of one minute to verbally label the picture. Her mother reported that Amber comprehends many of the pictures presented to her, but Amber was not able to expressively generate a label for them (examples: leaf, octopus).

Amber's lack of word finding was further demonstrated when she was asked to give synonyms for familiar words. She was unable to give many appropriate synonyms, but instead used a word to describe it. For example, when asked to give a synonym for *road,* she said, "This way." When asked to give a synonym for *steps,* she said, "Down."

Amber is estimated to use approximately 200 consistent words for expressive communication. She is learning to use augmentative and alternative communication in the form of activity-specific picture boards to indicate her wants and needs and to comment during daily activities and routines.

Phonology

In general, Amber's speech was moderately unintelligible. Administration of the *Goldman-Fristoe Test of Articulation,* however, revealed substitution of only two sounds (g/d, t/thumb), with other sounds being within normal limits for sounds in words. That is, Amber's unintelligibility is in connected speech rather than on the phonemic level.

Oral-Motor Examination

An oral peripheral examination revealed a tooth growing approximately one centimeter within the tooth arch or the hard palate. Lip pursing appeared distorted, with the orbicularis muscle appearing weaker on the right side. Amber was able to implode air, lateralize, and raise and lower her tongue. Her diadochokinetic rates were slow and labored.

▶ Diagnosis and Prognosis

As Amber has developed, her cognitive and receptive language skills, although delayed, have bypassed her ability to expressively communicate. Her difficulty producing functional verbal speech will continue to have a significant impact on her daily routines. This communication may consist of explanations of why she may be hurt, comments about the environment around her, and social interaction with peers during everyday activities such as going out into the community, interacting with peers, and communicating her medical needs to her family.

Amber's speech production deficits and word-finding difficulty hinder her ability to effectively and efficiently express herself to others. This inability to express herself has become very frustrating for both Amber and her communication partners. For example, when Amber becomes frustrated because she cannot effectively communicate her intended message, she was observed to sigh and say, "I just forgot." Her psychosocial and physical well-being are clearly affected by her poor expressive communication ability.

▶ Recommendations

It is very important that Amber's communication partners use the symbols on her picture communication board to communicate to her through the use of aided input to teach Amber the meaning of symbols. To use this strategy effectively, the communication partner participates in an activity with Amber and uses the communication board to describe and expand upon ideas. Through modeling of the use of symbols in this way, Amber will be able to expand her language system and develop ways to organize her vocabulary to efficiently increase the quality and rate of her communication.

It is also suggested that a visual schedule be used with Amber at school to prepare her for the events of the day. If Amber is prepared using pictures, she may better understand what is expected of her and refrain from some of her negative behaviors.

Other strategies that could be used to facilitate Amber's language development include recasts of her communication to correct forms and expansion of Amber's limited utterances using the picture communication board. Both of these strategies can be incorporated into natural interactions with Amber.

Amber should be continually assessed during intervention to see if the combination of the picture communication board and her verbal speech is meeting her communication needs. She should continue to see a speech-language pathologist to facilitate her use of the communication board for expressive language. The SLP should also continually monitor her use of an appropriate vocabulary and symbol set for functional communication. Intervention services should focus on helping Amber learn to use symbols for communication. The use of a voice output speech-generating device should not be ruled out, even though Amber currently uses some functional speech. Considerations should be made for Amber to use a voice output communication device to further enhance her language comprehension and the amount of vocabulary available to her at one time.

Appendix 17-C

Case Study 3: Speech-Language Evaluation

Name: Oscar
Sex: Male
Age: 3 years, 10 months

▶ Significant History

Oscar's prenatal and birth histories are remarkable, as he was born prematurely at 28 weeks.

His medical/health history is remarkable for asthma and ear infections. PE tubes were placed when he was two and a half. Oscar is diagnosed as having schizencephaly, an extremely rare developmental birth defect characterized by abnormal slits, or clefts, in the cerebral hemispheres of the brain.

Hearing and vision appear to be within normal limits. However, Oscar has not been formally tested for problems in these areas since birth.

Developmental milestones are delayed for motor and speech-language development. Oscar's physical abilities are a direct result of his diagnosis—Oscar is unable to walk and uses a wheelchair. He is unable to communicate functionally using verbal speech.

While Oscar's expressive speech-language development is significantly delayed, his receptive language and cognitive skills appear to be developing typically. Oscar has received speech/language therapy since infancy in an attempt to improve his oral-motor skills, with gains being noted in his increased ability to approximate some consonant sounds; this therapy was conducted through his state's early intervention program. Oscar's attempts at speech are somewhat unintelligible to family members and highly unintelligible to everyone other than his family members. He is currently using a 32-location voice output augmentative communication device. He receives speech/language therapy and music therapy once a week and occupational therapy and physical therapy twice a week.

There is no family history for speech-language disorders.

▶ Clinical Procedures

Assessment Tests

Mullen Scales of Early Learning

Peabody Picture Vocabulary Test–4th edition (PPVT-IV)

Vineland Adaptive Behavior Scales

MacArthur-Bates Communicative Development Inventory Words and Gestures

Clinical Assessment of Language Comprehension (CALC)

Sequenced Inventory of Communication Development (SICD-R)

Other

Informal observations at home

▶ Clinical Findings

General Observations

Oscar is a 3-year-old boy who enjoys social interaction with others, playing with toy trains, and reading books. He uses gestures, vocalizations, and eye-gaze to communicate. Oscar enjoys interactions with friends, family, and teachers. His ability to interact with others is significantly limited, however, owing to his lack of verbal communication ability.

Play

Oscar's functional play and social skills appear age appropriate. Both his cognitive skills and his social abilities appear to be areas of strength for Oscar, and they may continue to help his communication skills develop. Oscar exhibits extraordinary curiosity and perseverance when playing with toys. His manipulation and explorations of age-appropriate toys appear to be compromised only by his motor capabilities.

Nonverbal Communication

Oscar has successfully used 9-location and 32-location voice output augmentative communication devices to communicate in multiple environments, including home and private speech/language therapy. He uses his hand to directly access the device. He has progressed from using only 8 picture communication symbols available per activity overlay (playtime, book reading, snack time) to having as many as 32 picture communication symbols available per activity. Oscar appears to fully understand the concept of using a communication device. He primarily communicates nonverbally by pointing, focused eye-gaze, laughing, and vocalizations.

Receptive Language

When given the PPVT-IV test, Oscar received a standard score of 92, a percentile rank of 30, and an age equivalent of 38 months. He understands a range of vocabulary, including nouns, pronouns, shapes, and action and descriptive words. Overall, as reported by the SICD, Oscar demonstrates receptive language skills within the 48-month age range.

Expressive Language

Oscar demonstrates expressive language skills within the 12-month age range as reported by the SICD. He makes mostly vowel sounds, with some occasional consonants. He will occasionally imitate an "mmm" sound (to approximate "more"). Oscar's oral motor limitations due to his diagnosis of schizencephaly contribute to his expressive speech delay.

Oral-Motor Examination

Oscar is able to imitate a pucker, open his mouth, and smile (lip spread) when asked. He can slightly move his tongue forward. He has some drooling and pooling of saliva. He is beginning to make his vowels distinguishably long and short, yet shows difficulty with high/low pitch and producing the alveolar sounds /m, n, d/.

▶ Diagnosis and Prognosis

Oscar's prognosis for improved communication skills is excellent with ongoing speech-language therapy.

▶ Recommendations

It is recommended that Oscar continue to use a voice output SGD for expressive communication. Intervention services should focus on customization of vocabulary within a language-based strategy to build upon his comprehension of words and appropriate syntax.

Oscar may quickly become limited with 32 words per activity setting. He will require continual evaluation during intervention sessions to see if a more advanced dynamic display communication device would best meet his expressive language needs.

Oscar should continue to use his device consistently throughout daily routines and activities (e.g., home, school, community activities) and with a variety of communication partners (e.g., family, friends, therapists).

Oscar's family and other communications partners should provide consistent feedback on his communication needs as he grows so that the vocabulary available to him on his communication device grows with him over time.

Oscar should continue his school- and private-based speech/language interventions, with goals focusing on understanding and use of syntax in making sentences, early literacy skills, and speech production abilities. It will be important for current therapies to be coordinated and for therapists to be cognizant of Oscar's rapidly changing communication needs.

Glossary*

Accommodation A process in which individuals develop new schema to account for previously encountered information. For example, a child with an existing schema for "apples" encounters an orange. The child decides that the orange is not consistent with the concept of "apple" so a new schema for "orange" emerges.

Acculturation The process by which someone identifies with both the primary community (C1) in which he or she has been socialized and the broader majority community or host culture (C2).

Acoustic immittance measures Also known as tests of middle ear function; they include both tympanometry and acoustic reflex testing. These procedures, which give information about the presence or absence of middle ear pathology, are used in conjunction with the remainder of the audiometric test battery.

Acoustic reflex Part of the immittance test battery. This test involves the recording of the stapedius muscle activity.

Action words Words used to describe or demand an action. A class of words that refers to verbs.

Adaptation The process an individual uses to resolve a conflict between the way they currently understand a concept and conflicting/new information that has been received. Adaptation involves either assimilating the new information into an existing schema or accommodation.

Adoption age The length of time prior to adoption. The amount of time spent prior to adoption can affect the course of English language development.

Aided language stimulation An augmentative and alternative communication (AAC) intervention strategy in which the intervention facilitator (e.g., clinician, parent, teacher) points to picture symbols on a child's picture communication display in conjunction with ongoing spoken language stimulation.

American Sign Language A manual set of language symbols that are akin to spoken language symbols (e.g., semantics, grammar).

American Speech-Language-Hearing Association (ASHA) The professional, scientific, and credentialing association for more than 150,000 members who are speech-language pathologists, audiologists, and speech, language, and hearing scientists in the United States and internationally.

Applied behavior analysis (ABA) A behavioral system of intervention that is utilized to teach skills in humans, from toilet training to language; a combination of psychological and educational techniques that are utilized based on the needs of each individual child to measure behavior, teach functional skills, and evaluate progress. ABA therapists provide important services to children with autism to facilitate their difficulties in various areas of development.

Arcuate fasciculus The white matter tract of the brain that connects Broca's and Wernicke's areas, two areas of language processing.

Articulation The process of producing speech sounds.

Assessment The process of determining an individual's development, as well as his or her strengths and weaknesses, by interpreting his or her performance on formal tests, formal analyses, and informal observations within the context of his or her background history and reason for referral.

Assimilation The process by which someone in a new environment adopts and embraces the values, beliefs, and behaviors of the host culture (C2).

Asymmetrical When referring to audiological development, asymmetrical characterizes the profile of right and left ears differing in degree and (sometimes) type of hearing loss.

Attachment The bond or affective tie of infants to their parents.

Attention The ability of the child to focus on listening long enough to complete a task, such as understanding the content and meaning of what is said.

Attrition The process of losing a native language.

Attunement The ways in which internal emotional states are brought into communication within infant-caregiver interactions.

Auditory attention The cognitive control of attention directed toward a relevant auditory stimulus while simultaneously inhibiting attention toward irrelevant stimuli.

Auditory brain stem response audiometry A reliable, noninvasive, objective procedure that records neuroelectrical activity in response to sound. It is an indirect measure of hearing sensitivity.

---

* **Lynette Austin, PhD,** Assistant Professor, Department of Communication Sciences and Disorders, Abilene Christian University, and **Amy Hadley, EdD, CCC-SLP,** Associate Professor of Communication Disorders, The Richard Stockton College of New Jersey, contributed to this glossary.

Auditory closure The ability to fill in a missing or misspoken part of a word or message.

Auditory memory A type of memory that includes attention, listening, and recall. It is an essential ingredient for a child at the identification level and for the overall perception and processing of speech in general.

Auditory skills The foundational skills in which children will build many of their listening and communication skills. The development of the auditory skills typically occurs in four stages: detecting sounds, discriminating between sounds, identifying a sound, and comprehending a sound.

Auditory-based intervention Intervention that focuses on developing the listening and spoken language skills of individuals who are deaf or hard of hearing.

Augmentative and alternative communication (AAC) A multimodal intervention approach that uses forms of communication such as manual sign language, picture communication boards, and *speech-generating devices*, with the goal of maximizing the functional language and communication abilities of individuals who have severe communication impairments and little to no speech (ASHA, 2002).

Augmentative and alternative communication (AAC) assessment A critical component of AAC service delivery that can provide the foundation for basing intervention decisions for individuals requiring AAC intervention. It is conducted within a comprehensive, team-based assessment framework, often within various environments, and includes assessment of the AAC user, communication partners, environments, and the AAC system. The goal is to explore the range of appropriate AAC strategies, adaptations, devices, and services that may help a child fully participate in their environment(s) and enhance his or her functional communication with a variety of communication partners.

Augmentative and alternative communication (AAC) strategy The specific way or method in which AAC aids, symbols, and techniques are used to develop and/or enhance communication efficiency and effectiveness (e.g., language stimulation strategies, augmented input, aided language stimulation, communication-partner instruction, rate of communication enhancement strategies).

Augmentative and alternative communication (AAC) system An integrated set of components, including communication aids, symbols, strategies, and techniques, all working in concert to provide the maximum amount of support needed for an individual to fully communicate in all situations.

Augmentative and alternative communication (AAC) technique The way in which communicative messages are transmitted, such as direct selection or scanning.

Augmented communication input An augmentative and alternative communication (AAC) intervention strategy in which the intervention facilitator or communication partner uses both picture symbols and speech output produced by a speech-generating device (SGD) when the symbols are activated, in conjunction with ongoing spoken language during naturalistic and authentic daily activities. This strategy provides spoken and augmented language input to the child, models functional use of the SGD, and demonstrates to the AAC user that the SGD is an acceptable form for communicative interactions.

Autism spectrum disorder (ASD) A childhood disorder involving deficits in social, communication, play, and verbal behavior. ASD was first identified in 1943 by Leo Kanner, an American psychiatrist.

Autobiographical memory Episodic memory for personally experienced events (times, places, associated emotions, and other contextual who, what, when, where, why knowledge) and semantic memory for general knowledge and facts about the world.

Axon A part of the neuron that conducts information away from the cell body.

Axon terminals A part of the neuron that transmits information to other neurons.

Baby signs See *representational gestures*.

Background history An inventory of the child's past and current events and characteristics (e.g., reason for referral, events surrounding gestation and birth, medical and health status, points at which developmental milestones were met, genetic factors).

Basic-level terms The most general (or intermediate-level) terms in the hierarchy of semantic organization. These terms are generally acquired before other terms in the hierarchy. Also referred to as *ordinate-level terms*.

Beat gestures Manual movements that are produced with the rhythm of speech but do not convey semantic or deictic reference.

Behavioral (procedure) A procedure that requires a volitional response from a person.

Bottom-up approach An approach that is directed and planned, and typically employs a linear presentation in the sequence of easiest to most difficult. The therapist focuses on the child mastering one skill or skill level completely and then moves on to the next, more difficult level.

Bound morpheme A morpheme that cannot stand alone; it requires another morpheme, either free or bound, to complete it. Bound morphemes include most prefixes and suffixes. In the word "walked," "walk" is a free morpheme joined with the bound morpheme "-ed."

Breadth Breadth is how many words a test subject knows. In the clinical evaluation of children's vocabulary, we tend to focus on the breadth of words known to a child.

Broca's area The collective name for the Brodmann areas of the brain (BA) BA 44 and BA 45, located in the left frontal lobe.

Brodmann areas Regions of the cortex that were defined and numbered by neuroanatomist Korbinian Brodmann in the early 1900s.

Caudal When identifying brain structures in relation to one another, *caudal* refers to a structure that is "moving toward the tail."

Cell bodies The compact portion of the nerve cell containing the nucleus and surrounding cytoplasm, excluding the axons and dendrites. The cell bodies make up the gray matter of the brain. It can also referred to as the soma.

Central executor The component of working memory that allocates processing resources and attention to other components (visuo-spatial sketchpad, phonological working memory, episodic buffer).

Cerebellum The part of the brain that fine-tunes motor movement. It abuts the dorsal surface of the brainstem and connects to the brainstem via white matter tracts. The cerebellum regulates corrections in movement for coordination, posture, and motor movement learning. The cerebellum also activates for learning verbs and retrieving verbs from memory.

Cerebral cortex The cerebral cortex is the outermost layered surface of the brain that folds over the subcortical structures. The cerebral cortex has two subdivisions, or hemispheres, by the sagittal plane along the longitudinal fissure.

Child-directed speech Patterns of speech directed to babies and young children that are characterized by utterances that are shorter in length, simpler in grammatical complexity, slower in rate of speech, contextually redundant, and more perceptually salient than speech directed to older persons. Researchers suggest that the vocal and grammatical parameters of the primary linguistic data that are provided by the caretaker make semantic, syntactic, phonological, and pragmatic information more accessible to the young infant, who is innately wired to receive this information.

Classical conditioning Paradigm described by Pavlov, who discovered that dogs could be conditioned to salivate in response to a bell after pairing the bell with the presentation of food. Many concepts (e.g., stimulus response, paired association, stimulus generalization) are derived from this paradigm.

Cochlea A snail-shaped structure in the inner ear. It houses the sensory end organ of hearing (i.e., the organ of Corti).

Cochlear implant A surgical implant of electrodes within the cochlea that in turn provides the sensation of sound by electrically stimulating the auditory nerve.

Code switching The juxtaposition within the same speech exchange of passages belonging to two different grammatical systems. The switch can be intrasentential, within a sentence (Spanish-English switch: *Dame a glass of water. "Give me a glass of water."*), or it can be intersentential, across sentence boundaries (Spanish-English switch: *Give me a glass of water; tengo sed. "Give me a glass of water; I'm thirsty."*). The switches are not random, but rather are governed by constraints such as the free morpheme constraint and the equivalency constraint. Many people who are bilingual and/or bidialectal are self-conscious about their code switching and try to avoid it with certain interlocutors and in particular situations. In informal speech, it is a natural and powerful feature of a bilingual's/bidialectal's interactions.

Cognition In developmental psychology, a term used to refer to multiple processes such as memory, attention, perception, action, problem-solving, and imagery. In child development, a term used to refer to children's emerging ability to make sense of the world around them by interpreting input, integrating this information, and then producing planned actions.

Cognitive-constructivist Referring to the theoretical paradigm introduced by Jean Piaget, who described the developing human as being grounded in action—both observable and mental. The human infant was said to actively construct its knowledge through the use of invariant mechanisms, including the establishment of mental constructs or schemas, while engaging in sensory and motor activities.

Communication An act in which one person gives to or receives from another person information about that person's needs, desires, perceptions, knowledge, or affective states and includes speech, as well as other forms of expression such as body gestures, eye gaze, picture symbols, and printed words.

Communication aid A device used to transmit or receive messages during communicative exchanges. Aids range from simple non-electronic devices, such as picture symbol choice boards and head pointers, to high-technology electronic aids, such as dedicated speech-generating devices and laptop computers with speech synthesis software.

Communication partners Those individuals with whom the augmentative and alternative communication (AAC) user interacts; could include family, friends, peers, clinicians, teachers, and/or community workers.

Communicative competence The ability to use language(s) and/or dialect(s) and to know when and where to use which and with whom. This ability requires grammatical, sociolinguistic, discourse, and strategic competence. It is evidenced in a speaker's unconscious knowledge (awareness) of the rules/factors that govern acceptable speech in social situations.

Communicative profile A complete and individualized description of a child's strengths and needs in a variety of settings regarding the child's understanding and use of language, speech, oral-motor skills, and ability to communicate using nonconventional forms of communication such as gestures or sign language. It may be influenced by factors such as the child's cognitive development, communicative experiences, vocal and gestural production abilities, and comprehension skills.

Comprehension The process of turning an often highly complicated set of linguistic or nonlinguistic (or both) cues (e.g., signs, signals, or word combinations) into a meaningful message.

Comprehension (reading comprehension) The successful connection of statements and ideas in a text that leads to forming a coherent mental representation of the text; the reader is required to use prior knowledge to interpret information in the text and to construct a coherent mental representation or picture of what the text is about (Kendeou et al., 2005).

Comprehension level The comprehension of sound and its meaning; the final and most complicated stage of auditory development.

Conditioned play audiometry A method used to complete a hearing test on a young child. This method turns the hearing test into a listening game for the child; almost any toy or game will do. The idea is to condition the child to do something each time a sound is heard; this action can be dropping a block, putting a ring on a stick, or putting a piece in a puzzle, for example.

Conductive hearing loss A hearing loss that is the result of damage in the outer and/or middle ears. It is usually characterized by a decrease in the loudness of sound, but the clarity of speech typically remains intact. Conductive hearing loss is very often medically and/or surgically treatable. When it is caused by a condition such as otitis media, it fluctuates in severity, with some days much better or much worse than others.

Conductive mechanism The combination of the outer and middle ears. In its normal state, it is an air-filled environment. The conductive system as a whole (that is, the outer and middle ear together) has the job of gathering the sound (acoustic energy) from the environment, converting the sound (acoustic energy) into mechanical energy, and then delivering this mechanical energy to the inner ear.

Configuration the slow mapping process of adding phonological, semantic, and grammatical details to the word representation in long-term memory.

Consonants Sounds produced by partially or totally constricted vocal tract; classified by manner (degree and type of obstruction), place (location of obstruction), and voicing (whether vocal folds are vibrating).

Coordination/coregulation Ongoing mutual social referencing of the participants involved in social interactions.

Coronal plane An imaginary plane that slices the brain like a loaf of bread—behind both eyes, behind both ears, etc.

Corpus callosum A band of white matter that connects the left and right hemispheres of the brain by crossing midline between them.

Criterion-referenced measures Measures used to differentiate among levels of performance where no standardized measure of performance has been established.

Criterion-referenced tests Tests in which the speech-language pathologist evaluates the child's responses qualitatively, looking for any missing forms that can be targeted in therapy. The results of a child's performance on criterion-referenced measures are summed up as pass/fail scores, percentage correct, or performance rates; these scores indicate the child's level of mastery of a specific linguistic form.

Cultural bias Reduced or absent consideration of the examinee's experiential base as evidenced by the use of activities and items that do not correspond to the examinee's experiential base. This may lead to unfavorable performance on tasks and failure to represent the examinee's true skill or performance capabilities.

Cultural competence A person's knowledge and awareness of cultural and/or linguistic differences that may affect both the personal and professional experiences of the clinician with his or her clients.

Cultural diversity The exposure or immersion of an individual or group in more than one set of cultural beliefs, values, and attitudes. These beliefs, values, and attitudes may be influenced by race/ethnicity, sexual orientation, religious or political beliefs, or gender identification.

Cultural variables Shared and accepted factors that help a group define itself.

Culture The *explicit* behaviors and artifacts and *implicit* beliefs adopted by a person or group to define their social identity.

C-unit An independent clause and its modifiers. It is used to measure linguistic complexity.

Curriculum-based language assessment Assessment of a child's ability to use language to learn classroom material (Paul, 2005). It includes assessing a child's written work for the level of narrative development, grammaticality and complexity, use of diverse vocabulary, and use of figurative language.

Cycles phonological remediation approach An intervention developed for use with children who have highly unintelligible speech. The child is given quick but limited exposure to a target, and the speech-language pathologist typically returns to the pattern after a period of time. This allows for the child to internalize, sort, experiment with, and do self-rehearsal as a typically developing child does. Through this process, the child's sound system is reorganized. The child learns new rules to use in producing the sounds of the words of his language.

Deaf/hard of hearing A person presenting with a hearing loss who is typically unable to use his or her sense of audition as a means for daily communication. Individuals who are deaf/hard of hearing can derive benefit from hearing aids and use aural/oral speech for communication.

Deaf culture The culture of the deaf community, which has its own language (sign language) and its own accepted cultural norms. Hearing-impaired individuals who are members of the deaf community are, for the most part, isolated from the "hearing world." It is not surprising, therefore, that they are a separate and unique culture.

Decoding The process of translating orthographic symbols into phonemic symbols to decipher printed words; the core skill required in learning to read an alphabetic language.

Decontextualization The gradual distancing of a symbol from the original referent or learning context.

Deictic gestures Gestures that make reference to something in the environment (i.e., *showing, giving, pointing,* and *ritual request*). Also referred to as prelinguistic gestures because they emerge before the child speaks his or her first word.

Dendrites Parts of the neuron that receive/collect information from other neurons at their synapses.

Depth How well or how much a test subject knows about each word. Depth can also be thought of as richness of word knowledge.

Derivational morphemes Bound morphemes used to change the part of speech of a word.

Detection level The most basic level of sound awareness; it refers to the baby being able to detect the presence or absence of sound in the environment. In the normal-hearing infant, this is a clear-cut and uncomplicated process.

Development A gradual change in maturation over time that is described in terms of its typicality by comparisons with a normative sample.

Diagnostic intervention An informal means of assessing abilities when formal assessment (or diagnostic) measures are ineffective, invalid, or unable to be conducted in a timely fashion. The process involves implementation of intervention strategies and informal observation to determine the individual's strengths and needs and to determine the most appropriate course of intervention.

Dialect A neutral term used to describe a language variation. Dialects are seen as applicable to all languages and all speakers. All languages are analyzed into a range of dialects, which reflect the regional and social background of their speakers.

Dialectal variance The non-mainstream production of a language at the sound, word, or syntactic level.

Diencephalon A subcortical structure of the brain found rostral to the brainstem. The diencephalon includes the thalamus and the hypothalamus.

Disability A social construct perceived by those with an illness or disease.

Discourse competence The skills involved in the connection of a series of utterances to form a conversation and/or narrative.

Discrimination level The next higher level in difficulty in sound awareness beyond the detection level. With the discrimination level, children first master discrimination of the suprasegmental aspects of language before they master the segmental aspects.

Distributed neural network The connection of nodes of information across modalities that are represented throughout the brain.

Dorsal The dorsal surface of the brain refers to the upper surface and continues to the backside of the brain.

Dual-(differentiated-) language system hypothesis The assumption that children process individual languages through distinct language systems, thereby developing two differentiated mental representations of the languages from the onset of exposure.

Dynamic approach to assessment A more naturalistic approach to assessment, in which the speech-language pathologist examines a child's language and communication skills in natural contexts. It involves the observation of the child in routine activities, interacting with familiar people, manipulating objects, and playing with different toys alone and with others.

Dynamic assessment Assessment of not only what the child's current performance level is, but also how the child can learn. Because dynamic assessment provides information on the child's ability to learn, it provides the examiner with great insight for both identifying a language disorder and planning intervention.

Early communicative gestures Gestures that are part of routines, such as hand waving to say *good-bye* or nodding the head to say *no*.

Electrophysiologic (procedure) A procedure that does not require any active participation from the child. Such tests are unaffected by any degree of sleep or arousal and are not negatively affected by sedation. Further, they can be performed on anyone, aged pediatric through geriatric. These tests are the procedures of choice for screening hearing in the newborn infant population.

Emblems Conventional symbols such as the *high-five* to convey camaraderie, *okay* or *thumbs up* gestures to signal agreement, and the *hand across the throat* to signal stop. They are language-like in that they are abstract symbols.

Emergent account of language acquisition A theory that suggests that language acquisition is an emerging process by which children simultaneously integrate sources of acoustic, linguistic, social, and communicative information that they encounter within daily, naturally occurring interactions.

Emergentist coalition model A theory of word learning that proposes children take advantage of multiple environmental cues as well as innate cognitive biases to learn new words. With experience, these cues and biases work together and become more efficient in helping the child learn language.

Emotion A mental and physiological state associated with a wide variety of feelings, thoughts, and behaviors.

Empiricist theories Theories that explain language acquisition as a learned behavior; that children learn language through experience.

Encoding Basic and essential skill whereby the ear and auditory pathway (in a bottom-up fashion) physically receive and code sound, then send it upward toward the brain for eventual interpretation. Sound encoding is necessary and allows, for example, the perception and analysis of the acoustics of speech. In essence, children learn that sound has meaning and that they can produce sound for the purpose of communication in their environment.

Endogenous factors/intrinsic factors Factors within the child.

Engagement The human infant's ability to interact with others by utilizing joint attention, reciprocity, and intentionality.

Environmental controls Items that can be utilized to help an individual interact with his or her environment where he or she was previously unable to interact; examples include adapted toys and remote controls.

Epigenetics/epigenesist Epigenesis is the process in which genes react to environmental factors such as diet or toxins. Epigenetic marks decide which sets of genes may be expressed and which genes are not. Through epigenesis inheritable changes in genes can occur without a change in the DNA sequence.

Episodic buffer The component of working memory that integrates newly processed phonological, visual, and other modalities of information with old information from long-term memory prior to its storage in long-term memory.

Episodic memory Links that connect the emotional experience of an event with the what, when, and how of the event. This type of memory makes it possible for individuals to recollect happenings and events from their past and to use this information to project anticipated events into the future (Tulving, 1993). Episodic memory enables the individual to make predictions and, therefore, to infer in social interactions and in text comprehension.

Ethnic diversity Similar to *cultural diversity;* differences within and between groups of people already categorized by ethnicity.

Ethnic majority According to the U.S. Census Bureau (2000), those who identify as "white," connoting superiority.

Ethnic minority According to the U.S. Census Bureau (2000), all "nonwhites," suggesting inferiority.

Ethnicity An ever-changing cultural construct that forms the basis for a sense of social cohesion.

Ethnographic interviewing A personalized method of exploration that provides the clinician with an opportunity to obtain a deep, true, and naturalistic understanding of the behavior or culture under study. Through this process, the clinician listens to the behaviors and beliefs reported by the parent or caregiver, as obtained through a systematic and guided dialogue with the caretaker.

Eustachian tube Connects the middle ear space to the nasopharynx (or throat). Its primary functions are to provide the circulation of air to the middle ear cavity and the equalization of the pressure between the middle ear and the outside atmosphere.

Evaluation See *assessment.*

Event-related brain potentials (ERP) A technique that involves placing electrodes on a participant's scalp. The electrodes read electrical activity from the brain out through the scalp. Electrical activity from neurons is then transmitted to the computer and drawn as a waveform trace over time. Timing of the waveform, as well as amplitude (i.e., size) and direction (i.e., positive, negative) of the waveform, convey changes in activation.

Executive function Cognitive skill used to maintain attention on a task while searching through memories for solutions, selecting and organizing behaviors to execute, and monitoring the execution of these behaviors.

Exogenous factors/extrinsic factors Factors in the environment.

Expansion An intervention used when a child incorrectly produces a particular linguistic form; the speech-language pathologist then reinforces the correct production of the linguistic form by repeating the child's utterance, adding the missing grammatical markers or lexical items.

Expressive children Those children for whom general nominals account for less than 50% of their lexicon.

Extended optional infinitive account The hypothesis that the central deficit in specific language impairment (SLI) is in the part of grammar responsible for tense marking. According to this account, children with SLI go through an extended stage of mistakenly treating tense marking in main clauses as optional.

Facilitative play (indirect language stimulation) An intervention in which language is facilitated by utilizing toys or objects that draw the child's interest. It provides multiple opportunities for the child to map the nonlinguistic context onto words and sentences.

False belief The ability to recognize that others can have beliefs about the world that are diverging.

Fast mapping The process of linking a new word with its referent after a brief exposure.

Feedback "That annoying whistling" from hearing aids, which relatives and close friends of the hearing-impaired person may complain about.

Fine motor skills Movements involving smaller body muscles, such as the fingers and the muscles of the face that are used in speech (e.g., lip, tongue, and jaw movements). Mastering control of these muscles takes years. For example, it takes children at least age 5 years or later to learn to use all of the sounds of English correctly.

Fissure A very deep sulcus or groove in the brain.

Fluency The ability to read words without a conscious effort to sound out or blend them; it includes the ability to group words into meaningful phrases and to read with prosody, intonation, and stress.

Focused stimulation An intervention in which the child is bombarded with the target form in a variety of contexts. The child is exposed to multiple exemplars of a specific linguistic target (e.g., a word, a morpheme) within meaningful communicative contexts. Following exposure, the child is provided with opportunities to produce the targeted linguistic form. The therapy session is arranged with materials that would encourage spontaneous productions of the target forms following the speech-language pathologist's repeated models.

Formal testing One type of procedure used to evaluate the child's development. The child's performance is summed to a raw score and often statistically converted to a standard score or percentile so that the child's performance can be compared to a normative or criterion-referenced data set. Some formal tests evaluate a particular developmental domain (e.g., vocabulary); others contain a variety of subtests that sample several developmental domains (e.g., PLS-5).

Free morpheme The smallest unit of language that carries meaning and can exist independently.

Frequency The number of cycles of vibration per second.

Frontal lobe The part of the brain that contains structures involving the primary motor cortex, premotor and supplementary motor, Broca's area (left hemisphere), and prefrontal cortex

Function words Words referring to items that serve a grammatical function in relating to other content words (e.g., *what, is, for, to*).

Functional ability As it relates to hearing, a consequence of *many* factors; "degree" of loudness loss is just one of them. Other factors involved in determining the person's level of function include pre- or post-lingual onset of hearing loss, age of onset for post-lingual losses, speech-understanding ability, successful use of a hearing aid, speech reading skills, and cognitive abilities.

Functional communication context The discourse contexts in which the child communicates that are part of daily living activities (e.g., conversation, explaining an academic topic, defending a position, communicating needs in the classroom).

Functional core hypothesis A hypothesis stating that words are overextended to novel exemplars based on the shared actions or functions of objects rather than the perceptual features of the referents.

Functional magnetic resonance imaging (fMRI) A brain imaging technique that monitors the change in cell metabolism while processing stimuli. Oxygen levels in the blood change with neuronal activity as blood flow increases with task demand. The fMRI then yields a map of blood flow throughout regions of the brain.

General nominals Words referring to all members of a category. They include word classes such as objects, substances, animals, people, letters, numbers, pronouns, and abstractions.

Gesture-spoken language match combination A situation in which gesture and spoken language are produced at the same time and both modalities convey the same information.

Gesture-spoken language mismatch combination A situation in which gesture and spoken language are produced at the same time and each modality conveys different information. Mismatch combinations are often produced when children talk about concepts that they are still in transition of learning.

Give gesture A deictic gesture in which the child hands off an object to a communicative partner.

Government binding-principles and parameters A theory developed by Noam Chomsky in 1981 that describes the idiosyncratic parameters of particular languages as well as universal principles across languages.

Grammatical competence Knowledge and awareness of phonological, syntactic, and lexical skills.

Grammatical specific language impairment (SLI) A distinct subtype of language impairment characterized by persistent receptive and expressive language impairments that are restricted to core grammatical operations.

Grapheme A written symbol (letter) that represents a phoneme (sound).

Gray matter The part of the brain that is densely packed with cell bodies.

Gross motor skills Movements involving large muscles of the body, such as the arms and legs. Examples include rolling over, sitting unsupported, and walking. Acquisition of these skills occurs in an orderly, predictable process that usually precedes mastery of fine motor skills.

Gyrus A "hill" on the outer cortex of the brain.

Hearing aid An externally worn device for amplifying sound.

Hearing technologies Devices including traditional hearing aids, implantable devices, and cochlear implants.

Heritage Cultural variables that are most valued and are passed on from generation to generation.

Hierarchical organization of the lexicon The systematic organization of the lexicon such that the relationship between members of a category can be characterized as superordinate (e.g., animal), ordinate (e.g., dog, cat, pig, cow), and subordinate (e.g., collie, poodle).

High-frequency sensorineural hearing loss A hearing loss in which the person's ability to hear high frequencies is not merely "somewhat poorer," but rather "a lot poorer." At the same time, hearing for the lower frequencies is often intact.

Horizontal development The range of abilities or communicative functions within a particular developmental level.

Iconic gesture See *representational gestures*.

Identification level The point at which the child is able to identify or label an item; this can be by naming the item or pointing to it.

Illness An individual's *experience* of that condition.

Imitation An intervention in which the child receives a visual prompt (such as a picture or a toy) that provides him or her with an incentive to verbalize. The speech-language pathologist then provides a verbal model and asks the child to imitate the target form. The child's response is reinforced by verbal praise or by a token.

Impedance Resistance or opposition to the flow of energy.

Impedance mismatch The difference in the resistance properties of the air-filled middle ear and of the fluid-filled inner ear.

Inattention The inability to attend to a stimulus.

Incidental teaching procedure An intervention in which toys are strategically placed to elicit specific linguistic or communicative forms.

Independent (individualistic) A cultural orientation that stresses independence, self-reliance, and individual liberty; one's personal goals take priority over the goals of the group.

Indeterminate errors/responses A type of word retrieval error that provides no discernable relationship with the target (e.g., "I don't know" or "thing").

Index of Productive Syntax (IPSyn) A method of evaluating the grammatical complexity of language in preschool children. Language development is assessed in four separate areas of language knowledge and structure: noun phrases, verb phrases, questions/negations, and sentence structures. IPSyn requires the identification of 56 specific language structures in a corpus of 100 child utterances.

Individual family service plan (IFSP) A plan that recommends the delivery of services in naturalistic environments (e.g., in the child's home or in childcare facilities). It includes information about the child's physical, cognitive, social, emotional, and communicative development, and about his or her family, including its resources, concerns, and priorities. The IFSP also provides information about the services needed for the child, their frequency and intensity, and the expected outcomes.

Individualized education plan (IEP) A plan that states the child's strengths and weaknesses, the goals and objectives for therapy, the type of services the child needs, and the amount of time each week that services will be provided.

Individuals with Disabilities Education Act (IDEA) Federal legislation that requires states to provide children with a free, appropriate public education.

Inferior parietal lobule A posterior area of the brain that stores phonological information related to words.

Information processing A theoretical perspective that explains the human acquisition of information in a way that is analogous to the working of a computer, in that information is considered to be processed serially and/or simultaneously.

Information processing speed The speed or efficiency with which the brain performs basic cognitive operations; in effect, how quickly a person can react to incoming information.

Initiating behavior request (IBR) A type of protoimperative in which the infant uses eye contact and gestures to initiate attention coordination with another person to elicit aid in obtaining an object or event. IBR is used less for social purposes, but more for instrumental purposes.

Initiating joint attention (IJA) A type of protodeclarative in which the infant uses eye contact and/or deictic gestures (pointing or showing) to spontaneously initiate coordinated attention with a social partner. The infant is seeking interaction with another simply for the sake of sharing an experience.

Innate biases Intrinsic tendencies or preferences that children use to pair a newly heard word with the referent in their environment. Also referred to as *constraints* or *principles* of word learning.

Intellectual Disability (ID) A disability that impacts an individual's cognitive skills (such as reasoning, problem-solving, and planning).

Intentionality Purposive motivation that drives language acquisition.

Intentionality model Bloom and Tinker's (2001) model of the interaction between two domains of development—affect and cognition—in the young child. In this model, the development of the form, content, and use of language is embedded in engagement (i.e., the social-emotional development of the child) and effort (i.e., the cognitive development of the child).

Interactionist perspective A perspective derived from a range of perspectives that are either cognitive or social, placing equal emphasis on preexisting information that the child brings to learning and the role of environmental input on the child.

Interdependent (collective) A cultural orientation that stresses interdependence among members of a group or society and the importance of the goals/desires of the group over the goals/desires of the individual.

Interpreter A person specially trained to transpose oral or signed text from one language to another.

Interrupted language development Exposure to two different languages due to adoption with acquisition of one at a later age. Acquisition differs from typical monolingual children in that the interruption due to adoption lends itself to expressive language lags despite learning their second language relatively quickly.

Intervention The process of facilitating development to age-appropriate or developmentally appropriate levels.

Joint attention (JA) The process of sharing one's experience of observing an object or event by following gaze or pointing gestures.

Language (1) A complex and dynamic rule system of conventional symbols that is used in various modes for thought and communication (e.g., spoken, signed, written) and is generative. Rules govern five separable domains: pragmatics, phonology, morphology, semantics, and syntax. At the same time, these domains evolve within specific historical, social, and cultural contexts. (2) A socially shared code of symbols—written, spoken, or signed—that serves a communicative function. The symbols incorporated into a language have no inherent meaning but instead are arbitrary. Because competent users of the same language share a grammatical (rule-governed) system for generating new and allowable sentences, regardless of mode, it is presumed that they can meaningfully communicate with one another.

Language acquisition theories Theories about how children acquire language; usually attributed to biological or environmental influences.

Language assessment Systematic evaluation of an individual's language skills to determine strengths and weaknesses. Assessment may include both formal measures such as standardized tests and informal measures such as interviews and observations.

Language comprehension The ability to understand what is said so that the person can function as a listener in conversational exchanges. It provides an essential foundation on which individuals can build language production.

Language delay A situation in which a child exhibits typical development in all other areas except for language.

Language deviance A situation in which the child's language development is not just slower than that of the typically developing child but is different in some qualitative way.

Language difference A rule-governed language form (i.e., dialect) that deviates in some way from the standard language used by the mainstream culture.

Language disability A language disability may result from impairments in receptive language abilities, expressive language abilities, or both.

Language disorder (impairment) An impairment in comprehension and/or use of spoken language, written language, and/or some other symbol system. The disorder may involve (1) the form of language (phonologic, morphologic, and syntactic systems), (2) the content of language (semantic system), and/or (3) the function of language in communication (pragmatic system), in any combination (ASHA, 1993, p. 40).

Language diversity Patterns of linguistic differences inherent within and across populations, including second language acquisition processes, dialects, and bilingualism, where an individual or group has had significant exposure to more than one language or dialect.

Language input The exposure to written or spoken language. The input enables the learner to integrate the language they are exposed to into linguistic knowledge.

Language interference The ability to apply knowledge from one language (L1) to another language (L2).

Language intervention Remediation focusing on areas of weakness in language skills. Intervention may take a variety of forms including direct therapy as well as parent training and collaboration with other professionals serving the child.

Language learning disability (LLD) A learning disability marked by difficulty with speaking, listening, reading, and/or writing. The individual faces learning challenges as a result of impairment in the language domain. The challenges do not result from cognitive deficits, neurological impairment, sensory impairment, or social deprivation.

Language loss The apparent loss (attrition) of functional vocabulary and/or utterances in a language due to reduced exposure.

Language mixing Use of a linguistic structure from one language in place of a structure in another language; observed in the production of early bilinguals during periods in their development.

Language modality The manner in which language is utilized, specifically listening, speaking, reading, and writing.

Language production The ability to express information so that the person can function as a speaker in conversational exchanges.

Language sampling A technique for the assessment of bilingual children whereby naturalistic utterances are collected, transcribed, and analyzed.

Language transfer The use of a linguistic rule from one language that affects the production of structures in the other language for a period of time in development.

Language transparency The use of a linguistic structure from one language as a replacement for a structure in the other language for a period of time in development.

Language-ego permeability Beliefs about how language should be used or produced; a sense of 'boundaries" for what is acceptable language use and what is not; a sense for when language output is being degraded or changed. Individuals may have varying levels of tolerance for nonstandard forms of the language (e.g., language borrowing, code switching).

Language-use patterns The way that language is used given the context of discourse.

Late bloomers Children with slow expressive vocabulary growth during the toddler years who catch up to their typically developing peers by the end of their preschool years.

Late talkers Children with slow expressive vocabulary growth during the toddler years who do not catch up to their typically developing peers. Their delays eventually transcend vocabulary to difficulty with grammar.

Learning disability A learning challenge in which an individual's academic performance does not meet the potential suggested by their intellectual ability. A physical disability or a sensory deficit alone (e.g., hearing or visual impairment) does not constitute a learning disability. Learning disabilities are often manifested in the school environment as persistent difficulty with educational tasks involving reading, writing, and/or mathematics.

Left anterior front lobe An area of the cortical brain responsible for motor function related to language.

Lexeme A word's label or form (in contrast to the semantics or meaning of the word) that is comprised of a sequence of phonemes.

Lexical bootstrapping The notion that lexical and grammatical development are inseparable. Children use their accumulating knowledge of individual words to construct the grammar of their language.

Lexical representation The word form stored in memory; a sequence of phonemes that make up the lexeme.

Lexical-semantic network The connection of nodes of phonological, lexical, and semantic information across modalities that are represented throughout the brain.

Linguistic account Causal explanation for SLI that highlights the difficulties children have with learning grammar.

Linguistic bias Reduced or absent consideration of the examinee's linguistic differences during testing; typically a result of prescriptive beliefs of language development and production.

Linguistic construction A syntactic template that is paired with a conventionalized semantic and pragmatic content. Constructions are often associated with specific speech acts, such as asking a question or making a promise. Constructions vary with respect to their complexity, ranging from single words to complex sentences.

Listening The act of comprehending language through the aural modality.

Listening and spoken language The modalities in which oral language can be interpreted and expressed as receptive and expressive language.

Literacy The ability to identify, understand, interpret, create, communicate, and compute using printed and written materials associated with varying contexts. Literacy involves a continuum of learning in enabling individuals to achieve their goals, to develop their knowledge and potential, and to participate fully in their community and wider society.

Literacy artifacts Representations of print that enrich a child's environment.

Literacy socialization The social and cultural aspects of reading that a child acquires by being a member of a literate society.

Localization The location of the sound source in the environment.

Longitudinal fissure A fissure that runs along the dorsal aspect of the brain.

Mand-model procedure A technique in which the speech-language pathologist mands (explicitly directs the child, "Tell me what this is"), or provides the child with a choice ("Is the ball red or blue?") and then provides the child with the model.

Mastery The threshold when a child uses a particular linguistic form (e.g., the *-ing* morpheme) consistently and accurately 90% of the time when it is required or expected to be used.

Mean length of utterance (MLU) A measure of linguistic productivity in children. It is usually calculated by collecting 100 utterances from a child and dividing the number of morphemes by the number of utterances. A higher MLU is taken to indicate a higher level of language proficiency.

Mental representation Knowledge that is stored, or represented, in memory.

Mental states The state of mentality one is in. Language has the ability to influence mentalities and specific mentalities can predict behavior.

Metalinguistic skills The ability to think about language.

Metapragmatics The ability to be aware of the pragmatic functions related to speech.

Middle ear transformer function Functionality in which the ear is able to overcome the impedance mismatch.

Milestones Expected ages or time frames during which certain skills emerge or are acquired.

Minimalist program The most recent version of Chomsky's theory, in which the description of the language faculty includes only a representation of meaning and a recursive element called "merge" that provides the mechanism for joining words and phrases.

Mixed hearing loss A hearing loss that results from simultaneous damage to both the conductive and the sensorineural pathways.

Modeling An intervention technique in which the targeted linguistic form/behavior is presented to the child by the speech-language pathologist in a naturalistic context.

Modifiers Words referring to properties or qualities of things or events, such as attributes, states, locations, or possessives.

Morpheme The smallest unit of language that carries meaning.

Morphology A domain of language that encompasses the rules of the smallest unit of language that expresses meaning (e.g., plural *-s*, root word).

Multiple disabilities A general term for a combination of two or more impairments occurring at the same time; it can apply to children with a broad range of impairments in cognitive development, expressive and receptive communication, and physical ability.

Naming explosion See *vocabulary spurt*.

Naming insight See *vocabulary spurt*.

Natural partitions hypothesis A hypothesis proposing that concrete nouns promote more rapid learning than other word classes, particularly verbs, because they allow for greater transparency of the mapping between lexical and semantic information.

Nature perspective A perspective derived from rationalist philosophy that emphasizes the internal wiring of the child for perception and learning.

Neighborhood density A measure of how many words or neighbors that a target word has in memory when only one phoneme varies.

Neuron Nerve cell that transmits electrical signals.

Nominal insight See *vocabulary spurt*.

Nonverbal communication The nonlinguistic behaviors that may accompany verbal interactions. Gestures, proximity, eye contact, and touch, for example, may have substantial meaning in social interactions.

Norm-referenced measures Tests that look at each language as a separate entity and do not assess the relationship between two languages.

Novel name-nameless category (N3C) Principle stating that a novel word will be taken as the name for a previously unnamed object.

Nurture perspective A perspective derived from empiricist philosophy that relies primarily on observable phenomena to explain learning.

Obligatory context The context in which a particular language form is expected to occur. For example, if a child is referring to more than one object, the plural -*s* morpheme would be considered obligatory in that it must be used to convey the meaning of "more than one."

Occipital lobe Lobe of the brain that contains the primary visual cortex and the visual association cortex.

One-child policy Chinese policy limiting the number of children allowed to a family to one.

Operant conditioning Paradigm described by B. F. Skinner, who discovered that a rat's behavior could be shaped by systematically presenting a reinforcing stimulus to the successive approximations until ultimately the target behavior is produced. Concepts such as reinforcement, punishment, and schedule of reinforcement are derived from this paradigm.

Ordering of word classes The order of nouns, in subject (S) and object (O) positions, and verbs (V).

Ordinate terms See *basic-level terms.*

Organ of Corti The end organ of hearing.

Orientation The degree to which a person orients himself or herself toward the considerations of a collective body (e.g., a family, ethnic group) or toward individual achievement and motivation.

Orthographic Referring to print.

Ossicular chain Collective name for the bones in the ear: the malleus (hammer), incus (anvil), and stapes (stirrup).

Otitis media An inflammation of the middle ear; a middle ear infection.

Otoacoustic emissions (OAE) An electrophysiologic procedure that is based on the principle that a normal and healthy cochlea not only hears sound, but can also produce sound. OAEs can be spontaneously present or evoked. An *evoked* OAE occurs when a sound has been sent into the ear, and in response the ear produces a sound and sends it back out; this response can be recorded. *Spontaneous* OAEs are spontaneously present.

Overactivity A level of activity that is too high or greater than normal.

Overextension A type of word retrieval error that is characterized by a word being used too broadly to refer to referents that may be similar in perceptual feature or function.

Overgeneralization errors Errors that involve children's use of words in grammatical constructions in ways that are not conventional in their language community. Children may overgeneralize morphological patterns, for example, by saying *goed* instead of *went*, and they may overgeneralize syntactic patterns, for example, by saying *She broomed the floor.*

Parallel talk An intervention in which the speech-language pathologist describes the child's actions.

Parietal lobe Brain structure that stores phonological information related to words.

Performance assessment procedures Methods by which the speech-language pathologist evaluates a child's language knowledge, abilities, and achievements in a more naturalistic manner. One of the most common procedures is language sampling.

Perisylvian language zone Area of the brain surrounding the left lateral fissure; highly involved in language processing.

Perseverative errors A type of word retrieval error that is characterized by the repetition of a previously said word within a relatively short time interval.

Personal-social words Words that express affective states and social relationships, such as assertions (e.g., *no, yes, want*) and social expressive words (e.g., *please, ouch*).

Pervasive developmental disorder not otherwise specified (PDD-NOS) A classification used to account for those children who appear to represent "atypical autism." A child diagnosed with PDD-NOS presents with a pervasive impairment in social interaction and communication skills or stereotyped patterns of behavior, interests, or activities that do not meet the criteria for autistic disorder because of late age at onset, atypical symptoms, or subthreshold symptoms.

Phenotype An observable behavior or symptom when a gene is expressed.

Phoneme The smallest arbitrary unit of sound in a given language that can be recognized as being distinct from other sounds in the language.

Phonemic awareness The ability to consciously reflect on and manipulate the sounds in words without visual reference. Includes the blending, segmenting, and manipulation of individual phonemes.

Phonetically consistent forms (PCF) Stable vocalizations used to reference a specific event, object, or situation; not true words.

Phonological awareness An individual's knowledge or sensitivity to the sound structure of words (Pullen & Justice, 2003); the explicit awareness that words in the language are composed of syllables and phonemes (i.e., consonants and vowels) (Catts, 1991). At the emergent literacy level, it is reflected in activities such as rhyming, word play, and phonological corrections (van Kleeck & Schuele, 1987); additional representative skills include listening, alliteration, syllabication, and phonemic awareness.

Phonological development Acquisition of the speech sounds and patterns of a language.

Phonological deviations Speech sound changes, including omissions, substitutions, assimilations, and syllable-structure/context-related changes.

Phonological errors A type of word retrieval error that is characterized by similar phonological makeup to that of the target lexeme (e.g., *chicken* for *kitchen* or *miracleride* for *merry-go-round*).

Phonological intervention A remediation process that focuses on reorganizing the child's phonological system by helping the child learn to produce and acquire phonological patterns.

Phonological loop The component of working memory where speech-based input is encoded, maintained, and manipulated.

Phonological patterns Accepted groupings of sounds and word structures within an oral language.

Phonological short-term memory Responsible for temporarily storing and processing verbal information.

Phonology A domain of language that encompasses the rules of the sound system of the language; one of the five components of language. It is important for morphology, syntax, and semantics.

Phonotactic probability The frequency with which a sound or sound sequence occurs in the language.

Phrenology A study of behavior and the brain that maps abilities onto brain areas through the characteristics of the skull, such as the size of bulges.

Point gesture A deictic gesture that is characterized by an extension of the arm from the body and the index finger from the hand in the direction of a target (e.g., object, picture, event).

Planum temporale A brain structure in the Sylvian fissure along the temporal lobe. The left planum temporale is longer than on the right hemisphere, thereby allotting more cortex to processing behind the primary auditory cortex.

Pragmatics (1) A domain of language that encompasses the rule system for the use of language form and content. (2) The ability to get things done with gestures and words; the use of language in a social context.

Prelexical forms See *phonetically consistent forms (PCF)*.

Preschool specific language impairment (SLI) An impairment in which the child typically has a performance IQ within normal limits, normal hearing acuity, no behavioral or emotional disorders, and no gross neurological deficits, but presents with significant deficits in language production and/or comprehension (Leonard, 1998).

Primary intersubjectivity Infants' ability to use and respond to eye contact, facial affects, vocal behavior, and body posture in one-to-one interactions with caregivers; it occurs early in life (0–6 months).

Primary language impairment A language deficit that cannot be accounted for by a peripheral sensory deficit (e.g., hearing loss), a motor deficit (e.g., cerebral palsy), a cognitive deficit (e.g., mental retardation), a social or emotional impairment (e.g., autism spectrum disorders), harmful environmental conditions (e.g., lead poisoning or drug abuse), and gross neurological deficit (e.g., traumatic brain injury or lesions). It is often presumed to be due to impaired development or dysfunction of the central nervous system (Leonard, 1998).

Primary sensory areas The primary cortical areas that receive sensory input stimuli including taste, olfaction, touch, hearing, and vision.

Principle of conventionality A word learning bias that the child uses in word learning; it states that there are culturally agreed-upon names for things and these do not change.

Principle of extendibility A word learning bias that the child uses in word learning; it states that a word does not refer to only one object. Rather, a word refers to a category of objects, events, or actions that share similar properties.

Principle of mutual exclusivity A word learning bias that the child uses in word learning; it states that if an object already has a name, it cannot be referred to by another name.

Principle of reference A word learning bias that the child uses in word learning; it states that words but not other sounds label objects, actions, and events.

Principles of word learning See *innate biases*.

Probabilistic patterns Correlations between co-occurring linguistic elements, such as speech sounds, syllable sequences, and word combinations. Language learners are highly sensitive to recurrent patterns in the speech they hear, and they more readily process highly frequent patterns. Probabilistic patterns may involve either adjacent elements (see *sequential dependency*) or non-adjacent elements.

Procedural memory system The neural system underlying long-term memory of skills and procedures, or "how to" knowledge. Procedural memory is not easily verbalized and can be used without consciously thinking about it. This system supports statistical learning of complex patterns learned over time, such as sequences of linguistic elements.

Processing account Causal explanation for SLI that highlights the difficulties children have in processing speed and/or efficiency.

Prosody Suprasegmental aspects of speech such as stress, juncture, and intonation.

Protowords See *phonetically consistent forms (PCF)*.

Pull out A language intervention used with school-age children that can be provided by the speech-language pathologist on an individual basis or in small groups outside the classroom.

Pure tone An individual frequency of sound.

Push in A language intervention in which, to facilitate the child's participation in classroom activities, the speech-language pathologist may provide the therapy in the classroom.

Quick incidental learning (QUIL) Learning that occurs when children learn the meaning of a new word with minimal overt support (no direct teaching of the new word) but with multiple cues available to guide learning.

Race A construct that classifies humanity based on arbitrary biological or anatomical features and/or nebulous geographical boundaries. It is often misinterpreted and forms the basis for social blights such as racism and discrimination.

Rationalist theories Theories that explain language as an innate ability in humans; children are biologically programmed to acquire language.

Reading The act of decoding and comprehending language from written text.

Recasting An intervention that is similar to expansion but in which the speech-language pathologist changes the type of utterance (e.g., from a statement to a question) or changes the voice or the mood in which the utterance is being produced.

Referencing (1) The act of labeling; (2) an individual's ability to interpret other persons' attitudes toward what they are attending to.

Referential children Those children for whom general nominals account for more than 50% of their lexicon.

Referential language learners Children are classified as *referential language learners* if general nominals account for more than 50% of their total vocabulary.

Representational gestures Iconic gestures that convey some aspect of the referent's meaning. The meaning conveyed by representational gestures might be the form of an object, the function of an object, the path or quality of an action, or the spatial relationship between two objects expressed by a preposition.

Resonance properties The physical properties of an object that result in a natural tendency for it to vibrate at a particular frequency.

Resonant frequencies The natural frequency of an object set into vibration with the maximum amplitude depending on the physical parameters of the vibrating object.

Responding to joint attention (RJA) A situation in which the infant follows the direction of gaze, head turn, and or point gesture of another person.

Reverberation Sound bouncing off hard surfaces creating an echo-like effect that is then amplified through a hearing device, causing a smearing of sound.

Ritual request A deictic gesture that conveys an infant's want or need for something by reaching with open hand or moving an adult's hand to the referent of interest.

Rostral When identifying brain structures in relation to one another, *rostral* means "moving toward the head."

Sagittal plane An imaginary plane that slices the brain down the middle into hemispheres so that each eye and each ear falls on either side of the cut, and the nose would slice down the middle.

Scaffolds A teaching tool consisting of "help" that a child is given during learning (e.g., a model of a target behavior, cues, prompts).

Scheme A mental concept that individuals formulate to help them understand and organize information. For example, a child's initial scheme of "apple" may be "a round, red fruit."

Scripted play An intervention which a child and the speech-language pathologist enact a play routine based on common scripts with which the child is familiar (Olswang

& Bain, 1991). These scripts can range from daily routines such as a morning routine (e.g., waking up, brushing teeth, eating breakfast) to special-occasion scripts (e.g., planning a birthday party). These routines offer conventionalized, predictable contexts in which the speech-language pathologist can teach turn-taking, conversational skills, new linguistic forms such as vocabulary, grammatical morphology (such as verb tensing), and higher-level functions such as planning and problem solving.

Secondary intersubjectivity A triadic pattern of communication in which the infant relates to another person in relation to an object or event.

Secondary language impairment A language disorder that is associated with and presumed to be caused by factors such as sensory (hearing loss) or cognitive impairments (mental retardation). The language disorder can be part of a syndrome, which is the presence of multiple abnormalities in the same individual that are all caused by or originated from the same source.

Segmental Referring to such speech elements as phonemes, morphemes, and syllables.

Self-talk An intervention in which the speech-language pathologist describes his or her own actions.

Self-teaching hypothesis A situation in which "each successful decoding encounter with an unfamiliar word provides an opportunity to acquire the word-specific orthographic information that is the foundation of skilled word recognition. A relatively small number of [successful] exposures appear to be sufficient for acquiring orthographic representations … [in] this way, phonological recoding acts as a self-teaching mechanism or built-in teacher enabling a child to independently develop both [word]-specific and general orthographic knowledge" (Share, 1995).

Semantic errors A type of word retrieval error that is characterized by a taxonomic/hierarchical or thematic relationship with the target lexeme (e.g., *pig* for *cow*, or *animal* for *cow*).

Semantic feature hypothesis A hypothesis that states children classify and organize referents in terms of perceptual features such as size, shape, animacy, and texture.

Semantic representation The meaning information about a lexeme stored in memory. Semantic representations are multimodal and encompass learning from all sensory systems.

Semantics A domain of language that encompasses the rule system for the meaning of language.

Sensitive period The time when a child is particularly receptive to certain kinds of environmental experiences, increasing his or her ability to learn particular skills. The sensitive period is an ideal time for a child to learn.

Sensorimotor morphemes See *phonetically consistent forms (PCF)*.

Sensorineural hearing loss A hearing loss that is the result of damage to the inner ear and/or auditory nerve.

Sensorineural mechanism A function of the body that involves both the inner ear and the auditory nerve.

Sensory association areas Areas of the brain surrounding the primary sensory areas where various senses are interpreted into a meaningful experience.

Sequential-bilingual A person characterized by exposure to a second language after developing a level of fluency in the first language skills. Different linguistic components are believed to be affected by differing ages of acquisition (example: phonological representations in adults). Also known as *successive bilingualism.*

Sequential dependency The likelihood that one linguistic element will follow another in sequence. Language learners form expectations about which linguistic elements are likely to follow others.

Service delivery A factor that influences the success of the language-impaired child; determined by the resources of the particular school district, as well as by the school district's underlying philosophy regarding bilingual and special education.

Shape bias The tendency to extend words based on shared perceptual features of the original referent and novel exemplar.

Show gesture A deictic gesture in which a child holds an object in view of his or her partner to engage him in an interaction but does not hand over the object.

Simple view of reading The most widely accepted theory of reading that defines reading comprehension as the product of decoding and linguistic comprehension.

Simple view of writing A current theory of writing that suggests that text generation is the product of transcription and executive functions.

Simultaneous-bilingual A person characterized by concurrent exposure to two languages from an early age before the person has achieved a high level of fluency, dominance, or proficiency in either language; highly sensitive to the age of the language learner, as well as amount and quality of input provided in each language.

Slow mapping The extended period of word learning that enriches the lexical-semantic representation of a word after it has been fast mapped.

Social-cognitive perspectives Approaches to language acquisition that emphasize the interaction between the child's innate skills and his or her social experiences with others. In contemporary views, the child's requisite cognitive abilities allow him or her to process information, while pre-formed concepts for entities in the world serve as the basis for word learning and language development. The child's ability to infer the referential intentions of others is key to the language-learning process.

Social-emotional development An aspect of development that concerns a child's interest in bonding with others in the environment. It is related to language development in that a child who is related to others, and therefore engaged with others in meaningful activities, is ready to respond to stimuli and learn.

Social-pragmatic perspectives Approaches to language acquisition that focus on the child's development of the communicative functions or intentions of language, speaker-listener roles, the conversational rules of discourse, nonlinguistic means of communication, and the way that form and content shift based on the linguistic and nonlinguistic aspects of the context.

Sociolinguistic/sociocultural competence The use of language and communication rules appropriate in one's language and cultural group.

Sociological assessment model A process of assessment that considers that language learning is a complex process interrelated with personal, cultural, and experiential rules and expectations. Assessment must consider all of these factors to better inform the examiner as to the language experiences, motivations, and skills of the individual client.

Soma The cell body of the neuron that integrates electrical signals.

Sound encoding A basic and essential skill whereby the ear and auditory pathway physically receive and code sound, and then send it on its way toward the brain for eventual interpretation.

Sound system development Acquisition of the sounds of language.

Speaking The act of producing language through the oral modality.

Specific language impairment (SLI) Condition in which children demonstrate significant language-learning difficulties in the absence of cognitive, hearing, oral-motor, emotional, or environmental deficits.

Specific nominals Words referring to a specific exemplar of a category, whether or not it is a proper name (e.g., *mommy, daddy,* pet's name).

Speech-generating device (SGD) A computerized/electronic communication aid that produces speech. It displays pictures that represent what the individual wants to say or express. When a specific picture is pressed on the SGD, it generates speech in a digitized (recorded) or synthesized (computerized) form for the communication partner to hear.

Speech-language pathologist (SLP) A professional who is trained in the assessment and treatment of disorders in the areas of speech (articulation, voice, fluency), language, cognition, and eating/swallowing.

Speech mechanism The six major organs/subsystems that are used in the production of speech.

Speech recognition score A score that represents the percentage of speech that is understood when a speech signal is made sufficiently loud for the child; it is a measure of the clarity of speech.

Speech recognition threshold The softest level at which the child can recognize speech 50% of the time.

Speech sound disorders Problems producing the sounds of a language.

Spontaneous language sampling The process of eliciting and recording discourse-level communication from an individual for formal analysis.

Stage theories Theories that are useful in understanding the developmental changes children go through as they become proficient readers.

Standardized tests (norm-referenced measures) Standardized tasks that compare individual performance to performances of a defined population. These measures tend to examine the languages of a bilingual speaker as a separate construct, and they provide limited information as to the relationship between the two languages.

Standardized (norm-referenced) tests Tests that rank the child's abilities against the performance of age-matched children with typical language development.

Statistical (or probabilistic) learning The ability of infants to track statistics in the language they hear, such as the distribution of sounds in words, and the order of words in phrases. Statistical learning is supported by domain-general associative learning mechanisms and enables the child to discover the building blocks of linguistic structure.

Strategic competence The strategies used by the bilingual person to compensate for breakdowns in communication that may result from imperfect knowledge of the rules, fatigue, memory lapses, distraction, and anxiety.

Subcortical Structures of the brain that are under or buried within the cerebral cortex.

Subordinate terms Specific exemplars of ordinate terms (e.g., *collie* is a subordinate term in relation to *dog*).

Sulcus Valleys or grooves in the brain.

Superior longitudinal fasciculus The white matter tract arcuate fasciculus, which connects Broca's and Wernicke's areas, two areas of language processing.

Superordinate terms The broadest class of basic terms (e.g., *animal, transportation/vehicles*).

Suprasegmental Referring to such speech elements as pitch, prosody, rhythm, stress, and inflection.

Suprathreshold A level that is louder than the "barely detectable" threshold level.

Surface account The notion that, due to processing limitations, children with specific language impairments have difficulties perceiving inflections of brief duration, such as the past tense -*ed* and the third person singular -*s*. Incomplete processing of morphemes of low perceptual salience means that fewer of these morphemes are fully processed, which leads to a delay in the acquisition of these forms.

Symbols Items used to represent vocabulary. Symbols may be either unaided (e.g., signs, manual gestures, and facial expressions) or aided (e.g., actual objects, pictures, line drawings, and printed words); they range from arbitrary to transparent.

Syntactic bootstrapping The idea that children use the syntactic knowledge they have acquired to help them learn what words mean. For example, a child might use the constructions in which a novel verb is used to make inferences about the possible meaning of the verb.

Syntactic productivity Knowledge that the grammatical constructions of a language may be extended to new vocabulary. Children may demonstrate syntactic productivity by using a newly introduced word in a construction that they have never heard it used with, or by using the grammatical structure of a sentence to make inferences about the meaning of a newly introduced word.

Syntax A domain of language that encompasses the rule system for the sentence-level structure of language that marks relationships between words and ideas.

Temperament The combination of mental, physical, and emotional traits of children that affect their behavior.

Temporal lobe Area of the brain that contains BA 22, which is a *primary auditory cortex*.

Text generation The production of written language at the word, sentence, and text (or paragraph) levels.

Theory of mind (ToM) The ability to attribute mental states—beliefs, intents, desires, pretending, knowledge, and so on—to oneself and others, and to understand that others have beliefs, desires, and intentions that are different from one's own.

Threshold The softest level required for a person to just be able to detect the presence of the sound half of the time; that is, the level where 50% of the time the person hears the sound and 50% of the time he or she does not.

Time delay procedure An intervention technique in which the speech-language pathologist anticipates the child's needs or desires and intentionally waits for the child to initiate an action.

Traditional (developmental) approach to assessment An assessment technique that relies almost exclusively on age expectations and normative data. It includes checklists of age-expected behaviors to which infants and toddlers are compared to or measured against.

Traditional assessment model An imitation of the psychological model of assessment. This view suggests that language is a self-contained domain that can be analyzed apart from other domains (i.e., cognitive and emotional domains).

Transcription skills Part of the translation component of the writing process and includes handwriting and spelling abilities.

Transdisciplinary play-based assessment The assessment of not only language and communication skills, but also social-emotional, cognitive, and sensory-motor abilities. The assessment is implemented by a team that includes the parents and professionals from various disciplines (i.e., speech-language pathologists, occupational therapists, physical therapist, psychologist). The context of the assessment is play activities that vary depending on the child and the areas being evaluated. This approach is natural and follows the child's attentional needs.

Transformational Generative Grammar The original 1957 theory put forth by Chomsky, which described the innate knowledge of the native speaker-hearer of a language as including knowledge in the three main components of language—syntax, semantics, and phonology.

Translator A person trained to transpose written text from one language to another.

Traveling wave The wave in the cochlear fluid created by sound that entered the inner ear as mechanical energy.

Treatment See *intervention.*

Triggering A precursor language event that can lead to the integration of linguistic concepts. In word learning, triggering signals that a new sound sequence is a new word to be learned.

Tympanic membrane The eardrum.

Tympanometry An assessment method that provides an objective look at middle ear function (or middle ear *dysfunction*, as the case may be). During this test, a graph known as a tympanogram is created; it provides information that helps determine if middle ear pathology is present (e.g., an ear infection or punctured eardrum).

Underextension Use of a word to refer to only one exemplar of a referent (e.g., *dog* refers only to the family dog, not to other dogs).

Unilateral hearing loss A hearing loss that affects one ear only. It may be the result of conductive, sensorineural, or mixed pathology.

Unitary language system view A perspective suggesting that children exposed to two languages simultaneously process those languages through the same system, only to have the languages become separated over time.

Ventral The underside of the brain.

Verbal communication Discourse; the use of spoken utterances as means for relaying ideas.

Verbal working memory capacity The limited capacity of the language processing system. The human information processing system has a limited pool of resources available to perform linguistic computations; performance deteriorates when processing demands exceed the available resources.

Vertical development Increasing hierarchical development associated with increasing age and cognitive understanding.

Visual misperception errors A word retrieval error that shares perceptual features with the intended target but has no semantic or phonological relationship with the intended target (e.g., *lollipop* for a *balloon*).

Visual reinforcement audiometry (VRA) An assessment method that combines sound with toys that light up and relies on the child's localization behaviors. The procedure involves conditioning the child to search for the sound when it is heard. When the child hears the sound and localizes it, he or she is rewarded with the toy lighting up.

Visuo-spatial sketchpad The component of working memory that manipulates visual information for visual recognition and orientation of stimuli.

Vocabulary The words people must know to communicate effectively; exists in both oral and written modes.

Vocabulary spurt A discernable rapid increase in the number of words a child is learning and using; typically occurs after the child has acquired his or her first 50 words, between 18 and 24 months of age.

Vowels Sounds in which the tongue typically does not come in contact with any of the other articulators during production. Vowels are always voiced and typically are not nasalized. Additionally, they are created with a relatively open vocal tract and have no point of constriction.

Wernicke's area Area of the brain located on BA 22 known to be activated during language comprehension tasks.

White matter tracts Many axons traveling together.

Whole-object bias A word learning bias that the child uses in word learning; it guides the child to infer that the word label refers to the entire object and not just a part, an attribute, or its motion.

Word-finding difficulty The momentary inability to retrieve already known words from the lexicon.

Word learning constraints See *principles of word learning.*

Word retrieval errors Production of the wrong lexeme when naming a referent; such errors are often logically related to the word that was targeted.

Word-specific formulae Rote-learned combinatory patterns that are tied to specific lexical items.

Word spurt See *vocabulary spurt.*

Working memory The memory system that is involved in active, online processing of information. It allows for temporary storage of information while it is being manipulated or processed.

World Health Organization Organization that directs and coordinates international health within the United Nations.

Writing The act of producing language in the written modality.

Writing process (planning, translating, revising) The process of producing written text that includes the components of planning, translating, and revising. *Planning* is the generation and organization of ideas. *Translating* is the production of written text that includes both transcription skills (handwriting and spelling) and text generation at the word, sentence, and text levels.

References

American Speech-Language-Hearing Association (ASHA). (1993). *Definitions of communication disorders and variations.* Rockville, MD: American Speech-Language-Hearing Association.

American Speech-Language-Hearing Association (ASHA). (2002). *Communication development and disorders in multicultural populations: Readings and materials.* Retrieved from www.asha.org/about/leadership-projects/multicultural/readings/OMA_fact_sheets.htm

Bloom, L., & Tinker, E. (2001). The intentionality model and language acquisition. *Monographs of the Society for Research in Child Development, 66*(4), 267.

Catts, H. W. (1991). Facilitating phonological awareness: Role of speech-language pathologists. *Language, Speech, and Hearing Services in Schools, 22,* 196–203.

Leonard, L. (1998). *Children with specific language impairment.* Cambridge, MA: MIT Press.

Kendeou, P., Lynch, J. S., van den Broek, P., Espin, C., White, M., & Kremer, K. E. (2005). Developing successful readers: Building early narrative comprehension skills through television viewing and listening. *Early Childhood Education Journal, 33,* 91–98.

Olswang, L., & Bain, B. (1991). Intervention issues for toddlers with specific language impairments. *Topic (Topics) in Language Disorders, 11,* 69–86.

Paul, R. (2005). *Language disorders from infancy through adolescence: Assessment and intervention.* St. Louis, MO: Mosby-Year Book.

Pullen, P. C., & Justice, L. M. (2003). Enhancing phonological awareness, print awareness, and oral language skills in preschool children. *Intervention in School and Clinic, 39,* 87–98.

Share, D. L. (1995). Phonological recoding and self-teaching: Sine qua non of reading acquisition. *Cognition, 55*(2), 151–218.

Tulving, E. (1993). What is episodic memory? *Current Directions in Psychological Science, 2,* 67–70.

United States Bureau of the Census. (2002). *U.S. Census of Population and Housing.* Washington, DC: GPO.

van Kleeck, A., & Schuele, C. (1987). Precursors to literacy: Normal development. *Topics in Language Disorders, 7,* 13–31.

Index

gestures, 99, 103
hearing assessment, 70
language comprehension, 91
literacy skills, 219
speech sound disorders, 205
joint attention, 38
autism spectrum disorders, 125
horizontal development of, 122
perlocutionary stage, 150
prelinguistic skills of, 8
temperament, 116
theory of mind, 114
visual impairment and, 126
and vocalization, 121
joint story reading, 306
Josephine case study, 20–22
cultural competence, 263
gestures, 99, 103
hearing assessment, 70
language comprehension, 91
language impairments, 297, 300
literacy skills, 219
morphology and syntax
development, 182
speech sound disorders, 206

K

*Khan-Lewis Phonological Analysis, 2nd
Edition,* 203

L

labial assimilation, 198
labiodentals, 194
language
assessment, 10, 35
awareness, 211
biological basis for, 28–29
case studies, 18–25
child's background history, 11–12
clinical practice of speech-language
pathology, 14–16
definition of, 5–7
delays, 11
developmental milestones, 8–9
development of, 3–25
disorder, SLI, 127–128
domains of, 5–7
formal testing, 13–14
goal setting and interventions, 16–18
modalities of, 225–226
as modular skill, 30
receptive *vs.* expressive, 7
speech-language pathologists, 9–11
spontaneous language
sampling, 12–13
stages of communication, 7–8
language acquisition, 115

language acquisition device (LAD), 29
language acquisition theories, 28
language comprehension
assessment and measurement
of, 86–90
case studies, 91–92
context, role of, 75–78
language production and, 85–86
normal child development
strategies, 78–83
overview, 75
question comprehension, 86
research, importance of, 74–75
single words, 83–84
language development of
children, 282–283
language disorder interventions
case study, 44–46
child development, 42–43
cognitive interactionist theory, 35–37
intentionality model, 41
nature perspective theory and, 31–32
nurture perspective theory
and, 33–34
social-pragmatic models, 39
language-ego permeability, 264
Language Environment Analysis (LENA)
System, 79
language impairments
assessment procedures, 304–306
autism spectrum disorders, 302–303
in children, genes, 250
gestures and, 104–106
intellectual developmental
disorder, 303–304
intervention strategies, 306–308
language delay, 295
language deviance, 295
language difference, 295–296
language disability, 295
language disorder, overview, 294–295
late talkers, 296–297
literacy skills, 218
language input, 286
language interference, 282
language intervention, 32, 34
language learning disability
(LLD), 299–301
language loss, 267
language sampling, 305
language skills for children with
auditory devices
auditory system, 314–318
hearing loss, customized intervention
for children, 318–325
overview of, 314
language theories, overview of, 28
language transfer, 267
language transparency, 248
language-use patterns, 264
larynx, 192

lateral sound, 194
late talkers, 152, 296–297
morphology development, 181–188
lax vowels, 194
learned helplessness, 337
learning disabilities
case study, 234–235
diagnosing, 295
overview, 299–301
learning readiness, 100–102
Lenneberg, Eric, 28
lexeme, 6, 157
lexical development
bilingual language development, 267
connectionist accounts, 160–161
emergent coalition model, 156–157
expressive *vs.* referential language
learners, 154–155
illocutionary stage, 150–151
innate biases, 155–156
later development, 165–166
locutionary stage, 151–152
naming errors, 162–164
neighborhood density, 160
nouns, 152–154
over-and underextension, 162
overview, 150
perlocutionary stage, 150
phonotactic probability, 160
specific language impairment
(SLI), 298
word classifications, 153
word learning, 157–159
working memory, 164–165
lexical information, 6
lexical-semantic
representations, 159–160
lexical variety, 230
licensing, 9
limited-English proficient (LEP), 261
linguistic awareness, 212
linguistic-based interventions, 204–205
linguistic competence, 29
linguistic creativity, 29–30
linguistic, defined, 8
linguistic diversity. *See* cultural
competence
linguistic information, comprehension
and, 75–78
linguistic variables, cultural
differences, 264–265
linguistic verbs, 180
lips, 192
liquids, 194, 197
listening devices, auditory
system, 316–317
listening skills, 225
listening skills development
comprehension level, 64
detection level, 63
discrimination level, 63–64